PERIOPERATIVE MEDICINE

Hospital Medicine: Current Concepts
Scott A. Flanders and Sanjay Saint, *Series Editors*

PERIOPERATIVE MEDICINE

Medical Consultation and Co-Management

Edited by

AMIR K. JAFFER, MD, SFHM
University of Miami Miller School of Medicine

PAUL J. GRANT, MD, SFHM
University of Michigan Health System

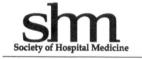

Hospitalists. Transforming Healthcare.
Revolutionizing Patient Care.

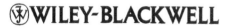

A JOHN WILEY & SONS, INC., PUBLICATION

Published by John Wiley & Sons, Inc., Hoboken, New Jersey
Published simultaneously in Canada

For general information on our other products and services or for technical support, please contact our
Customer Care Department within the United States at (800) 762-2974, outside the United States at
(317) 572-3993 or fax (317) 572-4002.

Wiley also publishes its books in a variety of electronic fOn1lats. Some content that appears in print
may not be available in electronic fonnat8. For more information about Wiley products, visit our web
site at www.wiley.com.

Library of Congress Cataloging-in-Publication Data:

Perioperative medicine / [edited by] Amir K. Jaffer, Paul Grant.
    p. ; cm.
Includes bibliographical references and index.
ISBN 978-0-470-62751-8 (pbk. : alk. paper)
I. Jaffer, Amir K. II. Grant, Paul, 1974-
[DNLM: 1. Perioperative Care. 2. Perioperative Period. WO 178]
617–dc23

                      2012026724

Printed in the United States of America

To my parents for their love, prayers, and support that helped me achieve my goal of becoming a doctor. This book and other aspects of my academic career would not be possible without the patience, unwavering love, and support of my wife Hajra and my wonderful children Saniya and Salman.

Amir K. Jaffer

To my parents, Douglas and Margaret Grant, who have inspired and motivated me throughout my entire medical career with unwavering love and encouragement.

Paul J. Grant

CONTENTS

PART III *POSTOPERATIVE CARE AND CO-MANAGEMENT BY SURGERY TYPE*

PART IV *COMMON POSTOPERATIVE CONDITIONS*

PREFACE

Perioperative medicine is an increasingly essential component of clinical practice for both hospitalists and hospital-based internists in the United States today. In a 2012 survey of attendees at the Society of Hospital Medicine Annual Meeting Precourse on this topic, over 90% were involved in co-management of surgical patients. With our aging population, patients are living longer and undergoing more surgeries than ever before. It is estimated that over 100,000 procedures are performed daily in the United States today. The associated costs of surgery and its complications also continue to increase significantly. It is projected that surgery-related adverse events cost the health system over $50 billion. These events need to be minimized through evidence-based strategies and interventions.

The first edition of our book *Perioperative Medicine: Medical Consultation and Co-Management* is envisioned to be a comprehensive textbook to help the internist, hospitalist, anesthesiologist, allied health professional, fellow, resident, and medical student manage the various aspects of medical care of the surgical patient. The focus is on both the preoperative and postoperative medical management of the surgical patient. This book is not intended to help guide intraoperative management. Rather, it focuses on systems, operations, and quality of perioperative care, assessment of patient and system-specific preoperative risk, evidence-based strategies that minimize risk, and management of common postoperative conditions. We also address important operational and system issues surrounding the development and implementation of both preoperative clinics and medical consultation services. In today's era of decreasing reimbursement, we have additionally focused on documentation, coding, billing, and payment issues, which are increasingly vital components of clinical practice. To facilitate access to the content, our book is divided into four main sections: Part I: Systems of Care, Quality, and Practice Management; Part II: Assessing and Managing Risk by Organ System or Special Population; Part III: Postoperative Care and Co-Management by Surgery Type; and Part IV: Common Postoperative Conditions.

As the Accountable Care Act is implemented, we must focus more and more on practicing high-quality, safe evidence-based perioperative care at the lowest cost. Therefore, patient care must be of the highest value across the whole perioperative spectrum. In addition, the principles of modern perioperative medicine may help us modify some long-standing traditions with limited benefit that can be eliminated from our current practice. We believe this book will arm you with a wealth of cutting-edge, evidence- and value-based knowledge that you can start using in your practice right away, and serve as a reference for years to come.

It is also our hope that this book will continue to enhance the overall quality of perioperative care you deliver. It was developed for you and we welcome comments and feedback regarding this first edition, as well as suggestions to improve future editions.

ACKNOWLEDGMENTS

We want to thank the series editors, Sanjay Saint and Scott Flanders, for their vision for this special series and for their trust in us. We especially want to thank all the contributing authors, as well as Thomas Moore and the Wiley staff for their assistance throughout the process of putting this book together. Finally, a special thanks to Ila Gold and Sarah Quadri for assisting during various stages of this book. The book would not be possible without all of you!

Amir K. Jaffer, MD, SFHM
(ajaffer@med.miami.edu)

Paul J. Grant, MD, SFHM
(paulgran@med.umich.edu)

CONTRIBUTORS

Uzma Abbas, MD
Assistant Professor of Clinical Medicine
Division of Hospital Medicine
Department of Medicine
University of Miami Miller School of Medicine
Medical Director, UM Hospitalist Service
University of Miami Hospital

Aijaz Ahmed, MD
Associate Professor of Medicine
Division of Gastroenterology and Hepatology
Stanford University School of Medicine

Kamal S. Ajam, MD
Clinical Assistant Professor
Wake Forest University Baptist Medical Center
Department of Anesthesiology
Carolinas Pain Institute

M. Chadi Alraies, MD, FACP
Clinical Assistant Professor of Medicine
Cleveland Clinic Lerner College of Medicine of Case Western Reserve University
Department of Hospital Medicine
Institute of Medicine, The Cleveland Clinic

Daniel Berland, MD, FACP, ABAM
Clinical Assistant Professor
Departments of Medicine and Anesthesiology
University of Michigan Health System

Nikolay Buagev, MD
Fellow, Trauma & Surgical Critical Care
Jackson Memorial Hospital

Aldo Pavon Canseco, MD
Assistant Professor of Clinical Medicine
Division of Hospital Medicine
University of Miami Miller School of Medicine

Michael P. Carson, MD
Associate Clinical Professor of Medicine
Assistant Clinical Professor of Obstetrics, Gynecology & Reproductive Sciences
UMDNJ—Robert Wood Johnson Medical School
Director of Research/Outcomes
Jersey Shore University Medical Center

Seema Chandra, MD
Assistant Professor of Clinical Medicine and Pediatrics
Division of Hospital Medicine
Department of Medicine
University of Miami Miller School of Medicine

Carol E. Chenoweth, MD
Professor of Medicine
Division of Infectious Diseases
Hospital Epidemiologist
University of Michigan Health System

Vineet Chopra, MD, FACP, FHM
Assistant Professor of Medicine
Department of Internal Medicine
University of Michigan Health System

Steven L. Cohn, MD, FACP
Director, Medical Consultation Service
University of Miami Hospital
Professor of Clinical Medicine
Division of Hospital Medicine
Department of Medicine
University of Miami Miller School of Medicine

Daniel Fleisher, MBA
Healthcare Management Engineering
University of Miami Health System

James B. Froehlich, MD, MPH, FACC
Associate Professor of Medicine
Director of Vascular Medicine
Director of Anticoagulation Clinic
University of Michigan Health System

Tong J. Gan, MD, FRCA
Professor of Anesthesiology and Vice-Chairman for Clinical Research
Department of Anesthesiology
Duke University Medical Center

Gregory C. Gardner, MD, FACP
Gilliland-Henderson Professor of Medicine
Division of Rheumatology
Adjunct Professor of Orthopaedics and Rehabilitation Medicine
University of Washington

Jeffrey J. Glasheen, MD, SFHM
Associate Professor of Medicine
Department of Medicine
Hospital Medicine Section
University of Colorado Anschutz Medical Campus

Paul J. Grant, MD
Assistant Professor of Medicine
Director, Perioperative and Consultative Medicine
Division of General Medicine
University of Michigan Health System

Fahim A. Habib, MD, FACS
Attending Trauma Surgeon
Ryder Trauma Center
Director of Critical Care
University of Miami Hospital
Assistant Professor of Surgery
DeWitt Daughtry Department of Surgery
University of Miami

Naeem Haider, MD
Clinical Assistant Professor
Department of Anesthesiology
University of Michigan Health System

Darrell W. Harrington, MD, FACP
Chief, Division of General Internal Medicine
Department of Medicine
Harbor-UCLA Medical Center
Associate Professor of Medicine
David Geffen School of Medicine at UCLA

Amir K. Jaffer, MD, FHM
Professor of Medicine
Chief, Division of Hospital Medicine
Department of Medicine
University of Miami Miller School of Medicine

Peter G. Kallas, MD
Assistant Professor of Medicine and Anesthesia
Medical Director, Perioperative Medicine
Northwestern University Feinberg School of Medicine

Siva S. Ketha, MD
Senior Associate Consultant
Division of Hospital Medicine
Mayo Clinic

Elias A. Khawam, MD
Consultation Liaison Psychiatry
Cleveland Clinical Lerner College of Medicine

Maninder S. Kohli, MD, FACP
Vice-Chair
Department of Medicine
Hinsdale Hospital

Ajay Kumar, MD, FACP, SFHM
Chief, Division of Hospital Medicine
Hartford Hospital

Tina P. Le, BS
Department of Anesthesiology
Duke University Medical Center

Joshua D. Lenchus, DO, RPh, FACP, SFHM
Associate Professor of Medicine
Division of Hospital Medicine
Department of Medicine
University of Miami Miller School of Medicine
Associate Program Director
Jackson Memorial Hospital Internal Medicine Residency

Dimitriy Levin, MD
Assistant Professor of Medicine
Department of Medicine
Hospital Medicine Section
University of Colorado Anschutz Medical Campus

Peter K. Lindenauer, MD, MSc, FACP
Associate Professor of Medicine
Director, Center for Quality of Care Research
Tufts University School of Medicine
Department of General Medicine
Baystate Medical Center

Xiao Liu, MD, PhD
Assistant Professor of Medicine
Tufts University School of Medicine
Academic Hospital Medicine Program
Division of General Internal Medicine/Geriatric
Baystate Medical Center

Brian F. Mandell, MD, PhD, MACP, FACR
Professor and Chairman of Academic Medicine
Department of Rheumatic and Immunologic Disease
Cleveland Clinical Lerner College of Medicine

Efren C. Manjarrez, MD, SFHM
Assistant Professor of Clinical Medicine
Associate Chief, Division of Hospital Medicine
Department of Medicine
Associate Chief Patient Safety and Quality Officer for Uhealth
University of Miami Miller School of Medicine

Paul Martin, MD
Professor of Medicine
Chief, Division of Hepatology
University of Miami Miller School of Medicine

Karen F. Mauck, MD, MSc
Consultant and Assistant Professor of Medicine
Division of General Internal Medicine
Department of Medicine
Mayo Clinic and Mayo Clinic College of Medicine

Mark G. McKenney, MD
Professor of Surgery
DeWitt Daughtry Department of Surgery
University of Miami Miller School of Medicine

Donnal L. Mercado, MD, FACP
Division of Endocrinology
Department of Medicine
Baystate Medical Center
Associate Clinical Professor
Tufts University School of Medicine

Franklin Michota, MD, FACP, FHM
Associate Professor of Medicine
Cleveland Clinical Lerner College of Medicine at Case Western Reserve
University

Katayoun Mostafaie, MD
Division of General Internal Medicine
Harbor-UCLA Medical Center
Assistant Professor of Medicine
David Geffen school of Medicine at UCLA

Lena M. Napolitano, MD, FACS, FCCP, FCCM
Professor of Surgery
Division Chief, Acute Care Surgery
Associate Chair, Department of Surgery
Department of Surgery
Director, Trauma and Surgical Critical Care
University of Michigan Health System

Kurt Pfeifer, MD, FACP
Associate Professor of Medicine
Division of General Internal Medicine
Associate Program Director
Internal Medicine Residency
Medical College of Wisconsin

James C. Pile, MD, FACP, SFHM
Associate Professor of Medicine
Divisions of Hospital Medicine and Infectious Diseases
MetroHealth Medical Center Campus of Case Western Reserve University

Leo Pozuelo, MD, FACP, FAPM
Section Head, Consultation Liaison Psychiatry
Cleveland Clinical Lerner College of Medicine

Marc A. Rozner, PhD, MD
Professor .
Anesthesiology & Perioperative Medicine
UT MD Anderson Cancer Center

Christina Gilmore Ryan, MD
Assistant Professor, General Internal Medicine
Assistant Professor, Neurological Surgery (Joint Appointment)
University of Washington

Sunil K. Sahai, MD
Associate Professor of Medicine
Department of General Internal Medicine
Medical Director, Internal Medicine Perioperative Assessment Center
University of Texas, MD Anderson Cancer Center

Emily K. Shuman, MD
Instructor of Medicine
Division of Infectious Diseases
Weill Cornell Medical College

Eric Siegal, MD, SFHM
Critical Care Medicine
Aurora St. Luke's Medical Center
Assistant Professor of Medicine
University of Wisconsin School of Medicine and Public Health

Barbara Slawski, MD, MS, FACP
Associate Professor of Internal Medicine and Orthopaedic Surgery
Chief, Section of Perioperative and Consultative Medicine
Director, Froedtert Memorial Lutheran Hospital Pre Admission Testing Clinic
Medical College of Wisconsin

Gerald W. Smetana, MD
Division of General Medicine and Primary Care
Beth Israel Deaconess Medical Center
Associate Professor of Medicine
Harvard Medical School

Andres F. Soto, MD
Medical Director Aventura Hospitalist
Aventura Hospital and Medical Center

Mihaela Stefan, MD, FACP
Assistant Professor of Medicine
Baystate Medical Center
Department of General Medicine
Tufts University School of Medicine

Anjala V. Tess, MD
Department of Medicine
Beth Israel Deaconess Medical Center
Assistant Professor of Medicine
Harvard Medical School

Charuhas V. Thakar, MD, FASN
Chief, Section of Nephrology
Cincinnati VA Medical Center
Associate Professor of Medicine
University of Cincinnati

Rachel E. Thompson, MD, FHM
Director, Medicine Consult Service
Assistant Professor, General Internal Medicine
Harborview Medical Center
Assistant Professor, Neurological Surgery (Joint Appointment)
University of Washington

David Wesorick, MD
Clinical Assistant Professor
Department of Internal Medicine
University of Michigan Medical School

Christopher Whinney, MD, FACP
Clinical Assistant Professor of Medicine
Department of Hospital Medicine
Cleveland Clinic Lerner College of Medicine

Jessica Zuleta, MD, FHM
Assistant Professor of Clinical Medicine
Division of Hospital Medicine
Department of Medicine
University of Miami Miller School of Medicine

PART 1

SYSTEMS OF CARE, QUALITY, AND PRACTICE MANAGEMENT

CHAPTER 1

HOSPITALIST AS A MEDICAL CONSULTANT

Siva S. Ketha and Amir K. Jaffer

INTRODUCTION

Medical consultation is an integral part of an Internal Medicine or a Hospital Medicine practice. Internists and hospitalists are often asked to evaluate a patient prior to surgery. The medical consultant may be seeing the patient at the request of the surgeon, or they may be a member of the primary care team assessing the patient prior to consideration for a surgical procedure. The timing of the consultation may vary from days to weeks prior to a planned elective surgical procedure and sometimes a few hours before an urgent procedure. The former is usually performed in a preoperative clinic or in an internist's office. The latter situation is frequently encountered in a hospitalist practice. Irrespective of the timing, the general objective of this evaluation is to determine the risk to the patient from the proposed procedure and from the patient's own known and unknown comorbidities and to recommend interventions to minimize these risks. This objective is accomplished by identifying comorbid disease conditions and risk factors for medical complications of surgery, optimizing the medical management of these conditions, recognizing and treating the potential complications, and working together with the surgical and anesthesia colleagues to form an efficient and effective perioperative care team.

Internists and hospitalists, especially individuals who have recently completed training, may not always be well acquainted with the process of medical consultation.[1] This is often because of inadequate exposure to the intricate nuances of medical consultation during residency training. However, medical consultation is an important component of both the outpatient internal medicine practice and the hospitalist practice. Therefore, it is worthwhile to develop an optimal consultation technique. This will also increase the likelihood that the recommendations of the consultant are implemented.

The focus of this chapter is on the general principles of medical consultation and specifically on the optimal interaction/communication between referring physicians and the medical consultant.

Perioperative Medicine: Medical Consultation and Co-Management, First Edition.
Edited by Amir K. Jaffer and Paul J. Grant.
© 2012 Wiley-Blackwell. Published 2012 by John Wiley & Sons, Inc.

ADVANTAGES OF MEDICAL CONSULTATION

Medical consultation is a widely prevalent practice. However, there is no evidence to show that this practice is associated with a decrease in perioperative morbidity and mortality. In fact in a recent, large population-based cohort study conducted by Wijeysundera et al., preoperative medical consultation was associated with significant, albeit small, increases in mortality and hospital stay after major elective noncardiac surgery. This study did have several limitations including the fact that it was an observational study and the mortality increase was small.[2]

But there is evidence showing that internists identify medical conditions that are related to surgical outcome and often recommend potentially lifesaving interventions for these conditions. In addition, medical consultants occasionally cancel or delay surgery so that medical conditions can be optimized.[3] In another study by Devereaux et al., it was found that medical consultants frequently recommended perioperative changes in the use of cardiac medications.[4] If the medical consultant makes evidence-based recommendations, then it is reasonable to conclude that consultation will improve the care of the surgical patient if such recommendations are followed. The effect of medical consultation on the length of stay is unclear. Phy et al. demonstrated a reduction in the length of stay and fewer minor complications when a hospitalist was part of the care team for patients after hip fracture surgery.[5] Macpherson et al. reported a decrease in the length of stay when an internist performed a postoperative medical management in patients who had undergone elective cardiothoracic surgery.[6] However, a more recent study by Auerbach in 2007 showed similar or increased costs and length of stay for patients who had a consultation from a generalist.[7] The authors of this study concluded that perioperative medical consultation produces inconsistent effects on the quality of care. Both this study and the other limited observational evidence are fraught with limitations and biases, and good randomized clinical trials are difficult to do in this area to study the true impact of medical consultation.

GENERAL PRINCIPLES OF MEDICAL CONSULTATION

Goldman et al. laid out the general principles of an effective medical consultation in 1983.[8] These principles are often referred to as the "Ten Commandments" of medical consultation and they are as follows:

I: Determine the Question

All too often consultants meticulously recapitulate the case and offer detailed recommendations but fail to address the question for which the consultation was called. It is important to respond to the specific question asked.

II: Establish Urgency

The consultant must determine whether the consultation is emergent, urgent, or elective and provide a timely response.

III: Look for Yourself

Confirm the history and physical exam, and check the test results.

IV: Be as Brief as Appropriate

Limit the number of recommendations.

V: Be Specific

It is recommended that the consultations should be brief and goal oriented. The impressions and differential diagnosis should be expressed concisely in order of likelihood.

VI: Provide Contingency Plans

Consultants should try to anticipate potential problems, such as what kind of postoperative complications might be expected in a particular patient. A brief description of therapeutic options to be employed should these problems arise is appropriate.

VII: Honor Thy Turf (or Thou Shalt Not Covet Thy Neighbor's Patient)

In general, consultants should play a subsidiary role. They should address the problem for which they were called and avoid running arguments in and out of the medical record with other services, especially if the problem lies outside their domain.

VIII: Teach with Tact

Requesting physicians appreciate brevity and clarity, but they also appreciate consultants who make an active effort to share their expertise and insights without condescension.

IX: Talk Is Cheap and Effective

It is crucial to have a direct conversation with the primary physician after a consultation has been performed. This is especially true if the recommendations are urgent or controversial.

X: Follow-Up

Consultants should recognize the appropriate time to fade gracefully into a background role, but that time is almost never the same day that the consultation note is signed.

A consultation is a request made to another physician to give his or her opinion (given their expertise in the field) on the diagnosis or management of a particular patient. The requesting clinician may seek consultation for preoperative risk assessment for surgery and anesthesia, advice on diagnostic problems or management issues in the perioperative period, confirmation of a plan or assessment and reassurance, or documentation for medical legal reasons. In general when a consultation is requested, the role of the consultant should be defined through communication with the referring physician. In a recent study by Salerno et al., it was found that surgeons more often desire "co-management" by internists in which the internist is asked to assume the management of specific aspects of the patient's care including order writing.[9] However, unless there is a preexisting arrangement for co-management, the surgeon needs to explicitly communicate this to the medical consultant.

Consultations should be requested in doubtful or difficult cases, or when they enhance the quality of medical care. The referring physician should always send a formal written or verbal consult request to the consulting physician unless a verbal description of the case has already been given.

Effective communication is the key to the art of medical consultation. The way in which the question or information is phrased can influence the consultant's response. For example, a request for "management of medical conditions" will generate a completely different response as opposed to a request for "management of postoperative hypertensive urgency." Ideally, the requesting physician should clearly state the questions to be answered by the consultant. However, this is often not the case. For example, Lee et al. found that there was disagreement between the primary physician and the consultant about the primary reason for consultation in 14% of cases.[10] A study by Kleinman et al. found that among preoperative cardiology consultations, over half of the consult requests were for "evaluation," 40% for "medical clearance," and no specific reason was noted for 5%.[11] In such instances, the consultant should directly communicate with the requesting physician to get a better sense of his or her needs in this regard. Given the high frequency of misunderstanding between consultants and referring physicians, direct communication is important and likely will prevent misinterpretation.

The consultant should always discuss potentially controversial recommendations with the primary team. It is not good practice to leave inflammatory notes in the chart. If the consultant identifies areas of concern distinct from the original reason for the consult, it is recommended that they discuss this with the primary team and seek their permission before discussing this in the chart. Conflicts of opinion should be resolved by a second consultation or withdrawal of the consultant.

Traditionally, consultative advice should be specific to the question asked. However, Salerno et al. found that only 41% of surgeons believed that internal medicine consultants should limit themselves to a specific question.[9] Consults should be performed in a timely fashion.[12] It is very useful if the requesting service indicates whether the consult is emergent, urgent, or routine to allow the consultant to respond accordingly.

The attending physician has overall responsibility for the patient's treatment and is in charge of the patient's care. The consultant physician should not assume the primary care of the patient without the consent of the referring physician. The medical consultant should be able to anticipate potential problems and make succinct therapeutic recommendations.[13] As a consultant, the physician should restrict advice to his or her area of expertise. For internists, this usually includes general internal medicine or cardiology and various aspects of perioperative medicine. It is not advisable to make recommendations regarding the type or route of anesthesia.

The consultant should make clear and concise recommendations regarding the management of the problem at hand. These immediate concerns must be evaluated in terms of their severity, the planned surgical procedure, the patient's perioperative risk, and the need for further testing or intervention. It is crucial to avoid making a long list of recommendations about all of the patient's issues as this might decrease the compliance with the recommendations.

Quite often, patients are interested in knowing the consultant's opinion at the end of the consultation visit. Unless the consultant is the patient's primary care physician, he or she should not express an opinion as to whether surgery should proceed. The final decision is best made by the surgeon in conjunction with the patient. The consultant does have the right to share his or her recommendations with the patient in the presence of the surgeon.

When the consultant's expertise is no longer necessary for the care of the patient, he or she should relay this to the primary team and write a note indicating that they are signing off the case. The sign-off note should ideally indicate appropriate recommendations and arrangements for follow up of the medical problems once the patient leaves the hospital.

PREOPERATIVE MEDICAL EVALUATION

A commonly stated purpose of a preoperative consultation request is to "clear" a patient for surgery.[14] As we have indicated before, the role of the internist or hospitalist is to outline the risks and interventions to help decrease this risk. We do not "clear" patients but in such referrals, the consultant can presume that the request is to provide a comprehensive preoperative evaluation. The consultant should avoid the use of the phrase "cleared for surgery." Instead, they should quantify the risk of potential complications from the procedure and propose a plan for risk reduction. This is accomplished by identifying all the risk factors (cardiac and pulmonary morbidity) and their severity, and making recommendations for optimizing the medical management of these risk factors. Risks are specific to the individual patient, the type of procedure proposed, and the type of anesthesia selected. If no such risks are identified, then the consultant's final statement could categorize this risk as low, intermediate, or high for the proposed surgery.

Another important aspect of preoperative medical consultation is management of perioperative medications. The medical consultant should make recommendations about the perioperative management of the patient's usual outpatient medications.[15] The consultant should also identify potential complications of the procedure (venous thromboembolism [VTE], wound infection, etc.) and make appropriate recommendations to prevent their occurrence. Many surgeons view postoperative VTE prophylaxis and surgical wound infection prophylaxis as their domain. But consultants who notice that optimal VTE and surgical wound prophylaxis is not being given should consider providing recommendations.

In summary, the medical consultant should be able to identify the pertinent medical problems, integrate this information with the physiologic stressors of anesthesia and surgery, anticipate potential perioperative problems, assess a patient's risk and need for further interventions, and communicate effectively with the surgeon and anesthesiologist.

CO-MANAGEMENT

The field of medical consultation has changed significantly since Goldman et al. published the Ten Commandments of Effective Consultation. It is common practice these days, for the consultant to step beyond the usual role of consultant and actively manage medical conditions by ordering tests and initiating therapies, which involves writing orders in the medical record—a practice known as co-management. With the increasing prevalence of the hospitalist model of care, co-management has also become commonplace. Co-management is seen most often in orthopedic surgery patients, but other surgical subspecialties are starting to request this type of service.[16–18] One advantage of the co-management model is that the medical consultant writes

TABLE 1.1. Modified 10 Commandments of Effective Consultation

	Commandment	Meaning
1.	Determine your customer.	Ask the requesting physician how you can best help them if a specific question is not obvious; they may want co-management.
2.	Establish urgency.	The consultant must determine whether the consultation is emergent, urgent, or elective.
3.	Look for yourself.	Consultants are most effective when they are willing to gather data on their own.
4.	Be as brief as appropriate.	The consultant need not repeat in full detail the data that were already recorded.
5.	Be specific, thorough, and descend from thy ivory tower to help when requested.	Leave as many specific recommendations as needed to answer the consult but ask the requesting physician if they need help with order writing.
6.	Provide contingency plans and discuss their execution.	Consultants should anticipate potential problems, document contingency plans, and provide a 24-h point of contact to help execute the plans if requested.
7.	Thou may negotiate joint title to thy neighbor's.	Consultants can and should co-manage any facet of patient care that the requesting physician desires; a frank discussion defining which specialty is responsible for what aspects of patient care is needed.
8.	Teach with tact and pragmatism.	Judgments on leaving references should be tailored to the requesting physician's specialty, level of training, and urgency of the consult.
9.	Talk is essential.	There is no substitute for direct personal contact with the primary physician.
10.	Follow-up daily.	Daily written follow-up is desirable; when the patient's problems are not active, the consultant should discuss signing off with the requesting physician beforehand.

orders thereby guaranteeing compliance with recommendations. A potential disadvantage of this practice is duplicate or conflicting orders if the consultant or surgeon is not knowledgeable of all orders in the chart.

In order to accommodate for these changing trends in the practice of consultative medicine, Salerno et al. have proposed minor modifications to the original "Ten Commandments of Effective Consultation" by Goldman et al.[8,9] The proposed changes have been presented in Table 1.1. These modified commandments recommend focusing less on defining a specific question for the consult and more on direct verbal communication about how the consultant might be able to help the requesting physician. If a co-management relationship is desired, then the consultant should take a proactive role in the management of the medical problems and in writing orders. They also recommend that the consultant need not worry about offering multiple recommendations relevant to the patient's care especially if the referral is from a surgeon Furthermore, the consult should provide explicit instructions on where he or she or an on-call colleague can be reached if the patient's clinical condition deteriorates. This more involved and interactive approach may be more apt for hospitalists and surgical subspecialists. This topic is discussed in more detail in Chapter 2.

REFERENCES

1. Devor M, Renvall M, Ramsdell J. Practice patterns and the adequacy of residency training in consultation medicine. *J Gen Intern Med.* 1993;8(10):554–560.
2. Wijeysundera ND, Austin PC, Beattie S, Hux JE, Laupacis A. Outcomes and processes of care related to preoperative medical consultation. *Arch Intern Med.* 2010;170(15):1365–1374.
3. Clelland C, Worland RL, Jessup DE, East D. Preoperative medical evaluation in patients having joint replacement surgery: added benefits. *South Med J.* 1996;89(10):958–960.
4. Devereaux PJ, Ghali WA, Gibson NE, et al. Physicians' recommendations for patients who undergo noncardiac surgery. *Clin Invest Med.* 2000;23(2):116–123.
5. Phy MP, Vanness DJ, Melton LJ, 3rd, et al. Effects of a hospitalist model on elderly patients with hip fracture. *Arch Intern Med.* 2005;165(7):796–801.
6. Macpherson DS, Parenti C, Nee J, Petzel RA, Ward H. An internist joins the surgery service: does comanagement make a difference? *J Gen Intern Med.* 1994;9(8):440–444.
7. Auerbach AD, Rasic MA, Sehgal N, Ide B, Stone B, Maselli J. Opportunity missed: medical consultation, resource use, and quality of care of patients undergoing major surgery. *Arch Intern Med.* 2007;167(21):2338–2344.
8. Goldman L, Lee T, Rudd P. Ten commandments for effective consultations. *Arch Intern Med.* 1983;143(9):1753–1755.
9. Salerno SM, Hurst FP, Halvorson S, Mercado DL. Principles of effective consultation: an update for the 21st-century consultant. *Arch Intern Med.* 2007;167(3):271–275.
10. Lee T, Pappius EM, Goldman L. Impact of inter-physician communication on the effectiveness of medical consultations. *Am J Med.* 1983;74(1):106–112.
11. Kleinman B, Czinn E, Shah K, Sobotka PA, Rao TK. The value to the anesthesia-surgical care team of the preoperative cardiac consultation. *J Cardiothorac Anesth.* 1989;3(6):682–687.
12. Horwitz RI, Henes CG, Horwitz SM. Developing strategies for improving the diagnostic and management efficacy of medical consultations. *J Chronic Dis.* 1983;36(2):213–218.
13. Sears CL, Charlson ME. The effectiveness of a consultation. Compliance with initial recommendations. *Am J Med.* 1983;74(5):870–876.
14. Katz RI, Cimino L, Vitkun SA. Preoperative medical consultations: impact on perioperative management and surgical outcome. *Can J Anaesth.* 2005;52(7):697–702.

15. Cygan R, Waitzkin H. Stopping and restarting medications in the perioperative period. *J Gen Intern Med.* 1987;2(4):270–283.

16. Batsis JA, Phy MP, Melton LJ, 3rd, et al. Effects of a hospitalist care model on mortality of elderly patients with hip fractures. *J Hosp Med.* 2007;2(4):219–225.

17. Roy A, Heckman MG, Roy V. Associations between the hospitalist model of care and quality-of-care-related outcomes in patients undergoing hip fracture surgery. *Mayo Clin Proc.* 2006; 81(1):28–31.

18. Huddleston JM, Long KH, Naessens JM, et al. Medical and surgical comanagement after elective hip and knee arthroplasty: a randomized, controlled trial. *Ann Intern Med.* 2004;141(1):28–38.

CHAPTER 2

CO-MANAGEMENT OF THE SURGICAL PATIENT

Eric Siegal

BACKGROUND

Co-management is generally defined as shared responsibility, authority, and account-ability for the management of a hospitalized patient.[1] The co-managing physician assumes a broader mandate than the traditional medical consultant, whose role is generally limited to a specific problem and who defers authority to the attending physician. In practice however, co-management varies substantially depending on a hospital's culture, the organization of its medical staff, and the personalities of the providers involved. Even within a single hospital, co-management often varies from service to service depending on the expectations of the individual physicians, the types of patients to be managed, and the level of skill or experience of the providers involved. Consequently, the term "co-management" encompasses models of care ranging from those indistinguishable from traditional medical consultation to those where the co-manager all but replaces the attending physician.

Co-management arrangements generally develop in one of three ways. They may evolve as a logical extension of long-standing working relationships between hospitalists and surgeons. Alternatively, they may be instituted by fiat, when a chief medical officer or department chair mandates co-management to address service, quality, or other performance deficiencies. Finally, co-management may develop seemingly accidentally; a classic example is the hospitalist service that initially admits a few patients with hip fractures but evolves to assume responsibility for nearly every orthopedic inpatient, irrespective of diagnosis.

Co-management has become integral to the practice of Hospital Medicine. At least 85% of hospital medicine groups (HMGs) provide co-management, and demand for this service continues to grow.[2] Many forces have driven the dramatic expansion of hospitalist co-management. Reflecting global hospital trends, surgical inpatients have become older, sicker, and more medically complex, necessitating greater involvement of physicians with expertise in the management of patients with acute and chronic medical illnesses. Surgeons, seeking to restrict their scopes of practice,

Perioperative Medicine: Medical Consultation and Co-Management, First Edition.
Edited by Amir K. Jaffer and Paul J. Grant.
© 2012 Wiley-Blackwell. Published 2012 by John Wiley & Sons, Inc.

reduce call burdens, and allocate greater time to performing procedures, have increasingly off-loaded inpatient management duties to hospitalists. Many HMGs have actively sought co-management to increase market share, demonstrate institutional value, and strengthen relationships with key stakeholders within the hospital. Hospital administrators have promoted co-management to reduce medical complications, standardize care, improve compliance with regulatory and quality metrics, and improve financial performance through better documentation, resource utilization, and patient throughput. Finally, to comply with increasingly stringent house staff workload restrictions, academic and teaching hospitals are turning to hospitalist co-management as a work reduction strategy.

Hospitalist co-management was initially conceived as a means to coordinate and improve the care of high-risk, medically complex surgical patients. Over time however, the scope of surgical co-management has broadened considerably. Hospitalists are increasingly assuming primary responsibility for surgical patients, and surgeons are choosing to serve as consultants. As a result, co-management now increasingly positions hospitalists as the de facto attending physicians for patients with acute surgical diagnoses, irrespective of their medical comorbidities.[3]

EVIDENCE

The evidence supporting the impact of hospitalist co-management on quality, efficiency, and cost of care is limited and mixed. Small cohort and retrospective studies indicate that hospitalist co-management of surgical patients modestly reduces length of stay (LOS) and cost without adversely impacting quality or outcomes.[4,5] There is very little empiric evidence to show that co-management actually improves quality of care or patient outcomes.[6] The only prospective, randomized trial of surgical co-management demonstrated that hospitalist co-management of orthopedic patients undergoing joint replacement surgery decreased the incidence of minor complications, such as the incidence of urinary tract infections, but had no impact on major complications or mortality.[7] Recent studies also suggest that hospitalist co-management appears to be most beneficial when it is targeted to surgical and specialty patients who have complex medical or care coordination issues.[4,8,9] Taken as a whole, the evidence to date tells us relatively little about how, when, where, or why surgical co-management is most effective. What is clear is that for the foreseeable future, the evolution and proliferation of co-management will continue to rapidly outstrip any evidence base. Hospitalist leaders will have to rely primarily on personal experience, anecdote, and advice from peers to determine when and how to provide effective surgical co-management.

RISKS AND BENEFITS

Based on published and anecdotal evidence, it appears that at minimum, well-designed and -managed co-management arrangements improve hospital performance, increase staff and physician satisfaction, and leverage limited surgical resources. However, the dramatic expansion of co-management suggests that there is widespread belief that co-management has a net positive impact on hospital operations and patient outcomes across a broad spectrum of patients, diagnoses, and services. It is therefore particularly important to recognize that while co-management can be beneficial, it also carries significant risks.

Complexity

Adding an additional physician to care that was historically rendered by a single surgeon or specialist increases the complexity of the care. As a rule, as a system becomes more complex, it becomes more sophisticated and adaptable, but also more prone to breakdowns and errors. Adding a co-managing physician to the care of a surgical patient increases the likelihood of miscommunication, duplication of effort, unclear accountability, and misappropriated responsibility, all of which may generate confusion, frustration, or errors. For the medically complex surgical patient, it is reasonable to assume that adding complexity is a reasonable trade-off for the medical expertise and oversight afforded by a hospitalist. The same may not hold true for surgical patients who are otherwise healthy or medically straightforward.

Scope of Practice

As the scope of co-management broadens to establish hospitalists as primary managers of surgical patients, there is growing risk that hospitalists will overstep their training and competencies. Over a decade ago, surveyed hospitalists reported mismatches between their training and their actual scope of practice, notably in acute neurology, neurosurgery, orthopedics, surgery, and psychiatry.[10,11] There is reason to be concerned that under the guise of co-management, hospitalists are managing patients for whom they are untrained and unqualified to provide care. Hospitalist co-management is also particularly susceptible to "mission creep." A term coined by the American military, mission creep describes the inadvertent evolution of a mission beyond its original intent, often with disastrous consequences. Mission creep is particularly germane to hospitalist co-management; hospitalists who initially co-manage a carefully selected subset of neurosurgical patients may inadvertently expand coverage to other neurosurgical patients that they are neither trained nor qualified to manage.

Inconsistent Delivery

Due to the absence of formal training or mandated certification in Hospital Medicine, the hospitalist workforce is highly variable. Within a single HMG, hospitalists may possess widely different skills, abilities, and comfort with co-managing acutely ill surgical patients. A hospitalist who can competently manage patients with acute intracranial hemorrhages may hand off to a partner who is unable to provide the same level of care. Such inconsistencies make it difficult to standardize care, create gaps in coverage, damage working relationships, and ultimately compromise patient safety.

Career Dissatisfaction

In well-designed co-management arrangements, hospitalists and specialists work equitably under clearly and mutually defined rules of engagement. They share responsibility for patients, collaborate to improve care, and learn from each other. However, it is easy for this relationship to become inequitable. Surgeons may expect hospitalists to shoulder the "undesirable" portions of inpatient care, such as cross coverage, family meetings, and discharge management. Hospital administrators may tacitly or overtly expect their financially subsidized hospitalists to accept any and all co-management referrals, irrespective of whether they are clinically appropriate. If these behaviors become ingrained, they cement a perception of hospitalists as subordinate members of the care team and may accelerate hospitalist job dissatisfaction and burnout.

Understaffing

As a rapidly growing specialty, Hospital Medicine faces critical and ongoing mismatches between the demand for and availability of qualified hospitalists. The erosion in popularity of general internal medicine and family medicine training has further undermined the pool of future hospitalists. As a consequence, many hospitalist programs will remain understaffed for the foreseeable future. Adding co-management services to understaffed hospitalist programs may destabilize programs, compromise care, and hasten staff turnover.

ELEMENTS OF SUCCESSFUL CO-MANAGEMENT PROGRAMS

Although there is no single path to developing successful co-management programs, successful programs do appear to share several common features. The participants have a clear sense of mission and a shared definition of success. They engage their stakeholders and define clear responsibilities and expectations for all parties. They proactively identify the potential weaknesses of the program and address them before they become problems. They understand the resources necessary to develop and sustain the program, and they work to ensure that the successes are replicated. Finally, they continually reexamine the program, strengthening relationships, building on successes, and addressing failures.

The six key elements of successful co-management are the following:

1. Identify the stakeholders and define their expectations.
2. Ask the tough questions.
3. Clarify roles and responsibilities.
4. Obtain resources and support.
5. Measure performance.
6. Revisit the relationship.

Identify the Stakeholders and Define Their Expectations

The first step to successful co-management is to clarify goals, identify the key stakeholders, and ascertain their expectations and assumptions for the relationship and its outcomes:

Identifying the Stakeholders

- Who is driving the co-management relationship? Is it being internally driven by the hospitalists and/or surgeons, or is it an external party, such as a hospital administrator?
- Identify the primary stakeholders. There should be at least one influential champion from the HMG, the surgical practice, and the hospital administration to develop and support the relationship. Once these stakeholders have been defined, determine if they are equally engaged, empowered, and supportive.
- Identify the secondary stakeholders. The co-management program may affect nursing staff, case managers, pharmacists, emergency departments, or other ancillary services, and they should be engaged to gain buy-in and solicit input.
- Identify and reach out to the skeptics. At absolute minimum, it will define who needs extra attention as the process unfolds. Often, skeptics raise legitimate concerns that may not be apparent to the champions.

Define the Expectations

- What are the primary reasons for providing co-management? Is the main goal to improve quality, increase efficiency, extend the reach of overstretched surgeons, or something else? Do all stakeholders share and support these expectations?
- What specific benefits do the HMG, hospital, and surgeons expect to realize as a result of this relationship? Will all parties benefit from the relationship? Who stands to gain or lose from success or failure?

Ask the Tough Questions

Once the expectations have been clearly defined, it is imperative to reality test them. While there is nothing wrong with setting "stretch" goals, the expectations have to be achievable and the benefits have to outweigh the costs. If the goals are overly ambitious, it is far better to reset them up front rather than after the program has failed to meet expectations. Second, it is important to question whether all of the appropriate stakeholders are involved and whether they are sufficiently engaged and influential to overcome obstacles as they arise. Once reasonable expectations have been set and the stakeholders have been vetted, it is helpful to ask specific questions about clinical and logistical risks posed by providing co-management:

Clinical Risks

- Are the hospitalists uniformly qualified to do the work? If not, how will they become qualified?

- Are there specific circumstances or diagnoses that should preclude co-management?
- Once the hospitalists begin co-management, how and when should the hospitalist call in the surgeon? Are there circumstances that mandate immediate or accelerated response from the surgeon?

Logistical Risks

- Is the HMG adequately staffed to provide this co-management service? If not, how might providing co-management impact other service lines, hospitalist morale, or quality of care?
- If staffing is an issue, can the HMG recruit qualified personnel, drop other duties, and/or phase in the program as staffing permits?

Clarify Roles and Responsibilities

As a precondition to effective co-management, it is vital to clarify roles, identify responsibilities for each aspect of care, and predetermine how disagreements over the content or process of care will be adjudicated. Hospital nurses, pharmacists, and other staff must have clear and consistent policies defining which responsibilities are the domains of the hospitalist versus the surgeon. Hospitalists and surgeons should also determine who will manage disposition and discuss postdischarge planning with patients and families. Finally, hospitalists and surgeons should have a mechanism for adjudicating inevitable disagreements over care. At best, failure to proactively address these issues frustrates hospital staff, patients, and families. At worst, it can lead to serious clinical errors that can harm patients and increase malpractice exposure. It is vital to address the "rules of engagement" before co-management begins and to insist on their consistent application by all parties.

Patient Selection and Scope of Practice

- Is every surgical patient appropriate for medical co-management? If not, what are the inclusion criteria?
- How will co-managed and non-co-managed patients be identified to differentiate them to physicians and hospital staff?
- Which specific clinical issues are the responsibilities of the hospitalist versus the surgeon? Do they overlap and if so, who makes the final call?

Delegation of Responsibilities

- Who should be called when a problem arises? Does this change dependent on the time of day, type of problem, or the acuity of the situation?
- What happens if the surgeon and hospitalist disagree over a care issue? Who makes the final call? Is there a mechanism for adjudicating such disputes?
- What is the hospitalist's role in the admission and discharge process? Who will write the history and physical examination and discharge summary, rec-

oncile medications, communicate with the primary care physician, and arrange follow-up? If this is a shared process, who does what?

- What are the expectations for communication between the hospitalist and the specialist? Does the surgeon expect a call every time a hospitalist sees a new patient, or vice versa?

Obtain Resources and Support

As a rule, surgical co-management is financially advantageous for surgeons, who can reallocate time previously spent on medical management (which is included in their surgical bundled payment) to increasing procedural volume or seeing more patients in the outpatient clinic. The same financial benefits may not exist for hospitalists. The overwhelming majority of HMGs require external financial support, reflecting the undervaluation of cognitive evaluation and management (E&M) codes as well as the inability to bill for much of the care coordination, patient education, and discharge management inherent to co-management. Furthermore, with its recent elimination of consultation codes, the Centers for Medicare and Medicaid Services (CMS) has eliminated co-managing hospitalists' ability to bill an initial high-value initial E&M code, further eroding the financial viability of co-management.

Although the finances of co-management vary considerably depending on payer mix, patient complexity, and the efficiency of the hospital, HMGs should generally assume that the financials of co-management do not differ substantially from any other book of business offered in the hospital. To avoid unpleasant financial consequences, the parties involved should address the financial implications of co-management:

- Is there a consistent and predictable volume of patients to be co-managed?
- Will the hospitalist bill as the attending physician or as a consultant, and how will this impact the financials?
- To what extent is the hospitalist expected to provide services that are unbillable, such as education, care management, or communication? Who will pay for this?
- What happens if both the hospitalist and surgeon address the same clinical issues and can only submit a single bill between the two of them?
- Will the added workload positively or negatively affect the efficiency and productivity of the physicians involved? Can midlevel providers deliver some of the care, and how will this affect the bottom line?
- If co-management positively impacts the hospital's bottom line, will those savings be used to offset the cost of the program?

Ultimately, support for co-management should be construed more broadly than just financials. Stakeholders should also determine whether additional resources are necessary to facilitate the goals of co-management. For example, if reducing LOS is a key expectation, it may be necessary to allocate additional case management resources to expedite hospital discharge. If the goal is to improve medication reconciliation at discharge, hospitalists may need improvements to the electronic health record or support from a hospital pharmacist. Additionally, hospitalists may require dedicated workspace or computer terminals on busy surgical units to facilitate efficient workflow. In the end, resources should be allocated to maximize the likelihood of the program achieving its goals.

Measure Performance

The fifth critical factor in building and maintaining a successful co-management service is to determine whether the program is actually delivering the expected results. Demonstrating success, especially early on, generates and maintains enthusiasm for the program, facilitates continuous improvement, makes it easier to replicate success in future endeavors, and justifies ongoing financial support. Early recognition of missed goals or errors creates confidence in the process and reduces the risk of serious harm to patients.

Measures should reflect outcomes that are realistically achievable, are specific, and can be reliably measured. Sample measures might include the following:

Financial

- Impact of focused physician documentation on hospital diagnostic related group (DRG) coding and revenue capture
- Impact on LOS and subsequent increase in patient throughput
- Impact on hospitalist and/or surgeon direct clinical productivity
- Impact on hospital costs due to changes in resource utilization

Quality

- Adherence rates to quality standards, such as deep vein thrombosis (DVT) prophylaxis, time to antibiotic administration, or medication reconciliation at discharge
- Thirty-day readmission rates
- Complication rates (iatrogenic infections, ICU transfers)
- Incidence of medication errors

Other

- Patient satisfaction scores (e.g., Press Ganey survey data)
- Hospital staff satisfaction or retention
- Surgeon satisfaction scores

Revisit the Relationship

Finally, it is vital to build a regular regime of reevaluation into the relationship. Over time, the previously enthusiastic stakeholder may become jaded, while the skeptic may become a convert. Problems that are initially thought to be trivial may fester if not proactively addressed. The three most important questions to ask are whether the program's goals are being met, whether the stakeholders are happy with the program and how the program is impacting patient care. It is far better to proactively look for problems than to wait for it to blow up.

Finally, put the basic agreements about the program in writing. Although every aspect of the program does not need to be memorialized, putting the key points on paper forces clarity, reduces legal exposure, and minimizes the occurrence of memory lapses.

REFERENCES

1. Siegal E. Just because you can doesn't mean that you should: a call for the rational application of hospitalist comanagement. *J Hosp Med*. September 2008;3(5):398–402.
2. Society of Hospital Medicine. The Society of Hospital Medicine 2005–2006 Survey: The Authoritative Source on the State of the Hospital Medicine Movement. Published by the Society of Hospital Medicine, 2006. Executive summary available at http://www.hospitalmedicine.org/AM/Template.cfm?Section=Survey&Template=/CM/ContentDisplay.cfm&ContentID=14352. Accessed September 2 2008.
3. Gesensway D. Feeling pressure to admit surgical patients? Hospitalists work to set limits on co-management arrangements. Today's Hospitalist. January 2008.
4. Pinzur MS, Gurza E, Kristopaitis T, et al. Hospitalist-orthopedic co-management of high-risk patients undergoing lower extremity reconstruction surgery. *Orthopedics*. Jul 2009;32(7):495.
5. Phy MP, Vanness DJ, Melton LJ, et al. Effects of a hospitalist model on elderly patients with hip fracture. *Arch Intern Med*. Apr 11 2005;165:796–801.
6. Auerbach AD, Rasic MA, Sehgal N, Ide B, Stone B, Maselli J. Opportunity missed: medical consultation, resource use, and quality of care of patients undergoing major surgery. *Arch Intern Med*. Nov 26 2007;167(21):2338–2344.
7. Huddleston JM, Long KH, Naessens JM, et al. Medical and surgical comanagement after elective hip and knee arthroplasty: a randomized controlled trial. *Ann Intern Med*. Jul 6 2004; 141(1):28–38.
8. Southern WN, Berger MA, Bellin EY, Hailpern SM, Arnsten JH. Hospitalist care and length of stay in patients requiring complex discharge planning and close clinical monitoring. *Arch Intern Med*. Sep 24 2007;167(17):1869–1874.
9. Simon TD, Eilert R, Dickinson LM, Kempe A, Benefield E, Berman S. Pediatric hospitalist comanagement of spinal fusion surgery patients. *J Hosp Med*. Jan 2007;2:23–29.
10. Plauth WH, Pantilat SZ, Wachter RM, Fenton CL. Hospitalists' perceptions of their residency training needs: results of a national survey. *Am J Med*. Aug 15 2001;111:247–254.
11. Glasheen JJ, Epstein KR, Siegal E, Kutner J, Prochazka AV. The spectrum of community-based hospitalist practice: a call to tailor internal medicine residency training. *Arch Intern Med*. Apr 9 2007;167(7):727–728.

CHAPTER 3

IMPROVING THE QUALITY AND OUTCOMES OF PERIOPERATIVE CARE

Mihaela Stefan and Peter K. Lindenauer

INTRODUCTION

Nearly a decade after the publication of "Crossing the Quality Chasm: A New Health System for the 21st Century,"[1] improving the quality, safety, and value of the U.S. healthcare system continues to be a major objective for both payers and providers. Spending on hospital care in the United States now consumes approximately 32% of the healthcare budget,[2] and yet the average Americans has only a 50% chance of receiving care that is recommended in clinical guidelines.[3] In its landmark reports,[1,4] the Institute of Medicine identified many strategies that might be used to help close this gap, ranging from greater use of information technology to making scientific evidence more useful and accessible to clinicians. Two of the most significant recommendations were the promotion of greater transparency regarding the system's performance on safety, evidence-based practice, and patient satisfaction, and the enactment of changes to the payment system to better reward quality.

In this chapter, we describe the rationale and drivers of today's public reporting programs, review approaches to measuring the quality of perioperative and surgical care, examine the evidence concerning the benefits of public reporting programs, and discuss some of the reasons why these programs remain controversial.

HOW PUBLIC REPORTING COULD IMPROVE QUALITY OF CARE AND PATIENT OUTCOMES

Berwick et al.[5] described two interrelated pathways through which transparency might improve quality of care and lead to better patient outcomes, which they called the selection and change pathways (Figure 3.1).

Perioperative Medicine: Medical Consultation and Co-Management, First Edition.
Edited by Amir K. Jaffer and Paul J. Grant.

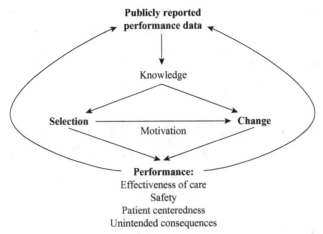

Figure 3.1.   Two pathways through which transparency might lead to improved hospital value. From Berwick et al.[5] and Hannan et al.[12]

Selection

Through this pathway, patients, physicians, and healthcare plans might use information about performance to preferentially choose providers with better quality. This shift would lead to higher quality of care at the population level as a greater percentage of patients are cared for at institutions with better outcomes. On a superficial level, this mechanism appears relatively straightforward: A patient requiring bypass surgery would only need to look up the performance of the different hospitals in their area and choose the surgeon or hospital with the best outcomes. Unlike the change pathway described below, selection does not depend on hospitals to make any changes in care in order for public reporting to have a beneficial effect on health outcomes.

Change Pathway

Public release of performance data might lead to better quality of care by stimulating or catalyzing improvement efforts of providers. Creating awareness of a hospital's performance, especially if that performance is poor, may appeal to the professionalism of physicians, nurses, and hospital administrators, motivating them to engage in quality improvement (QI) activities that can lead to changes in practice that ultimately improve care. Additionally, the threat that patients or referring providers might use performance data to influence their decisions about where to receive care or direct their patients is another potential motivation for QI through the change pathway. What distinguishes the change pathway from the selection pathway is that change is the fundamental driver for better outcomes.

APPROACHES TO MEASURING QUALITY

Donabedian[6] described three domains—structure, process, and outcomes—through which quality of care can be assessed, and this classic model continues to guide many contemporary efforts to measure and report the quality of health care across a wide range of practice settings.

Structure refers to the characteristics of the settings in which providers deliver health care, including material resources (e.g., electronic medical records), human resources (e.g., staffing in the intensive care unit), and organizational structure. A primary advantage of structural measures of quality is that they are generally easy to measure, and to the extent that there is good evidence to support the connection between the structure and patient outcomes, they can be assumed reliable indicators of quality.

An example of a contemporary structurally oriented reporting system is the Leapfrog Group online posting of hospital ratings based on surgical volumes for high-risk procedures (http://www.leapfroggroup.org) (Figure 3.2).

Processes of care refer to what is actually done to the patient,[7] such as whether thromboprophylaxis measures are ordered for surgical patients.

In contrast to many structural measures of quality, process measures are often highly actionable—in that, they can be directly influenced by care process redesign and, unlike outcome measures of quality, do not depend on risk adjustment to make comparisons across hospitals.

Health outcomes are the direct result of a patient's health status as a consequence of contact with the healthcare system, such as rates of mortality, readmissions or complications, or patient satisfaction. An example of an outcomes-oriented reporting system is the annual report of institution-specific hospital-acquired infection rates published by Pennsylvania Health Care Cost Containment Council

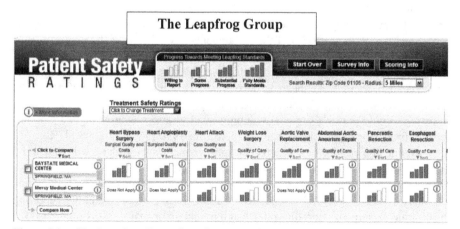

Figure 3.2.   The Leapfrog Group (http://www.leapfroggroup.org).

(http://www.phc4.org) and risk-adjusted mortality rate and readmission rate (http://www.hospitalcompare.hhs.gov).

Numerous web sites currently offer patients the ability to compare hospitals on multiple aspects of healthcare quality. Table 3.1 gives a summary of the most important current reporting initiatives that measure surgical quality of care.

The most important web site engaged in public reporting of healthcare quality in the United States is known as Hospital Compare and is operated by the Centers for Medicare and Medicaid Services (http://www.hospitalcompare.hhs.gov/). Hospital Compare is a consumer-oriented reporting service, which provides performance rates on quality measures on four clinical conditions and surgery. The clinical measures reported on Hospital Compare focus on four medical conditions and on surgical care. As of 2010, Hospital Compare includes eight performance measures centered on surgical quality, which address surgical antibiotic prophylaxis, glycemic control postcardiac surgery, venous thromboembolism prophylaxis, and continuation of beta-blockers during the perioperative period (Table 3.2).

EVIDENCE FOR PUBLIC REPORTING EFFECTS ON SELECTION BY PATIENTS AND PROVIDERS

Impact on Patient Selection

Whether or not the selection pathway leads to better health outcomes depends on the willingness and ability of patients and referring physicians to find, interpret, and act on information about quality of care to choose the best physician or hospital.

Evidence suggests that consumers strongly support public reporting of healthcare providers' performance, and they perceive large differences between hospitals and physicians. In its 2008 update on consumers' views of patient safety and quality information from the Kaiser Family Foundation, roughly half of Americans believe that there are *large* differences in the quality of care provided by hospitals and physicians in their local area. In contrast, only 7–10% of those surveyed reported that they had used publicly available performance data to make healthcare-related decisions, and the majority (94%) of the respondents never heard of the major government initiative around hospital quality—the Hospital Compare web site. Although consumers' use of publicly reported performance data remains low, their recognition of the value of these data appears to have grown over time. Between 1996 and 2008, the same Kaiser Family Foundation Survey reported that the percentage of Americans who would prefer a surgeon with high-quality ratings over a surgeon who has treated friends or family more than doubled from 1996 (20%) to 2008 (47%).

While the results of these recent surveys suggest a greater willingness by patients to use publicly reported data to make healthcare decisions, empirical evidence of such decision making is lacking. In a survey of patients who had undergone coronary bypass surgery in Pennsylvania in 1988,[8] only 2% said that public reporting of hospital or surgeon mortality rates had a moderate or major effect on their decision making, and just 12% were even aware of the existence of public reports. Eight years later, 11% of patients sought information about hospitals before deciding on

TABLE 3.1. Most Important Current Reporting Initiatives for Surgical Hospitals' Quality

Rating service	Types of surgeries scored	Structure measures	Process measures	Outcome measures	Patient population
Hospital Compare	All surgeries				All patients
Surgical Care Improvement Project (SCIP)			Antibiotic use Thromboprophylaxis Beta-blockers use Glycemic control after cardiac surgery		
Leapfrog	CABG, PCI AAA repair Pancreatic resection Esophagectomy Aortic valve replacement Bariatric surgery High-risk deliveries	CPOE ICU staffing Procedure volumes	Safe-practice scores	Risk-adjusted mortality for CABG	All patients
Healthgrades	Cardiac Vascular Orthopedic Abdominal Transplant	Presence of newborn ICU	Leapfrog safe-practice scores	Length of stay Survival Complications Patient safety indicators Cost	Medicaid Medicare
US News	ENT Cardiac Orthopedic Neurosurgery Urology	Nurse staffing Magnet hospital Key technologies Trauma center	Reputation based on physicians surveyed	Mortality index Patient safety index	Medicare

CABG, coronary artery bypass graft; PCI, percutaneous coronary intervention; AAA, abdominal aortic aneurysm; ENT, ear, nose, and throat; CPOE, computerized physician order entry.

TABLE 3.2. Surgical Care Improvement Project (July 2008 through June 2009)

Hospital process of care measure	United States average (%)	Massachusetts average (%)	% for Baystate Medical Center	% for Mercy Medical Center	% for Hartford Hospital
% of surgery patients who *were taking beta-blockers* before surgery, who were kept on the beta-blockers during perioperative period	87	94	90% of 174 patients[2]	90% of 105 patients	93% of 112 patients
% of surgery patients who were given *an antibiotic at the right time* (within 1 h before surgery) to help prevent infection	91	95	99% of 895 patients[2]	95% of 422 patients	92% of 452 patients
% of surgery patients whose doctors ordered *treatments to prevent blood clots* after certain types of surgeries	88	93	100% of 404 patients	98% of 435 patients	99% of 248 patients

The percentage includes only patients whose history and condition indicate the treatment is appropriate (http://www.hospitalcompare.hhs.gov).

elective major surgery.[9] Nevertheless, two recent systematic reviews[10,11] concluded that there is limited evidence that public reporting affect patients' choices of physicians and hospitals.

Why Transparency Has Had Limited Effects on the Selection of Hospitals by Patients   There are a number of plausible explanations for why both past and current transparency initiatives have had little to no effect on patients' choice of which hospital to seek care. First, health care is complex, and before arriving in the emergency department, many patients do not know what is actually wrong with them. For example, the patient with abdominal pain goes to the hospital to both have the cause of the pain *diagnosed*, and to have it treated, and without knowing that the cause of the pain is an inflamed appendix, it would be difficult to use a hospital rating web site to identify the best institution to have the appendix removed. Furthermore, patients frequently rely on physicians to act on their behalf when making a choice between hospitals or surgeons. Second, patients are often not in a position to make choices of a hospital. For an emergent admission, patients may have little or no choice but to go to the nearest hospital. Third, often there are only few hospital providers in a local market, so patients have limited choices to find hospitals, which are close to home. Finally, in elective settings, patients typically choose a physician whose admitting privileges dictate hospital choice. Lastly, despite significant advances in quality measurement and reporting, performance data remain limited to only a few conditions, and different web sites produce conflicting results.

Impact on Referring Providers

Public reporting might influence the selection of hospitals and surgeons by referring providers; however, this requires that providers have confidence in the accuracy of the reports and have enough options to choose from. Hannan et al. surveyed New York cardiologists regarding the state cardiac surgery report and found that despite the fact that the majority found the report easy to understand and at least somewhat accurate, only 38% said that changed their referral patterns.[12] The available evidence suggest that primary care physicians' decisions for referral is more influenced by personal knowledge of the specialist or previous experience rather than by data about quality or performance.[13]

Impact on Market Share

Several studies have found minimal changes in hospital market share after the public reporting of mortality data. Jha and Epstein examined the New York State Cardiac Surgery Reporting System data from 1989 to 2002 and found no evidence that performance was associated with subsequent change in hospitals' market share.[14]

EVIDENCE THAT PUBLIC REPORTING IMPROVES QUALITY OF CARE

Effects on QI Activity

A recent systematic review[11] concluded that public reporting is an effective method of stimulating QI. A landmark study by Hibbard et al. is representative of the results.[15] This survey-based investigation measured the number of QI activities in cardiac and obstetric care undertaken by 24 Wisconsin hospitals that were included in an existing public reporting system and compared them with the number undertaken by 98 other Wisconsin hospitals that received either a private report on their own quality performance or no quality report at all. The study found that the hospitals that participated in public reporting were engaged in significantly more QI activities than were the hospitals receiving private reporting or no reporting.

In one of the very few randomized trials of public reporting of the quality of hospital care for patients, Tu and colleagues evaluated whether the public release of data on cardiac quality indicators led hospitals to undertake QI activities that improve healthcare processes and patient outcomes. The Enhanced Feedback for Effective Cardiac Treatment (EFFECT)[16] study evaluated patients admitted with acute myocardial infarction (AMI) or congestive heart failure (CHF) at 86 Canadian hospitals that were randomized to receive early (the intervention group) or late feedback (the control group) of a public report card on their baseline performance. The authors found that hospitals in the early feedback group were significantly more likely to engage in QI activities related to cardiac care (73.2% of early feedback group vs. 46.7% of delayed feedback group for AMI care and 61.0% of early feedback group vs. 50.0% of delayed feedback group for CHF care).

Effects on Outcomes

In contrast, the evidence concerning the effects of public reporting on patient outcomes is less consistent. The 2008 systematic review by Fung et al. identified 11 studies that addressed this issue in the hospital setting: Five found that public reporting had a positive effect on patient outcomes, while six demonstrated a negative effect or no effect.[11] One particularly well-studied example of public reporting is the New York State Cardiac Surgery Reporting System, which was established in 1989 as the first statewide program to produce annual data for public dissemination on risk-adjusted death rates following coronary artery bypass grafting (CABG), by hospital and by surgeon. The program was associated with a significant decline of risk-adjusted mortality from 4.17% to 2.45% during the first 3 years.[17] Nevertheless, other states that did not have public reporting systems in place experienced similar reduction,[18] although one study found that the decrease in mortality after CABG was greater in New York than for the United States as a whole.[19]

HOW TRANSPARENCY PROGRAMS MIGHT REDUCE HEALTHCARE COSTS

In general, it is challenging to identify an obvious mechanism through which improvements in process of care measures, mortality rates, or satisfaction might result in lower healthcare spending. However, if greater transparency resulted in improvements in readmission rates, healthcare-associated infections, or other complications of hospitalization, large savings could be realized. The study by Zhan and Miller identified those cases that were likely to be medical injuries resulted from failure in the process of care in a hospital.[20] Regarding postoperative complications, the study found a significant excess in cost of $57,727 for postoperative sepsis, $53,500 for postoperative respiratory failure and $21,700 for postoperative thromboembolism. In theory, publicly reporting these data should stimulate research regarding circumstances and risk factors associated with these medical injuries and prompt hospitals to develop strategies to prevent them, consequently reducing healthcare cost.

UNINTENDED CONSEQUENCES

Efforts to promote greater transparency of hospital quality can have unintended effects, including overuse, teaching to the test, gaming, adverse selection (or cherry picking), and misuse of the data by patients.

Overuse

In 2003, the Infectious Diseases Society of America updated its guidelines on community-acquired pneumonia to recommend that patients receive antibiotics within 4 h of hospital admission. This recommendation was adopted as an incentive-linked performance measure by Centers for Medicare and Medicaid Services (CMS). Kanwar et al. studied the impact of this guidelines-based incentive and found that after its implementation, more patients received antibiotics in a timely fashion but there was an increase in the proportion of patients without pneumonia who were given antibiotics unnecessarily.[21] Other quality measures that are at risk for overuse and misuse include prophylaxis for deep vein thrombosis, glycemic control measures, and immunization.

"Teaching to the Test"

In the context of public reporting initiatives, concerns about "teaching to the test" refers to a situation in which hospitals might invest limited resources in an area subject to reporting, while neglecting other more important areas that might yield greater clinical benefit.

Gaming

Gaming refers to those situations in which participants find ways to maximize measured results without actually improving care. For example, hospitals might attempt to improve their "performance" simply by focusing on documentation and coding practices. While no additional patients will experience better outcomes, the hospitals' performance appears to improve.

Adverse Selection or "Cherry Picking"

In this scenario, a provider might reject the sickest patients or might select patients based on the likelihood of a positive outcome or compliance with treatment protocols rather than need. For example, Pennsylvania cardiologists expressed difficulty in finding cardiovascular surgeons for high-risk patients after CABG report was introduced.[22]

Causing Patients to Make Poor Choices

Rothberg et al. assessed the level of agreement regarding hospital quality for four conditions across five web sites that produce hospital rankings. They found that the sites evaluated different measures of structure, processes, and outcomes, and reached different conclusions about which hospitals performed best and which performed poorly. Leonardi had a similar conclusion examining six Internet rating programs of surgical care and outcomes.[23] He found that the web sites were inconsistent in their level of detail and rating; the government and nonprofit services were more accessible and transparent with their data, but the proprietary sites had procedure-specific data, which were more complete.[23] Additionally, it is possible that patients will use publicly available quality measures to make inferences about the quality of care for conditions that are not the focus of measurement and reporting effort. Yet it is unclear whether the same factors that lead one hospital to achieve good outcomes in cardiac surgery will necessarily make it a good choice for a patient in need of bowel resection. In such circumstances, it is possible that use of report cards to choose a hospital for a condition not subject to reporting will lead patients to make poor choices.

METHODOLOGICAL CHALLENGES IN PUBLIC REPORTING

Measure Selection

Identifying process measures of quality that are grounded in strong evidence is a critical step in achieving the support of clinicians and ultimately improving patient outcomes. Yet more than 20 years after the term evidence-based medicine was coined,[24] most of medicine remains based on therapies for which evidence is limited or nonexistent. This has created an important obstacle in the development of new process measures. Furthermore, even for those treatments for which the evidence is clear, variation in processes of care across hospitals explains only a small fraction of the difference in patient outcomes. One explanation is that while process measures are valuable in that they provide directly actionable information that can be used to target gaps in care quality, outcomes such as mortality and readmission are influenced by many factors that are independent of existing process measures.

Risk Adjustment

The limitation of the process measure-based approach to measuring hospital quality is one of the factors that have led to resurgence in the use of outcome measures such as complications, mortality, and readmission rates. Yet unlike the case with process measures, in order to compare outcomes across hospitals, it is necessary to adjust for differences in patient case mix. An important limitation of risk adjustment is that it is only capable of reducing the effect of differences in measured characteristics of patients but remains subject to residual confounding by unmeasured patient factors. Without appropriate adjustment for patient severity of illness, hospitals with the highest mortality rates are likely to be those that treat the sickest patients, not the ones that provide the poorest care.[25] For those designing quality transparency programs, risk adjustment is an important challenge and still a matter of controversy.

The Problem with Small Sample and Low Event Rates

Conditions and procedures included in public reporting programs must provide sufficient case volumes and event rates to make it possible to discriminate between performers with some degree of certainty. In the setting of surgical outcomes, Dimick et al.[26] examined whether the seven surgical procedures for which mortality has been promoted as a quality indicator (CABG surgery, repair of abdominal aortic aneurysm, pancreatic resection, esophageal resection, pediatric heart surgery, craniotomy, hip replacement) are performed frequently enough to reliably identify hospitals with increased mortality rates. He determined the minimum caseload necessary to reliably detect increased mortality rates and found that, with the exception of CABG, the operations for which surgical mortality has been advocated as a quality indicator are generally not performed with sufficient frequency to identify a hospital whose mortality rate was twice the national average, even using a 3-year sample of cases. This study suggests that developing surgical or perioperative quality measures based on mortality rates is inherently problematic.

FUTURE DIRECTIONS

While public reporting of hospital quality increases transparency and makes hospitals more accountable for their performance, the evidence that it results in better quality of care or patient outcomes is limited, and to date, patients have not truly embraced public reporting programs as a way of choosing which hospital to seek care. By necessity, hospital report cards only provide information on the measures selected for inclusion and provide only a partial picture of overall care quality. Increasing the value of public reporting will depend on a variety of factors, including developing new measures, choosing relevant conditions for reporting, increasing awareness among patients and referring physicians, and better linking hospital performance to payment. With regard to development of new measures, the CMS has outlined plans to increase the number of publicly reported measures to more than 70 by 2010 and more than 100 by 2011. While this will provide information about a greater number of conditions, there is also the risk that patients may be overwhelmed by the added complexity. The development of new outcome measures are a particular priority because patients and payers ultimately care more about the result of their care than how these results were achieved. However, outcome measurement should expand beyond mortality and readmission to include functional status and quality of life. Ideally, programs should use a mix of measures, including outcomes, process, and structural and patient experience. Yet the cost and logistic challenges of collecting these kinds of data have generally limited their application to the research setting. The conditions that are publicly reported need to have clinical significance (impact on quality and length of life) and be relevant to a large number of consumers.

One of the important objectives within public reporting is to make patients more aware of the value and availability of information about quality. While patients are generally enthusiastic about the accountability provided by quality transparency, the main reason for their limited use appears to be the complexity of the information.[27] The literature suggests that the format design and type of data presented can influence the understanding of the measures used in reports. Furthermore, there are data presentation strategies that improve comprehension among patients and if utilized, would likely increase the use of quality care indicators and the efficacy of reporting efforts.[28,29] Consumers find performance measures most useful when the information is presented as grades or ratings, and when there are enough—but not too many—categories of performance (four to five categories are usually most effective). This year, the Society for Thoracic Surgeons (STS) in collaboration with

Consumers Union, will start to publish a ranking system for cardiac surgeons and programs offering CABG (www.consumerreprots.org/health). The grading will be easy to comprehend by consumers (1- to 3-star rating system) and will address five areas: overall performance, patients' survival, avoidance of complications, and extent to which the program follow the recommended surgical best practices and to which recommended medications are used.

A successful public reporting program requires the information presented to be consistent and accurate. Engaging providers in designing the quality reporting program will increase participation (in voluntary transparency initiatives), help ensure clinical and practical relevance of the measures, and increase acceptance by providers of the program's measures and methods. The National Surgical Quality Improvement Program, although not yet publicly available is one example in this direction; it is a national, risk-adjusted, peer-controlled program with audited data collection.

Partnership between different organizations to collect accurate and timely data may lead to consolidation of the number of Internet rating sites and improvement of the quality, transparency, and accessibility of the data presented.

CONCLUSION

While evidence that greater transparency about the quality of health care is being used by patients, or has lead to better outcomes, is limited, there is little debate that patients and payers have a right to know the quality of care they are receiving. Because transparency is a core value of democratic societies, there remains a pressing need to invest in the development and implementation of better and more sophisticated measures of quality.

REFERENCES

1. Committee on the Quality of Healthcare in America. *Crossing the Quality Chasm: A New Health System for the 21st Century*. Washington, DC: National Academy Press; 2001.
2. Hartman M, Martin A, McDonnell P, Catlin A. National health spending in 2007: slower drug spending contributes to lowest rate of overall growth since 1998. *Health Aff (Millwood)*. Jan–Feb 2009;28(1):246–261.
3. McGlynn EA, Asch SM, Adams J, et al. The quality of health care delivered to adults in the United States. *N Engl J Med*. Jun 26 2003;348(26):2635–2645.
4. Kohn LT, Corrigan JM, Donaldson MS. *To Err Is Human: Building a Safer Health System*. Washington, DC: National Academy Press; 1999.
5. Berwick DM, James B, Coye MJ. Connections between quality measurement and improvement. *Med Care*. Jan 2003;41(1 Suppl):I30–I38.
6. Donabedian A. Evaluating the quality of medical care. *Milbank Mem Fund Q*. Jul 1966;44(3 Suppl):166–206.
7. Gustafson DH, Hundt AS. Findings of innovation research applied to quality management principles for health care. *Health Care Manage Rev*. Spring 1995;20(2):16–33.
8. Schneider EC, Epstein AM. Use of public performance reports: a survey of patients undergoing cardiac surgery. *JAMA*. May 27 1998;279(20):1638–1642.

9. Schwartz LM, Woloshin S, Birkmeyer JD. How do elderly patients decide where to go for major surgery? Telephone interview survey. *BMJ*. Oct 8 2005;331(7520):821.

10. Faber M, Bosch M, Wollersheim H, Leatherman S, Grol R. Public reporting in health care: how do consumers use quality-of-care information? A systematic review. *Med Care*. Jan 2009;47(1):1–8.

11. Fung CH, Lim YW, Mattke S, Damberg C, Shekelle PG. Systematic review: the evidence that publishing patient care performance data improves quality of care. *Ann Intern Med*. Jan 15 2008;148(2):111–123.

12. Hannan EL, Stone CC, Biddle TL, DeBuono BA. Public release of cardiac surgery outcomes data in New York: what do New York state cardiologists think of it? *Am Heart J*. Jul 1997;134(1): 55–61.

13. Forrest CB, Nutting PA, Starfield B, von Schrader S. Family physicians' referral decisions: results from the ASPN referral study. *J Fam Pract*. Mar 2002;51(3):215–222.

14. Jha AK, Epstein AM. The predictive accuracy of the New York State coronary artery bypass surgery report-card system. *Health Aff (Millwood)*. May–Jun 2006;25(3):844–855.

15. Hibbard JH, Stockard J, Tusler M. Does publicizing hospital performance stimulate quality improvement efforts? *Health Aff (Millwood)*. Mar–Apr 2003;22(2):84–94.

16. Tu JV, Donovan LR, Lee DS, et al. Effectiveness of public report cards for improving the quality of cardiac care: the EFFECT study: a randomized trial. *JAMA*. Dec 2 2009;302(21):2330–2337.

17. Hannan EL, Kumar D, Racz M, Siu AL, Chassin MR. New York State's Cardiac Surgery Reporting System: four years later. *Ann Thorac Surg*. Dec 1994;58(6):1852–1857.

18. Ghali WA, Hall RE, Ash AS, Rosen AK, Moskowitz MA. Evaluation of complication rates after coronary artery bypass surgery using administrative data. *Methods Inf Med*. Jun 1998; 37(2):192–200.

19. Peterson ED, DeLong ER, Jollis JG, Muhlbaier LH, Mark DB. The effects of New York's bypass surgery provider profiling on access to care and patient outcomes in the elderly. *J Am Coll Cardiol*. Oct 1998;32(4):993–999.

20. Zhan C, Miller MR. Excess length of stay, charges, and mortality attributable to medical injuries during hospitalization. *JAMA*. Oct 8 2003;290(14):1868–1874.

21. Kanwar M, Brar N, Khatib R, Fakih MG. Misdiagnosis of community-acquired pneumonia and inappropriate utilization of antibiotics: side effects of the 4-h antibiotic administration rule. *Chest*. Jun 2007;131(6):1865–1869.

22. Schneider EC, Epstein AM. Influence of cardiac-surgery performance reports on referral practices and access to care. A survey of cardiovascular specialists. *N Engl J Med*. Jul 25 1996;335(4): 251–256.

23. Leonardi MJ, McGory ML, Ko CY. Publicly available hospital comparison web sites: determination of useful, valid, and appropriate information for comparing surgical quality. *Arch Surg*. Sep 2007; 142(9):863–868; discussion 868–869.

24. Eddy DM. Clinical decision making: from theory to practice. Connecting value and costs. Whom do we ask, and what do we ask them? *JAMA*. Oct 3 1990;264(13):1737–1739.

25. Shojania KG, Forster AJ. Hospital mortality: when failure is not a good measure of success. *CMAJ*. Jul 15 2008;179(2):153–157.

26. Dimick JB, Welch HG, Birkmeyer JD. Surgical mortality as an indicator of hospital quality: the problem with small sample size. *JAMA*. Aug 18 2004;292(7):847–851.

27. Blendon RJ, DesRoches CM, Brodie M, et al. Views of practicing physicians and the public on medical errors. *N Engl J Med*. Dec 12 2002;347(24):1933–1940.

28. McGee J, Kanouse DE, Sofaer S, Hargraves JL, Hoy E, Kleimann S. Making survey results easy to report to consumers: how reporting needs guided survey design in CAHPS. Consumer Assessment of Health Plans Study. *Med Care*. Mar 1999;37(3 Suppl):MS32–MS40.

29. Hibbard JH, Peters E, Slovic P, Finucane ML, Tusler M. Making health care quality reports easier to use. *Jt Comm J Qual Improv*. Nov 2001;27(11):591–604.

CHAPTER 4

THE PREOPERATIVE EVALUATION: HISTORY, PHYSICAL EXAM, AND THE ROLE OF TESTING

Paul J. Grant

INTRODUCTION

A thoughtful preoperative evaluation is essential given the potential for significant risk in patients undergoing surgery. More than ever, the preoperative evaluation requires meticulous attention given the progressively complex and aging patient population. Furthermore, surgeons have become increasingly specialized, often making them ill-equipped to perform an adequate medical preoperative evaluation. The number of inpatient noncardiac surgeries has increased from the estimated 35 million that were performed in the United States in 2004,[1] making it important for clinicians to be competent in executing a comprehensive evaluation. In addition to assessing risk, the preoperative evaluation also provides an opportunity to optimize patient comorbidities and to detect any unrecognized disease that may lead to poor surgical outcomes.

The Joint Commission requires that all patients receive a preoperative history and physical examination within 30 days before surgery. However, they do not clearly define the elements of the evaluation. Subsequently, many clinicians order a battery of tests prior to surgery, which is problematic. It should be noted that the Centers for Medicare and Medicaid Services (CMS) does not pay for "routine" preoperative testing. A specific medical indication (patient sign or symptom) requires documentation before CMS will reimburse for the test.

This chapter will review the basics of the preoperative evaluation including the history and physical examination, in addition to advising when supplementary testing is indicated such as blood work, electrocardiograms (ECGs), and chest radiographs (CXRs). Preoperative cardiac stress testing and pulmonary function testing

Perioperative Medicine: Medical Consultation and Co-Management, First Edition.
Edited by Amir K. Jaffer and Paul J. Grant.

are addressed in other chapters in this textbook. It is important to note that despite a growing body of evidence, there are gaps in the perioperative literature. With limited data in the form of randomized controlled trials and observational studies, we often rely on guidelines, expert opinion, and consensus statements when evaluating our patients preoperatively.

THE BASICS OF THE PREOPERATIVE EVALUATION

The main components of the preoperative evaluation include a comprehensive history, a detailed physical exam, and *selected* additional testing.

The History

The patient history is the most important component of the preoperative evaluation. The vast majority of pertinent information will be obtained through the history, and decisions regarding additional testing are primarily based on the patient interview. The history should include the following elements.

History of Present Illness   This portion of the history can be kept rather brief. The details as to *why* the patient requires (or elects to have) surgery is of minor importance for the risk stratification process, and time is better spent on other areas of the preoperative evaluation. Knowing the type of surgery, its level of urgency, and the scheduled date are the most important aspects of this section.

Past Medical History   This is likely the most important component of the entire preoperative evaluation. A complete and accurate listing of all of the patient's major medical comorbidities requires detailed understanding and documentation. Although cardiac risk factors are often the focus of questioning (particularly the presence of any of the Revised Cardiac Risk Indices[2] [ischemic heart disease, congestive heart failure, diabetes requiring insulin therapy, stroke/transient ischemic attack, creatinine > 2 mg/dL]), it is also important to inquire about pulmonary risk factors (i.e., chronic obstructive pulmonary disease [COPD], cigarette use, advanced age) as perioperative pulmonary complications are equally as prevalent as cardiac events.[3] Lastly, it is important to ask if the patient's known comorbidities are well controlled. This is particularly true for nonurgent or elective surgeries. Examples include ensuring that a patient's blood pressure, diabetes, heart disease, rheumatologic disorder, and psychiatric illness are optimized prior to surgery.

Medications   Obtaining a complete and accurate list of medication names and dosages is essential during the preoperative evaluation. In addition to prescribed medications, it is imperative to ascertain if the patient is taking over-the-counter medications, vitamins, or herbal supplements. It is estimated that approximately one-third of preoperative patients take herbal medication.[4] Medications that effect bleeding (i.e., aspirin, nonsteroidal anti-inflammatory drugs [NSAIDs], and warfarin) require specific attention as they typically need to be discontinued several days prior to surgery.

Allergies   A complete list of patient allergies needs to be included in the pre-operative evaluation. Allergies to latex and anesthetic agents deserve specific questioning.

Surgical and Anesthetic History   Inquiring about a patient's previous experi-ence with surgery can provide valuable information. Bleeding complications, reac-tions to anesthesia, hemodynamic instability, and cardiopulmonary compromise that may have occurred during previous operations warrant careful assessment in addi-tion to a preoperative evaluation by an anesthesiologist.

Social and Family History   Patients who consume an excessive amount of alcohol or have a history of alcohol withdrawal (with delirium tremens being the most severe form) need to be identified prior to surgery so appropriate preventative measures can be employed. For patients who smoke cigarettes, the preoperative evaluation provides an opportunity for a "teachable moment" to counsel in smoking cessation. Any illicit drug use also needs to be ascertained given the possibility of drug toxicity, side effects, and withdrawal. A family history may address instances of venous thromboembolic disease, abnormal bleeding, or side effects to anesthesia in immedi-ate family members.

Review of Systems   A complete review of systems provides the opportunity to ensure that a patient's chronic medical comorbidities are optimized, and also to uncover any previously undiagnosed medical conditions. Inquiring about symptoms such as chest pain, shortness of breath, lower extremity edema, and palpitations is appropriate as a positive response would drive further testing. Furthermore, directed questioning in the review of systems will sometimes prompt the patient in remem-bering previous transient diagnoses such as venous thromboembolism, acute kidney injury, syncope, anemia, or transient ischemic attack.

Functional Capacity   It is important to assess a patient's functional capacity during the preoperative evaluation. This is typically done by asking the patient if they can perform various tasks or activities without symptomatic limitation. Fair evidence exists indicating that patients who are able to achieve a high functional capacity may experience fewer perioperative complications.[5] The American College of Cardiology Foundation/American Heart Association Perioperative Guidelines indicate that the ability to perform 4 metabolic equivalents (METs) or greater cor-relates with at least "fair" functional capacity, and the majority of these patients can proceed to surgery without further cardiovascular evaluation.[6] Four METs is often equated with the ability to climb up one to two flights of stairs without limitation.

The Physical Exam

Although a comprehensive physical exam is customary, focused attention is placed on information gained from the history. For example, patients with congestive heart failure warrant a careful examination of the heart, lungs, neck veins, and lower extremities to evaluate the level of disease compensation. Additionally, patients diagnosed with COPD require a careful pulmonary examination to ensure their disease is optimally managed.

Patients that describe a new symptom in the history should also be evaluated with an appropriate physical examination. Unexpected physical exam findings may also deserve further investigation depending on the urgency of the surgery. Examples may include a new heart murmur, lower extremity edema, or pulmonary wheezes. In the case of a cardiac murmur, it is important to determine its chronicity and whether the murmur is functional or structural. Virtually all murmurs should be evaluated by echocardiography if not previously performed as this can determine the severity of any underlying disease and alter perioperative management. Aortic stenosis increases the risk of perioperative mortality and nonfatal myocardial infarction irrespective of commonly used cardiovascular risk screening tools such as the Revised Cardiac Risk Index.[7]

Vital signs are routinely obtained as part of the preoperative examination. Several studies have shown that systolic blood pressures (SBPs) of less than 180 mm Hg and diastolic blood pressures (DBPs) of less than 110 mm Hg are not an independent risk factor for perioperative cardiovascular events.[6] However, the preoperative evaluation may provide a good opportunity to initiate hypertension treatment or optimize current therapy given the higher lifelong incidence of cardiovascular disease and stroke in patients with chronically elevated blood pressures. For significantly elevated blood pressures (i.e., SBP > 180 mm Hg and/or DBP > 110 mm Hg), the potential benefits of optimizing treatment need to be weighed against the risks of delaying surgery.

PREOPERATIVE TESTING

The literature is clear that clinicians have a tendency to order excessive tests prior to surgery. It is estimated that 60–70% of preoperative testing is unnecessary provided that an appropriate history and physical examination are performed.[8] Furthermore, the evidence suggests that the results of such testing are rarely used, and the chance of a test abnormality altering patient management is low.[9] The problems with ordering unnecessary tests are many. The more tests that are ordered will lead to more false-positive findings. This will often lead to additional testing that increases patient anxiety, cost, risk for surgical delay, and even patient risk if more invasive testing is performed in pursuing abnormal results. However, given results from a recent study in Canada, it is possible that the number of routine preoperative tests being ordered (ECGs and CXRs in this study) may be decreasing.[10]

A large randomized trial of 18,189 patients undergoing cataract surgery was performed to determine if routine preoperative testing would reduce the incidence of intraoperative and postoperative medical complications.[11] The mean age of the entire patient population was 73 years. The battery of preoperative testing obtained in one group consisted of a complete blood count, serum electrolytes, urea nitrogen, creatinine, glucose, and an ECG, while the other group had no routine preoperative testing. The overall rate of complications was the same in both groups, leading the authors to conclude that routine preoperative testing did not improve patient safety.

The results for this trial can likely be extrapolated to patients undergoing other low-risk procedures.

Physicians often fear medical–legal risk if routine preoperative testing is not obtained. But interestingly, it is estimated that 30–60% of unexpected abnormalities detected on preoperative tests are ignored.[12] Ignoring abnormal test results is certainly more likely to increase liability from a medical–legal standpoint, and is a practice that is strongly discouraged.

When used appropriately, testing does play a role in the preoperative evaluation. Silverstein and Boland developed a conceptual framework for evaluating the value of preoperative testing.[13] Their framework addresses four key principles:

1. Diagnostic efficacy (whether the test correctly identifies abnormalities)
2. Diagnostic effectiveness (whether the test changes the physician's diagnosis)
3. Therapeutic efficacy (whether the test changes patient management)
4. Therapeutic effectiveness (whether the test changes patient outcomes)

The more of these four principles that are present when considering a preoperative test indicates a more useful test. For example, preoperative pregnancy testing in the right patient population is considered a very useful test.[14] First, patients are often unreliable in knowing their pregnancy status with routine preoperative pregnancy screening being positive in up to 2.2% of tests. Furthermore, the history and physical exam are often inadequate to determine if a patient is pregnant. When using Silverstein and Boland's four principles outlined above, pregnancy testing would meet all of the criteria indicating that it is an effective preoperative test.

In general, preoperative testing may be able to identify factors that increase surgical risk when used appropriately. Testing can provide a means to better assess a patient's chronic disease, as well as establish a baseline value that may undoubtedly change or require monitoring in the postoperative setting. And of course, preoperatively testing is always indicated when evaluating undiagnosed signs and symptoms, as would be the case for nonsurgical patients.

LABORATORY TESTING

As mentioned above, the history and physical examination is the major driver in determining whether preoperative laboratory testing is indicated. In general terms, younger and healthier patients, in addition to those undergoing low-risk procedures, seldom require preoperative laboratory testing. However, there is reasonable data to suggest that this generalization could be extended to most surgical populations.

A comprehensive literature review that included a variety of patient populations found that the frequency of unsuspected abnormal laboratory results that influence patient management prior to surgery ranges from 0% to 2.6%.[9] The laboratory testing in this analysis included hemoglobin, white blood cell count, platelets, prothrombin time, partial thromboplastin time, electrolytes, renal function, glucose, liver function tests, and urinalysis.

A prospective single-center study in France included 3883 patients undergoing a variety of surgical procedures with either general or regional anesthesia.[15] The overall incidence of *selectively* performed tests that were abnormal was 30%. Of these, only 3% resulted in management consequences. After an analysis of these patients was performed by anesthesiologists as well as an automated method, only 7% of preoperative tests ordered were considered useful.

A smaller trial of 100 patients undergoing surgery with general anesthesia was prospectively audited using the medical record.[16] Preoperative screening laboratory testing was abnormal in 9.1% of results, and perioperative management was altered as a result of only two abnormal tests (0.3%). A total of eight perioperative complications occurred, none of which could have been predicted according to the authors. Interestingly, the laboratory results were present in the medical chart at the time of surgery in only 57% of the cases.

Some preoperative guidelines recommend using age as a criterion to obtain additional testing. Although older patients are statistically more likely to have abnormal laboratory results, it is controversial whether this is predictive of an increased risk for perioperative events. A prospective cohort study of patients aged 70 years or older undergoing noncardiac surgery was performed to evaluate the prevalence and predictive value of abnormal preoperative laboratory tests.[17] In 544 patients, the prevalence of abnormal results ranged from 0.7% to 12%; however, their ability to predict adverse outcomes was poor. Only surgical risk (as defined by the 1996 American Heart Association/American College of Cardiology) and an American Society of Anesthesiologists (ASA) class >2 were predictive of perioperative events. The authors concluded that routine preoperative testing based on age alone may not be indicated in geriatric patients, but rather selective testing as indicated by the history and physical examination.[17]

Patients with acceptable laboratory results within the previous 4 months are also unlikely to require additional testing if there has been no interval change in their clinical status. A retrospective cohort analysis using computerized laboratory data from a tertiary care Veterans Affairs Hospital assessed 1109 consecutive patients having elective surgery.[18] Only 0.4% of repeated laboratory tests at the time of surgery were outside a range considered to be acceptable for surgery. Furthermore, most of these abnormalities were predictable from the patient's history.

In summary, preoperative laboratory testing should be reserved for patients with a clinical indication based on the information obtained from the history and physical examination. Table 4.1 provides clinical situations when selective ordering of specific laboratory tests may be indicated prior to surgery.

THE ECG

The ECG is a routinely ordered test in the preoperative setting despite a lack of strong data in many patient populations. The prognostic value of a routine preoperative ECG in patients undergoing noncardiac surgery was retrospectively studied in 23,036 patients in The Netherlands.[19] Multivariate logistic regression analysis was

TABLE 4.1.   Recommendations for Selective Preoperative Laboratory Testing

Laboratory test	Potential indications
White blood cell count	Signs/symptoms of infection or myeloproliferative disorder
	Exposure to myelotoxic medications (i.e., chemotherapy)
Hemoglobin	Signs/symptoms of anemia
	Anticipated major intraoperative blood loss
Platelets	History of bleeding diathesis or myeloproliferative disorder
	History of advanced liver disease or alcohol abuse
	History of thrombocytopenia (i.e., ITP)
Prothrombin time (PT)	History of bleeding diathesis
	History of chronic liver disease or malnutrition
	Exposure to warfarin
	Long-term antibiotic exposure
Partial thromboplastin time (PTT)	History of bleeding diathesis
	Exposure to unfractionated heparin
Electrolytes	Renal insufficiency
	Medication exposure that can effect electrolytes (i.e., diuretics)
Glucose	Suspected diabetes mellitus
Renal function tests (BUN, Cr)	History of renal disease
	Exposure to medications that effect renal function
Serum aminotransferases (AST, ALT)	No indication; obtain liver *function* tests (i.e., PT, PTT, albumin, platelets) for patients with known/suspected liver disease

ITP, idiopathic thrombocytopenic purpura; BUN, blood urea nitrogen; Cr, creatinine; AST, aspartate aminotransferase; ALT, alanine aminotransferase.
Data from Smetana GW, Macpherson DS. The case against routine preoperative laboratory testing. *Med Clin North Am.* 2003;87:7–40.

applied to evaluate the relationship between ECG abnormalities and cardiovascular death. Although the preoperative ECG did not provide prognostic information for patients undergoing low-risk or low- to intermediate-risk surgery, an abnormal ECG was predictive of a greater incidence of cardiovascular death in higher-risk surgeries, particularly when patient risk factors were considered.

A similar analysis performed at two Canadian university hospitals used the electronic medical record to study 2967 noncardiac surgery patients greater than 50 years of age to determine independent predictors of postoperative myocardial infarction and all-cause in-hospital death.[20] Bundle branch blocks were identified as an independent risk for postoperative myocardial infarction and all-cause mortality; however, this did not improve prediction beyond risk factors identified in the patient history. Furthermore, a retrospective cohort-controlled study by Dorman et al. found that the presence of a bundle branch block was not associated with a high incidence of postoperative cardiac complications in 455 adult patients undergoing noncardiac, nonophthalmologic surgery.[21]

A retrospective study at Brigham and Women's Hospital in Boston aimed to determine if ordering an ECG could be targeted to patients likely to have an abnormality that would affect perioperative management.[22] Out of 1149 ECGs reviewed, 7.8% of patients had at least one significant abnormality. Of these, all but 0.44% could have been predicted by the presence of any of the following risk factors: age >65 years, congestive heart failure, high cholesterol, angina, myocardial infarction, and severe valvular disease.

Although age is a common criterion for obtaining a preoperative ECG, is it unclear if this is evidence based. It is true that older patients are more likely to have ECG abnormalities, but whether these abnormalities are predictive of postoperative complications is uncertain. A prospective observational trial of 513 patients aged 70 years or greater undergoing noncardiac surgery were studied by Liu et al.[23] Preoperative ECG abnormalities were common and seen in 75.2% of patients. However, the presence of these abnormalities was not associated with an increased risk of postoperative cardiac complications. Only an ASA class ≥3 or a history of congestive heart failure was predictive of cardiac events. The authors cautioned that obtaining a preoperative ECG on the basis of age alone may not be indicated.

The ASA attempted to develop a set of guidelines that included recommendations regarding the preoperative ECG. However, due to the lack of convincing data, they were only able to devise a "Practice Advisory Task Force" with the following opinions[24]:

- an ECG may be indicated for patients with known cardiovascular risk factors,
- recognize that ECG abnormalities are more common in patients who are older and have more cardiovascular risk factors,
- no consensus for a minimum age for a preoperative ECG could be determined.

In its 2009 preoperative guidelines,[6] the American College of Cardiology Foundation/American Heart Association provides recommendations for obtaining a preoperative ECG based on patient risk factors and type of surgery. These recommendations are summarized in Table 4.2.

In general, it is common practice to obtain a preoperative ECG for patients with known cardiovascular disease or risk factors. It is also reasonable to order an ECG for patients undergoing higher-risk procedures. It should be noted that pathologic Q-waves in contiguous ECG leads fulfill one of the criterion of the Revised Cardiac Risk Index,[2] which is an evidence-based, widely used, and validated cardiovascular risk stratification tool. Patients with a higher risk index may require altered preoperative management. Data from the Framingham study reveals that although unrecognized myocardial infarctions as defined by pathologic Q-waves are rare in patients younger than age 45 (0.65% in men, 0.26% in women), they increase significantly in patients 75–84 years of age (6% in men, 3.4% in women).[25] Lastly, having a baseline ECG may prove to be valuable for comparison should a patient develop postoperative complications such as hemodynamic instability, chest pain, or shortness of breath.

TABLE 4.2. Preoperative Resting 12-Lead ECG Recommendations by the American College of Cardiology Foundation/American Heart Association 2009 Preoperative Guidelines

Recommendation class	Patient population (level of evidence)
Class I—ECG should be obtained	≥1 clinical risk factor[a] undergoing vascular surgery (B)
	Known CAD, PAD, or CVD undergoing intermediate-risk surgery (C)
Class IIa—ECG is reasonable to obtain	No clinical risk factors[a] undergoing vascular surgery (B)
Class IIb—ECG may be considered	≥1 clinical risk factor[a] undergoing intermediate-risk surgery (B)
Class III—ECG should not be obtained	Asymptomatic patients undergoing low-risk surgery (B)

Levels of evidence: B = data derived from a single randomized trial or nonrandomized studies; C = only consensus opinion of experts, case studies, or standard of care.
[a] Clinical risk factors: ischemic heart disease, compensated or prior heart failure, diabetes mellitus, renal insufficiency, and cerebrovascular disease.
ECG, electrocardiogram; CAD, coronary artery disease; PAD, peripheral artery disease; CVD, cerebrovascular disease.
Source: Fleisher LA, Beckman JA, Brown KA, et al. 2009. ACCF/AHA focused update on perioperative beta blockade incorporated into the ACC/AHA 2007 guidelines on perioperative cardiovascular evaluation and care for noncardiac surgery: a report of the American College of Cardiology Foundation/American Heart Association Task Force on Practice Guidelines. *J Am Coll Cardiol.* 2009;54:e13–e118.

THE CXR

The practice of obtaining a routine preoperative CXR appears to date back to World War II as a means to detect tuberculosis.[26] Despite being one of the more expensive preoperative tests, there is limited evidence that the CXR will alter preoperative management. Although an abnormal CXR has been shown to be predictive of postoperative pulmonary complications, numerous trials have demonstrated that imaging rarely provides any additional information beyond what can be determined by the history and physical examination.[9]

A large prospective multicenter pilot study enrolled 6111 patients to assess the influence of a routine preoperative CXR on anesthetic management prior to elective surgery.[27] Abnormal CXRs were reported in 18.3% of patients, but abnormal results altered anesthetic management in only 5.1% of patients. Factors associated with patients requiring altered management included male sex, age >60 years, ASA class ≥3, and the presence of respiratory diseases.

In a meta-analysis of 21 studies assessing the value of routine preoperative CXRs, only 10% were abnormal, and in only 1.3% were the abnormalities considered unexpected.[28] Moreover, the unexpected CXR abnormalities were of significant importance to affect management in only 0.1% of the patients. A more recent systematic review also assessed the value of screening preoperative CXRs in addition to reporting on postoperative pulmonary complications.[29] The authors found that although diagnostic yield increased with age, most of the CXR abnormalities consisted of chronic disorders. Furthermore, the proportion of patients who had a change in perioperative management was low, and postoperative pulmonary complications were similar between patients who had a preoperative CXR and those who did not.

The preoperative pulmonary evaluation seldom requires more than a complete history and physical examination. However, when a new symptom is reported, a previous diagnosis is uncertain, or a patient presents with decompensation of their chronic lung disease, it is reasonable to obtain a preoperative CXR. Procedure-related risk factors for postoperative pulmonary complications, such as surgical procedures within the thorax or close to the diaphragm, may also impact the decision to obtain a CXR. Preoperative pulmonary guidelines from the American College of Physicians state that a preoperative CXR may be helpful for patients older than 50 with known cardiopulmonary disease who are undergoing upper abdominal, thoracic, or abdominal aortic aneurysm surgery.[30]

CONCLUSION

The preoperative evaluation requires a comprehensive assessment in order to accurately risk-stratify patients in addition to achieving medical optimization. In the majority of cases, this can be accomplished by obtaining a thorough history and a complete physical examination. Only selective use of additional preoperative testing is recommended as justified by specific findings in the history and physical examination. Additional studies such as laboratory tests, ECG, and CXR should only be obtained if it will influence perioperative management.

REFERENCES

1. DeFrances CJ, Podgornik MN. *2004 National Hospital Discharge Survey*. Advance data from vital and health statistics; no. 371. Hyattsville, MD: National Center for Health Statistics; 2006. Available from: http://www.cdc.gov/nchs/data/ad/ad371.pdf. Accessed February 22, 2011.
2. Lee TH, Marcantonio ER, Mangione CM, et al. Derivation and prospective validation of a simple index for prediction of cardiac risk of major noncardiac surgery. *Circulation*. 1999;100:1043–1049.
3. Fleischmann KE, Goldman L, Young B, Lee TH. Association between cardiac and noncardiac complications in patients undergoing noncardiac surgery: outcomes and effects on length of stay. *Am J Med*. 2003;115:515–520.
4. Ang-Lee MK, Moss J, Yuan CS. Herbal medicines and perioperative care. *JAMA*. 2001;286:208–216.
5. Reilly DF, McNeely MJ, Doerner D, et al. Self-reported exercise tolerance and the risk of serious perioperative complications. *Arch Intern Med*. 1999;159:2185–2192.
6. Fleisher LA, Beckman JA, Brown KA, et al. 2009 ACCF/AHA focused update on perioperative beta blockade incorporated into the ACC/AHA 2007 guidelines on perioperative cardiovascular evaluation and care for noncardiac surgery: a report of the American College of Cardiology Foundation/American Heart Association Task Force on Practice Guidelines. *J Am Coll Cardiol*. 2009;54:e13–e118.

7. Kertai MD, Bountioukos M, Boersma E, et al. Aortic stenosis: an underestimated risk factor for perioperative complications in patients undergoing noncardiac surgery. *Am J Med.* Jan 1 2004; 116(1):8–13.

8. Garcia-Miguel FJ, Serrano-Aguilar PG, Lopez-Bastida J. Preoperative assessment. *Lancet.* 2003;362:1749–1757.

9. Smetana GW, Macpherson DS. The case against routine preoperative laboratory testing. *Med Clin North Am.* 2003;87:7–40.

10. Thanh NX, Rashiq S, Jonsson E. Routine preoperative electrocardiogram and chest x-ray prior to elective surgery in Alberta, Canada. *Can J Anaesth.* 2010;57:127–133.

11. Schein OD, Katz J, Bass EB, et al. The value of routine preoperative medical testing before cataract surgery. *N Engl J Med.* 2000;342:168–175.

12. Roizen MF. More preoperative assessment by physicians and less by laboratory tests. *N Engl J Med.* 2000;342:204–205.

13. Silverstein MD, Boland BJ. Conceptual framework for evaluation laboratory tests: case-finding in ambulatory patients. *Clin Chem.* 1994;40:1621–1627.

14. Hepner DL. The role of testing in the preoperative evaluation. *Cleve Clin J Med.* 2009;76(Suppl 4):S22–S27.

15. Charpak Y, Blery C, Chastang CL, et al. Usefulness of selectively ordered preoperative tests. *Med Care.* 1988;26:95–104.

16. Johnson RK, Mortimer AJ. Routine pre-operative blood testing: is it necessary? *Anaesthesia.* 2002;57:914–917.

17. Dzankic S, Pastor D, Gonzalez C, Leung JM. The prevalence and predictive value of abnormal preoperative laboratory tests in elderly surgical patients. *Anesth Analg.* 2001;93:301–308.

18. Macpherson DS, Snow R, Lofgren RP. Preoperative screening: value of previous tests. *Ann Intern Med.* 1990;113:969–973.

19. Noordzij PG, Boersma E, Bax JJ, et al. Prognostic value of routine preoperative electrocardiography in patients undergoing noncardiac surgery. *Am J Cardiol.* 2006;97:1103–1106.

20. Van Klei WA, Bryson GL, Yang H, Kalkman CJ, Wells GA, Beattie WS. The value of routine preoperative electrocardiography in predicting myocardial infarction after noncardiac surgery. *Ann Surg.* 2007;246:165–170.

21. Dorman T, Breslow MJ, Pronovost PJ, Rock P, Rosenfeld BA. Bundle-branch block as a risk factor in noncardiac surgery. *Arch Intern Med.* 2000;160:1149–1152.

22. Correll DJ, Hepner DL, Chang C, Tsen L, Hevelone ND, Bader AM. Preoperative electrocardiograms: patient factors predictive of abnormalities. *Anesthesiology.* 2009;110:1217–1222.

23. Liu LL, Dzankic S, Leung JM. Preoperative electrocardiogram abnormalities do not predict postoperative cardiac complications in geriatric surgical patients. *J Am Geriatr Soc.* 2002;50:1186–1191.

24. Practice advisory for preanesthesia evaluation: a report by the American Society of Anesthesiologists Task Force on Preanesthesia evaluation. *Anesthesiology.* 2002;96:485–496.

25. Kannel WB, Abbott RD. Incidence and prognosis of unrecognized myocardial infarction. An update on the Framingham study. *N Engl J Med.* 1984;311:1144–1147.

26. Sagel SS, Evens RG, Forrest JV, Bramson RT. Efficacy of routine screening and lateral chest radiographs in a hospital-based population. *N Engl J Med.* 1974;291:1001–1004.

27. Silvestri L, Maffessanti M, Gregori D, Berlot G, Gullo A. Usefulness of routine pre-operative chest radiography for anaesthetic management: a prospective multicenter pilot study. *Eur J Anaesthesiol.* 1999;16:749–760.

28. Archer C, Levy AR, McGregor M. Value of routine preoperative chest x-rays: a meta-analysis. *Can J Anaesth.* 1993;40:1022–1027.

29. Joo HS, Wong J, Naik VN, Savoldelli GL. The value of screening preoperative chest x-rays: a systematic review. *Can J Anaesth.* 2005;52:568–574.

30. Qaseem A, Snow V, Fitterman N, et al. Risk assessment for and strategies to reduce perioperative pulmonary complications for patients undergoing noncardiothoracic surgery: a guideline from the American College of Physicians. *Ann Intern Med.* 2006;144:575–580.

CHAPTER 5

PERIOPERATIVE MEDICATION MANAGEMENT

Christopher Whinney

BACKGROUND

Operative treatment of disease has a tremendous yet unrecognized impact on modern medical systems. An estimated 33 million patients undergo surgery in the United States annually. Serious adverse events occur in over 1 million of these patients, at an estimated cost of $25 billion annually. With the aging population, it is anticipated that surgical referrals will increase by 25%, costs by 50%, and costs of perioperative complications by 100%.[1] Given these staggering numbers, it is imperative that clinicians involved with patients undergoing surgery know the basics of perioperative diagnosis and management.

A key component to delivery of quality perioperative care is the management of the patient's chronic medication regimen. Surgical patients—many of whom are elderly—are commonly on multiple medications, have renal or hepatic disease that can alter drug metabolism, and may not be adequately educated about their medication regimens.

In addition, the increasing surgical burden that comes with an aging population, along with rising expectations for functional recovery, has likewise elevated the importance of perioperative medication management.

RELEVANCE

Not surprisingly, a significant proportion of patients presenting for surgery take medications for chronic conditions. However, a retrospective study showed an odds ratio for postoperative complications of 2.7 when patients were taking medications unrelated to the procedure. This was particularly notable for patients taking cardiovascular drugs or agents that act on the central nervous system, if patients were NPO ("nothing by mouth") for more than 24 h before surgery, and if the operation was more than 1 h in duration.[2] These findings could reflect destabilization of

Perioperative Medicine: Medical Consultation and Co-Management, First Edition.
Edited by Amir K. Jaffer and Paul J. Grant.
© 2012 Wiley-Blackwell. Published 2012 by John Wiley & Sons, Inc.

the disease processes for which the patients were taking chronic medications that required interruption.

Stopping a chronic medication for a surgical procedure raises the possibility that its resumption could be overlooked, especially since medical errors are particularly common in the transition between healthcare settings following hospital discharge. A population-based cohort study among all elderly patients discharged from hospitals in Ontario, Canada, over a 5.5-year period found that 11.4% of patients undergoing elective surgery did not resume their indicated chronic warfarin therapy within 6 months after its presurgical discontinuation.[3] Although 6-month rates of unintended failure to resume therapy were lower for statins (4%) and ophthalmic beta-blocker drops (8%), these findings underscore that drug discontinuation always carries a risk that therapy might not be resumed as indicated.

Surgery also elicits a significant stress response and a challenge to homeostasis manifested by increased sympathetic tone and release of pituitary hormones, which can affect metabolism of chronic medications. In addition, surgery (especially gut-related procedures) can disrupt the absorption of oral drugs due to villous atrophy, diminished blood flow to the gut, edema, mucosal ischemia, and diminished motility from postoperative ileus and use of narcotics.[4]

The evidence base surrounding the management of medications in the perioperative period is sparse at best. Recommendations in this area rely largely on other forms of evidence including expert consensus, case reports, *in vitro* studies, recommendations from pharmaceutical companies, and other known data (pharmacokinetics, drug interactions with anesthetic agents, and effects of the agent on the primary disease and on perioperative risk). That being said, we need to make reasonable recommendations for medication management in this arena.

GENERAL GUIDELINES

Several general principles can be applied in managing perioperative medications. First, medications with significant withdrawal potential that do not negatively affect the procedure or anesthesia administration should be continued during the perioperative period. Examples of this include beta-blockers and alpha-blockers such as clonidine. Second, medications that increase surgical risk and are not essential for short-term quality of life should be discontinued during the perioperative period. If a medication does not fall clearly into one of these categories, then one must rely on physician judgement, based on the stability of the condition being treated and anesthetic and surgical concerns. Consultation with your hospital pharmacist, surgeon, and/or anesthesiologist is a reasonable approach when questions arise in this vein.

SPECIFIC MEDICATION CLASSES

Antiplatelet Agents

Aspirin, nonsteroidal anti-inflammatory drugs (NSAIDs), thienopyridine, and non-thienopyridine drugs all have effects on the platelet and can therefore be termed "antiplatelet" agents. Antiplatelet agents such as aspirin and thienopyridines (clopidogrel, ticlodipine, prasugel) are an integral part of management of coronary, cerebral, or peripheral vascular disease for maintenance of vessel patency and event risk reduction. NSAIDs are also ubiquitous for pain and inflammation control; however, they also increase the risk of postoperative bleeding. For most patients who are on aspirin for primary prevention purposes and on NSAIDs for symptomatic relief, short-term discontinuation of these agents perioperatively does not lead to increased adverse outcomes; therefore, it is reasonable to discontinue them 7–10 days prior to elective surgery.

For patients taking aspirin therapy for secondary prevention with a concomitant risk for potential withdrawal phenomenon of increased platelet aggregation, consider the risks of continuing (bleeding) versus the benefits of continuing (antithrombosis). BéLisle and Hardy[5] noted an approximately 300 cc increase in perioperative blood loss in a review of 50 studies of cardiac surgery patients; no increase in transfusion requirement was noted.

A meta-analysis of 474 studies showed that the use of aspirin increased intraoperative bleeding by a factor of 1.5, without increasing risk of morbidity or mortality.[6] Neilipovitz et al.[7] studied patients undergoing peripheral vascular surgery who continued aspirin therapy, and found a decreased perioperative mortality rate and increased life expectancy, with an increase in non-life-threatening hemorrhagic complications.

Oscarsson et al.[8] recently published a randomized controlled trial comparing the continuation of aspirin 75 mg (given 7 days preoperatively until 3 days postoperatively) with a placebo group. Two hundred twenty patients were enrolled who were undergoing intermediate- or high-risk surgery, and all had at least one Revised Cardiac Risk Index (RCRI) criteria. Of note, the authors chose to exclude patients with intracoronary stents due to an interim publication of a guideline change. There were 109 patients in the aspirin group and 111 patients received placebo. Four patients (3.7%) in the aspirin group and 10 patients (9.0%) in the placebo group had elevated troponin T levels in the postoperative period ($P = 0.10$). Twelve patients (5.4%) had a major adverse cardiac event (acute myocardial infarction, severe arrhythmia, cardiac arrest, or cardiovascular death) during the first 30 postoperative days. Two of these patients (1.8%) were in the aspirin group and 10 patients (9.0%) were in the placebo group ($P = 0.02$). The absolute risk reduction for major adverse cardiac events was 7.2% and the relative risk reduction was 80%. No increased bleeding was noted, but the study was not powered to evaluate bleeding complications. The study was limited in that the authors planned to recruit 540 patients based on power calculations but stopped at 220 patients due to the difficulty in finding eligible patients for inclusion. In addition, new published recommendations regarding perioperative guidelines for antiplatelet agents were released at that time, which suggest continuing aspirin through the perioperative period.[9]

There is some literature evidence of a rebound phenomenon with ASA withdrawal, and it is known that the trauma of surgery creates a prothrombotic and proinflammatory state.

Thus, for noncardiac and nonvascular surgeries, if there is no clear increased risk of consequential bleeding in these patients (i.e., urologic surgery or neurosurgery who are at increased bleeding risk), then aspirin should be continued through the perioperative period according to the American College of Cardiology/American Heart Association (ACC/AHA) and the European Society of Cardiology (ESC), as well as several other authors.[9–11]

For patients who require dual antiplatelet therapy with aspirin and clopidogrel for a recently placed drug-eluting stent (DES) in a coronary artery or arteries, the risks for adverse events is significantly increased. Premature discontinuation of dual antiplatelet therapy tremendously increases the risk for early and late stent thrombosis, which has a case fatality rate of 45% and a 70% rate of myocardial infarction. A science advisory from the ACC/AHA in association with other professional medical societies recommends that patients with drug-eluting coronary artery stents should remain on combination aspirin and clopidogrel for a minimum of 1 year.[12] Therefore, elective surgery should be deferred at least 1 year in this patient population if at all possible, until more data surrounding the perioperative management of DESs becomes available.

When patients require elective, urgent, or emergent surgery and they have had a recent DES placed (less than 1 year), then decision making becomes more complicated. Collet and Montalescot[13] suggested an algorithm for post-DES patients who require surgery. This involves the surgeon and anesthesiologist assessing the bleeding risk, the cardiologist evaluating the risk of stent thrombosis, and all three devising an individual management plan. If there is a major risk of both stent thrombosis and bleeding, surgery should be postponed for at least 6–12 months post-DES. Table 5.1 elucidates the decision making. If this is not possible, aspirin use should be continued and clopidogrel therapy stopped 5 days before surgery. If the bleeding risk is small and there is a major risk of stent thrombosis, then dual antiplatelet therapy should be continued in the perioperative period.

Some cardiologists have begun to recommend the use of short-acting glycoprotein IIb/IIIa inhibitors as bridging therapy perioperatively to reduce the likelihood of stent thrombosis. Limited literature exists in this regard. Savonitto et al.[14] did a phase II trial of the short-acting GPIIb/IIIa receptor blocker tirofiban as a bridging mechanism to prevent DES thrombosis with clopidogrel discontinuation while mitigating bleeding risk during urgent surgery. Thirty patients with a DES implanted a median duration of 4 months prior to surgery were bridged with tirofiban. No cases of death, myocardial infarction, stent thrombosis, or surgical reexploration due to bleeding were noted; one major and one minor bleeding episode (based on thrombosis in myocardial infarction [TIMI] criteria) were noted. Of note, 14 patients continued aspirin throughout the perioperative period. This trial had no control group, and the small number of patients led to a wide confidence interval (CI) (0–11.6%) for events, limiting any definitive conclusions. If such a therapy is to be considered, it should be done in close collaboration with cardiology and anesthesia.

Cardiovascular Medications

In general, cardiovascular medications should be continued throughout the perioperative period as they treat and stabilize conditions such as coronary artery disease, congestive heart failure, and cardiac arrhythmias. Beta-adrenergic antagonists are predominantly used for cardiac risk reduction, blood pressure management, and

TABLE 5.1. Recommendations of the SFAR (French Society of Anesthesiology and Intensive Care) Regarding Management of Oral Antiplatelet Therapy in Patients with Drug-Eluting Stents Undergoing Surgery

Drug-eluting stent		Bleeding risk related to surgery (should be evaluated with the surgeon and the anesthesiologist)		
		Major	Intermediate	Minor
Risk of acute stent thrombosis (should be evaluated with the cardiologist)	Major	Postpone surgery until 6 months up to 1 year after DES implantation *if impossible* Stop aspirin and stop clopidogrel 5 days prior to surgery, or stop aspirin and clopidogrel 10 days max prior to surgery and initiate alternative therapy	Postpone surgery until 6 months up to 1 year after DES implantation *if impossible* Maintain aspirin and stop clopidogrel 5 days prior to surgery	Maintain dual OAT
	Moderate	Stop aspirin and clopidogrel 5 days prior to surgery, or stop aspirin and clopidogrel 10 days max prior to surgery and initiate alternative therapy	Maintain aspirin and stop clopidogrel 5 days prior to surgery	Maintain dual OAT or maintain aspirin and stop clopidogrel 5 days prior to surgery

Bleeding risk assessment
Major: cannot be performed with OAT
Moderate: can be performed with aspirin
Minor: can be performed with aspirin and clopidogrel
In all cases, surgery should be postponed at least 6 weeks after any acute coronary syndrome if possible.

Acute DES thrombosis risk assessment
Major: implantation <6 months or patient requiring prolonged dual OAT patient or patients with high-risk features
Moderate: implantation >6 months

OAT, oral antiplatelet therapy; DES, drug-eluting stent.
From Collet J-P, Montalescot G. *Eur Heart J Suppl.* 2006;8(Suppl G):G46-G52. Used with permission.

arrhythmias. These agents, especially beta1-selective agents, have been extensively studied for their potential in perioperative cardiovascular risk reduction, and are a controversial topic in medical and anesthesia circles. This debate is discussed in Chapter 9. However, due to the potential for clinical withdrawal and tachycardia, patients already taking beta-blockers should be continued on them in the perioperative period, with substitution of intravenous (IV) formulations if they are unable to tolerate oral medications.

Alpha-antagonists such as clonidine are also used commonly for antihypertensive effects. These should also be continued in the perioperative period as they have a clear propensity for withdrawal and rebound hypertension. Topical and IV formulations are available for when patients are unable to tolerate oral medications.

Calcium channel blockers are also generally safe to continue in the perioperative period. If these are prescribed for hypertension or for heart rate control (such as diltiazem for atrial fibrillation), then they should be continued. However, they are not essential as there are many parenteral formulations of antihypertensive agents at the disposal of the anesthesiologist, and strict blood pressure control is not necessary or even desired intraoperatively. Since anesthesia induction induces vasodilatation, which can lead to hemodynamic instability, some blood pressure elevation is acceptable and even preferred.

Antiarrhythmic drugs should be continued throughout the perioperative period. Agents such as digoxin and amiodarone have long half-lives, so they can either be given or withheld on the morning of surgery. If prolonged NPO status is anticipated then parenteral doses of these agents can be administered. Class IA agents such as quinidine, procainamide, and disopyramide can be given orally; if a patient is NPO, then IV procainamide is available. Some agents such as flecainide or sotalol do not have parenteral alternatives, so parenteral beta-blockers, verapamil, or digoxin may be used if arrhythmias ensue. For ventricular arrhythmias, parenteral lidocaine or amiodarone is a good therapeutic option.

Diuretics are typically withheld on the morning of surgery due to concerns for volume depletion and electrolyte disruption although limited literature exists in support of this practice.

Angiotensin-converting enzyme (ACE) inhibitors and angiotensin receptor blockers (ARBs) are used for hypertension and for afterload reduction in heart failure, and have significant long-term mortality benefits. However, they are associated with hypotension with induction of anesthesia, often requiring intraoperative vasopressor therapy. The literature does support a benefit of perioperative ACE inhibition toward decreased mortality, but these studies do not note whether these agents were stopped prior to surgery, how far in advance they were stopped, and how quickly they were restarted postoperatively if they were discontinued. Rosenman et al.[15] conducted a random-effects meta-analysis from five studies totaling 434 patients evaluating the consequences of continuing versus withholding ACE inhibitors and ARBs in the perioperative period. Patients receiving an immediate preoperative ACE/ARB dose were more likely to develop hypotension requiring vasopressor therapy (relative risk [RR] 1.50, 95% CI 1.15–1.96); however, no further conclusions regarding major cardiac events or mortality could be made due to insufficient data. More studies are needed in this area, but given the available data, this author's practice is to discontinue ACE inhibitors on the morning of surgery, and ARBs at least 24 h before surgery if possible, due to their longer half-life.

Statins (HMG Co-A reductase inhibitors) have clear associations with perioperative mortality benefit by randomized trials and epidemiologic data. The reduction in vascular events with statin exposure is likely attributed to their pleiotropic effects such as plaque stabilization, reduction in inflammation, and decreased thrombogenesis. Previous concerns for increased risk of rhabdomyolysis are not well founded, as these were based on scant individual case reports with marked confounding. Therefore, statins should be taken on the morning of surgery and continued in the postoperative period as much as possible.

Pulmonary Medications

Patients with asthma or chronic obstructive pulmonary disease should continue their inhaled steroids, beta-agonists, and anticholinergic agents in the perioperative period as usual. If patients develop bronchospasm, then nebulized versions of the above agents can be administered. Theophylline and parenteral aminophylline are used for systemic beta-agonist activity, but these agents have been associated with tachycardia and proarrhythmic potential without clear benefit over inhaled beta-agonist therapy. Oral or parenteral corticosteroids can be administered for acute exacerbations requiring systemic anti-inflammatory therapy if the surgery is urgent in nature. Leukotriene inhibitors do not appear to have interactions with anesthetics and can be continued perioperatively.

Medications for Diabetes

Patients with diabetes are at increased risk for perioperative morbidity and mortality predominantly from infections and from cardiovascular events. Available data indicate that tight glycemic control in the perioperative period is associated with decreased mortality, length of critical care unit stay, and wound infections in cardiac surgery patients. However, the degree of glycemic control required in critically and noncritically ill patients is not clear, and the risks of hypoglycemia may be more prominent than previously considered. Recently, the recommendations for control of hyperglycemia have been revised by the American Association of Clinical Endocrinologists (AACE) and the American Diabetes Association (ADA): Treat when blood glucose levels exceed 180 mg/dL and aim for glucose levels of below 180 mg/dL in critically ill patients and below 140 mg/dL in noncritically ill patients.[16] The goals of glycemic management around surgery are to achieve the above glycemic targets, to avoid clinically significant hyper- and hypoglycemia, to maintain electrolyte and fluid balance, and prevent diabetic ketoacidosis in type 1 diabetics.

Oral hypoglycemic medications should be withheld in advance of surgery due to the patient's NPO status. Sulfonylureas should be held on the morning of surgery only. Metformin should be held on the morning of surgery as well; however, if the planned procedure requires IV contrast or has potential for hemodynamic instability with diminished renal perfusion, then consider withholding the drug 1–2 days in advance of surgery. Thiazolidinediones can lead to fluid retention and should be held in advance of surgery. Some advocate withholding it for several days; however, this is probably not necessary if no clear evidence of volume overload is present. GLP-1 agonists (such as exenatide) can slow gastric motility and should be held on the day of surgery. DPP-4 inhibitors (incretin enhancers) do not cause significant hypoglycemia so they can be continued, but they are probably not helpful as they primarily influence postprandial glycemic control.

Patients on intermediate-acting insulin should take at least one-half to two-thirds of their usual dose the night before and on the morning of surgery, as approximately one-half of insulin is used for non-nutrient metabolic needs. Consideration should be given to administering full dose intermediate- or long-acting insulin (such as glargine). Insulin coverage should be anticipatory and dosed for basal coverage (with long-acting and intermediate-acting agents) and mealtime doses with additional units for coverage as needed (with short- or rapid-acting insulin). "Sliding scale" insulin alone is insufficient and has been shown to lead to unacceptable rates of both hyper- and hypoglycemia. Insulin administration should also mirror the route and frequency of nutrient intake; continuous feedings require more continuous insulin administration (such as with an insulin drip or long-acting subcutaneous agent), whereas intermittent feedings require intermittent insulin doses for mealtimes or bolus feedings. More details as to management of insulin therapy in the perioperative period are covered in Chapter 11.

Corticosteroids

The hypothalamic–pituitary–adrenal (HPA) axis is critical for generating an appropriate stress response in the perioperative period. Patients taking exogenous steroids have a potential risk of secondary adrenal insufficiency, typically characterized by adrenal cortical atrophy and insufficient adrenocorticotrophic hormone secretion. Exogenous steroids suppress corticotropin-releasing hormone (CRH) and pituitary adrenocorticotropic hormone (ACTH) release, and steroid withdrawal could thus precipitate adrenal crisis. Individual patient response to exogenous steroids is quite variable, and the frequency of true perioperative adrenal crises is quite rare.

Marik and Varon[17] did a systematic review involving 315 patients who underwent 389 procedures in two randomized controlled trials and five cohort studies. Patients who received their usual daily dose of steroids (not stress doses) prior to and during elective procedures manifested no hypotensive episodes; only two patients became hypotensive when steroids were stopped preoperatively. Some authors feel that the current trend of stress dose steroids in the perioperative period is excessive. However, current recommendations[18] suggest that any patient who has received an equivalent of 20 mg/day of prednisone for greater than 5 days is at risk for suppression of the HPA axis within the last 12 months. Similarly, equivalent doses of prednisone 5 mg (or less) for any period of time will usually not suppress the HPA axis, and therefore, no stress doses are needed. When patients take between 5 and 20 mg of exogenous steroids daily or take an every-other-day dose, then it is recommended to either test the patient with an ACTH stimulation test or to simply administer the steroids. In the interest of time and convenience, and that short-term steroids quickly tapered back to baseline will probably have little deleterious effect,

TABLE 5.2.   **Recommendations for Perioperative Steroid Administration**

Procedure	Emergent surgery	Elective or urgent surgery
MINOR (local anesthesia, <1 h)	25 mg IV hydrocortisone or equivalent	No empiric steroids; if clinical suspicion of AI, give 25 mg IV hydrocortisone intraoperatively
MODERATE (general, vascular, orthopedic procedures)	50 mg IV hydrocortisone or equivalent	Preop short ACTH stimulation test[a]: no steroids if negative; if positive or suspect AI, 50 mg IV hydrocortisone
MAJOR (larger, prolonged surgeries, coronary artery bypass grafting [CABG])	100 mg IV hydrocortisone or equivalent	Preop short ACTH stimulation test[a]: no steroids if negative; if positive or suspect AI, 100 mg IV hydrocortisone

Continue steroid dosing every 8 h for 48 h; consider endocrine consultation if prolonged need for steroids.

[a] The short ACTH stimulation involves administration of 250 μg IV synthetic ACTH (cosyntropin) followed by a plasma cortisol collection in 30 min. A plasma cortisol concentration of more than 18–20 mg/dL is consistent with normal adrenal function.
ACTH, adrenocorticotropic hormone; AI, adrenal insufficiency; IV, intravenous.
Source: Kohl BA and Schwartz S. Surgery in the patient with endocrine dysfunction. *Med Clin North Am.* 2009;93:1031–1047. Used with permission.

this author's customary practice is to administer the stress dose steroids with a rapid taper. Table 5.2 has the recommended dosing of stress dose steroids based on clinical suspicion of adrenal insufficiency, home steroid dosing, and the urgency and severity of the procedure. If patients have clinical suspicion of adrenal insufficiency (hyperkalemia, hyponatremia, hypertension, eosinophilia), then appropriate steroid replacement should be assessed and administered as outlined in Table 5.2. Patients with known adrenal insufficiency should be administered stress dose steroids without further testing.

Herbal Medications

Herbal medications are used by up to one-third of patients undergoing surgery. These agents are often perceived by the public as being natural and therefore completely safe; however, they are not regulated by the Food and Drug Administration (FDA) as they are considered food supplements. This means these agents may contain variable amounts of the active ingredient in addition to other compounds. On the other hand, prescription medicines are often perceived as artificial and therefore less safe, despite rigorous standards from the FDA for dosing and safety.[19] Clinicians must be mindful to specifically inquire about herbal preparations and over-the-counter medications as many patients may not even consider these to be "medications." These agents in general should be discontinued at least 1 week prior to surgery, preferably 2 weeks. Table 5.3 highlights the eight most common herbal medications used by patients presenting for surgery, and includes the potential perioperative complications.

TABLE 5.3. Pharmacologic Effects and Perioperative Management Recommendations of Commonly Used Herbs

Herb	Relevant pharmacologic effects	Perioperative concerns	Preoperative discontinuation
Ginseng	Hypoglycemia; inhibits platelet aggregation (may be irreversible); increased PT-PTT in animals	Hypoglycemia; increased bleeding risk; decreased anticoagulation effect of warfarin	Stop 7 days before surgery
Ephedra (ma huang)	Increased heart rate and blood pressure through direct and indirect sympathomimetic effects	MI and stroke risk through tachycardia and hypertension; ventricular arrhythmias with halothane; depletes endogenous catecholamine stores and may cause intra-op hemodynamic instability; life-threatening interaction with MAOIs	Stop at least 24 h before surgery
Garlic	inhibits platelet aggregation (may be irreversible); increased fibrinolysis; equivocal blood pressure lowering activity	Increased bleeding risk especially in conjunction with other antiplatelet agents	Stop 7 days before surgery
Gingko	Inhibits platelet-activating factor	Increased bleeding risk especially in conjunction with other antiplatelet agents	Stop 36 h before surgery
Kava	Sedation, anxiolysis	Increased sedative effect of anesthetics; potential for addiction, tolerance, and withdrawal	Stop at least 24 h before surgery
St. John's wort	Inhibition of neurotransmitter uptake	Many drug–drug interactions through induction of cytochrome P450 enzymes (cyclosporine, steroids, warfarin, benzodiazepines, calcium channel blockers and others), decreased digoxin levels	Stop 5 days before surgery
Echinacea	Activation of cell-mediated immunity	Allergic reactions; immune suppression	No data

PT-PTT, prothrombin time–partial thromboplastin time; MI, myocardial infarction; MAOIs, monoamine oxidase inhibitors.
Source: Ang-Lee MK, Moss J, Yuan C-S. Herbal medicines and perioperative care. *JAMA.* 2001:286:208–216. Used with permission.

Psychiatric Medications

Psychiatric medications are routinely continued perioperatively, as decompensation of psychiatric conditions should be avoided if possible. Agents such as selective serotonin reuptake inhibitors (SSRIs), the newer serotonin–norepinephrine reuptake inhibitors (SNRIs), and benzodiazepines are safe to continue. Some concern exists for perioperative arrhythmias in conjunction with tricyclic antidepressants (TCAs), but the literature does not support this concern. Monoamine oxidase (MAO) inhibitors are now used much less frequently, but are still employed for refractory depressive disorders. These agents lead to an accumulation of biogenic amines in the central nervous system, which can lead to a hypertensive crisis if used with indirect sympathomimetics, or a serotonin-like syndrome when used with meperidine or dextromethorphan. However, anesthesia may be performed safely if meperidine is avoided and only direct-acting sympathomimetics, such as phenylephrine, are used.

When patients remain NPO for a period of time postoperatively, continuing psychiatric medications may be difficult as few of them have alternative routes of administration.

In Europe, IV TCAs such as clomipramine and imipramine have been studied as well as the IV SSRI citalopram and the dual-acting mirtazapine. Parenteral amitriptyline and imipramine are FDA approved for intramuscular use but are not commercially available. No antidepressants have been marketed for rectal preparation; however, a transdermal preparation of the MAO inhibitor selegiline has received FDA approval, and studies should be forthcoming in the medically ill patient. Currently, the hospitalist has the option of dispensing SSRIs in liquid preparation form and mirtazapine in a dissolvable oral tablet in order to facilitate absorption in the NPO patient.

Both haloperidol and fluphenazine have long-acting depot preparations that are given monthly and every 2 weeks, respectively. IV haloperidol, although not approved by the FDA for IV use, is the most common IV antipsychotic used in the hospital setting. It is well tolerated, and progressive dosing guidelines have been published for the agitated patient.

Of the atypical antipsychotics, short-acting forms of intramuscular olanzapine and ziprasidone are available. A long-acting preparation of risperidone (Consta®, Janssen Pharmaceutical, Titusville, NJ) is used as maintenance treatment. Olanzapine has an oral dissolvable tablet form (Zydis®, Eli Lilly, Indianapolis, IN), which can be used for the NPO patient. The only FDA-approved parenteral mood stabilizer is a preparation of valproic acid (Depacon, Abbot Laboratories, N. Chicago, IL), which can be given intravenously.

Anticoagulation Management

Over 2 million Americans currently take anticoagulant agents for prevention or treatment of thromboembolic events. As the population ages, so will the frequency of surgical procedures, and consequently, clinicians will need to manage perioperative anticoagulation more frequently. Discontinuation of anticoagulation leaves patients unprotected from thromboembolic risk for several days around the time of surgery. However, aggressive anticoagulation in the perioperative period may increase bleeding risk.[20] Thus, clinicians must consider the indication for long-term anticoagulation and extrapolate the risk for thrombotic events compared with the risk for bleeding events (Table 5.4).

In weighing risks and benefits, consider both the patient characteristics and the procedure characteristics. Some procedures, such as cataract extractions, trab-

TABLE 5.4. Risk Stratification of Which Patients on Warfarin Should Receive Perioperative Bridging

High risk for thromboembolism: bridging advised

Known hypercoagulable state as documented by a thromboembolic event and one of the following:

- Protein C deficiency
- Protein S deficiency
- Antithrombin III deficiency
- Homozygous Factor V Leiden mutation
- Antiphospholipid-antibody syndrome

Hypercoagulable state suggested by recurrent (two or more) arterial or idiopathic venous thromboembolic events[a]

Venous or arterial thromboembolism in prior 1–3 months

Rheumatic atrial fibrillation

Acute intracardiac thrombus visualized by echocardiogram

Atrial fibrillation plus mechanical heart valve in any position

Older mechanical valve model (single-disk or ball-in-cage) in mitral position

Recently placed mechanical valve (<3 months)

Atrial fibrillation with history of cardioembolism

Intermediate risk for thromboembolism: bridging on a case-by-case basis

Cerebrovascular disease with multiple (two or more) strokes or transient ischemic attacks without risk factors for cardiac embolism

Newer mechanical valve model (e.g., St. Jude) in mitral position

Older mechanical valve model in aortic position

Atrial fibrillation without a history of cardiac embolism but with multiple risks for cardiac embolism[b]

Venous thromboembolism >3–6 months ago[c]

Low risk for thromboembolism: bridging not advised

One remote venous thromboembolism (>6 months ago)[c]

Intrinsic cerebrovascular disease (e.g., carotid atherosclerosis) without recurrent strokes or transient ischemic attacks

Atrial fibrillation without multiple risks for cardiac embolism

Newer-model prosthetic valve in aortic position

[a] Not including primary atherosclerotic events, such as stroke or myocardial infarction due to cerebrovascular or coronary disease.
[b] For example, ejection fraction <40%, diabetes, hypertension, nonrheumatic valvular heart disease, transmural myocardial infarction within the preceding month.
[c] For patients with a history of venous thromboembolism undergoing major surgery, consideration can be given to postoperative bridging therapy only (without preoperative bridging).
Reprinted, with permission, from Rosenman et al.[15]
Source: Jaffer AK, Brotman DJ, Chukwumerije N. When patients on warfarin need surgery. *Cleve Clin J Med.* 2003; 70:973–984. Reproduced with permission.

eculectomies, gastrointestinal endoscopic procedures without biopsies, uncomplicated tooth extractions, superficial skin procedures, and joint and soft tissue
aspirations/injections do not require cessation of therapeutic anticoagulation in most
cases. More invasive procedures typically have higher bleeding risks and anticoagulation will typically need to be discontinued prior to the procedure. The challenge
then becomes how large a window of time unprotected from thrombosis or embolism
is the treating clinician willing to tolerate. This becomes the decision-making point
for bridging therapy with a shorter-acting anticoagulant (unfractionated heparin or
low-molecular-weight heparin [LMWH]) to minimize this unprotected window
of time.

High-risk patients have up to a 10% rate of thromboembolism per year and
are typically managed with bridging therapy as the concern for a thromboembolic
event outweighs the perceived bleeding risk. This involves discontinuation of warfarin 5–6 days before surgery and initiating therapeutic dosing of subcutaneous
LMWH or IV unfractionated heparin when the patient's international normalized
ratio (INR) falls below the therapeutic range. The bridging agent is stopped immediately prior to surgery (from 6 to 24 h prior, depending on the type of heparin used),
and anticoagulation is resumed as soon as possible postoperatively.[11] Figure 5.1
describes this process in detail.

Low-risk patients have an annual arterial thromboembolic risk of less than
5%, or a monthly venous thromboembolism (VTE) risk of less than 2%. As the
perioperative bleeding risk with bridging therapy outweighs the thromboembolic
risk in these patients, bridging therapy is not indicated. Warfarin can be discontinued
approximately 5 days prior to surgery, and resumed postoperatively when the bleeding risk related to surgery is minimal.

Intermediate-risk patients have an annual arterial thrombotic event risk
between 5% and 10%, and a monthly VTE risk between 2% and 10%. These patients
may have comparable risks of bleeding and thromboembolism, so individual patient
and procedure factors must be assessed on a case-by-case basis in these patients.

Assessment of thromboembolic risk perioperatively is not simply achieved by
taking the yearly risks and dividing by 365 to obtain a daily risk. Surgery creates a
prothrombotic milieu that can increase VTE risk by 100-fold, and discontinuation
of warfarin has been associated with biochemical evidence of rebound hypercoagulability.[21] Therefore, even in low- and intermediate-risk patients, appropriate VTE
prophylaxis measures should still be applied, even if bridging therapy is not indicated. In addition, consider the consequences of the thromboembolic event being
averted by bridging. While arterial events are less frequent, they cause significantly
more death and disability when they do occur (20–30% mortality and 30–40% rate
of disability, compared with combined rates of 5–10% for VTE and 3–13% for
bleeding events).

IV unfractionated heparin and LMWH are typically used for bridging therapy,
although controversy exists related to the use of LMWH in patients with mechanical
heart valves. The prescribing information (package insert) for enoxaparin states that
use for "thromboprophylaxis in pregnant women with mechanical prosthetic heart
valves has not been adequately studied."[22] This refers to the study where two of eight
pregnant women receiving enoxaparin developed valvular thrombosis leading to
maternal and fetal death, whereas none of four patients receiving unfractionated

Preoperatively

Ensure patient does not have any contraindications to LMWH bridging such as:
- allergy to LMWH
- history of HIT
- severe thrombocytopenia
- extremes of weight (severely underweight of overweight)
- creatinine clearance <15 mL/min (weight-based dosing if 15–30 mL/min)
- poor patient reliability
- inability to administer injections

Provide bridging instructions:
- stop warfarin 5 days before surgery (if INR 2–3)
- stop warfarin 6 days before surgery (if INR 3–4.5)
- start LMWH* 36 h after last warfarin dose
- administer last dose of LMWH 24 h prior to procedure†
- check INR on morning of surgery to ensure <1.5 and in some cases <1.2

Postoperatively

- restart LMWH* approximately 24 h post procedure or consider thromboprophylaxis dosing of LMWH on post-op day 1 if patient is at high risk for bleeding (discuss with surgeon)
- restart warfarin at patient's usual dose on the evening of the surgical day
- check INR daily until patient is discharged and periodically thereafter until INR is therapeutic
- check CBC on post-op days 3 and 7 to monitor platelets
- discontinue LMWH when INR is therapeutic for two consecutive days

Figure 5.1. Perioperative bridging strategy using low-molecular-weight heparin (LMWH). *Enoxaparin 1 mg/kg q12h or 1.5 mg/kg q24h or dalteparin 120 U/kg q12h or 200 U/kg q24h or tinzaparin 175 U/kg q24h. †Take full dose if using twice daily LMWH dosing, take two-third dose if using once daily LMWH. HIT, heparin-induced thrombocytopenia; INR, international normalized ratio; CBC, complete blood count. From Grant PJ, Brotman DJ, and Jaffer AK. Perioperative anticoagulant management. *Med Clin North Am.* 2009;93:1105–1121. Reproduced with permission.

heparin developed valve thrombosis. In the two deaths, anti-Factor Xa levels were subtherapeutic at some intervals during treatment; subsequent studies note that the physiology of pregnancy can affect the pharmacokinetics of enoxaparin, leading to lower anti-Factor Xa levels. Therefore, if enoxaparin is to be used in pregnant patients for any reason, anti-Factor Xa levels should be monitored and kept between 0.5 and 1.2 anti-Factor Xa units. Nevertheless, unfractionated heparin should be used for any pregnant patients with mechanical heart valves requiring bridging therapy.[20]

Excluding pregnant patients, several studies have documented the safety of LMWH for bridging patients with mechanical heart valves. Ansell[23] reviewed data on 461 patients from 10 studies; three patients had transient ischemic attacks and no patients had strokes or valve thrombosis.

SUMMARY

Management of medications in the perioperative period is critical in order to maintain stability of medical comorbidities and sustain quality of life during a time of altered hemostasis. In general, the clinician should continue medications with significant withdrawal potential, stop medications that increase surgical risk and are not essential for short-term quality of life, and use clinical judgement if neither of these criteria clearly apply.

Decisions about antiplatelet agents and anticoagulants should be made based on risk of operative bleeding and risk of thrombosis related to the condition for which they are prescribed. Most cardiovascular medications are safe and efficacious and should be continued, with the potential exception of diuretics and ACE/ARBs which should be held in volume-depleted states or for patients with acute kidney injury. Pulmonary medications are safe and steroids should typically be continued with stress dosing reserved for high-risk patients or high-risk procedures. Psychiatric medications are generally safe and should be continued during the perioperative period with few exceptions.

REFERENCES

1. Jaffer A, Michota F. Why perioperative medicine matters more than ever. *Cleve Clin J Med.* 2006;73(Suppl 1):S1.
2. Kennedy JM, et al. Polypharmacy in a general surgical unit and consequences of drug withdrawal. *Br J Clin Pharmacol.* 2000;49:353–362.
3. Bell CM, et al. Potentially unintended discontinuation of long-term medication use after elective surgical procedures. *Arch Intern Med.* 2006;166:2525–2531.
4. Pass SE, Simpson RW. Discontinuation and reinstitution of medications during the perioperative period. *Am J Health Syst Pharm.* 2004;61:899–914.
5. BéLisle S, Hardy JF. Hemorrhage and the use of blood products after adult cardiac operations: myths and realities. *Ann Thorac Surg.* 1996;62(6):1908–1917.
6. Burger W, Chemnitius JM, Kneissl GD, Rucker G. Low-dose aspirin for secondary cardiovascular prevention—cardiovascular risks after its perioperative withdrawal versus bleeding risks with its continuation—review and meta-analysis. *J Intern Med.* 2005;257:399–414.
7. Neilipovitz DT, Bryson GL, Nichol G. The effect of perioperative aspirin therapy in peripheral vascular surgery: a decision analysis. *Anesth Analg.* 2001;93(3):573–580.
8. Oscarsson A, et al. To continue or discontinue aspirin in the perioperative period: a randomized, controlled clinical trial. *Br J Anaesth.* 2010;104:305–312.
9. Fleisher LA, Beckman JA, Brown KA, et al. ACC/AHA 2007 guidelines on perioperative cardiovascular evaluation and care for noncardiac surgery: a report of the American College of Cardiology/American Heart Association Task Force on Practice Guidelines. *Circulation.* 2007;116:e418–e499.
10. Poldermans D, Bax JJ, Boersma E, et al. Guidelines for pre-operative cardiac risk assessment and perioperative cardiac management in non-cardiac surgery. The Task Force for Preoperative Cardiac

Risk Assessment and Perioperative Cardiac Management in Non-Cardiac Surgery of the European Society of Cardiology (ESC) and endorsed by the European Society of Anaesthesiology (ESA). *Eur Heart J.* 2009;30:2769–2812.

11. Grant PJ, Brotman DJ, Jaffer AK. Perioperative anticoagulant management. *Med Clin North Am.* 2009;93:1105–1121.
12. Grines CL, et al. Prevention of premature discontinuation of dual antiplatelet therapy in patients with coronary artery stents: a science advisory from the American Heart Association, American College of Cardiology, Society for Cardiovascular Angiography and Interventions, American College of Surgeons, and American Dental Association, with representation from the American College of Physicians. *J Am Coll Cardiol.* 2007;49(6):734–739.
13. Collet JP, Montalescot G. Premature withdrawal and alternative therapies to dual oral antiplatelet therapy. *Eur Heart J.* 2006;8(Suppl G):G46–G52.
14. Savonitto S, et al. Urgent surgery in patients with a recently implanted coronary drug-eluting stent: a phase II study of "bridging" antiplatelet therapy with tirofiban during temporary withdrawal of clopidogrel. *Br J Anaesth.* 2010;104:285–291.
15. Rosenman DJ, et al. Clinical consequences of withholding versus administering renin-angiotensin-aldosterone system antagonists in the preoperative period. *J Hosp Med.* 2008;3:319–325.
16. Moghissi ES, Korytkowski MT, DiNardo M, et al. American Association of Clinical Endocrinologists and American Diabetes Association consensus statement on inpatient glycemic control. *Endocr Pract.* 2009;15:353–369.
17. Marik PE, Varon J. Requirement of perioperative stress doses of corticosteroids: a systematic review of the literature. *Arch Surg.* 2008;143(12):1222–1226.
18. Kohl BA, Schwartz S. Surgery in the patient with endocrine dysfunction. *Med Clin North Am.* 2009;93:1031–1047.
19. Ang-Lee MK, Moss J, Yuan C-S. Herbal medicines and perioperative care. *JAMA.* 2001; 286:208–216.
20. Jaffer AK, Brotman DJ, Chukwumerije N. When patients on warfarin need surgery. *Cleve Clin J Med.* 2003;70:973–984.
21. Kearon C, Hirsh J. Management of anticoagulation before and after elective surgery. *N Engl J Med.* 1997;336(21):1506–1511.
22. Product Information: Enoxaparin (Lovenox). Sanofi-Aventis, Bridgewater, NJ, 2011.
23. Ansell JE. The perioperative management of warfarin therapy. *Arch Intern Med.* 2003; 163:881–883.

CHAPTER 6

DEVELOPING, IMPLEMENTING, AND OPERATING A PREOPERATIVE CLINIC

Seema Chandra, Daniel Fleisher, and Amir K. Jaffer

WHY A PERIOPERATIVE SYSTEM MAKES SENSE

This chapter focuses on the design and implementation of a multidisciplinary preoperative clinic in the academic setting. While the creation of a new clinic at any hospital or institution is a difficult and time-consuming endeavor, our experience at the University of Miami in the past year has resulted in a robust, jointly governed clinic, which has evaluated over 3000 patients prior to surgery in the first year of operations.

The preoperative clinic, whether it is run by anesthesia alone or by anesthesia and internal medicine, provides multiple services to the hospital. Not only does the clinic risk-stratify the patients prior to surgery, thus flagging individuals who would benefit from testing, preoperative consultation, or medical optimization preoperatively, but it also serves as a clearinghouse for all surgeries to ensure compliance with regulatory agencies' requirements (Joint Commission on Accreditation of Healthcare Organizations [JCAHO], American Health Care Organization [AHCA], and others). Additionally, by completing necessary preanesthesia evaluations and history and physicals prior to the day of surgery, time is saved on the morning of surgery, potentially leading to fewer delayed cases or same-day cancellations. For example, at the Cleveland Clinic, surgical delays have been decreased by 49% through the use of a comprehensive preoperative center.[1] Finally, the preoperative clinic often introduces the patient to the surgical facility and orients them to the routines of surgery. This can play a significant role in allaying patient fears and concerns prior to surgery and improving overall patient satisfaction.

In our review of preoperative clinics, we found that the primary financial value associated with implementing a preoperative program is the *indirect revenue*

Perioperative Medicine: Medical Consultation and Co-Management, First Edition.
Edited by Amir K. Jaffer and Paul J. Grant.

generated by reducing surgical cancellations and delays, rather than direct revenues associated with preoperative consultations and diagnostic testing.[2] In presenting this to the hospital administration, the focus should be on understanding the potential benefits in terms of increasing surgical revenues and reducing costs associated with cancellations and delays. The most readily accessible and directly contributable metric is the rate of same-day cancellations, which often could be prevented by improved preoperative screening. Depending on the size and surgical volume of the hospital, a 2% reduction in same-day cancellations can often justify the cost of implementing a preoperative clinic. As will be highlighted later, adding collaboration with internal medicine can also add a revenue source via the preoperative medical consultation.

VARIOUS DELIVERY MODELS

Our group identified three models currently in use across the country at various preoperative centers:

- *Anesthesia-Run Clinic.* These clinics comprise the majority of preoperative clinics nationwide. These are usually hospital-run and generate no additional revenue for the facility as there is no separate consultative service provided to the patient. However, the expense of running the clinic is justified by corresponding decreased costs on the day of surgery. These clinics are potentially able to reduce delays on the morning of surgery because of the successful completion of the preanesthesia evaluation prior to the day of surgery. Additionally, this type of clinic plays an integral role in ensuring regulatory compliance. Ideally, as higher-risk patients are identified, these patients could be flagged for further intervention or delay of surgery, thus reducing same-day cancellations. In general, the anesthesia-run clinic does not typically provide preoperative medical optimization; patients are generally referred back to their primary care physician (PCP) or sent for medical or specialty consultation.

- *Separate Internal Medicine and Anesthesia Clinics.* This model is found in a few centers and is perhaps exemplified at the Cleveland Clinic. All patients are screened and are triaged to one of the following: no preoperative assessment required until the day of surgery, anesthesia evaluation only, medicine evaluation only, or both medicine and anesthesia evaluation. This system can address all the goals of an anesthesia-only clinic and can also perform medical optimization of patients prior to surgery. Additionally, the medical clinic is able to bill for preoperative medical consultation and thus generate revenue. This system works well at a large academic medical center with a long history of interdisciplinary collaboration, but it does require significant infrastructure and resources as there are two separate clinics and two separate sets of physicians and midlevel providers.

- *Combined Internal Medicine and Anesthesia Clinic.* This hybrid model was chosen for our newly developed clinic at the University of Miami. This style of clinic maintains the advantages of the two separate clinics (ensuring regulatory compliance, completing preanesthesia evaluations, and providing medical optimization) but requires less infrastructure and support staff by combining the facilities. Additionally, the shared governance of the clinic has created a platform for increased collaboration between internal medicine and anesthesia in standardizing and streamlining the preoperative approach at our multiple surgical facilities.

The following pages will further describe the particulars of our development process at the University of Miami and help provide a framework for the development of preoperative clinics in general.

BUILDING THE TEAM

The UHealth Preoperative Assessment Center (UPAC) at the University of Miami was developed to optimize patients going for surgery at the University of Miami Hospital (an academic tertiary care center) and the University of Miami Sylvester Cancer Center. In preparing to create the initial project concept and business plan to present to the health system leadership, a cross-disciplinary team from the Departments of Medicine (division of hospital medicine), Anesthesia, and Surgery, and the Healthcare Management Engineering Office was created. This discovery task force consisted of representatives from the following:

- *Hospital Operations.* The chief nursing officers and nursing directors from the respective hospitals provided presurgical requirements for the operating rooms and recommendations for reducing surgical delays and cancellations.
- *Hospital Medicine.* The chief and physicians from the Division of Hospital Medicine established guidelines for preoperative evaluation, algorithms for preoperative testing and care, and recommendations for patient flow and staffing for the preoperative clinic.
- *Anesthesia.* The heads of Anesthesia established standardized preanesthesia guidelines and testing requirements.
- *Surgery.* Representatives from a cross section of surgical specialties provided input on methods for determining and communicating requirements for preoperative care.
- *Healthcare Management Engineering.* Managed the project team and documented process flows and business requirements.

The team met weekly to formulate the project concept and establish guidelines for the development of the preoperative center. The following guiding principles were established:

- Create a unified, patient-centric preoperative process for the UHealth System.
- Instill processes to improve patient safety and ensure operational effectiveness.
- Design a system that is financially viable.

PROJECT DEVELOPMENT

Following the work of the discovery team, smaller project work groups were created to develop detailed requirements for the business plan, which were reported to a project steering committee for review. These work groups included the following:

- *Operations.* Operational work flows, including preoperative screening at the surgeon's office, screening form submission, phone screen administration, and patient medical chart creation.
- *Clinical.* Clinical processes, including medical documentation, medical algorithms, preoperative assessment and planning, surgeon and anesthesiologist communications.
- *Revenue Cycle.* Revenue cycle setup, including scheduling, registration, billing, and collections.
- *Facilities.* Physical layout and equipment requirements for the preoperative clinic.
- *IT/Telecom.* Systems and telecommunications requirements.
- *Human Resources.* Clinic staffing, including position transfers and new position hiring.
- *Communications.* Internal and external marketing, including web site and brochures.

Each work group established requirements to incorporate into the project proposal. The following sections outline the key elements of the project development for the preoperative clinic.

Establishing Need

As stated in the introduction, we identified two possible sources of revenue for the clinic. The primary source was the indirect revenue generated by reducing surgical cancellations and delays. As our clinic also aimed to complete the preanesthesia evaluation prior to the day of surgery, there are also potentially decreased costs on the day of surgery as there is less time devoted to anesthesia evaluation on the day of surgery. Additionally, there were direct revenue sources identified such as the preoperative medical consultation, as well as the generation of diagnostic testing. In our facility, we also identified elements of patient satisfaction, which could be addressed by the creation of a preoperative clinic.

Process Flow

Once the need is established and the current challenges and opportunities are understood, the proposed process can be established. At the University of Miami, we implemented a universal screening process via questionnaires and nurse phone screens. Patients identified as having medical comorbidities that could benefit from evaluation were referred to UPAC or to their primary care provider. The UPAC anesthesiologist maintains oversight of this process and reviews all data, thus ensuring that even patients who did not come in for in-person evaluation at clinic still have the necessary testing on file in the surgical chart.

Forecasting Demand

The expected workload for the preoperative center was driven by anticipated surgical volumes, which were provided by Finance from each hospital's 5-year plan. These surgical volumes where then extrapolated into (1) consultations at UPAC, (2) consultations with PCPs, and (3) preoperative phone screens. The following methods were used for estimating volumes:

- *Consultations.* Based on the screening questionnaire developed and the patient populations at each hospital, it was initially estimated that 50% of patients would require a preoperative consultation. Of these, it was estimated that 80% would be referred to UPAC and 20% would be referred to their PCP or to a specialist. The following examples illustrate the calculations:
  - ○ UPAC Consultations: 50 surgeries/day × 50% require consultation × 80% referred to UPAC = 20 UPAC consultations/day;
  - ○ PCP Consultations: 50 surgeries/day × 50% require consultation × 20% referred to PCP = 5 PCP consultations/day.
- *Phone Screens.* It was estimated that 50% of patients would require only a preoperative phone screen. The calculation for daily phone screens is illustrated below:
  - ○ 50 surgeries/day × 50% requiring phone screen = 25 phone screens/day.

These extrapolations were used to estimate annual, monthly, and daily volumes for consultations and phone screens. The 80th percentile day was used for staffing and facility design, which is found by ranking daily volumes and finding the level where 80% fall either at or below. A common design mistake is to use the average day, which if used will result in the clinic being understaffed or undersized during 50% of operating days.

Staffing

The preoperative center would serve as both an outpatient clinic for preoperative consultations and diagnostic testing, as well as the work space for nurses to conduct patient phone screens and compile medical charts. Roles were established based on these work flows, and staffing levels where set for the roles based on the 80th percentile design day outlined in the previous section.

Facility Design and Outfitting

The design of the clinic was based on the requirement to function as both an outpatient clinic and as a work space for preoperative phone screens and chart preparation.

The following functional areas were incorporated into the design and outfitted with the listed equipment:

- *Reception Desk for Check-In.* Computers, phones, print/copy/fax machine, label printer
- *Patient Waiting Area.* Television, coffee machine, magazine rack
- *Vitals Stations.* Computer, [medical equipment], scale
- *Exam Rooms.* Computer, exam table, [medical equipment], biomedical waste disposal
- *Bariatric Exam Room.* Larger exam room with specialized exam table
- *Phlebotomy Room.* Blood draw chair, centrifuge, specimen refrigerator, electrocardiographic (EKG) machine
- *Checkout Stations.* Computers, label printers
- *Hospitalist/Anesthesiologist Workroom.* Workstations, computers, print/copy/fax machine
- *Nursing Workroom.* Workstations, computers, print/copy/fax machine, chart storage, file storage, kitchen area with sink/microwave/coffeemaker/refrigerator

Information Systems

The information systems requirements of the clinic will vary based on the current systems used by the health system. At the very least, the clinic will need the following functionality:

- access to view surgical scheduling,
- method to categorize patients by preoperative requirement (consult, phone screen, etc.),
- ability to create and maintain a work list of patients for consultation and phone screens,
- ability to schedule patients for preoperative consultations at the clinic.

Depending on the sophistication of your operating systems, especially if functioning with an electronic health record, you may also be able to create preoperative documentation electronically and distribute to surgeons and anesthesiologists electronically.

BUSINESS CASE DEVELOPMENT

The business plan for the UPAC was developed by the project manager in partnership with the Finance departments from the medical practice and the respective hospitals. The project value was evaluated based on direct revenues from consultations and diagnostic testing and expected reduction in surgical cancellations over expected operating expenses.

Business Case Outline

The business case should provide an overview of the project proposal with supporting financial data pertaining to projected revenues, direct and indirect cost savings, and expected operating expenses. Partner with your finance department to develop a 5-year EBIDTA analysis (earnings before interest, depreciation, and amortization), which should include financial performance measures including payback period, net present value (NPV), return on investment (ROI), and breakeven point. While the project plan should provide a more detailed description of the project requirements and rollout strategy, the business case should be a brief document (five pages or less) that succinctly outlines the project value and the capital and operating budgets required.

IMPLEMENTATION

Following project approval, the project manager and project teams will be responsible for managing the capital budget for the implementation, hiring new staff for the clinic, and integrating the clinic into operations. The same teams involved in the project proposal and business case development will likely transition onto project implementation teams, and will be joined by others from support areas throughout the organization who will be involved with the clinic setup, including the business office, information technology, human resources, health information management, and regulatory and compliance.

The following section outlines some of the key components in the project implementation phase. In most cases, the framework for the project has been outlined, but during project implementation, the detailed requirements are established.

Project Plan

The first step in project implementation is the development of a detailed project plan. The project plan should outline project categories, detailed tasks required in each category, owner(s) for each task, and the required completion date for each task. Please reference Table 6.1 at the end of this chapter for an example of a project plan outline.

Project Management

The project will typically be comprised of a core project team or steering committee, with working teams for the various functional groups. The project manager will be responsible for coordinating and overseeing progress of each of the working teams and reporting progress to the steering committee. In most cases, members of the project teams juggle project needs with their daily work requirements, so the project manager must carefully track individual progress to ensure adherence to the overall project plan.

Human Resources

Perhaps the most critical step in ensuring the success of the project is the recruitment and hiring of the clinic manager, which in the case of the University of Miami was a new nurse director. It is recommended that the clinic manager be hired 1–2 months prior to the opening of the clinic, allowing them to be involved in staff hiring, clinic setup, and training.

For the remaining staff, a careful inventory of current preoperative and surgical roles should be performed to determine if any functions will be transitioning to the preoperative clinic. In this case, new hires may be mixed with position transfers from other areas, which will not require position recruiting but will require human resources intervention.

Revenue Cycle Setup

As mentioned earlier, the added financial benefit of the internal medicine preoperative consultation is the ability to generate direct revenue. For this to happen, an actual consult must be sent from the surgeon to the preoperative center. In our institution, we facilitated this by use of standard language at the bottom of a questionnaire given by the surgeons to their patients in clinic, and we have enclosed our standard language in Table 6.2 at the end of this chapter.

Additionally, there are several managed care plans that do not permit medical consultation; we flag these patients on arrival to the preoperative center so that they do not receive any bills from the facility.

System Integration

The preoperative clinic will interact with a number of entities within the health system, including surgeon's offices for patient referrals, diagnostic services for patient testing, and hospital preanesthesia and surgical operations teams. Representatives from these organizations should be included in the project development, and lines of communication should be established for day-to-day operations post go-live. These would include establishing processes for accommodating add-on patients for preoperative consultations, referring preoperative clinic patients for same-day ancillary services (stress test, chest X-ray, etc.), and delivery of results for the preoperative consultation to surgeons and anesthesiologists in advance of surgery.

Communications

Once detailed operating plans have been finalized and a go-live date has been set, the final step is communicating plans to partner organizations throughout the health system. Below are some recommended forms of communication prior to opening:

- in-service presentations for surgeons, anesthesiologists, and hospital staff;
- lunch and learn sessions for surgical coordinators;
- open house for key partners and neighboring clinics;
- e-mail communications from health system leadership.

OPERATIONS

The operations of a successful preoperative center require a careful understanding of the dual role this clinic plays. The clinic, just like any other outpatient clinic, must function smoothly and allow the patient to progress through in a seamless fashion, minimizing delays and ensure all needed evaluations and testing are performed in a timely fashion. Additionally, the clinic must serve the needs of the hospital by decreasing delays and increasing efficiency in the operating rooms. Since the business case for most preoperative clinics rests on the indirect revenue generated by the facility, careful monitoring and evaluation of these metrics is critical to the ongoing success and funding of the project. At our facility, we have monthly and quarterly reviews of surgical delays and cancellations, and we are developing methods to measure patient satisfaction and patient outcomes (including length of stay, perioperative complications, etc.).

Additionally, there is an ongoing need for education with all the involved parties including surgeons, anesthesia providers, ancillary services, and hospital administration, and in our care, the nurse director has taken a lead in facilitating communication between these groups.

SUMMARY

The creation of a preoperative clinic is labor and time intensive, but can yield significant benefit to a hospital including decreased same-day cancellations, increased on-time surgical starts, and increased patient satisfaction. The more recent innovation of adding collaboration between medicine and anesthesia, either in separate clinics or a combined clinic, has the added benefits of providing preoperative medical optimization and generating direct revenue through consultation.

The keys to success include the following:

1. Having a multidisciplinary team from project design onward to ensure that all potential needs and challenges are anticipated, and to ensure buy-in from the involved parties, particularly surgeons, anesthesiologists, and hospital administration.

2. Prior to implementation, a clinic manager or director must be identified. This person is responsible for troubleshooting day-to-day challenges and ensuring communication between the project team and the referring physicians.

3. Adequate infrastructure (technology physical space, clinical equipment) and support must be devoted to the clinic prior to opening to ensure the ability to provide efficient and comprehensive care.

4. Ongoing monitoring and evaluation of the project to ensure that key metrics are being met and, if not, to prompt reengineering of the system as needed.

TABLE 6.1. Sample Project Plan Categories for a Preoperative Clinic Implementation

Category	Task	Owner(s)
Human resources	Current staff transition	Leadership/human resources
	New position hiring	Leadership/human resources
Clinical	Preoperative documentation	Hospital medicine/anesthesia
	Diagnostic testing guidelines	Hospital medicine/anesthesia
	Preoperative care algorithms	Hospital medicine/anesthesia
	Preanesthesia requirements	Anesthesia
Operational processes	Surgeons office referral	Surgeons' offices/clinic operations
	Clinic consultation	Clinical operations
	Phone screen	Clinical operations
	Surgical chart prep	Clinical operations
Revenue cycle	Scheduling	Business office
	Registration	Business office
	Insurance verification	Business office
	Charge capture	Business office
	Billing and collections	Business office
Information systems	Surgical patient tracking	Information technology
	Clinical systems	Information technology
	Scheduling system	Information technology
	Charge capture system	Information technology
Facility and equipment	Design	Architect
	Construction	Construction manager
	Medical equipment	Supply chain/procurement
	Office equipment	Supply chain/procurement
	IT (PCs, printers, copiers)	Information technology
	Telecom (phones, fax)	Telecommunications
Recurring accounts	Office supplies	Clinical operations
	Medical supplies	Clinical operations
	Blood draw pickup	Clinical operations
	Utilities	Clinical operations
	Television/cable	Clinical operations
	Housekeeping	Clinical operations
	Biomedical waste	Clinical operations
	Security	Clinical operations
Marketing	Brochures	Marketing/clinic operations
	Web site	Marketing/clinic operations
	Internal communications	Marketing/clinical operations

TABLE 6.2.   Sample Language for the Preoperative Medical Consult Request

To be completed by surgeon and/or designee

☐ If responding YES to <u>any</u> questions, a preoperative consultation with a physician is recommended (select one):

☐ Preoperative Center   ☐ Primary Care Physician   ☐ Specialist:
                                         (PCP)   _____

☐ If responding NO to <u>all</u> questions, patient will complete a phone screen with a registered nurse prior to surgery.

If requesting a consultation:

Based on a review of the patient's medical history and specific medical conditions outlined, a consultation with a qualified internist or specialist (as directed) is requested. This consultation is requested to minimize risks of developing complications as result of surgery and/or anesthesia.

_____   _____   ____/____/____   _____
Surgeon Name (PRINT)   Signature   Date   Time

REFERENCES

1. Jaffer AK, Brotman D. Perioperative care: an opportunity to expand and diversify the hospitalist's portfolio. *Hospitalist*. 2004;3:12–14.
2. Pollard JB, Zboray AL, Mazze RI. Economic benefits attributed to opening a preoperative evaluation clinic for outpatients. *Anesth Analg*. 1996;83:407–410.

CHAPTER 7

DEVELOPING, IMPLEMENTING, AND OPERATING A MEDICAL CONSULTATION SERVICE

Joshua D. Lenchus and Kurt Pfeifer

INTRODUCTION

The expanding role of hospitalists in many institutions has led to an increased inter-action with surgical and other nonmedical services. Some examples include participa-tion on rapid response and code teams, co-management of orthopedic surgery patients, and general medical consultation. At the same time, increasingly complex medical comorbidities in nonmedical hospitalized patients have heightened the need for medical specialists in their care. In this setting, proficiency in perioperative and consultative medicine becomes essential for the practitioner of hospital medicine. For centers with a large nonmedical hospital volume, development of local experts in this area coupled with consistently high demand for their services may promote, or even necessitate, the development of a medical consultation service. The following chapter details the planning and implementation of a medical consultation service.

DETERMINING NEEDS AND RESOURCES

The creation of any new service begins with a needs analysis. With respect to a medical consult service, the "customers" are the other services to which recommen-dations will be provided, with the patient as the ultimate beneficiary. This section details some of the initial considerations in setting up such a service.

Institutional Needs

Prior to determining how medical consultation might benefit an internal medicine department, the needs of the institution must be ascertained. Hospital and department

Perioperative Medicine: Medical Consultation and Co-Management, First Edition.
Edited by Amir K. Jaffer and Paul J. Grant.

TABLE 7.1. The Bricks of the Foundation of a Medical Consultation Service

Services provided: consultation versus co-management
Hours of operation
Response time
Order writing privileges and responsibilities
Primary contact person
Communication standards
Standardized order sets
Reporting structure
Funding

administration should be consulted for the following data: surgical volume, other nonmedical inpatient volume, complexity of inpatients, and the number of external versus internal referrals of inpatients. Surgical and nonmedical volume must be adequately high with sufficient medical complexity to warrant the creation of a medical consultation service and to generate enough revenue to meet goals (see further information later in this section). Information on the referral source of hospitalized patients also helps determine the need for a separate medical consultation service rather than utilizing patients' primary care providers. For example, a hospital with a large volume of external referrals will have many inpatients without an internist on staff at that site, making the use of a separate medical consultant service necessary.

Once the institution's needs are understood, the resources available for a medical consultation service can be verified and the roles of the service established. Table 7.1 identifies the major elements to be addressed in this area.

Type of Services Provided

The first step is deciding the type of service that will be provided. Strict consultation, co-management, or some combination will affect the service's structure. This is discussed in greater detail in Chapters 1 and 2. It is important to note the nuances of each when devising the service's blueprint. For the purpose of brevity, we will use the phrase "consult" to mean any of the above. For example, in some purely academic models, the service may only accept consults from nonmedical services, and provide specific recommendations addressing a particular issue, while others may provide 24-hour consultation and co-management. In some community settings, the service may provide similar consultation and include after-hours management of acute problems. In still other scenarios, the service can be crafted to consult for a predetermined group (e.g., orthopedic surgeons), providing a vast array of medical guidance and support. Yet others include among their responsibilities medical emergency calls such as participation on a rapid response team and/or "code team."

Although it is impossible to fully predict future utilization of a medical consultation program, attempts should be made to understand the nature of the majority of calls and the predominant patient population. At some institutions, the bulk of consult service requests are for blood pressure and glucose management, preoperative assessment, lab and electrocardiographic (EKG) abnormalities, altered mental status, and medical emergencies in the adult population. Teams may be consulted by a variety of nonmedical services who contact them at any time. Being prepared for the common problems will assist a program in developing algorithms and triage systems to effectively handle consult requests.

Expectations and Lines of Responsibility

Assuring an efficient medical consultation program requires clear establishment of consulting services' expectations for timeliness of consults, order-writing privileges, and primary contact personnel. Once a call is received, anticipated turnaround time should be agreed upon. While there is no standard answer to this question, institutional bylaws, and/or rules and regulations may specify one. Some facilities have policies that emergency consults should be seen as quickly as possible, urgent calls fielded within the hour, and routine questions addressed within 24 h. However, timelines may be individualized per facility, if not already done.

The question of order writing also needs to be answered from the outset. Will orders written by a consulting team be accepted at face value, or will they need to be cosigned or approved by the primary team? Again, institutional policies and procedures may prevail, but some have found that writing orders in the chart directly facilitates the timeliness of them being carried out. For instance, if consulted by a surgical team, they may be in the operating room by the time the consultant arrives to evaluate the patient, and they may not see the written recommendations until much later. Writing orders, accompanied by "if approved by primary team" or some similar statement, will result in the nurse calling the nonmedical team. In this way, the order is carried out quickly, and the team receives a secondary method of communication to attest to the consultant's presence. The alternative to writing orders in the chart is to simply document the recommendations in the progress note section and monitor the orders to see if they were carried out. Ultimately, the incorporation of advice frequently boils down to clear lines of responsibility and good communication.

The assignment of the primary contact for consultant care (e.g., house staff, midlevel practitioners, or faculty) should also be discussed. In teaching facilities, house staff can be the initial point of contact for consulting services, perform the consultation, and withhold questionable recommendations until the attending rounds on the patient. However, at some institutions, it may be logistically or politically inadvisable to have a training physician be the "face" of the consult service. Midlevel practitioners can perform similarly in some settings, and faculty can simply provide advice in real time. The real question is one of logistics and manpower—who will see the patients in a timely manner and be the primary source of communication? The use of midlevel practitioners and training physicians will be addressed later in this chapter.

Communication Standards

With multiple modalities of communication, some prefer that orders are written directly, and others may favor writing a note in the chart. In either case, as described above, this may not suffice for providing timely recommendations to services that may not see such documentation for a prolonged period. Technically savvy clinicians may use text messaging or mobile phones to contact the consulting team, but care must be taken not to violate the Health Insurance Portability and Accountability Act (HIPAA) restrictions in conveying patient-sensitive information through text or e-mail. These are typically acceptable methods to solicit a return call from the primary service, or direct them to review your documentation rather than convey the information itself. Of course, whenever possible, communication should occur face-to-face or over the phone, and the details of this communication (with whom and when) should be detailed in consultation notes. Such communication builds rapport with consulting services and confirms that your recommendations were received. Additionally, this two-way communication provides the opportunity for questions to be asked so as to minimize any potential for misunderstanding.

Standardized Order Sets

Once a consult program is conceived, the decision to implement specific algorithms, or order sets, for a variety of issues should be addressed. Many institutions use evidence-based guidelines for addressing different patient populations for a variety of surgical procedures and common inpatient problems. Examples include preoperative evaluation algorithms and protocols for treating hypertension in pregnant patients.

Funding

The issue of funding is never straightforward. If a facility's payer mix is "good" (e.g., more insured than noninsured patients), medical consultation may in fact pay for its own full-time employee. This may not be the case at some institutions, so they may opt to add responsibilities to their consultant. Some could choose to add bedside procedural performance in an effort to generate additional money and work relative value units (wRVUs). Still others may want to add consultant work at other sites on campus, and yet others may wish to include the consultant in staffing preoperative clinics. These decisions will be site specific and include a critical evaluation of the demand for the service, creating a realistic supply model (e.g., staffing), and arriving at a financially viable business plan to present as the medical consult service develops.

Implementation of a medical consultation program requires that the foundation be set, roles and responsibilities delineated, and a business plan presented and approved. In so doing, remember that communication is the key in customer service. In this regard, the goal is to communicate efficiently and effectively in order to build a strong positive reputation for providing valuable service. Constant reassessment should occur, and as a service gains in popularity, the workload will increase concomitantly. Hours and staffing issues may require adjustment; the service will never be stagnant.

It may be beneficial to assign a medical director, someone who serves as liaison or "point person" between the primary teams and those to whom the service will report. It is always an advantage to have an individual with whom others can relate, a face to which they can associate the service, and someone that others can approach with issues of concern. Aside from crafting schedules and being the consummate problem solver, this position adds a personal and accountable level to the service.

COLLABORATION WITH NONMEDICAL SERVICES

One of the greatest challenges in the creation of a successful medical consultation program is establishing effective collaboration with a broad range of very different clinicians, including anesthesiologists, physiatrists, neurologists, psychiatrists, and surgeons. Each nonmedical service has a unique patient population and specific needs for medical consultation. In some situations, the consultants may even find themselves in the role of mediator between medical and nonmedical services. One such example may be deciding if a patient requires transfer from a surgical service to a medical one. Navigating such landscapes requires great tact and excellent interpersonal skills that are inherent personality traits rather than learned skills. However, with application of a handful of general recommendations and an understanding of the common issues encountered in this collaborative model, internists can establish a mutually beneficial relationship with nonmedical services that results in high-quality patient care.

Regardless of the unique characteristics of one's institution or the types of nonmedical clinicians who will utilize a medical consultation service, establishing a strong collaborative relationship through effective communication is crucial. Unfortunately, in many centers, communication between different services is sporadic and only used to voice grievances rather than work together on system improvement. Several different techniques for opening communications with nonmedical services can be utilized (Table 7.2). All of these are effective for maintaining a healthy dynamic with nonmedical services, but during the initiation of a medical consultation program, meeting with leadership from these services and organizing focus groups with their clinicians is likely to be most useful.

Launching a medical consultation service should begin with meeting with leadership from the nonmedical services that would most benefit from general medicine assistance. The prospective leader of a medical consultation service must enter such discussions with a full understanding of what he or she can provide and how the nonmedical service will benefit. However, in order to establish mutual respect, the focus of the meeting should be determining how medical services can assist other

TABLE 7.2.   **Techniques for Establishing Communication with Nonmedical Services**

Survey nonmedical clinicians on their needs, expectations, and current level of satisfaction

Meet individually with service line chiefs or department chairs

Attend departmental meetings of nonmedical services

Organize focus groups of nonmedical clinicians

TABLE 7.3. Examples of Questions to Ask in Focus Groups with Nonmedical Clinicians

In what situations do you feel medical consultation would be most helpful to you?

What behaviors or practices from medical services have you found to be particularly effective?

What problems have you experienced working with medical services in the inpatient setting?

Would you prefer medical services to manage medical problems independent of you (co-management) or simply provide recommendations?

For what conditions would you not want assistance from the medical consultation service?

clinicians rather than explaining how nonmedical physicians need assistance from internists.

Service leadership can offer good insight on ways a medicine consult service can improve, but the most specific and useful information may come from focus groups conducted by nonmedical clinicians. Focus groups typically consist of 6–12 representatives of the nonmedical service who are asked several qualitative questions about clinical operations related in some way to general medicine. Questions should be focused enough to prevent tangential discussions but also open enough to allow interactive discussion (Table 7.3). Group members are allowed to answer questions in a collective and interactive manner while the group leader records responses and discussion. The results of focus groups can then be taken back to the nonmedical leadership to refine goals and expectations for the services to be provided by the medical consultation program.

While each institution will have unique aspects of the interaction between medical and nonmedical services, several common considerations are worth discussing and are included below. Knowledge of these will allow for more insightful discussions with nonmedical services as well as foster understanding and effective communication between general medicine and other specialties.

Surgical Specialties

For all surgical specialties, the greatest concerns related to medical care are poor outcomes, prolonged length of stay, and same-day surgery cancellations. Addressing the first two problems can be accomplished through medical care provided in either a traditional consultation role or in a co-management model. Different surgical specialties will have very different preferences, but it is critical for the medical consultation service to understand the specific expectations of each group. Addressing the issue of same-day surgery cancellations not only requires provision of excellent preoperative medical care but also establishing a good working relationship with anesthesiology (described below.)

Orthopedic Surgery

Medical consultation has been most strongly embraced by orthopedic surgery, and several studies have demonstrated positive outcomes from perioperative care provided by internists.[1-3] In most of these investigations, a medical co-management system was employed, and at many institutions, a system of automatic consultation for co-management of common medical comorbidities is utilized. When discussing collaboration with orthopedic surgery services, internists should inquire if the orthopedic service wishes to leave all nonsurgical management to the medical consultant and if a system of automatic consultation might streamline this process.

Anesthesiology

Anesthesiologists have a unique interface with both surgeons and medical services. They are ultimately responsible for many of a patient's perioperative outcomes yet their involvement in planning and care coordination typically occurs only shortly before and after surgery. Frustrations can arise on all sides if the anesthesiologist disagrees with management decisions made by medical and/or surgical services. This is particularly true when the anesthesiologist cancels a surgery on a patient previously "cleared" by their medical colleagues. The medical consultant has the opportunity to greatly improve the relationship between all three services and reduce same-day cancellations. By meeting with your institution's anesthesiologists, a medical consultation service can determine what standards they expect for preoperative evaluation and documentation. Simply agreeing on a set of indications for preoperative testing, guidelines for preoperative medication management, or a template for preoperative history and physicals may go far in improving relationships. Furthermore, it is important to follow one of Goldman's Ten Commandments of medical consultation—"honor thy turf."[4] Medical consultants should focus on general medicine problems and not provide recommendations on the type of anesthesia or intraoperative monitoring since these are in the domain of anesthesiology. With continuous communication and feedback with anesthesiology, a medical consultation program can become an invaluable part of perioperative care at an institution.

Other Nonmedical Specialties

Many other nonmedical specialties have primary responsibility for the care of hospitalized patients, and their comfort with managing medical comorbidities is highly variable. For some, such as psychiatry, co-management of all medical problems is likely desired. Conversely, physiatrists and neurologists at many institutions are quite secure in their ability to manage many common medical conditions. Thus, for any other nonmedical service, it is extremely important to determine specific expectations of the medical consultant, including order-writing responsibilities, call instructions, and overnight availability.

CONSULTATION VERSUS CO-MANAGEMENT

This topic is discussed in more detail in Chapters 1 and 2. Briefly, these are two separate concepts that need to be considered by any medical consult service. While traditional consultation has a historical basis and is typically offered to any nonmedical service, co-management is a more recent mode of patient care and has been implemented effectively at institutions across the country.[1,5–8] The basic premise in consultation-only is that a patient is seen for a specific reason, similar to the role surgical consultants play for internists. For example, if a consultation is requested for a patient with uncontrolled hypertension, the internist takes ownership of that particular issue by providing the primary team direction until it is under control, including recommendations for hospital discharge.

At present, co-management is most commonly found with orthopedic surgeons. A typical example would be a patient with multiple medical comorbidities who is admitted to the hospital with a hip fracture. The surgeon's role is to perform surgery while the internist addresses all of the patient's medical issues. This model is akin to a super consultant. That is, the internist becomes the primary caregiver for all of the patient's medical needs, whether acute or chronic. This is in contrast to the traditional consultant model where the internist would only be called for a specific medical issue, address it, and then sign off.

COORDINATION WITH A PREOPERATIVE EVALUATION CLINIC

A natural partnership between medical and surgical services can be developed with the creation of an on-site preoperative clinic. A preoperative clinic can decompress the hospital with patients who will undergo surgery at some future time by performing the assessment once discharged. The operation of the clinic can be even more effective if its staff includes an anesthesiologist, medical assistant, and secretary among its complement, in addition to the internist. At the clinic, the patient can be evaluated, appropriate tests can be ordered, the results can be reviewed, and the patient can be provided with the necessary documentation regarding his or her operative risk. Having access to the patient's prior medical records will alleviate duplicate testing, making the journey to the operating suite faster and less costly. This model has the potential to decrease the risk of same-day surgery cancellations, something that will be looked on favorably by surgeons and hospital administration.

ROLE OF MIDLEVEL CARE PROVIDERS AND TRAINEES

As previously mentioned, other clinicians can be the "first responders" to the call for consultation. However, it is imperative to specify roles, responsibilities, and expectations as they will be the initial point of contact with the "customer," or primary team. Many of the issues raised above should be addressed (i.e., from which services are consults acceptable, timeliness of response, and ability to write orders). If midlevel providers will be assisting during the day, it is important to determine how consults will be handled after hours if the service operates around the clock. A benefit for including such practitioners is the ability to increase the service's capacity. Rules governing midlevel providers are dependent on individual state laws (promulgated by the respective boards) and specific hospital bylaws. In some areas, nurse practitioners (NPs), for example, are independently licensed providers who may effectively see patients on their own, working under a protocol established by a physician. Physician assistants (PAs) always require physician supervision in the hospital setting. Another benefit to employing NPs and PAs is their ability to independently bill without the patient needing to be seen by an attending, but at a reduced physician rate.

In academic facilities, trainees can be a useful workforce. At some institutions, a medical resident is on call for 24 h every day. Consults are initially fielded by the resident; he/she gathers some basic information from the primary team before visiting the patient. Once a history is obtained and a physical exam is performed, the resident discusses the case with the consult attending, soliciting answers to any questions, and documenting the service's recommendation. If this is done after hours, the attending will see the patient on the following day.

When incorporating trainees, it is critical to ensure that the Accreditation Council for Graduate Medical Education (ACGME) requirements are met. For internal medicine, the ACGME Residency Review Committee (RRC) states that residents must gain experience in the role of a medical consultant during their training. However, there are strict guidelines for the creation of a curriculum and its components. Examples include limits on the number of hours a resident may work and a prescribed amount of time off between shifts and over the course of 4 weeks, among others. Specific curricular development is beyond the scope of this chapter. While some have opted to develop their own, others have used online resources such as that available from the Society of Hospital Medicine (http://shmconsults.com), which provides comprehensive consultative medicine modules that can be viewed for free, with the ability to obtain continuing medical education credit for licensed physicians.

MEASUREMENT OF SUCCESS

Ultimately, a medical consultation program must demonstrate its value to an institution and its funding departments. Various measures have been previously reported in studies of medical consultation programs and are metrics that should be utilized during the initiation of the consult service (Table 7.4). Many of these outcomes are tracked at institutions for other purposes and can be obtained without much investment

TABLE 7.4. Outcome Measures to Determine the Impact of a Medical Consultation Service

Length of stay

Hospitalization costs

Incidence of complications (i.e., acute kidney injury, congestive heart failure)

Utilization of special resources (i.e., blood products)

Incidence of same-day surgery cancellations

of additional time or money. In order to best determine the impact of a medical consultation service, data for each outcome prior to the service's initiation should be obtained for comparison. Although these "hard" outcomes are important to measure, some of the greatest gains made by a medical consultation program will be intangible and represented by increased satisfaction among nonmedical clinicians and other healthcare staff. Therefore, satisfaction surveys of these groups should also be employed to gather data supporting the continuation or growth of the service.

CONCLUSION

The development and implementation of a medical consultation service is a worthwhile venture. This process requires initial data gathering, interaction with peers to determine service-specific needs (i.e., traditional consultations and/or co-management), securing funding, creating staffing models, and measuring outcomes. While there is no universally applicable model, thoughtful planning in design and execution need to be undertaken. The reward is an efficient service that can serve as a role model for other hospital services. It provides the benefits of collaboration with other services, fostering strong communication, and accomplishing safe and effective patient care.

REFERENCES

1. Huddleston JM, Long KH, Naessens JM, et al. Hospitalist-Orthopedic Team Trial Investigators. Medical and surgical comanagement after elective hip and knee arthroplasty: a randomized, controlled trial. *Ann Intern Med.* 2004;141(1):28–38.
2. Batsis JA, Phy MP, Melton LJ, III, et al. Effects of a hospitalist care model on mortality of elderly patients with hip fractures. *J Hosp Med.* 2007;2(4):219–225.
3. Pinzur MS, Gurza E, Kristopaitis T, et al. Hospitalist–orthopedic co-management of high-risk patients undergoing lower extremity reconstruction surgery. *Orthopedics.* 2009;32(7):495.
4. Goldman L, Lee T, Rudd P. Ten commandments for effective consultations. *Arch Intern Med.* 1983;143:1753–1755.
5. Whinney C, Michota F. Surgical comanagement: a natural evolution of hospitalist practice. *J Hosp Med.* 2008;3(5):394–397.
6. Phy MP, Vanness DJ, Melton LJ, III, et al. Effects of a hospitalist model on elderly patients with hip fracture. *Arch Intern Med.* 2005;165(7):796–801.
7. Fisher AA, Davis MW, Rubenach SE, Sivakumaran S, Smith PN, Budge MM. Outcomes for older patients with hip fractures: the impact of orthopedic and geriatric medicine cocare. *J Orthop Trauma.* 2006;20(3):172–180.
8. Friedman SM, Mendelson DA, Bingham KW, Kates SL. Impact of a comanaged Geriatric Fracture Center on short-term hip fracture outcomes. *Arch Intern Med.* 2009;169(18):1712–1717.

CHAPTER 8

PERIOPERATIVE MEDICINE: CODING, BILLING, AND REIMBURSEMENT ISSUES

Jessica Zuleta and Seema Chandra

INTRODUCTION

Historically, preoperative assessments performed the day prior or the day of surgery have led to poor utilization of healthcare resources as manifested by indiscriminate use of preoperative diagnostic testing, operating room cancellations and delays for medical reasons, and prolonged length of hospital stays. In 2005, surgical expenditures comprised 29% of the overall $1.9733 trillion healthcare spending and 4.6% of the gross domestic product.[1] In light of our increasing healthcare spending, payers in our healthcare system have implemented cost-containment measures. These measures directly affect current coding, billing, and reimbursement practices of our healthcare system.

BACKGROUND

In 1992, Medicare transitioned our physician reimbursement system from the traditional "customary, prevailing, and reasonable charges" to the current fee-for-service based on Hsiao's resource-based relative value (RBRV) system.[2,3] The transition allowed Medicare, our nation's largest public payer, to decouple Medicare payment rates from physician charges and align them with the resources needed to perform levels of service as designated by the American Medical Association's (AMA) five-digit Current Procedural Terminology (CPT) codes. Upon implementation of the RBRV system, Medicare was able to decelerate growth of spending on physician services: from 1985 to 1991, spending on physician services grew at an annual rate of 10.8%; from 1992 to 2000, it grew at an annual rate of 4.7.[2] Based on Medicare's

Perioperative Medicine: Medical Consultation and Co-Management, First Edition.
Edited by Amir K. Jaffer and Paul J. Grant.
© 2012 Wiley-Blackwell. Published 2012 by John Wiley & Sons, Inc.

moderate success in containing cost, commercial payers adopted Medicare's fee schedule in 1993.

Under the current RBRV system, 52% of the total RVU (relative value unit) value reflects the degree of physician work required to perform various levels of service designated by CPT codes. The reimbursement relationship between RVUs and CPT codes is reviewed every 5 years by the AMA/Specialty Society RVS Update Committee (RUC).[4] The depth of a physician's evaluation during a patient encounter is reflected by the extent of documentation in the patient's chart. In turn, the extent of documentation defines the evaluation and management (E/M) code submitted to payers for financial reimbursement. In light of the influence documentation has on reimbursement, requirements have been standardized by the American Medical Society. Physicians need to be familiar with documentation requirements to ensure that their documentation accurately reflects the degree of physician work and use of healthcare resources elicited by individual patient encounters. Appropriate and thorough documentation of patient encounters facilitates timely reimbursement from Medicare and commercial insurance payers.

In 1966, the AMA developed the CPT system of terminology as a means of reporting medical, surgical, and diagnostic services to public and private health insurance programs in a uniform language. By standardizing communication in the medical record and among agencies handling insurance claims, the CPT system of terminology allowed medical and surgical services to be catalogued and tracked for statistical and actuarial purposes. The implementation of the CPT system was so well received that, from 1983 through 1987, the Centers for Medicare and Medicaid Services (CMS) gradually expanded its use of CPT terminology. CMS currently mandates the use of CPT via its Healthcare Common Procedure Coding System (HCPCS) for reporting services for Medicare Part B, for state Medicaid agencies reporting in the Medicaid Management Information System, and for reporting outpatient hospital surgical procedures. Furthermore, the Health Insurance Portability and Accountability Act (HIPAA) of 1996 requires the use of both CPT and HCPCS in reporting physician services, physical and occupational therapy services, radiological procedures, clinical laboratory tests, medical diagnostic procedures, hearing and vision services, and transportation services such as ambulance transport. With the support of the federal government, AMA CPT has become the most widely used and preferred coding system of healthcare services in the United States by both public and private payers.

Currently, the CPT codebook is divided into six sections of healthcare services: E/M, anesthesiology, surgery, radiology, pathology and laboratory, and medicine. E/M services are a reflection of the "content" of the services provided. It is the documentation of the service content that is crucial to both the selection of the appropriate E/M service level and the financial reimbursement for patient service. Documentation in the medical records serves three main purposes: it serves as a means of communication among healthcare providers, it provides tangible evidence of patient care, and it is a means of justifying billing claims. E/M service documentation has three requisite components: the history, the physical exam, and the medical decision-making portion. The breadth and documentation complexity of each of these three individual components influences the appropriateness of selected E/M level of services.

DOCUMENTATION

Reimbursement for preoperative consultative services is equally dependent on the degree of documentation and level of coding submitted to healthcare payers. Preparing a patient for surgery generates three important documents: the surgical history and physical, the medical preoperative consultation report, and the preanesthesia evaluation. Preoperative consultation has distinct "rules of engagement." First, a medical preoperative consult must be initiated by a formal referral; it may come in the form of a written or verbal solicitation from the surgeon, requesting a preoperative evaluation for a patient. Next, the physician performing the consultation is then required to both acknowledge the source and context of the consultation request and to communicate his or her professional evaluation and recommendations to the requesting party. This reciprocal communication to the surgeon may take the form of either a letter of consultation or a copy of the preoperative encounter's comprehensive progress note.[5]

CMS and AMA have jointly established two equally acceptable sets of documentation guidelines: the 1995 guidelines and the 1997 guidelines. The main distinguishing factor between the two guidelines is the physical exam documentation. Regardless of the documentation guidelines selected, the three key elements of E/M service need to be taken into consideration when selecting an E/M level.[6,7] The first key element is history; there are four types of history and four sub-elements to the history (Table 8.1). The extent of documentation for each sub-element defines the type of history obtained from the patient. All patient encounters must begin with a chief complaint describing the reason for the patient encounter in the patient's own words.

The history of present illness (HPI) is a chronological description of the development of the chief complaint. It utilizes eight descriptive elements: location, quality, severity, duration, timing, context, modifying factors, and associated signs and symptoms. There are only two kinds of HPI: brief or extended. The brief HPI requires the documentation of ≤ 3 out of 8 elements of the HPI while the extended HPI requires either ≥ 4 elements of the HPI or commentary on the status of ≥ 3 chronic/active conditions.

The review of systems (ROS) is an inventory of standardized body systems used to identify and clarify signs and/or symptoms the patient may be experiencing or has experienced prior to the evaluation. There are 14 recognized body systems

TABLE 8.1. **History Component**

Type of history	Chief complaint	History of present illness	Review of systems	Past family and/ or social history
Problem focused	Required	Brief	N/A	N/A
Expanded problem focused	Required	Brief	Problem pertinent	N/A
Detailed	Required	Extended	Extended	Pertinent
Comprehensive	Required	Extended	Complete	Complete

N/A, not applicable.

for the ROS. As noted in Table 8.1, there are three types of ROS: problem pertinent, extended, or complete. A problem pertinent ROS expands on the problem presented in the chief complaint, while the extended ROS addresses the body system referenced in the chief complaint along with two to nine additional relevant body systems. The complete ROS queries the body system addressed in the chief complaint and 10–13 of the remaining body systems.

The final sub-element of the history is the past, family, and/or social history (PFSH). The past history encompasses prior illnesses, operations, injuries, and treatments; the family history addresses family-related medical events, diseases, and hereditary conditions. Meanwhile, the social history incorporates an age-appropriate review of past and current activities. The depth at which PFSH is explored and documented defines if it is a pertinent PFSH or a complete PFSH. All forms of new patient encounters, initial outpatient or inpatient visits, and consults require documentation of PFSH.

The second key element of an E/M level of service is the physical examination. The extent of physical exam documentation influences the level of E/M service performed. There are four levels of physical examination: problem focused (PF), expanded problem focused (EPF), detailed (Det), and comprehensive (Comp). The physical exam guidelines are tools of documentation that determine the level of examination performed. Although there are two exam guidelines (1995 and 1997 guidelines), both are equally recognized by CMS and AMA. The 1995 guidelines allow for greater variation of documentation but the phrase "abnormal" must be expounded upon within the *affected* body area or organ system. However, within an *unaffected* body area or organ system, the phrase "negative" or "normal" is acceptable. All general multisystem exams must detail findings of at least 8 of 12 organ systems. On the other hand, the 1997 exam guidelines center around 11 standardized examination templates that are either single-organ system examinations or the comprehensive general multisystem exam. The overriding theme of these 1997 templates is the standardized documentation requirements stipulated for the selected exam template.

 The final key element of an E/M level of service is the medical decision making (MDM). There are four levels of MDM defined by the number of diagnoses or management options, the amount and complexity of data reviewed, and the risk of complications and morbidity/mortality involved with the presenting problem, diagnostic procedures, and management options (Table 8.2). There are two key

TABLE 8.2. Medical Decision-Making Component

Number of diagnoses/ management options	Amount/complexity of data reviewed	Risk of complications and/or morbidity and mortality	Type of MDM
Minimal	Minimal or none	Minimal	Straightforward (SF)
Limited	Limited	Low	Low complexity (LCx)
Multiple	Moderate	Moderate	Moderate complexity (MCx)
Extensive	Extensive	High	High complexity (HCx)

points to keep in mind with MDM. To qualify for any given MDM level, two of three elements in the MDM table must be met or exceeded. Overall risk is determined by the highest level of risk in the presenting problem, the diagnostic procedure, or the management options.

CODING, BILLING, REIMBURSEMENT

Once an E/M level of service is established, the CPT code is chosen. Selection of a CPT code is dependent on location of service (inpatient or outpatient), type of visit (new/initial or established/subsequent visit), and type of service (visit or consultation) (Table 8.3). Sometimes more than 50% of a patient encounter is dominated by

TABLE 8.3.   E/M Services

Req. # of components	E/M level	History	Exam	MDM	Time (min)
E/M: outpatient					
3/3 outpatient new visit	99201	PF	PF	SF	10
	99202	EPF	EPF	SF	20
	99203	Det	Det	LCx	30
	99204	Comp	Comp	MCx	45
	99205	Comp	Comp	HCx	60
2/3 outpatient subsequent visit	99211	Minimal	Minimal	Minimal	5
	99212	PF	PF	SF	10
	99213	EPF	EPF	LCx	15
	99214	Det	Det	MCx	25
	99215	Comp	Comp	HCx	40
3/3 outpatient consult	99241	PF	PF	SF	15
	99242	EPF	EPF	SF	30
	99243	Det	Det	LCx	40
	99244	Comp	Comp	MCx	60
	99245	Comp	Comp	HCx	80
E/M: inpatient					
3/3 initial hospital care	99221	Det/Comp	Det/Comp	SF/LCx	30
	99222	Comp	Comp	MCx	50
	99223	Comp	Comp	HCx	70
2/3 subsequent hospital visit	99231	PF	PF	SF/LCx	15
	99232	EPF	EPF	MCx	25
	99233	Det	Det	HCx	35
3/3 consult (non-Medicare)	99251	PF	PF	SF	20
	99252	EPF	EPF	SF	40
	99253	Det	Det	LCx	55
	99254	Comp	Comp	MCx	80
	99255	Comp	Comp	HCx	110

SF, straightforward; LCx, low complexity; MCx, moderate complexity; HCx, high complexity.

face-to-face (floor time if in an intensive care unit) counseling or coordination of care. Under these circumstances, documentation of time and description of the encounter are the deciding factors for select E/M services. Be mindful that encounter descriptions should communicate what transpired during a counseling session and narrate the activities central to care coordination.

As of January 1, 2010, the patient's health insurance coverage also influences the CPT code ultimately submitted for preoperative reimbursement. Medicare no longer recognizes AMA CPT consultation codes in any venue but Telehealth G-codes.[8] However, it does continue to recognize new/initial visit codes. This policy change affects preoperative consultations conducted on Medicare patients, including Medicare secondary payers (MSPs). When a patient has both primary commercial health insurance and MSP, the reimbursement issue can be challenging. On the one hand, consultative physicians may submit the appropriate E/M consultative code to the primary commercial payer, then resubmit the same consultative E/M code along with the amount paid by the commercial payer to Medicare with the understanding that Medicare will then determine whether further payment is due for the visit. The second option, involves the submission of two E/M codes for the same visit. The first E/M consultation code is submitted to the commercial primary payer, while the second E/M code submitted to Medicare is appropriate to the setting of care and level of patient complexity for Medicare billing; the second E/M code submitted must be accompanied by a report stating the amount paid by the commercial insurance. Once Medicare has the appropriate E/M code supported by documentation and the amount paid by the commercial payers, then it will rule on whether further payment is due.[5]

If AMA CPT consultation codes are submitted after January 1, 2010, then the billing claim will not be denied but will be returned stating that Medicare uses another E/M code for reporting and payment of the service rendered. This allows physicians and billing specialists to rectify the submission error. Therefore, since the claims are not denied, providers cannot utilize advance beneficiary notices (ABNs) in lieu of submitting the correct CPT codes to Medicare.[9] However, if the primary payer is Medicare, then the only recognized billing codes for preoperative evaluations will be either initial hospital visit (99221–99223), new office visit (99201–99205), or established outpatient visit (99211–99215). The level of service and documentation required for each of these encounters has not changed.

Although CMS maintains that elimination of consultation codes is a budget neutral move. The potential loss of revenue from consultation code elimination can be theoretically be offset by the increased RVUs assigned to all new/established outpatient visits, a higher Medicare allowable (MCA) payment for each visit, and increased reimbursement for global surgical charges. CMS has projected the percent redistribution of consultation codes to new/established visits but terms this redistribution as anticipated destination codes; it is not to be construed as a CMS crosswalk between consult codes and inpatient/outpatient encounters. The documentation requirements of previously recognized consultation codes do not equitably crosswalk to the projected destination codes' documentation requirements. For example, 70% of level 3 inpatient consult codes (99253) are anticipated to map to level 2 new

TABLE 8.4. Centers for Medicare and Medicaid Services (CMS) 2010 Consultation Destination Codes

2009 CMS reimbursement (consultation codes)	2009 WRVUs (consultation codes)	Traditional inpatient consultation codes	2010 CMS inpatient destination codes[a]	2009 WRVUs (destination codes)	2009 CMS reimbursement (destination codes)	2010 WRVUs (destination codes)	2010 Medicare allowable (MCA) reimbursement (destination codes)
	1	99251	99221 70%	1.88	~$99.49	1.92	$106.90
	1.5	99252	99221 35%				
			99222 35%	2.56	~$135.90	2.61	$142.95
~$128.14	2.27	99253	99222 70%				
~$184.89	3.29	99254	99222 35%	3.78	~$199.75	3.86	$208.43
			99223 35%				
~$225.56	4	99255	99223 70%				

[a] Percentage indicates the expected 2010 distribution of traditional inpatient consultation codes to inpatient codes. WRVUs, work-related value units.

inpatient visit (99222). However, documentation for E/M level 99253 requires a *detailed* history, *detailed* physical exam, and *low* complexity MDM, while level 99222 documentation requires a *comprehensive* history, *comprehensive* physical exam, and *moderately* complex MDM. Physicians providing preoperative evaluations need to be cognizant of the added documentation requirements of patient encounters recognized by CMS in lieu of consultation codes. If the documentation of an inpatient preoperative visit does not support the selection of the projected 2010 CMS destination code, then CMS recognizes that the most appropriate E/M code may indeed be a subsequent visit and not a new inpatient. CMS payment processors will not penalize physicians for selecting a subsequent visit E/M for a new preoperative visit as long as the documentation supports the selected E/M level visit code submitted for reimbursement (Table 8.4).

FUTURE

In the horizon, there are two coding and billing issues yet to be addressed. First, historical precedent suggests it is simply a matter of time before commercial payers follow CMS' policy on consultation codes. Therefore, providers are advised to keep abreast of private payer policies with regard to consultation codes. It is unclear when this will happen, but it is anticipated to occur in the near future. The second issue is the inflammatory topic of bundled payments for hospitals and physicians. As of 2007, the Medicare Payment Advisory Commission (Medpac) has advocated bundle payments to curb inefficient utilization of healthcare resources.[10] The rationale behind implementation of bundled payments is to promote shared accountability and collaboration between hospitals and physicians. It is hoped that bundled payments will be a financial incentive for hospitals and physicians to improve their collective performance. Under bundled payments, Medicare would pay a fixed predetermined amount to both hospital and its physicians on staff to provide care covered by Medicare during a patient's admission; this episode of care may be defined as the hospital stay and 30 days after discharge.[11] Currently, there are pilot studies for selected conditions being conducted across the nation to provide seed data on whether bundling payments will have a sufficiently positive impact on our healthcare system to stimulate more efficient use of resources. In the wake of the new healthcare reform bill, answers to the above two issues will be forthcoming. Regardless of the answers, appropriate documentation of services and selection of CPT codes will maximize physician reimbursement in the upcoming healthcare reform climate.

REFERENCES

1. Munoz E, Munoz W, 3rd, Wise L. National and surgical health care expenditures, 2005–2025. *Ann Surg*. 2010;251(2):195–200.
2. Hariri S, et al. Medicare physician reimbursement: past, present, and future. *J Bone Joint Surg Am*. 2007;89(11):2536–2546.
3. Hsiao WC, et al. The resource-based relative value scale. Toward the development of an alternative physician payment system. *JAMA*. 1987;258(6):799–802.

4. Association, A.M. AMA/Specialty Society RVS Update Process available at http://www.ama-assn. org/ama1/pub/upload/mm/380/rvs_booklet_07.pdf, A.M. Association, Editor. 2009, Chicago.

5. CMS. *Revisions to Consultation Services Payment Policy.* Web ed. MLN Matters. Vol. MM6740. 2009, Centers for Medicare and Medicaid Services.

6. CMS. *1995 Documentation Guidelines for Evaluation and Management Services.* Web ed. MLN Products. 1995, Centers for Medicare and Medicaid Services. 1–15.

7. CMS. *1997 Documentation Guidelines for Evaluation and Management Services.* Web ed. MLN Products. 1997, Centers for Medicare and Medicaid Services. 1–51.

8. CMS. *Revisions to Consultation Services Payment Policy*, D.o.H.H.S. (DHHS), Editor. 2009, Centers for Medicare & Medicaid Services (CMS).

9. CMS. *Questions and Answers on Reporting Physician Consultation Services.* Web ed. MLN Matters. Vol. SE1010. 2010, Centers for Medicare & Medicaid Services. 12.

10. Mutti A, Lisk C. *Moving toward bundled payments around hospitalizations.* 2007. pp. 1–21. Available at http://www.medpac.gov/transcripts/1107_bundling_hosp_AM_pres.pdf.

11. Hackbarth G, Reischauer R, Mutti A. Collective accountability for medical care—toward bundled Medicare payments. *N Engl J Med.* 2008;359(1):3–5.

PART II

ASSESSING AND MANAGING RISK BY ORGAN SYSTEM OR SPECIAL POPULATION

CHAPTER 9

ASSESSING AND MANAGING CARDIOVASCULAR RISK

Vineet Chopra and James B. Froehlich

INTRODUCTION AND EPIDEMIOLOGY

Although there has been considerable advancement in operative interventions and anesthetic techniques, coronary artery disease (CAD) continues to remain an important cause of complications during noncardiac surgery. In the 234 million people that undergo major noncardiac surgery each year, perioperative cardiac events cause a significant number of perioperative deaths and increase both hospital stay and long-term mortality.[1,2] The risk of a perioperative cardiac event is a dynamic interplay between the patient's condition prior to surgery, the presence of comorbidities that affect cardiac status, and the stress and duration of the planned surgical procedure.[3] This chapter will discuss the principles and practices of estimation and reduction of perioperative cardiac risk.

From a physiologic perspective, perioperative cardiac events occur due to (1) mismatch in the oxygen demand : supply ratio (due to flow-limiting lesions in one or more coronary arteries), (2), rupture of coronary plaque (related to vascular inflammation precipitated by surgical stress), or (3) a combination of these factors.[4] Given the near linear correlation between CAD and its associated comorbidities with age, elderly patients are at increased risk of developing perioperative cardiac events. Furthermore, the elderly are almost four times more likely to require surgical intervention than the rest of the population.[5] The 2005 U.S. National Hospital Discharge Survey reported that the largest increase in surgical procedures over the past decade occurred in middle-aged and elderly cohorts (Figure 9.1).[6] Thus, we are faced with a veritable epidemic of older adults often with coronary disease that are increasingly likely to undergo surgical procedures.

Addressing this concern, there exist several evidence-based guidelines that systematically identify strategies to ameliorate perioperative cardiac events.[27,28,40,41] Unfortunately, the evidence shows that our observance of established guidelines is poor, even though adherence to these guidelines improves outcomes.[7] For instance,

---

Perioperative Medicine: Medical Consultation and Co-Management, First Edition.
Edited by Amir K. Jaffer and Paul J. Grant.

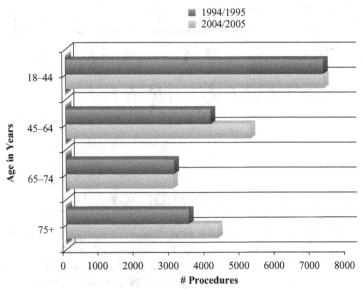

Figure 9.1.   Change in number of discharges for surgical procedures by age group: 1994/1995 versus 2004/2005. Adapted from DeFrances et al.[6] See color insert.

one study found that only 41% of patients with peripheral artery disease (PAD) received guideline-recommended medical therapy such as statins and beta-blockers.[8] Implementation of the guidelines improves outcomes and conserves precious resources. Thus, an opportunity exists to improve the quality of perioperative cardiac care.

IMPORTANT ELEMENTS OF THE CLINICAL HISTORY

The interval prior to surgery provides pause to review important elements that may impact operative outcome. The clinical history is the foundation of this evaluation and should focus on the following:

(A) detection of significant ischemic heart disease;
(B) evaluation of the stability of known CAD;
(C) assessment of comorbidities known to influence perioperative outcomes;
(D) review of prior surgical interventions and complications (if any);
(E) appraisal of functional status.

Detection of Significant Ischemic Heart Disease

An important goal of the perioperative evaluation is to detect the presence of significant, undiagnosed heart disease. It is thus imperative for the consultant to obtain an accurate and complete review of systems with regard to the cardiovascular system. For instance, has there been unexplained or persistent chest pain or pressure, shortness of breath, or lower extremity edema? Has the patient suffered prior cerebrovascular events such as stroke or transient ischemic attacks? Are there telltale signs of peripheral vascular disease such as claudication, rest pain, erectile dysfunction, or loss of hair in the lower extremities?

Evaluation of the Extent and Stability of CAD

In patients with known ischemic heart disease, it is important to determine if a patient has undergone recent cardiac testing or revascularization. Several retrospective studies have shown that prior revascularization (either coronary artery bypass grafting or percutaneous coronary intervention within the past 5 years) in the absence of cardiac symptoms, offers protection with respect to surgical risk and may obviate the need for preoperative testing.[9,10]

Assessment of Comorbidities Known to Influence Perioperative Outcomes

The perioperative history must also lend itself to the detection and quantification of other important comorbidities that affect perioperative cardiac risk. For instance, does the patient suffer from insulin-requiring diabetes? Is there a history of renal insufficiency? It is important to state that traditional cardiovascular risk factors, such as tobacco use, hypertension, or hyperlipidemia (though pertinent in the development of CAD), have not been found to influence perioperative cardiac events.

Review of Prior Surgical Interventions and Complications

Prior perioperative events can help the consultant predict and clarify risk in problematic territories. For instance, did the patient experience postoperative chest pain, pulmonary edema, or a significant cardiac arrhythmia? Were there intra- or postoperative electrocardiographic (EKG) changes suggesting underlying CAD? Conversely, the absence of cardiac events in the context of recent surgery provides some reassurance that the patient has an adequate cardiopulmonary reserve to withstand surgical intervention.

Assessment of Functional Status

An accurate appraisal of functional capacity is an important element of the perioperative history. Functional status is measured in metabolic equivalents (METs); those able to achieve a higher functional capacity experience fewer perioperative complications.[11] The American College of Cardiology (ACC)/American Heart Association's (AHA) Perioperative Guidelines state that a functional status of 4 METs (the ability to climb two flights of stairs or run at a slow pace), is predictive of fair functional capacity and precludes further cardiac testing. Assessment of capacity can become difficult in the elderly, obese, or arthritic patient, and thus, reliable risk indices must be used to augment the interpretation of functional capacity if the baseline is unclear.

PHYSICAL EXAMINATION

Just as history is dedicated to discovering factors that may adversely affect surgery, the physical exam should be directed to confirm and complement historical concerns. Does inspection of the precordium reveal a displaced point of maximal cardiac impulse? Is there evidence of jugular venous distention suggestive of elevated filling pressures? On palpation, is there diastolic shock or parasternal heave indicating pulmonary hypertension or right ventricular strain? Careful auscultation of the chest should be performed to identify important cardiac findings such as extra heart sounds or rales suggesting pulmonary edema and/or decompensated heart failure? Are there clinically detectable cardiac murmurs (especially flow-limiting murmurs such as aortic stenosis) that may require echocardiographic assessment?

The physical exam should also assess vascular health in other territories. For example, the abdominal exam should focus on the detection of abdominal or reno-vascular bruits much as the neck exam should search for carotid bruits. Evaluation of the lower extremities for edema, pulses, and stigmata of vascular disease is equally necessary.

PERIOPERATIVE TESTING

An understanding of perioperative physiology may help elucidate the role of perioperative testing for cardiovascular disease. While it was initially presumed that most perioperative events occurred due to flow-limiting CAD, autopsy results of patients suffering fatal perioperative cardiac events showed that almost 40–50% did not have obstructive coronary disease.[12] These patients suffered coronary thrombosis possibly due to a heightened vascular and systemic inflammatory state resulting in invasion of coronary plaque by circulating monocytes/macrophages.[13,14] Such areas of "vulnerable plaque" are nearly impossible to detect via current testing methods as they appear remarkably innocent on coronary angiography and remain innocuous on stress testing. Thus, cardiac testing in the perioperative setting does not permit the identification of vulnerable plaque. Stress tests and coronary angiography detect cardiac ischemia only in areas where there is significant coronary stenosis, a pathology that does not account for all perioperative cardiac events.

A review of the studies evaluating the performance of cardiac testing in the perioperative period reveals a striking congruence of results. Irrespective of whether the test employed was perfusion imaging, treadmill EKG, or dobutamine echocardiography, perioperative stress tests are plagued by average sensitivity and poor specificity. Therefore, a negative stress test carries a high negative predictive value, but a positive stress test correlates poorly with perioperative cardiac events. Recent studies pooled the prognostic value of six diagnostic tests and found a combined sensitivity of 83% (95% confidence interval [CI] 77–92%) and a specificity of 47%

(95% CI 41–57%) for myocardial perfusion imaging; the positive and negative predictive values were 11% and 97%, respectively.[15,16] Similarly, stress echocardiography has a high negative predictive value (between 90% and 100%) but poor positive predictive value (between 25% and 45%) implying that the postsurgical probability of a cardiac event is low despite wall motion abnormalities.[17]

Who should receive cardiovascular testing in the preoperative setting? To answer this, we must recognize that perioperative testing provides refinement of a clinically determined likelihood of cardiac events. Thus, patients at low risk do not benefit from testing, as their management is not affected by test results. Similarly, patients at high risk suffer a higher incidence of cardiac events and stand to benefit from the implementation of risk-reduction strategies, not from further testing. One might conclude it is justified to limit testing to those patients at intermediate cardiac risk. This strategy has been repeatedly tested in the literature with little success. Boersma et al. showed that irrespective of whether intermediate-risk patients underwent preoperative stress testing prior to vascular surgery, immediate or long-term cardiac outcomes were not changed. Instead, clinical risk scoring predicted perioperative complications with accuracy.[18] In DECREASE, Poldermans et al. randomized patients at risk of adverse outcome to receive cardiac stress testing versus revascularization prior to noncardiac surgery. Importantly, all patients received beta-blockers (bisoprolol) titrated to heart rate and blood pressure in the perioperative setting. At 30 days, there was no observed difference in death or myocardial infarction (MI) between groups (1.8% vs. 2.3%, odds ratio [OR] 0.78l, 95% CI 0.28–2.1; $P = 0.62$).[19] Thus, even via a strategy targeting intermediate-risk patients, preoperative testing does not appear beneficial. Given the available literature, routine perioperative testing or treatment is no longer recommended and should be restricted to ACC/AHA Class I indications (Table 9.1).

PREDICTING PERIOPERATIVE CARDIOVASCULAR RISK

Given the low positive predictive value of cardiovascular stress testing, calculating perioperative cardiovascular risk has largely fallen to clinical risk prediction methodologies. The American Society of Anesthesiologists (ASA) was the first to develop a classification system to assess clinical risk in 1963 (Table 9.2).[20] The most important shortcoming of this system was that almost every patient scored a "2" or a "3," offering little precision with respect to cardiac risk. The Goldman risk score was derived empirically by identifying which demographic and clinical variables were associated with cardiac events using multivariable analysis across 1001 patients (Table 9.3). Risk factors most associated with cardiac adverse events included active heart failure, recent MI, malignant arrhythmias, aortic stenosis, and/or underlying comorbid disease. The investigators devised a scoring method weighing each of these factors to predict the likelihood of cardiac complications (Table 9.4).[21]

In subsequent years, the Goldman risk score was refined by Detsky et al. and L'Italien and colleagues.[22,23] L'Italien identified five variables in patients undergoing vascular surgery that were most strongly associated with cardiac events (increasing age, presence of diabetes requiring treatment, a history of angina, a history of

TABLE 9.1. Cardiac Conditions Warranting Evaluation and Treatment before Noncardiac Surgery

Condition	Clinical examples
Unstable coronary syndrome(s)	Unstable angina (CCS class III or IV)
	Acute myocardial ischemia or infarction
	Recent myocardial infarction (>7 days but ≤1 month)
Decompensated heart failure	NYHA functional class IV symptoms
	New-onset heart failure or newly detected heart failure
	Decompensated heart failure (pulmonary edema, PND, rales, etc.)
Significant atrial arrhythmias	Symptomatic bradycardia
	High-grade atrioventricular block
	Mobitz type II block
	Third-degree atrioventricular block
	Supraventricular arrhythmias with rapid ventricular rate at rest (≥100 beats/min)
	Atrial fibrillation with rapid ventricular rate at rest (≥100 beats/min)
Ventricular arrhythmias	Newly recognized or detected ventricular tachycardia
	Ventricular fibrillation
Severe valvular disease	Severe aortic stenosis (AVA ≤ 1.0 cm^2 or mean gradient ≥40 mm Hg)
	Symptomatic mitral stenosis (e.g., with heart failure or presyncope)

AVA, aortic valve area; CCS, Canadian Cardiovascular Society; NYHA, New York Heart Association; PND, paroxysmal nocturnal dyspnea.
From Fleisher et al.[27]

TABLE 9.2. American Society of Anesthesiology Physical Status Classification System

Risk class	Clinical profile	Detailed description and examples
I	Normal	No organic or physiologic disturbance, healthy with good exercise tolerance. Excludes the very young and very old.
II	Mild systemic disease	Well-controlled disease of one body system, no functional limitations. Examples include hypertension, diabetes mellitus, COPD, and mild obesity.
III	Severe systemic disease *No Threat to Life*	Disease involving more than one system with some functional limitations. Examples include congestive heart failure, prior MI, stable angina, and chronic renal failure.
IV	Severe systemic disease *Threat to Life*	Disease that is severe, poorly controlled, end-stage, and a constant threat to life. Examples include end-stage COPD, unstable angina, severe aortic stenosis, and recent stroke.
V	Moribund patient, ≤24 h of life expectancy	Disease that is likely to terminate life within 24 h (without surgical intervention), at imminent risk of death. Examples include severe sepsis, multiorgan failure, and DIC.
VI	Brain death	A brain-dead patient whose organs may be removed for harvesting/donation purposes.

Adapted from the American Society of Anesthesiology.[20]
COPD, chronic obstructive pulmonary disease; MI, myocardial infarction; DIC, disseminated intravascular coagulation.

TABLE 9.3. Goldman Risk Scoring System

Clinical parameters		Risk points
Demographic	Age > 70	5
	MI within 6 months	10
Cardiac examination	Signs of CHF (S3, JVD)	11
	Aortic stenosis	3
EKG variables	Arrythmia [other than sinus, PACs]	7
	5 or more PVCs per minute	7
Clinical variables	General medical conditions (any one or a number of the following)[a]	3
Surgical variables	Emergent surgery	4
	Peritoneal, thoracic, or aortic surgery	4

[a] General medical conditions include $pO_2 < 60$; $pCO_2 > 50$; K < 3; $HCO_3 < 20$; BUN > 50; Creat > 3; elevated SGOT; chronic liver disease; bedridden.
Adapted from Goldman et al.[21]
CHF, congestive heart failure; JVD, jugular venous distention; PACs, premature atrial contractions; PVCs, premature ventricular contractions; BUN, blood urea nitrogen; SGOT, serum glutamic oxaloacetic transaminase.

TABLE 9.4. Postoperative Outcomes Based on Goldman's Risk Score

Point range	Risk group	Complications (%)	Deaths (%)
0–5	I	4 (0.7%)	1 (0.2%)
6–12	II	15 (5%)	5 (2%)
13–25	III	15 (12%)	3 (2%)
>25	IV	4 (22%)	10 (56%)

Adapted from Goldman et al.[21]

myocardial infraction or Q-waves on EKG, and/or a history of heart failure). Lee and colleagues further improved on these data and created the Revised Cardiac Risk Index (RCRI), a risk model derived from multivariate analysis of retrospectively gathered clinical information (from 2893 patients in a derivation cohort undergoing elective major noncardiac surgery). The model was prospectively validated in 1422 patients from the same institution. Lee's RCRI identified six clinical parameters (Table 9.5) that are independently associated with adverse perioperative outcome (Figure 9.2).[24]

It is important to summarize two key aspects of these methodologies. First, despite all of our operative developments and advancements, there is a striking similarity across 50 years of perioperative trial data in the variables most associated with cardiac events. Second, clinical risk-prediction techniques provide far greater accuracy and insight in determining cardiac risk and event rates than do tests, as they identify patients likely to develop unstable coronary disease in the perioperative setting rather than find "stable" CAD. Lee's RCRI appears to be the best tool available today for forecasting perioperative cardiac events and continues to excel in discriminating high- from low-risk patients since its publication in 1999.[25]

TABLE 9.5. Lee's Revised Cardiac Risk Index

Clinical variable	Point
History of ischemic heart disease	1
Intraperitoneal, intrathoracic, or supra-inguinal vascular surgery	1
History of congestive heart failure	1
Prior transient ischemic attack or stroke	1
Preoperative treatment with insulin	1
Serum creatinine >2.0	1

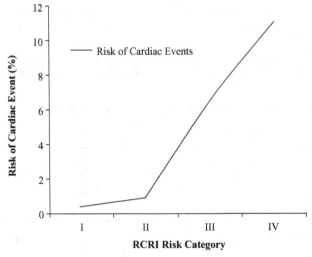

Figure 9.2. Risk of cardiac events by Revised Cardiac Risk Index class. Class I = zero points; Class II = 1 point; Class III = 2 points; Class IV = 3 or more points. Adapted from Lee et al.[24] See color insert.

THE ACC/AHA PERIOPERATIVE GUIDELINES

The ACC/AHA guidelines on perioperative cardiovascular evaluation for noncardiac surgery were first published with the goal of organizing a growing body of literature within perioperative medicine.[26] Importantly, it provided an algorithmic approach integrating clinical assessment and testing to mitigate cardiac events. Since the publication of the original guideline, much has been learned about perioperative cardiac events and their incongruous relationship to obstructive CAD. Notably, some studies confirmed the value of clinical risk prediction, while others failed to show improvement in cardiac outcomes via stress testing or revascularization.[15-17] These data prompted revisions to the original guidelines.[27]

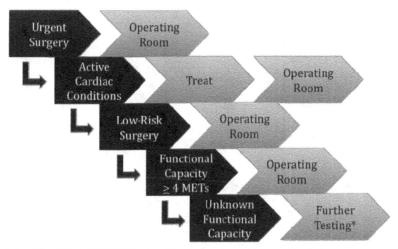

Figure 9.3.   Simplified ACC/AHA algorithm for perioperative cardiac risk assessment and care. *Based on risk factors and risk of surgery. Adapted from Fleisher et al.[28] See color insert.

In its latest iteration, the 2009 ACC/AHA Perioperative Guidelines incorporates recent data regarding perioperative beta-blockade and outlines strategies for reducing perioperative cardiac events by identifying and targeting those that stand to benefit most from interventions. The paradigm has also shifted to identifying those groups that do not require further cardiac testing or treatment.[28] The ACC/AHA Guidelines feature an algorithm that represents a stepwise approach to perioperative assessment (Figure 9.3). Patients who face urgent or emergent surgery, those undergoing low-risk surgeries, and those with reasonable functional capacity without symptoms of cardiac disease require no further testing. On the other hand, patients with active Class I ACC/AHA conditions should have surgery deferred and undergo urgent cardiovascular evaluation (Table 9.1). Patients with poor or unknown functional status or those that face an intermediate-risk surgery should be stratified via the use of clinical risk-prediction tools, such as RCRI. Patients with low RCRI scores need not undergo further testing. Conversely, patients with an RCRI ≥3 or with an unclear functional status facing high-risk surgery should undergo cardiac testing and/or medical treatment owing to their higher risk of perioperative cardiac events.

INTERVENTIONS TO LOWER PERIOPERATIVE CARDIAC RISK

An exciting area of development over the past decade has been the increasing investigation of therapies directed to lowering perioperative risk.

Perioperative Revascularization

The Coronary Artery Surgical Study (CASS) is the largest retrospective study examining the effect of preoperative revascularization on subsequent cardiac events.[29] Among 1961 patients undergoing noncardiac surgery, CASS found fewer postoperative deaths (1.7% vs. 3.3%; $P = 0.03$) and MIs (0.8% vs. 2.7%; $P = 0.02$) in those undergoing revascularization compared with medical therapy. However, in the only prospective randomized controlled study to evaluate the effect of prophylactic revascularization prior to noncardiac surgery (Coronary Artery Prophylaxis Study [CARP]), McFalls et al. showed that there was no benefit from coronary bypass grafting with respect to either immediate or long-term outcomes among 510 high-risk patients undergoing vascular surgery compared with medical therapy alone.[30] Subsequent studies of CASS showed that the observed benefit may have been due to the enrichment of the CASS cohort by patients with poor left ventricular ejection fraction, peripheral arterial disease, and three-vessel CAD, all of whom stood to benefit from revascularization.[31] Furthermore, the study analysis was post hoc and did not consider the cumulative risk of cardiac and subsequent noncardiac surgery. Even in patients deemed at high risk for cardiac events, a recent study affirmed no apparent benefit from preoperative revascularization.[32]

The failure of revascularization to improve cardiac outcomes has also been reported in several large studies outside of the operative context. In the Clinical Outcomes Utilizing Revascularization and Aggressive Drug Evaluation (COURAGE) study, there was no difference with respect to death or MI between those undergoing percutaneous coronary intervention and optimal medical therapy versus medical therapy alone.[33] Importantly, COURAGE included many patients with ischemia documented on noninvasive testing. The Bypass Angioplasty Revascularization Investigation in Diabetes-2 (BARI 2-D) study also showed no advantage of revascularization over intensive medical therapy among diabetics with stable CAD.[34] What about patients with demonstrable ischemia? The DECREASE-V study randomized patients with active ischemia (detected via stress echocardiography) slated to undergo vascular surgery to revascularization versus medical treatment.[35] All patients received bisoprolol titrated to achieve a resting heart rate of 60–65 beats/min. The study found no difference in 30-day outcomes in either arm and reported a nonstatistically significant trend toward decreased mortality or MI at 30 days in the medically managed cohort. Thus, the literature has consistently shown that revascularization is without benefit, even in high-risk patients undergoing vascular surgery and cannot be justified as a preoperative risk-reducing measure.[30,32,35]

Perioperative Beta-Blockers

In their seminal study, Mangano et al. administered 50–100 mg (depending on predefined hemodynamic parameters) of oral atenolol to 200 randomized subjects with or at risk for CAD immediately before induction of anesthesia and found increased event-free survival at 6-month, 1-year, and 2-year intervals.[36] Poldermans et al. followed closely with DECREASE-I, reporting that patients undergoing vascular surgery with clinical evidence of ischemia (wall-motion abnormalities detected by

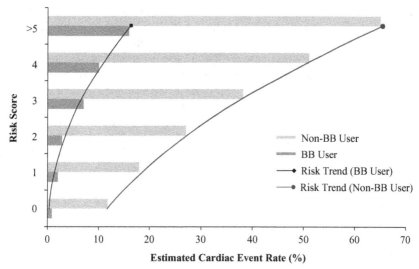

Figure 9.4.   Association between beta-blocker (BB) use and cardiac events in patients undergoing vascular surgery (risk trend). Adapted from Boersma et al.[37] See color insert.

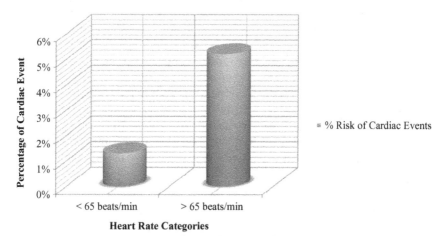

Figure 9.5.   Relationship between heart-rate reduction and perioperative events. Adapted from Poldermans et al.[19] See color insert.

dobutamine stress echocardiography) treated with carefully titrated perioperative bisoprolol 2.5 mg orally experienced fewer cardiac events than control.[37] Importantly, reduction of cardiac complications occurred irrespective of clinical risk and was more evident among those with abnormal stress tests (Figure 9.4). Subsequent analysis of observational data by Poldermans et al. confirmed that the benefit of beta-blockers was directly related to perioperative heart-rate reduction, with an event rate of 1.3% in those whose heart-rate was controlled to ≤65 beats/min versus 5.2% in those with heart rates ≥65 beats/min (Figure 9.5).[19] Lindenauer et al. analyzed the benefit of perioperative beta-blockers according to RCRI score across 782,969 Medicare beneficiaries and found that patients with low RCRI scores may experience no benefit and possibly harm associated with perioperative intraoperative bradycardia and hypotension from this treatment.[38] They also observed an association between beta-blocker use and lowered mortality in subjects at high risk of cardiac events. These findings called for a strategic approach incorporating clinical risk and heart-rate control when applying perioperative beta-blockade.

Results form the Perioperative Outcomes Ischemia Study Evaluation (POISE) study called into question the routine use of beta-blockers.[39] In POISE, 8351 patients were randomized to either 200 mg long-acting metoprolol daily or placebo. The trial protocol specified that Toprol-XL be administered as a 100 mg oral dose 2–4 h prior to surgery, followed by a second dose of 100 mg 6 h postoperatively, provided that heart rate was ≥45 beats/min and systolic blood pressure was ≥100 mm Hg. The regimen was continued at 200 mg daily. POISE showed cardiac benefit form beta-blockade; however, every cardiac event prevented occurred at the expense of increased mortality, sepsis, and ischemic stroke.

Given these cautionary data, the 2009 ACC/AHA Focused Update on Perioperative Beta-Blockers narrowed the Class I indications of perioperative beta-blockade only to those already receiving this therapy.[40] However, POISE provided several valuable lessons. First, in every case, beta-blockers should only be offered with close attention to hemodynamic parameters. Second, they should be initiated between 7 and 30 days prior to surgery with dose titration to target a resting heart rate between 60 and 70/min, maintaining systolic blood pressures >100 mm Hg.[41,42] Third, among those receiving beta-blockers, treatment must be continued throughout the perioperative period, substituting intravenous agents if oral intake is not possible. Finally, postoperative tachycardia should not reflexively call for higher doses of beta-blockers, but investigation and treatment of the underlying cause (e.g., pain, hypovolemia, infection, etc.). The optimal duration of beta-blocker therapy cannot be derived from the presently available data; however, the occurrence of delayed cardiac events and late benefits is incentive to continue these agents for months postoperatively.[35–38]

Perioperative Statins

Several observational studies have implied a protective benefit of statin therapy in patients undergoing noncardiac surgery. Lindenauer et al. reported that perioperative statin users had a lower crude mortality (2.13% vs. 3.02%, $P \leq 0.001$), after adjusting for covariates and propensity score (OR 0.62; 95% CI 0.58–0.67).[43] In another retrospective study, Ward et al. found that statin use was associated with lower all-cause mortality, cardiovascular mortality, MI, and stroke (6.9% vs. 21.1%, $P = 0.008$) in patients undergoing vascular surgery.[44]

In 2004, Durazzo et al. were the first to show that 20 mg of perioperative atorvastatin reduced cardiac events in 100 patients undergoing major vascular surgery (26% vs. 8%; $P = 0.31$). Notably, this effect was seen at immediate follow-up and persisted at 180 days.[45] In the recent double-blinded, placebo-controlled DECREASE-III study, Schouten et al. found that 80 mg fluvastatin significantly reduced death from cardiovascular causes (4.8% vs. 10.1%, heart rate [HR] 0.47; 95% CI 0.24–0.93; $P \leq 0.01$) and postoperative myocardial ischemia (10.8% vs. 19.0%, HR 0.55; 95% CI 0.34–0.88; $P \leq 0.01$) in 497 vascular surgery patients when started 37 days prior to surgery. Importantly, the study also found significant attenuation of inflammatory markers (C-reactive protein and interleukin-6), implying that statins may have exerted their beneficial effect through inflammatory pathways. In their study, fluvastatin was well tolerated without significant adverse effects.[46]

There exist no formal recommendations for perioperative statin use at this juncture. However, studies have shown that perioperative discontinuation of statins among patients maintained on this therapy may produce a "rebound" phenomenon, leading to coronary events.[47] Therefore, continuing perioperative statins among those on this therapy appears appropriate. As no intravenous formulations of statins exist, statins with a long half-life (such as rosuvastatin, atorvastatin, and fluvastatin) should be used in the perioperative setting.

POSTOPERATIVE MONITORING AND MANAGEMENT

Postoperative monitoring and management are important components of ensuring positive cardiac outcomes after major noncardiac surgery.

Postoperative EKG Monitoring for ST-Segment Changes

EKG monitoring has long been the cornerstone of monitoring for postoperative cardiac events; conventional EKG monitoring for the detection of transient ST-segment changes has frequently been used as a surrogate marker of cardiac ischemia in clinical trials.[30,36,37] Despite this widespread use, the data on postoperative EKG monitoring are mixed, and recent studies have questioned the ability of EKG monitoring alone to adequately detect ischemia across all spectrums of cardiac risk.[48,49] Several studies report a higher incidence of perioperative cardiac events when EKG changes occur postoperatively. In addition, the duration of ST-segment change correlates with perioperative MI.[50] Thus, in an isolated high-risk cohort, continuous EKG monitoring for ST-segment changes may be helpful.[51] However, the utility of routine postoperative continuous ST-segment monitoring is of questionable value in patients at low-intermediate risk and cannot be routinely recommended. Further studies are needed to define the optimal strategy and target populations that may benefit from this intervention.

Postoperative Biomarkers

A biomarker is a characteristic that can be objectively measured and serves as an indicator of an abnormal biologic or pathologic process. In the postoperative setting, cardiac troponins T and I (cTnT and cTnI) have been used as biomarkers of myocardial ischemia. Existing evidence, though limited, suggests that even small increases in cTnT in the perioperative period portend a worse cardiac prognosis.[52] There is currently no algorithm or strategy that defines which populations should receive biomarker monitoring in the postoperative setting. This appears to be a monitoring method that (like ST-segment monitoring) is best used in high-risk cohorts. Biomarkers such as CRP, BNP, or NT-pro BNP may have a role in identifying vulnerable patients at risk of cardiac events beyond clinical risk prediction tools.[53,54] For instance, a meta-analyses by Karthikeyan et al. (reviewing nine studies and 3281 patients) found that a single preoperative measurement of BNP or NT-proBNP served as a powerful, independent predictor of perioperative cardiac events during the 30 days after noncardiac surgery.[55] Such results are promising, but further studies testing and developing strategies that help define the target population, application, and implications of biomarker testing are necessary before we can routinely include biomarker data in the prevention of perioperative cardiac events.

PERIOPERATIVE QUALITY INDICATORS

The continuation of perioperative beta-blockers in those already on this therapy is a quality measure endorsed by the Centers for Medicare and Medicaid Services (CMS). Should we expand this metric? We argue against this. The benefit from beta-blockers lies in a strategy targeting those already on this therapy or those with demonstrable ischemia—an exceedingly narrow range of patients. In this subset, achieving the optimal drug dose and hemodynamic balance is dynamic, complex, and difficult to reduce to a single model. This degree of "granularity" may not be captured by a standardized measure and may result in the use of beta-blocker therapy in populations where harm results. The Surgical Care Improvement Project (SCIP) CARD2 quality metric endorses the perioperative continuation of beta-blockers in those already receiving this therapy.[56] This narrow measure echoes the ACC/AHA recommendations and is justifiable. Given the heterogeneity of the evidence, adoption of metrics beyond this seems untimely and unwise.

PATIENT EDUCATION

Perioperative consultants form the front line in educating patients about cardiac risk and the potential for harm from surgical intervention. By synthesizing the totality of patient and surgical risk in the context of surgical necessity, the perioperative consultant is able to provide an accurate statement regarding surgery. Patients should be advised that there is little value in routine testing; rather, it is the quality of perioperative testing that matters most. Furthermore, it is imperative that the perioperative consultant educate their patient on the importance of compliance with their beta-blocker and statin treatment in the perioperative setting (up to and including the morning of surgery) with specific attention to the dangers of premature discontinuation of these drugs prior to surgical intervention. It is only through such a partnership that patient satisfaction and provider potential will be fully realized. The discontinuation and cessation of antiplatelet therapy and patient education is discussed in Chapter 5.

SUMMARY

The assessment and management of perioperative cardiac risk involves a fundamental understanding of perioperative physiology, the integration of clinical history and physical examination, and the selective application of testing and risk-reducing therapies to populations where benefit from these interventions clearly exists. The literature has shown no additional value and the potential for harm from routine perioperative stress testing, unless such testing is targeted toward specific patients. Clinical risk prediction tools outperform stress testing in predicting perioperative cardiac events and serve as the front line for informing cardiac risk. Subsequently, selective interventions based on clinical risk prediction may be considered as a "second tier" to optimize preoperative status.

The ACC/AHA Preoperative Guidelines present an evidence-based, algorithmic approach to perioperative evaluation and should be routinely implemented in this setting. Questions as to who should receive postoperative monitoring and whether biomarkers provide insight beyond clinical risk prediction methodologies represent new and upcoming areas of research in perioperative management that are likely to further impact this rapidly evolving area. Patient education is a fundamental role of the perioperative consultant and a mutual partnership through this period will undoubtedly lead to positive outcomes.

REFERENCES

1. Fleischmann KE, Goldman L, Young B, Lee TH. Association between cardiac and noncardiac complications in patients undergoing noncardiac surgery: outcomes and effects on length of stay. *Am J Med.* Nov 2003;115(7):515–520.
2. Landesberg G, Shatz V, Akopnik I, et al. Association of cardiac troponin, CK-MB, and postoperative myocardial ischemia with long-term survival after major vascular surgery. *J Am Coll Cardiol.* Nov 5 2003;42(9):1547–1554.
3. Poldermans D, Hoeks SE, Feringa HH. Pre-operative risk assessment and risk reduction before surgery. *J Am Coll Cardiol.* May 20 2008;51(20):1913–1924.
4. Zaman AG, Helft G, Worthley SG, Badimon JJ. The role of plaque rupture and thrombosis in coronary artery disease. *Atherosclerosis.* Apr 2000;149(2):251–266.
5. Naughton C, Feneck RO. The impact of age on 6-month survival in patients with cardiovascular risk factors undergoing elective non-cardiac surgery. *Int J Clin Pract.* May 2007;61(5):768–776.
6. DeFrances CJ, Cullen KA, Kozak LJ. National Hospital Discharge Survey: 2005 annual summary with detailed diagnosis and procedure data. *Vital Health Stat 13.* Dec 2007;(165):1–209.
7. Cabana MD, Rand CS, Powe NR, et al. Why don't physicians follow clinical practice guidelines? A framework for improvement. *JAMA.* Oct 20 1999;282(15):1458–1465.
8. Hoeks SE, Scholte Op Reimer WJ, van Gestel YR, et al. Medication underuse during long-term follow-up in patients with peripheral arterial disease. *Circ Cardiovasc Qual Outcomes.* Jul 2009;2(4):338–343.
9. Gottlieb A, Banoub M, Sprung J, Levy PJ, Beven M, Mascha EJ. Perioperative cardiovascular morbidity in patients with coronary artery disease undergoing vascular surgery after percutaneous transluminal coronary angioplasty. *J Cardiothorac Vasc Anesth.* Oct 1998;12(5):501–506.
10. Hassan SA, Hlatky MA, Boothroyd DB, et al. Outcomes of noncardiac surgery after coronary bypass surgery or coronary angioplasty in the Bypass Angioplasty Revascularization Investigation (BARI). *Am J Med.* Mar 2001;110(4):260–266.

11. Nelson CL, Herndon JE, Mark DB, Pryor DB, Califf RM, Hlatky MA. Relation of clinical and angiographic factors to functional capacity as measured by the Duke Activity Status Index. *Am J Cardiol*. Oct 1 1991;68(9):973–975.
12. Cohen MC, Aretz TH. Histological analysis of coronary artery lesions in fatal postoperative myocardial infarction. *Cardiovasc Pathol*. May–Jun 1999;8(3):133–139.
13. Monahan TS, Shrikhande GV, Pomposelli FB, et al. Preoperative cardiac evaluation does not improve or predict perioperative or late survival in asymptomatic diabetic patients undergoing elective infrainguinal arterial reconstruction. *J Vasc Surg*. Jan 2005;41(1):38–45; discussion 45.
14. Muller JE, Kaufmann PG, Luepker RV, Weisfeldt ML, Deedwania PC, Willerson JT. Mechanisms precipitating acute cardiac events: review and recommendations of an NHLBI workshop. National Heart, Lung, and Blood Institute. Mechanisms Precipitating Acute Cardiac Events Participants. *Circulation*. Nov 4 1997;96(9):3233–3239.
15. Kertai MD, Boersma E, Bax JJ, et al. A meta-analysis comparing the prognostic accuracy of six diagnostic tests for predicting perioperative cardiac risk in patients undergoing major vascular surgery. *Heart*. Nov 2003;89(11):1327–1334.
16. Etchells E, Meade M, Tomlinson G, Cook D. Semiquantitative dipyridamole myocardial stress perfusion imaging for cardiac risk assessment before noncardiac vascular surgery: a meta-analysis. *J Vasc Surg*. Sep 2002;36(3):534–540.
17. Shaw LJ, Eagle KA, Gersh BJ, Miller DD. Meta-analysis of intravenous dipyridamole-thallium-201 imaging (1985 to 1994) and dobutamine echocardiography (1991 to 1994) for risk stratification before vascular surgery. *J Am Coll Cardiol*. Mar 15 1996;27(4):787–798.
18. Boersma E, Poldermans D, Bax JJ, et al. Predictors of cardiac events after major vascular surgery: role of clinical characteristics, dobutamine echocardiography, and beta-blocker therapy. *JAMA*. Apr 11 2001;285(14):1865–1873.
19. Poldermans D, Bax JJ, Schouten O, et al. Should major vascular surgery be delayed because of preoperative cardiac testing in intermediate-risk patients receiving beta-blocker therapy with tight heart rate control? *J Am Coll Cardiol*. Sep 5 2006;48(5):964–969.
20. Owens WD, Felts JA, Spitznagel EL, Jr. ASA physical status classifications: a study of consistency of ratings. *Anesthesiology*. Oct 1978;49(4):239–243.
21. Goldman L, Caldera DL, Nussbaum SR, et al. Multifactorial index of cardiac risk in noncardiac surgical procedures. *N Engl J Med*. Oct 20 1977;297(16):845–850.
22. Detsky AS, Abrams HB, Forbath N, Scott JG, Hilliard JR. Cardiac assessment for patients undergoing noncardiac surgery. A multifactorial clinical risk index. *Arch Intern Med*. Nov 1986;146(11): 2131–2134.
23. L'Italien GJ, Cambria RP, Cutler BS, et al. Comparative early and late cardiac morbidity among patients requiring different vascular surgery procedures. *J Vasc Surg*. Jun 1995;21(6):935–944.
24. Lee TH, Marcantonio ER, Mangione CM, et al. Derivation and prospective validation of a simple index for prediction of cardiac risk of major noncardiac surgery. *Circulation*. Sep 7 1999;100(10): 1043–1049.
25. Ford MK, Beattie WS, Wijeysundera DN. Systematic review: prediction of perioperative cardiac complications and mortality by the Revised Cardiac Risk Index. *Ann Intern Med*. Jan 5 2010; 152(1):26–35.
26. Eagle KA, Brundage BH, Chaitman BR, et al. Guidelines for perioperative cardiovascular evaluation for noncardiac surgery. Report of the American College of Cardiology/American Heart Association Task Force on Practice Guidelines. Committee on Perioperative Cardiovascular Evaluation for Noncardiac Surgery. *Circulation*. Mar 15 1996;93(6):1278–1317.
27. Fleisher LA, Beckman JA, Brown KA, et al. ACC/AHA 2007 guidelines on perioperative cardiovascular evaluation and care for noncardiac surgery: a report of the American College of Cardiology/American Heart Association Task Force on Practice Guidelines (Writing Committee to Revise the 2002 Guidelines on Perioperative Cardiovascular Evaluation for Noncardiac Surgery) developed in collaboration with the American Society of Echocardiography, American Society of Nuclear Cardiology, Heart Rhythm Society, Society of Cardiovascular Anesthesiologists, Society for Cardiovascular Angiography and Interventions, Society for Vascular Medicine and Biology, and Society for Vascular Surgery. *J Am Coll Cardiol*. Oct 23 2007;50(17):e159–e241.

28. Fleisher LA, Beckman JA, Brown KA, et al. 2009 ACCF/AHA focused update on perioperative beta blockade incorporated into the ACC/AHA 2007 guidelines on perioperative cardiovascular evaluation and care for noncardiac surgery. *J Am Coll Cardiol.* Nov 24 2009;54(22):e13–e118.

29. Eagle KA, Rihal CS, Mickel MC, Holmes DR, Foster ED, Gersh BJ. Cardiac risk of noncardiac surgery: influence of coronary disease and type of surgery in 3368 operations. CASS Investigators and University of Michigan Heart Care Program. Coronary Artery Surgery Study. *Circulation.* Sep 16 1997;96(6):1882–1887.

30. McFalls EO, Ward HB, Moritz TE, et al. Coronary-artery revascularization before elective major vascular surgery. *N Engl J Med.* Dec 30 2004;351(27):2795–2804.

31. Rihal CS, Eagle KA, Mickel MC, Foster ED, Sopko G, Gersh BJ. Surgical therapy for coronary artery disease among patients with combined coronary artery and peripheral vascular disease. *Circulation.* Jan 1 1995;91(1):46–53.

32. Garcia S, Moritz TE, Goldman S, et al. Perioperative complications after vascular surgery are predicted by the Revised Cardiac Risk Index but are not reduced in high-risk subsets with preoperative revascularization. *Circ Cardiovasc Qual Outcomes.* Mar 2009;2(2):73–77.

33. Boden WE, O'Rourke RA, Teo KK, et al. Optimal medical therapy with or without PCI for stable coronary disease. *N Engl J Med.* Apr 12 2007;356(15):1503–1516.

34. Frye RL, August P, Brooks MM, et al. A randomized trial of therapies for type 2 diabetes and coronary artery disease. *N Engl J Med.* Jun 11 2009;360(24):2503–2515.

35. Poldermans D, Schouten O, Vidakovic R, et al. A clinical randomized trial to evaluate the safety of a noninvasive approach in high-risk patients undergoing major vascular surgery: the DECREASE-V Pilot Study. *J Am Coll Cardiol.* May 1 2007;49(17):1763–1769.

36. Mangano DT, Layug EL, Wallace A, Tateo I. Effect of atenolol on mortality and cardiovascular morbidity after noncardiac surgery. Multicenter Study of Perioperative Ischemia Research Group. *N Engl J Med.* Dec 5 1996;335(23):1713–1720.

37. Poldermans D, Boersma E, Bax JJ, et al. The effect of bisoprolol on perioperative mortality and myocardial infarction in high-risk patients undergoing vascular surgery. Dutch Echocardiographic Cardiac Risk Evaluation Applying Stress Echocardiography Study Group. *N Engl J Med.* Dec 9 1999;341(24):1789–1794.

38. Lindenauer PK, Pekow P, Wang K, Mamidi DK, Gutierrez B, Benjamin EM. Perioperative beta-blocker therapy and mortality after major noncardiac surgery. *N Engl J Med.* Jul 28 2005; 353(4):349–361.

39. Devereaux PJ, Yang H, Yusuf S, et al. Effects of extended-release metoprolol succinate in patients undergoing non-cardiac surgery (POISE trial): a randomised controlled trial. *Lancet.* May 31 2008;371(9627):1839–1847.

40. Fleischmann KE, Beckman JA, Buller CE, et al. 2009 ACCF/AHA focused update on perioperative beta blockade. *J Am Coll Cardiol.* Nov 24 2009;54(22):2102–2128.

41. Poldermans D, Bax JJ, Boersma E, et al. Guidelines for pre-operative cardiac risk assessment and perioperative cardiac management in non-cardiac surgery: the Task Force for Preoperative Cardiac Risk Assessment and Perioperative Cardiac Management in Non-Cardiac Surgery of the European Society of Cardiology (ESC) and endorsed by the European Society of Anaesthesiology (ESA). *Eur Heart J.* Nov 2009;30(22):2769–2812.

42. Dunkelgrun M, Boersma E, Schouten O, et al. Bisoprolol and fluvastatin for the reduction of perioperative cardiac mortality and myocardial infarction in intermediate-risk patients undergoing non-cardiovascular surgery: a randomized controlled trial (DECREASE-IV). *Ann Surg.* Jun 2009;249(6):921–926.

43. Lindenauer PK, Pekow P, Wang K, Gutierrez B, Benjamin EM. Lipid-lowering therapy and in-hospital mortality following major noncardiac surgery. *JAMA.* May 5 2004;291(17):2092–2099.

44. Ward RP, Leeper NJ, Kirkpatrick JN, Lang RM, Sorrentino MJ, Williams KA. The effect of preoperative statin therapy on cardiovascular outcomes in patients undergoing infrainguinal vascular surgery. *Int J Cardiol.* Oct 10 2005;104(3):264–268.

45. Durazzo AE, Machado FS, Ikeoka DT, et al. Reduction in cardiovascular events after vascular surgery with atorvastatin: a randomized trial. *J Vasc Surg.* May 2004;39(5):967–975; discussion 975–966.

46. Schouten O, Boersma E, Hoeks SE, et al. Fluvastatin and perioperative events in patients undergoing vascular surgery. *N Engl J Med.* Sep 3 2009;361(10):980–989.

47. Williams TM, Harken AH. Statins for surgical patients. *Ann Surg.* Jan 2008;247(1):30–37.

48. Biagini A, L'Abbate A, Testa R, et al. Unreliability of conventional visual electrocardiographic monitoring for detection of transient ST segment changes in a coronary care unit. *Eur Heart J.* Oct 1984;5(10):784–791.

49. Leung JM, Voskanian A, Bellows WH, Pastor D. Automated electrocardiograph ST segment trending monitors: accuracy in detecting myocardial ischemia. *Anesth Analg.* Jul 1998;87(1):4–10.

50. Landesberg G, Luria MH, Cotev S, et al. Importance of long-duration postoperative ST-segment depression in cardiac morbidity after vascular surgery. *Lancet.* Mar 20 1993;341(8847):715–719.

51. Fleisher LA. Real-time intraoperative monitoring of myocardial ischemia in noncardiac surgery. *Anesthesiology.* Apr 2000;92(4):1183–1188.

52. Priebe HJ. Perioperative myocardial infarction—aetiology and prevention. *Br J Anaesth.* Jul 2005;95(1):3–19.

53. Tsimikas S, Willerson JT, Ridker PM. C-reactive protein and other emerging blood biomarkers to optimize risk stratification of vulnerable patients. *J Am Coll Cardiol.* Apr 18 2006;47(8 Suppl):C19–C31.

54. Rodseth RN, Padayachee L, Biccard BM. A meta-analysis of the utility of pre-operative brain natriuretic peptide in predicting early and intermediate-term mortality and major adverse cardiac events in vascular surgical patients. *Anaesthesia.* Nov 2008;63(11):1226–1233.

55. Karthikeyan G, Moncur RA, Levine O, et al. Is a pre-operative brain natriuretic peptide or N-terminal pro-B-type natriuretic peptide measurement an independent predictor of adverse cardiovascular outcomes within 30 days of noncardiac surgery? A systematic review and meta-analysis of observational studies. *J Am Coll Cardiol.* Oct 20 2009;54(17):1599–1606.

56. Cardiac CMS. Measures: Surgical Care Improvement Project (SCIP), Quality Measure 2 (SCIP-CARD-2): surgical patients on a beta-blocker prior to arrival that received a beta-blocker during the perioperative period. 2010. The Joint Commission Web Site. Available at http://manual.jointcommission.org/releases/Archive/TJC2010B1/MIF0059.html. Accessed January 21, 2010.

CHAPTER 10

ASSESSING AND MANAGING PULMONARY RISK

Gerald W. Smetana

EPIDEMIOLOGY

The three greatest sources of medical morbidity and mortality after major surgery are pulmonary, cardiac, and thromboembolic complications. While clinicians routinely consider thromboembolic prophylaxis and cardiac risk before high-risk noncardiac surgery, the preoperative evaluation must also include an assessment of the risk of postoperative pulmonary complications (PPCs) and recommendations for strategies to reduce this risk. This is often neglected. Ample evidence in the literature indicates that clinically important pulmonary and cardiac complications occur with similar frequency after major surgery. For example, in a study of 8930 patients undergoing hip fracture repair, serious pulmonary, cardiac, and thromboembolic complications occurred in 2.6%, 2.0%, and 1.0% of patients, respectively.[1] Similar findings resulted from a study of the 3970 patients used to develop the Revised Cardiac Risk Index.[2]

In the past two decades, clinicians have become more aware of this risk, and the required assessment has evolved from one of expert opinion to an evidence-based discipline. Awareness of the importance of preoperative pulmonary evaluation has, for example, prompted the American College of Physicians (ACP) to issue a new guideline to improve clinical care and minimize practice variation.[3] For purposes of risk assessment, important PPCs include pneumonia, respiratory failure, atelectasis, and exacerbation of underlying disease. As the risk factors for each are similar, and based on limitations in the available source literature, we will consider these together rather than separately. In this chapter, we discuss the factors from clinical evaluation that increase the risk of PPC, the limited role for testing, and strategies to reduce this risk. The risk factors and prevention strategies for pulmonary embolism differ and are thus discussed separately (Chapter 32).

HISTORY

The clinical history is the single most important element of the preoperative pulmonary evaluation. A careful history that considers both patient- and procedure-related

Perioperative Medicine: Medical Consultation and Co-Management, First Edition.
Edited by Amir K. Jaffer and Paul J. Grant.
© 2012 Wiley-Blackwell. Published 2012 by John Wiley & Sons, Inc.

risk factors will accurately estimate PPC risk for most patients before noncardiac surgery. The physical examination serves most often to confirm the history, and testing plays an even smaller role in the preoperative pulmonary assessment. Risk factors for PPC differ from those of cardiac and thromboembolic complications and place more emphasis on procedure-related risk factors.

Patient-Related Risk Factors

The most rigorous assessment of the impact of potential patient-related risk factors for PPC comes from a systematic review that forms the backbone of the above-mentioned ACP guideline (Table 10.1).[4] Novel conclusions from a careful review of the literature included recognition of the importance of age as a risk factor and the failure of obesity as a risk factor.

TABLE 10.1. Selected Patient- and Procedure-Related Risk Factors from the ACP Guideline

Risk factor	Odds ratio for PPC	95% confidence interval
Patient-related risk factors		
Age		
• 50–59	1.50	1.31–1.71
• 60–69	2.09	1.65–2.64
• 70–79	3.04	2.11–4.39
• ≥80	5.63	4.63–6.85
ASA classification ≥2	4.87	3.34–7.10
Congestive heart failure	2.93	1.02–8.03
Total functional dependence	2.51	1.99–3.15
COPD	2.36	1.90–2.93
Cigarette use	1.40	1.17–1.69
Procedure-related risk factors		
Surgical site		
• Aortic	6.90	2.74–17.36
• Thoracic	4.24	2.89–6.23
• Any abdominal	3.01	2.43–3.72
• Upper abdominal	2.91	2.35–3.60
• Neurosurgical	2.53	1.84–3.47
Emergency surgery	2.21	1.57–3.11
Surgery > 3 h	2.26	1.47–3.47
General anesthesia	1.83	1.35–2.46

Adapted from Smetana et al.[4]
ACP, American College of Physicians; PPC, postoperative pulmonary complications; ASA, American Society of Anesthesiologists; COPD, chronic obstructive pulmonary disease.

The most important patient-related risks are advanced age and a high American Society of Anesthesiologists' (ASA) classification score.[5] Age confers an independent risk beginning at age 50; the PPC risk climbs with each subsequent decade such that an otherwise healthy individual ≥80 years of age has a greater than fivefold increase in PPC risk when compared with a patient <50 years of age. This is in contrast to cardiac risk assessment where age drops out of the analysis after adjustment for comorbidities more common with advanced age.[6] While advanced age, by itself, does not prohibit safely proceeding to major noncardiac surgery, its presence should prompt a careful consideration of the indications for the planned surgery and an appropriate informed consent discussion with the patient regarding pulmonary risk.

The ASA classification is an integrative score of 1–5 based on the clinician's impression of the overall burden of medical comorbidities.[5] This is highly reliable between observers and proves to be one of the most important predictors of PPC risk. Definitions in this classification scheme are (1) a normal healthy patient, (2) a patient with mild systemic disease, (3) a patient with severe systemic disease, (4) a patient with severe systemic disease that is a constant threat to life, and (5) a moribund patient who is not expected to survive without the operation. According to the ACP review, for example, the odds of developing a PPC are 4.87-fold greater for patients who are at least ASA class 2 as compared with those who are ASA class 1 (Table 10.1).

As expected, chronic obstructive pulmonary disease (COPD) is an important patient-related risk factor (odds ratio [OR] 2.93). The risk becomes higher with increasing disease severity as estimated by exercise capacity and functional impairment. In contrast to COPD, asthma is not a risk factor for PPC.[7] However, this applies only to patients whose asthma is well controlled by virtue of being wheeze free and with a forced expiratory volume in 1 s (FEV_1) or peak flow of at least 80% of predicted or personal best. Cigarette use, after controlling for COPD and other comorbidities, is a weak risk factor (OR 1.33).

Obstructive sleep apnea (OSA) is a novel risk factor for airway complications in the immediate postoperative period and also for PPCs.[8] It has been uncertain whether preoperative screening patients for OSA, among patients who are not known to have the disease, improves perioperative outcomes. The STOP questionnaire[9] consists of four questions using this mnemonic: (1) do you *snore* loudly?, (2) do you often feel *tired*, fatigued, or sleep during the daytime?, (3) has anyone *observed* you to stop breathing during your sleep?, and (4) do you have or are you being treated for high blood *pressure*? A recent trial used the STOP questionnaire to screen patients for OSA before surgery.[10] Using an Apnea–Hypopnea Index (AHI), a measure of OSA severity, of >15, the sensitivity and specificity for the STOP questionnaire as a diagnostic test were 74% and 53%, respectively. PPC rates (but not total complication rates) were significantly higher among patients with a high-risk STOP score (34% vs. 11%, $P < 0.05$). This study suggests that screening for OSA with a simple tool may help to identify high-risk patients and to rationally allocate resources for risk-reduction strategies. The value of preoperative screening for OSA may be particularly high among patients undergoing bariatric surgery. The incidence of OSA (either known or previously undetected) among bariatric surgery patients in one study was 77%.[11]

Congestive heart failure (CHF) proves, surprisingly, to be a stronger risk factor (OR 2.93) than COPD. It is also one of the principal risk factors for postoperative cardiac complications.[6]

Obesity would intuitively appear to increase risk due to a propensity for hypoventilation after surgery. However, the literature has quite consistently shown that obesity is not a risk factor for PPCs and should not be considered when estimating risk. This appears to hold true even for patients with morbid obesity, such as those undergoing bariatric surgery.[12] This is not to say that clinicians should ignore this factor when performing a preoperative evaluation as obesity is a risk factor for venous thromboembolic complications (see Chapter 32). Other patient-related risk factors include functional dependence (the need for help in performing activities of daily living), weight loss, impaired sensorium, and corticosteroid use.

Procedure-Related Risk Factors

The single most important risk factor for PPC is surgical site. This proves more important than any patient-related risk factor and should be the first consideration when estimating PPC risk for a particular patient. Certain procedures are inherently high risk, even for otherwise healthy or low-risk patients (Table 10.1). The rule that risk increases with proximity of the surgical incision to the diaphragm remains generally true. The highest risk procedures are aortic (OR 6.90), thoracic (OR 4.24), abdominal (OR 3.01), and neurosurgical (OR 2.53). This indicates that even healthy patients are at high risk for complications when undergoing a high-risk procedure.

Other procedure-related risks include emergency surgery and surgery lasting more than 3 h. General anesthesia may be a risk factor, but evidence derived from high-quality randomized controlled trials is mixed, and its impact on PPC risk remains controversial.[13]

PHYSICAL EXAMINATION

The physical examination only rarely uncovers a risk factor that escaped detection after careful history taking. The patient with, for example, COPD or CHF would usually be identified by a history of dyspnea or effort intolerance. However, occasionally a prolonged expiratory phase, wheezes, or decreased breath sounds on examination would be the first evidence of COPD. When present, these factors substantially increase PPC risk.[14]

Even when the diagnosis of COPD or CHF is apparent after history taking, the examination often serves to estimate severity of the underlying disease. PPC risk most likely correlates with severity of COPD or CHF as estimated by physical examination, but this has not been well studied. An examination of the upper airway and posterior pharynx is an important part of the anesthesiologist's preoperative examination but is less helpful for the hospitalist when estimating traditional PPC risk. The remainder of the general medical examination remains an important element of the preoperative evaluation (see Chapter 4) but provides no further refinement of PPC risk.

TESTING

Testing to estimate PPC risk could potentially serve several roles. One would be to further refine risk for patients at intermediate risk for PPC after clinical evaluation. Another would be to establish a prohibitive value (e.g., of lung function) below which the risk of surgery would be unacceptably high. Finally, testing could potentially more accurately predict risk than clinical evaluation and thus be warranted before certain high-risk surgeries. However, none of these three potential rationales has proven true after a careful review of the literature.

Spirometry is the test for which there is the greatest intuitive appeal, and the most evidence in the literature. While it is true that a low FEV_1 ($FEV_1 < 50\%$ predicted) or low FEV_1/forced vital capacity ratio (FEV_1/FVC ratio <70%) generally confers higher PPC risk, most of these patients would not escape clinical detection. That is, the history and physical examination would establish a diagnosis of COPD and an estimate of its severity. Most commonly, the spirometric values simply confirm the estimate of severity that is already apparent. Few studies have evaluated the incremental value of spirometry when compared with clinical evaluation. For example, in the 2006 ACP guideline, among four studies that used multivariable analysis to determine the independent value of spirometry, only one study found FEV_1 to be a stronger predictor than clinical risk factors.[4] In addition, there is no evidence that there is a prohibitive threshold of FEV_1 below which surgery is contraindicated. The ACP guideline recommended the use of spirometry as a preoperative test for patients in whom the reason for dyspnea or effort intolerance is uncertain after clinical evaluation (i.e., cardiac vs. pulmonary vs. deconditioning) and in those with COPD or asthma only if it is uncertain whether their airflow obstruction is maximally reduced before elective surgery.

Chest radiography is another commonly performed preoperative test. The belief that a preoperative chest radiograph serves as an important baseline in the event that a postoperative study is required is untested and probably untrue. Whether baseline abnormalities consistent with COPD or CHF independently predict PPC risk is uncertain. In the ACP guideline, two small studies suggested an independent value (OR 4.81, confidence interval [CI] 2.43–9.55) when added to clinical evaluation, but this was based on a small number of patients. Most studies of chest radiographs have evaluated the impact on preoperative management rather than the risk of PPC. In a review of eight studies of preoperative chest radiographs ($n = 14,650$), while 23.1% of all studies were abnormal, only 3.0% of studies influenced perioperative management.[15] Still, hospitalists need to decide when to obtain a preoperative chest radiograph despite the mixed results from the literature. Pending future studies, the ACP has suggested this study for patients with known cardiopulmonary disease and for those over age 50 years who are planning upper abdominal, thoracic, or aortic surgery.[4]

Unexpectedly, a simple blood test has better test characteristics than either chest radiography or spirometry to predict PPC risk. Low serum albumin (<3.5 g/dL) is an independent predictor of PPC risk.[4,16] For a patient at intermediate risk of PPC after clinical evaluation, measurement of serum albumin may help to refine risk. Impaired renal function (serum creatinine >2.1 mg/dL [7.5 mmol/L]) is an independent predictor although whether clinicians should routinely measure renal function in high-risk surgeries is unknown.

Cardiopulmonary exercise testing (CET) provides an objective estimate of exercise capacity. The principal results from CET are maximum oxygen uptake (VO_{2max}) and ventilatory anaerobic threshold (VAT). The preponderance of research into the value of CET as a preoperative test has focused on patients preparing for lung resection. However, there is a growing body of data regarding its role before noncardiothoracic surgery. In a recent review of the literature, VO_{2max} and, to a lesser degree, VAT predicted perioperative mortality and all postoperative complications.[17] However, most studies pooled all postoperative complications and did not specifically consider PPC. This test is not widely used in clinical practice but may prove helpful in the patient with intermediate or uncertain risk after clinical evaluation. For example, CET could refine the risk estimate in a patient with a history of poor exercise capacity for which the basis is uncertain.

PREDICTING RISK/GUIDELINES

It is not possible to estimate risk by adding or multiplying the impact of individual risk factors. However, it is possible to predict risk by considering the number of proven risk factors for a particular patient undergoing a particular type of surgery. The only published guidelines for preoperative pulmonary evaluation are those of the ACP in 2006. The ACP is currently in the process of updating these guidelines. Based on the strength of evidence, and using a modified version of the U.S. Preventive Services Task Force criteria, the ACP has applied letter grades to individual risk factors (Table 10.2). Risk factors earning a grade "A" are those for which there is good evidence from the literature to support the factor.[3] These include advanced age, ASA class ≥2, CHF, functional dependence, COPD, high-risk surgical site, general anesthesia, prolonged or emergency surgery, and serum albumin level <3.5 g/dL. In particular, clinicians should estimate risk for all patients undergoing high-risk surgery, and for those who are older, have multiple medical comorbidities, or have preexisting cardiopulmonary disease.

CLINICAL PREDICTION RULES (CPRs)

In contrast to estimation of cardiac risk, for which there is broad consensus on the value of the Revised Cardiac Risk Index as an important tool,[6] no published risk index is widely used to estimate PPC risk. However, among the published CPRs for PPC, the most carefully constructed and validated are those deriving from the Department of Veterans Affairs National Surgical Quality Improvement Program

TABLE 10.2.   Strength of Evidence for Risk Factors and Laboratory Test to Predict PPC Rates

Patient-related risk factor	Strength of recommendation	Procedure-related risk factor	Strength of recommendation
Advanced age	A	Aortic aneurysm repair	A
ASA class ≥2	A	Thoracic surgery	A
Functionally dependent	A	Abdominal surgery	A
COPD	A	Upper abdominal surgery	A
CHF	A	Neurosurgery	A
Impaired sensorium	B	Prolonged surgery	A
Abnormal chest exam	B	Head and neck surgery	A
Cigarette use	B	Emergency surgery	A
Alcohol use	B	Vascular surgery	A
Weight loss	B	General anesthesia	A
Diabetes	C	Perioperative transfusion	B
Obesity	D	Hip surgery	D
Asthma	D	GU/GYN surgery	D
Obstructive sleep apnea	I	Esophageal surgery	I
Corticosteroid use	I		
HIV infection	I	Laboratory tests	
Arrhythmia	I		
Poor exercise capacity	I	Albumin <35 g/L	A
		Chest radiograph	B
		BUN > 7.5 mmol/L (21 mg/dL)	B
		Spirometry	I

A. There is good evidence to support the particular risk factor or laboratory predictor.
B. There is at least fair evidence to support the particular risk factor or laboratory predictor.
C. There is at least fair evidence to suggest that the particular factor is not a risk factor or laboratory test does not predict risk.
D. There is good evidence to suggest that the particular factor is not a risk factor or the laboratory test does not predict risk.
I. There is insufficient evidence to determine if the factor increases risk or laboratory test predicts risk. Evidence is lacking, poor quality, or conflicting.
Adapted from Smetana et al.[4]
GU/GYN, urologic and gynecologic; BUN, blood urea nitrogen.

(NSQIP).[16,18,19] In contrast to the common approach of lumping all PPC together, the authors of these studies separately considered the risk factors for postoperative pneumonia and respiratory failure. In 2007, the authors published an updated respiratory failure index that included patients from selected academic medical centers as well as Veterans Administration hospitals.[19] Most of the important risk factors after multivariable analysis were similar to those identified for the ACP guideline. New risk factors in the NSQIP index, which did not appear in the ACP guideline, included high work relative value unit (RVU) (as a proxy for surgery complexity), sepsis,

TABLE 10.3. Clinical Prediction Rule: the Original Arozullah (NSQIP) Respiratory Failure Index

Risk factor	Point value	
Surgical site		
• Aorta	27	
• Thoracic	21	
• Neurosurgery, upper abdominal, or peripheral vascular	14	
• Neck	11	
Emergency surgery	11	
Serum albumin <3.5 g/dL	9	
Blood urea nitrogen >30 mg/dL	8	
Functionally dependent	7	
COPD	6	
Age		
≥70 years	6	
60–69 years	4	
Class	Point total	Respiratory failure risk[a]
1	≤10	0.5%
2	11–19	1.8%
3	20–27	4.2%
4	28–40	10.1%
5	>40	26.6%

[a] In validation cohort.
NSQIP, National Surgical Quality Improvement Program; COPD, chronic obstructive pulmonary disease.
Adapted from Arozullah et al.[16]

ascites, orofacial surgery, and hypernatremia. Lower risk was assigned to low serum albumin, functional dependence, and CHF than in the ACP guideline.

The updated respiratory failure index has 28 factors and is too complicated for use in clinical practice. The original NSQIP respiratory failure index is the simplest of the three tools and is the most clinically relevant CPR for clinicians who wish to determine a numerical risk estimate for postoperative respiratory failure (Table 10.3). A slightly more complicated CPR exists for postoperative pneumonia (not shown).[18] Figure 10.1 outlines an approach to risk assessment and intervention strategies to reduce the risk of PPC. Evidence supporting the risk reduction strategies follows.

MINIMIZING RISK

Hospitalists who perform preoperative pulmonary evaluations have two principal goals. The first is to estimate PPC risk for the given patient undergoing the planned

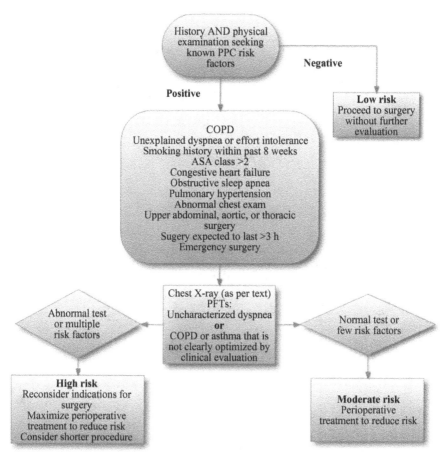

Figure 10.1. Approach to pulmonary risk assessment and management. PPC, postoperative pulmonary complication; COPD, chronic obstructive pulmonary disease; ASA, American Society of Anesthesiologists; PFTs, pulmonary function tests.

surgery. The second is to determine if the patient is in his or her best possible condition before surgery and to propose strategies to minimize PPC risk when appropriate. When considering the impact of specific risk-reduction strategies, it is important to evaluate high-quality randomized controlled trials of the intervention. In doing so, certain intuitive established interventions prove to be unhelpful or of minimal benefit, whereas unexpected finding establish novel interventions to be of value. Risk-reduction strategies tend to be generic: the selection of a particular strategy is guided by the overall risk, not the particular factors that contribute to increased risk.

The risk-reduction strategy for which there is the best evidence is lung expansion maneuvers; it was the only grade A intervention in the ACP guideline.[13] The physiology of PPC relates to a fall in lung volumes after surgery due to pain, splinting, and the effects of anesthesia itself. This drop in lung volumes after surgery leads

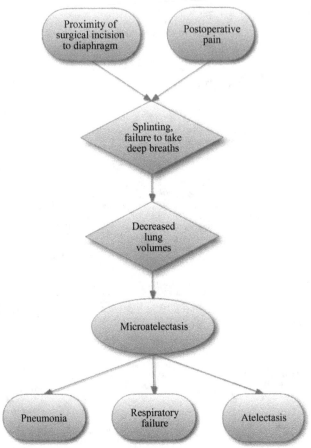

Figure 10.2.   Pathophysiology of postoperative pulmonary complications. Adapted from Smetana GW. Evaluation of preoperative pulmonary risk. In: Rose BD, editor. UpToDate. Wellesley: UpToDate. Available at http://www.uptodateinc.com.

to microatelectasis, which is then the substrate for clinically relevant PPC (Figure 10.2). Lung expansion maneuvers decrease the expected fall in lung volumes after surgery and thus can potentially interrupt this pathophysiologic process. Lung expansion maneuvers include (1) deep breathing exercises (a component of chest physical therapy), (2) incentive spirometry, (3) inspiratory muscle training, and (4) continuous positive airway pressure (CPAP). The literature supports all four of these strategies as effective tools to reduce PPC risk.

Incentive spirometry is comparable with deep breathing exercises; each reduces PPC rates by approximately one-half.[20] The combination of the two is no more effective than either one alone. Both strategies are probably more effective when teaching begins before surgery rather than in the postoperative period. CPAP is as effective as incentive spirometry and deep breathing exercises. However, it is resource intensive in terms of staffing requirements in the hospital and carries a small risk of barotrauma. It is best to reserve this for patients who are unable to perform the effort-dependent maneuvers.

Recently, a particularly intensive strategy of preoperative inspiratory muscle training has proven to be of particular value.[21] In a study of patients undergoing coronary artery bypass surgery, this strategy reduced rates of pneumonia by 60% and all PPC by 48%. The intervention group received daily training, 7 days per week, for at least 2 weeks before surgery. Training included inspiratory muscle training, education in active cycle breathing techniques, and forced expiration techniques. One session per week was supervised by a physical therapist. This intervention could be employed in clinical practice by an outpatient chest physical therapy or pulmonary rehabilitation clinic.

Another proven strategy is the selective, rather than routine, use of nasogastric tubes after abdominal surgery.[22] Selective means its use for symptoms such as nausea or distension. The mechanism for this observation is most likely a risk of microaspiration of gastric contents when a nasogastric tube is in place. The evidence for this strategy has grown since publication of the ACP guideline and would now earn a grade A level of evidence.

Postoperative pain is a contributing factor for hypoventilation and PPC after surgery near the diaphragm. Strategies to reduce postoperative pain could potentially improve ability to take deep breaths after surgery and therefore reduce PPC risk. The impact of such strategies on PPC rates has been the subject of debate. Authors of a recent systematic review have demonstrated that thoracic epidural analgesia reduces all PPC rates after coronary bypass (OR 0.41) and aortic (0.63) surgeries, and respiratory failure rates after abdominal surgery (OR 0.77).[23] Clinicians should routinely consider this intervention after these high-risk surgeries.

Whether general anesthesia confers a higher risk of PPC than neuraxial blockade (spinal or epidural anesthesia) has been controversial. A large meta-analysis published in 2000 reported that this was the case[24]; however, more recent well-designed randomized trials have not consistently made this observation. Among six observational trials that used multivariable analysis and qualified for inclusion in the ACP guideline, the OR for PPC associated with general anesthesia was 2.35. As other considerations often play a more important role when selecting anesthetic type, it is best for the hospitalist consultant to defer this decision to the anesthesiologist, rather than to offer a controversial recommendation that may put the anesthesiologist at medicolegal risk if a complication were to occur.

While an intuitively appealing strategy, it is uncertain whether laparoscopic surgery carries a lower risk of PPC than open abdominal surgery. Results in the literature are mixed and inconclusive. There are other, however, other well-established benefits of laparoscopic surgery including less postoperative pain and earlier return to full function. The use of long-acting neuromuscular blockers such as pancuronium increases the likelihood of postoperative residual neuromuscular blockade. This can decrease postoperative lung volumes and therefore increase the risk of PPC.[25,26]

The impact of cigarette cessation before surgery is uncertain. Clearly, the preoperative evaluation of the patient who smokes cigarettes offers a "teachable moment" to urge smoking cessation. However, many uncontrolled studies of cigarette cessation have found higher PPC rates among recent quitters within 1–2 months before surgery. The basis for this observation may be an increase in sputum production in the weeks after successful cigarette cessation. Two small randomized trials have attempted to resolve this question.[27,28] Overall PPC rates in these studies, however, were low, and the studies were underpowered to show a benefit from cigarette cessation. However, no increase in PPC rates occurred among successful quitters. Pending more definitive research, clinicians should recommend cigarette cessation if at least 2 months can elapse between the quit date and the elective surgery.

Several potential strategies do not reduce PPC risk and should not be performed solely for this concern. These include intraoperative use of right heart catheterization, and enteral or total parenteral nutritional support for patients who are malnourished or who have a low serum albumin.

POSTOPERATIVE MANAGEMENT

Several of the most effective strategies to reduce PPC rates begin in the postoperative period. Among those effective strategies discussed above, these include lung expansion maneuvers, epidural analgesia, and selective (rather than routine) use of nasogastric tubes after abdominal surgery. There is no evidence that systematic surveillance for PPC after high-risk surgery, with routine postoperative chest radiographs, improves outcomes. When PPC do occur, their treatment is the same as for patients who are not undergoing surgery.

QUALITY INDICATORS

Quality indicators play an important role in the development and maintenance of a high-quality, safe, hospitalist-based medical consultation program. Recognition of unexpectedly high PPC rates on, for example, a particular surgical floor or service, may prompt a root cause analysis to identify factors that contribute to this risk. The principal outcome-based quality indicator regarding pulmonary assessment would be PPC themselves: pneumonia, respiratory failure, atelectasis requiring treatment, and exacerbation of preexisting COPD or asthma. Postoperative pulmonary embolism has differing risk factors and effective preventive strategies; it would not be included among PPC for purposes of assessing outcomes.

Intermediate process measures are also important quality indicators. Their measurement may help to identify deviations from standards of care and prompt interventions to reduce practice variation. These include (1) cigarette cessation counseling for smokers before elective surgery, (2) use of lung expansion maneuvers after high-risk surgeries (abdominal, thoracic, and aortic), (3) proper implementation of postoperative analgesia, and (4) rates of nasogastric tube use after abdominal surgery.

PATIENT EDUCATION

Patient education plays only a small role in a comprehensive program to reduce PPC rates. Most interventions are the responsibility of the clinicians. However, patients can control several risk factors for PPC. These include active participation in a plan for preoperative smoking cessation (with at least 2 months before elective surgery), preoperative learning of planned postoperative lung expansion maneuvers (or participation in an inspiratory muscle training program if recommended), and prompt reporting to the responsible physician of any preoperative worsening of symptoms or lung function among patients with asthma or COPD. In addition, patients may learn the symptoms that may suggest a postoperative pulmonary complication and the need to proactively report such symptoms to nursing staff.

SUMMARY

PPCs are common, morbid, and contribute to prolonged length of stay and unplanned intensive care unit transfers. Risk factors are now well established and include both patient-related and procedure-related factors. Surgical site is the single most important predictor; other important factors include ASA classification, age, CHF, and COPD. Laboratory testing only rarely adds value to the clinical risk assessment. Routine spirometry does not refine the risk assessment or reduce PPC rates. Chest radiography may be helpful for patients with existing cardiopulmonary disease or unexplained dyspnea who are undergoing high-risk surgeries. For patients at high risk for PPC, effective strategies to reduce risk include preoperative inspiratory muscle training, smoking cessation if there is adequate time available before elective surgery, postoperative lung expansion maneuvers, postoperative epidural analgesia, and the selective use of nasogastric tubes after abdominal surgery. Quality indicators include overall PPC rates as well as rates of process measures including proven strategies to reduce risk.

REFERENCES

1. Lawrence VA, Hilsenbeck SG, Noveck H, Poses RM, Carson JL. Medical complications and outcomes after hip fracture repair. *Arch Intern Med.* Oct 14 2002;162(18):2053–2057.
2. Fleischmann K, Goldman L, Young B, Lee T. Association between cardiac and noncardiac complications in patients undergoing noncardiac surgery: outcomes and effects on length of stay. *Am J Med.* 2003;115:515–520.
3. Qaseem A, Snow V, Fitterman N, et al. Risk assessment for and strategies to reduce perioperative pulmonary complications for patients undergoing noncardiothoracic surgery: a guideline from the American College of Physicians. *Ann Intern Med.* 2006;144:575–580.
4. Smetana GW, Lawrence VA, Cornell JE. Preoperative pulmonary risk stratification for noncardiothoracic surgery: systematic review for the American College of Physicians. *Ann Intern Med.* 2006;144:581–595.
5. American Society of Anesthesiologists. ASA Physical Status Classification System. 2010. Available at http://www.asahq.org/clinical/physicalstatus.htm. Accessed Octorber 1, 2010.

6. Lee T, Marcantonio E, Mangione C, et al. Derivation and prospective validation of a simple index for prediction of cardiac risk of major noncardiac surgery. *Circulation.* 1999;100:1043–1049.

7. Warner DO, Warner MA, Barnes RD, et al. Perioperative respiratory complications in patients with asthma. *Anesthesiology.* 1996;85(3):460–467.

8. Hwang D, Shakir N, Limann B, et al. Association of sleep-disordered breathing with postoperative complications. *Chest.* 2008;133:1128–1134.

9. Chung F, Yegneswaran B, Liao P, et al. STOP questionnaire: a tool to screen patients for obstructive sleep apnea. *Anesthesiology.* May 2008;108(5):812–821.

10. Chung F, Yegneswaran B, Liao P, et al. Validation of the Berlin questionnaire and American Society of Anesthesiologists checklist as screening tools for obstructive sleep apnea in surgical patients. *Anesthesiology.* May 2008;108(5):822–830.

11. Sareli AE, Cantor CR, Williams NN, et al. Obstructive sleep apnea in patients undergoing bariatric surgery—a tertiary center experience. *Obes Surg.* Mar 2011;21(3):316–327.

12. Blouw EL, Rudolph AD, Narr BJ, Sarr MG. The frequency of respiratory failure in patients with morbid obesity undergoing gastric bypass. *AANA J.* Feb 2003;71(1):45–50.

13. Lawrence VA, Cornell JE, Smetana GW. Strategies to reduce postoperative pulmonary complications after noncardiothoracic surgery: systematic review for the American College of Physicians. *Ann Intern Med.* 2006;144:596–608.

14. Lawrence VA, Dhanda R, Hilsenbeck SG, Page CP. Risk of pulmonary complications after elective abdominal surgery. *Chest.* Sep 1996;110(3):744–750.

15. Smetana GW, Macpherson DS. The case against routine preoperative laboratory testing. *Med Clin North Am.* 2003;87:7–40.

16. Arozullah AM, Daley J, Henderson WG, Khuri SF. Multifactorial risk index for predicting postoperative respiratory failure in men after major noncardiac surgery. The National Veterans Administration Surgical Quality Improvement Program. *Ann Surg.* Aug 2000;232(2):242–253.

17. Smith TB, Stonell C, Purkayastha S, Paraskevas P. Cardiopulmonary exercise testing as a risk assessment method in non cardio-pulmonary surgery: a systematic review. *Anaesthesia.* Aug 2009;64(8):883–893.

18. Arozullah AM, Khuri SF, Henderson WG, Daley J. Participants in the National Veterans Affairs Surgical Quality Improvement Program. Development and validation of a multifactorial risk index for predicting postoperative pneumonia after major noncardiac surgery [update of Ann Intern Med. 2001 Nov 20;135(10):919–21]. *Ann Intern Med.* Nov 20 2001;135(10):847–857.

19. Johnson RG, Arozullah AM, Neumayer L, Henderson WG, Hosokawa P, Khuri SF. Multivariable predictors of postoperative respiratory failure after general and vascular surgery: results from the patient safety in surgery study. *J Am Coll Surg.* 2007;204(6):1188–1198.

20. Thomas JA, McIntosh JM. Are incentive spirometry, intermittent positive pressure breathing, and deep breathing exercises effective in the prevention of postoperative pulmonary complications after upper abdominal surgery? A systematic overview and meta-analysis. *Phys Ther.* Jan 1994;74(1):3–10; discussion 10–16.

21. Hulzebos E, Helders P, Favie N, de Bie R. Brutel de la Riviere A, van Meeteren N. Preoperative intensive inspiratory muscle training to prevent postoperative pulmonary complications in high-risk patients undergoing CABG surgery. A randomized clinical trial. *JAMA.* 2006;296:1851–1857.

22. Nelson R, Edwards S, Tse B. Prophylactic nasogastric decompression after abdominal surgery. *Cochrane Database Syst Rev.* 2007;(3):CD004929.

23. Liu SS, Wu CL. Effect of postoperative analgesia on major postoperative complications: a systematic update of the evidence. *Anesth Analg.* Mar 2007;104(3):689–702.

24. Rodgers A, Walker N, Schug S, et al. Reduction of postoperative mortality and morbidity with epidural or spinal anaesthesia: results from overview of randomised trials. *BMJ.* Dec 16 2000;321(7275):1493.

25. Berg H, Roed J, Viby-Mogensen J, et al. Residual neuromuscular block is a risk factor for postoperative pulmonary complications. A prospective, randomised, and blinded study of postoperative pulmonary complications after atracurium, vecuronium and pancuronium. *Acta Anaesthesiol Scand.* Oct 1997;41(9):1095–1103.

26. Murphy GS, Szokol JW, Marymont JH, Greenberg SB, Avram MJ, Vender JS. Residual neuromuscular blockade and critical respiratory events in the postanesthesia care unit. *Anesth Analg.* Jul 2008;107(1):130–137.
27. Moller AM, Villebro N, Pedersen T, Tonnesen H. Effect of preoperative smoking intervention on postoperative complications: a randomised clinical trial. *Lancet.* Jan 12 2002;359(9301):114–117.
28. Lindstrom D, Sadr Azodi O, Wladis A, et al. Effects of a perioperative smoking cessation intervention on postoperative complications: a randomized trial. *Ann Surg.* Nov 2008;248(5):739–745.

CHAPTER 11

ASSESSING AND MANAGING ENDOCRINE DISORDERS

David Wesorick

DIABETES AND HYPERGLYCEMIA

Introduction

A distinct set of skills and knowledge is required to successfully manage diabetes and hyperglycemia in the perioperative setting. As it pertains to diabetes management, the perioperative period is a time of chaos, with the patient experiencing changes in diet, medications, and insulin resistance. At the same time, the responsibility for managing the diabetes shifts from the patient to the healthcare team. This section will discuss the assessment and the perioperative management of the patient with diabetes and/or hyperglycemia.

Epidemiology

It has been estimated that close to 20% of patients undergoing surgery in the United States are known to have diabetes mellitus.[1] In addition, hyperglycemia often occurs after surgery in patients who were not previously known to have a diagnosis of diabetes.

History

A good medical history is the key to assessing diabetes in the perioperative setting.

Before surgery, the primary objective is to understand the patient's baseline metabolic control and management strategy. The history should include a detailed account of all of the following: the diabetes medications used, the frequency of blood glucose monitoring, the baseline glycemic control, the most recent hemoglobin A1c (HbA1c) level, the frequency of hypoglycemia, any signs of hypoglycemia

Perioperative Medicine: Medical Consultation and Co-Management, First Edition.
Edited by Amir K. Jaffer and Paul J. Grant.
© 2012 Wiley-Blackwell. Published 2012 by John Wiley & Sons, Inc.

unawareness, and recent events suggesting metabolic instability such as emergency room visits and/or hospitalizations. An assessment of possible diabetes-related complications, such as neuropathy, retinopathy, and nephropathy, is also appropriate, as is an assessment of cardiac risk.

Testing

Most patients with diabetes require limited testing in the preoperative setting. The preoperative laboratory evaluation for most patients with diabetes should include an HbA1c level (if not already performed in the last 3 months). A fasting glucose level is also appropriate for those patients that do not check their own blood glucose levels regularly. Other labs might include measures to assess chronic diabetes complications, such as a serum creatinine to assess renal function.

In the postoperative setting, regular bedside glucose testing should be performed for all diabetes patients, and for any patients noted to have significant hyperglycemia. Traditionally, glucose testing has been performed with each meal and at bedtime in patients that are eating regular meals, and at least four times daily in fasting patients. But the frequency of bedside glucose testing depends on several variables, including the type of nutrition that the patient is receiving and the stability of the patient's blood glucoses.

Patients who are found to have new hyperglycemia postoperatively should undergo HbA1c testing to help ascertain the degree of preoperative hyperglycemia. This can be helpful in differentiating undiagnosed diabetes from self-limited, stress-induced hyperglycemia, as discussed more below.

Management

Successful management of diabetes is predicated on stability and consistency, especially with respect to diet and medication management. In the perioperative setting, however, stability and consistency are often lost and the environment becomes one of relative chaos. Consistent carbohydrate intake becomes impossible as the patient fasts for the procedure; usual medications are held and new medications are added; and glycemic control is undermined by the counter-regulatory hormones that are released as a response to the stress of surgery. Surgical patients often require significant modifications of their diabetes medical regimens to safely bring them through the chaos of surgery.

There is very little evidence on which to base recommendations for medical management of diabetes in the perioperative setting. Therefore, most of the recommendations in this section are based on the opinions of experts and the extrapolation of knowledge gained in other realms of diabetes management.[1-7]

Preoperative Management

The goal of preoperative medical management of diabetes is to allow the patient to present for the operation with adequate glycemic control and, if possible, potential to maintain metabolic control through the entire operation.

The Preoperative Management of Oral Diabetes Medications Through experience, a general approach to the management of oral diabetes medications has emerged.[6] Oral diabetes medications are usually held perioperatively. Metformin is usually held in the perioperative setting, based on its potential to exacerbate the development of lactic acidosis, which might occur if the patient were to experience shock, hypoxemia, or renal failure. However, the risk of lactic acidosis occurring secondary to metformin therapy has been exaggerated, and a Cochrane Review was unable to show any increase in the risk of developing lactic acidosis in an analysis of over 59,000 patient-years of use.[8,9] Still, it is reasonable to hold metformin in the perioperative setting in cases where there is a risk of one of these complications. Metformin is usually resumed postoperatively when the patient is stable and resuming nutritional intake. Insulin secretagogues (e.g., sulfonylureas and meglitinides) should be held when a patient is fasting, as they may cause hypoglycemia if taken in the absence of carbohydrate nutrition. The management of thiazolidinediones (e.g., rosiglitazone and pioglitazone) in the perioperative setting is probably of little consequence clinically, as these medications have long half-lives, slow onset of action, and do not usually result in hypoglycemia. Most clinicians hold these medications while the patient is fasting, and resume them once the patient is able to resume oral intake. Alpha-glucosidase inhibitors (e.g., acarbose and miglitol) are only effective when the patient is taking carbohydrates via the enteral route, and are typically held during the fasting period as well. There is little experience on which to base the perioperative use of the newer incretin-based diabetes medications (e.g., exenatide, sitagliptin, pramlintide). Many clinicians manage these medications in a manner similar to other noninsulin agents, holding them on the day of surgery and restarting them once the patient is stable and eating postoperatively.

The Preoperative Management of Insulin Regular insulin and rapid-acting insulin analogues (e.g., aspart, lispro, glulisine) are typically used to provide nutritional coverage (i.e., insulin to cover the carbohydrates in the diet). When patients are fasting in preparation for surgery, these insulin preparations are generally held.

The management of intermediate- or long-acting insulin (e.g., NPH, detemir, glargine) in the preoperative period is somewhat more complex. In order to properly manage these insulins, the clinician must understand the role that they play in the patient's regimen. This requires a basic understanding of the principles of anticipatory, physiologic insulin prescribing (a.k.a. basal–bolus insulin).[1,5,6] If this insulin is used in combination with rapid/short-acting insulin in a physiologic regimen (where there is a mix of approximately half short/rapid-acting insulin and half intermediate/long-acting insulin), then it is likely that most of the intermediate/long-acting insulin represents true basal insulin, most of which the patient will require when fasting. However, when used alone (or with insufficient short-acting insulin), they provide both basal and a nutritional coverage (i.e., some part of the intermediate- or long-acting insulin is effectively covering carbohydrate intake).

The goal of management of intermediate- and long-acting insulin when a patient is fasting before surgery is to give the patient the needed basal insulin, but to avoid causing hypoglycemia by giving more insulin than the patient needs for basal coverage. It is important to remember that type 1 diabetes patients require basal insulin *at all times*, and withholding basal insulin in this population will lead to severe metabolic derangements, including diabetic ketoacidosis (DKA). Withholding basal insulin from type 2 diabetes patients can also be detrimental, leading to progressive hyperglycemia. This means that the clinician must make a recommendation that is really nothing more than an educated guess about how much basal insulin the person will require to achieve metabolic stability through the perioperative period. The clinician can usually offer reasonable recommendations by following a few simple rules:

> *Rule #1.* A clinician can decide if it is safe to give a patient's usual dose of intermediate- or long-acting insulin on the evening before surgery by inquiring about the patient's morning glucose levels. If these levels are stable, and usually >100 mg/dL, it is probably safe to give the patient's usual dose of insulin on the evening before surgery. Some experts would recommend small reductions in the evening dose of intermediate- or long-acting insulin in some patients, especially those patients who exhibit tight glucose control in the morning, and those who are having surgery late the following day.

> *Rule #2.* Morning doses of intermediate- or long-acting insulins are usually reduced during the preoperative fasting period to avoid inducing hypoglycemia. If the intermediate- or long-acting insulin is part of a regimen that includes a balance of nutritional insulin and basal insulin, it is appropriate to administer most (e.g., 75% or more) of that dose. However, if the intermediate- or long-acting insulin is being used alone, or the dose is >60% if the total daily dose of insulin, that insulin is also providing some nutritional coverage, and a more significant dose reduction may be appropriate during the fasting period (see Table 11.1).

> *Rule #3.* The dose of peaking, intermediate-acting insulin (NPH and, to a lesser degree, detemir) should generally be reduced in a fasting patient. The administration of this type of insulin leads to peak insulin levels that might be higher than true basal needs. Table 11.1 offers some recommendations for managing intermediate-acting insulin on the day of surgery.

Premixed insulins also deserve mention here. Premixed insulins pose special challenges because they contain regular insulin or rapid-acting insulin *in combination with* intermediate- or long-acting insulin. This means that it is impossible to use this type of insulin without giving a fixed ratio of both of these insulin types. As already mentioned, the fasting patient should typically not be treated with regular insulin or rapid-acting insulin, and so the management of these patients is sometimes difficult. Management options include prescribing a separate intermediate- or long-acting insulin (the most physiologic option, but requires the patient to fill a new

TABLE 11.1.   Guidelines[a] for Management of Intermediate- and Long-Acting Insulins on the Day of Surgery

Baseline insulin regimen	Recommendations for preoperative insulin management
Morning dose of glargine as part of a regimen that includes regular or rapid-acting insulin for nutritional coverage	Give approximately 75% of glargine[b] on the morning of surgery
Morning dose of glargine when it is the patient's only insulin (including use in combination with oral agents), or if glargine is >60% of the total daily insulin dose	Give approximately 50% of glargine on the morning of surgery
Morning dose of detemir or NPH	Give approximately 50% of detemir or NPH on the morning of surgery
Premixed insulin (any combination that includes a component of regular or rapid-acting insulin, i.e., "70/30" mixes)	Significantly reduce the dose or entirely avoid giving any mixed insulin to a fasting patient, as mixed insulin contains a component of fast-acting insulin that may result in hypoglycemia if not counterbalanced by nutritional intake
Insulin pump	The basal rate of the continuous subcutaneous insulin infusion can be continued through the night prior to surgery and on the day of surgery. Management of the insulin pump intraoperatively should be determined by the managing anesthesiologist.

[a] These guidelines are only intended to illustrate the application of the general principles of physiologic insulin discussed in the text, and recommendations for individual patients may vary. These recommendations assume that the patient will be fasting on the day of surgery, and that the patient's morning blood glucose is >100. Relative hypoglycemia in this setting may necessitate additional dose modifications. The patient's baseline glycemic control and the timing of surgery may also impact decisions about dosing of these insulins while fasting.
[b] If the glargine dose is >60% of the total daily dose of insulin, give approximately 50% of the usual dose.

insulin prescription), holding the insulin altogether without replacement (this options fails to provide basal insulin, but is acceptable for some type 2 patients), or giving the premixed insulin with a significant dose reduction.

A detailed discussion of subcutaneous insulin infusion (a.k.a., insulin pumps) is beyond the scope of this text. However, established insulin pump patients often have an accurate basal rate, and as a rule, pumps can be continued as basal insulin up to (and sometimes throughout) the surgery.

Postoperative Management

The Evidence Base for Postoperative Diabetes Management   There are two major questions that arise when managing diabetes or hyperglycemia in the postoperative setting: What is the optimal blood glucose for the patient? And, how can that level of metabolic control be achieved?

There has been a reasonable amount of clinical research addressing these questions in critically ill patients. In 2001, a study of over 1500 surgical ICU patients demonstrated a mortality benefit for patients who were managed with an intravenous (IV) insulin infusion with a blood glucose target of 80–110 mg/dL compared with the control group with a blood glucose target of 180–200 mg/dL.[10] However, other studies,[11-15] including the large (n = 6104), multicenter NICE-SUGAR study,[14] have not been able to reproduce these findings. The NICE-SUGAR study divided critically ill patients into two groups. The "tight control" group was managed with an IV insulin infusion with an aggressive glycemic target of 81–108 mg/dL (actual average mean glucose achieved: 118 mg/dL). The "loose control" group aimed for a glucose level of <180 mg/dL. Even with this less aggressive goal, two-thirds of the patients in the loose control group were treated with an IV insulin infusion (actual average glucose achieved: 145 mg/dL). In this study, the loose control group experienced a lower 90-day mortality and fewer episodes of hypoglycemia. As a result, many experts now recommend avoiding tight control (as defined in the NICE-SUGAR protocol) and recommend targets that are more consistent with the glucoses that were achieved in the loose control group.[16] An American Diabetes Association (ADA) and American Association of Clinical Endocrinologists (AACE) consensus statement recommends that the target glucose for critically ill patients should be 140–180 mg/dL.[17]

In critically ill patients, IV insulin infusions have become the method of choice for controlling blood glucoses.[18] This trend is based on clinical experience illustrating the practical advantages of insulin infusions in these patients. IV insulin infusions provide the most easily titrated and flexible insulin delivery method, but at the cost of requiring close monitoring and greater nursing resources.

Unfortunately, there are currently no prospective trials examining the optimal blood glucose level in noncritically ill surgical patients. Basic science research suggests that hyperglycemia has acute, adverse effects. For example, hyperglycemia in some models has been shown to cause neutrophil dysfunction, impairment of vascular endothelial function, alterations in the coagulation system, and gastroparesis, all of which may be detrimental in the postoperative setting.[1] Moreover, observational studies have shown an association between hyperglycemia and mortality in surgical and nonsurgical inpatients.[19-21] Other observational studies have demonstrated an association between surgical infections and hyperglycemia.[21-25] However, in the absence of prospective studies, it is uncertain whether the hyperglycemia actually contributes to the development of these undesirable outcomes, or is simply a marker of a more severely ill group of patients. With the exception of the ICU studies discussed above, there have not been prospective studies examining the effect of varying levels of glycemic control on hard outcomes in surgical patients. Therefore, there are limited data on which to base postoperative glycemic targets for this patient population. An ADA/AACE consensus statement recommends that the fasting blood glucose target for noncritically ill, hospitalized patients should be <140 mg/dL, and that random glucoses should be less than 180 mg/dL, based on the opinion of experts.[17] Given the lack of outcomes data supporting these targets, they

TABLE 11.2.   Summary of Inpatient Glycemic Goals and the Best Methods for Achieving them

Patient type	Glycemic target[a]	Method of control
Critically ill	140–180 mg/dL	Typically IV insulin infusion
Noncritically ill	<140 mg/dL (fasting) <180 mg/dL (random)	Typically subcutaneous insulin but will depend on patient circumstances and characteristics (see text and Table 11.3)

[a] Recommendations are based on expert opinion.

must be viewed as general guidelines, as opposed to hard targets. Moreover, individualization of these targets is appropriate, considering the patient's risk for hypoglycemia, functional and cognitive status, preferences, and life expectancy.[7] A summary of inpatient glycemic goals is shown in Table 11.2.

There is very little evidence defining precise methods for achieving glycemic control in noncritically ill patients. Recommendations about how to manage diabetes and hyperglycemia in the postoperative setting in these patients are based on expert opinion, and discussed in detail below.

An Overview of Postoperative Glycemic Management   The decision about how to best manage a patient with diabetes in the postoperative setting requires the careful consideration of several variables, including the severity of the patient's illness/surgery, the patient's level of stability, the patient's nutritional circumstances, the type of diabetes (1 or 2), and the degree of metabolic dysfunction present. An assessment of these variables can help the clinician decide if the patient can simply resume the preoperative diabetes medications after surgery, or if modifications will be necessary.

How Ill/Unstable Is the Patient?   Stable patients after minor surgery usually do not experience a severe counter-regulatory hormone response, and typically can resume a regular diet immediately after surgery. In most cases, these patients can be managed postoperatively by simply restarting the preoperative medical regimen. In contrast, patients undergoing major surgery often require a period of monitoring and recovery after surgery, and may experience more dramatic glycemic changes related to stronger counter-regulatory hormone responses. In these patients, oral diabetes medications are usually avoided, and a subcutaneous insulin regimen is often appropriate. Critically ill patients may experience rapid changes in stability, and their insulin regimens must be highly flexible. In these patients, the standard of care has become the use of IV insulin infusion therapy, when needed, to achieve reasonable blood glucose control.

Can the Patient Eat?   This question often mirrors the previous question, because the patients who are the most severely ill are the most likely to experience major changes in nutrition. Patients often experience interruptions in nutrition after surgery (e.g., to allow the resumption of bowel function after intra-abdominal surgery). These patients may fast for a period of several days and the postoperative diabetes management regimen must be fundamentally different than the preoperative regimen. Oral agents are usually inappropriate in this setting, and regular and rapid-acting insulins must be used with caution to avoid hypoglycemia. However, many of these patients will require a basal level of insulin to avoid severe metabolic disturbances. Some type 2 diabetes patients (e.g., those not on insulin preoperatively) might be managed through a period of fasting with the use of intermittent insulin injections (i.e., supplemental insulin, as discussed below). However, if these patients experience blood glucoses outside of the target range, more aggressive insulin regimens using basal insulin should be employed. Most type 2 diabetes patients who are treated with insulin in the preoperative setting will require some basal insulin postoperatively, even when fasting. Of course, type 1 diabetes patients always require a basal rate of insulin to avoid DKA, and these patients are often most easily managed via the use of an IV insulin infusion until stable nutrition can be resumed.

What Is the Patient's Current Glycemic Control?

Patients who have a dramatic loss of metabolic control in the postoperative setting may require intensive treatment. Generally, oral diabetes medications are not appropriate for rapidly intensifying treatment. There are no evidence-based rules for determining which levels of hyperglycemia require more intensive treatment in noncritically ill patients, but patients with severely deranged metabolic control are often treated with IV insulin infusions initially.

Table 11.3 presents an overview of postoperative diabetes management based on the patient's characteristics and clinical circumstances.

The Postoperative Management of Oral Diabetes Medications

As discussed above, oral agents are not well-suited to the management of unstable, fasting, or severely hyperglycemic patients postoperatively. These agents are slow acting and difficult to rapidly titrate. However, in patients who are stable, eating, and have no contraindication, the resumption of the oral home regimen may be appropriate.

The Postoperative Management of Subcutaneous Insulin

Insulin is the drug of choice for the treatment of most hyperglycemic patients in the postoperative setting. Insulin is indicated in the immediate postoperative setting for all patients that were using insulin preoperatively, and all patients who have postoperative blood glucose levels consistently out of the target range. Subcutaneous insulin is fast acting, easily titrated, and rarely contraindicated.

In some cases, the patient's home insulin regimen can simply be resumed in the postoperative setting. The patient's home regimen should be used when the patient is stable, tolerating his usual nutrition, and without significant glycemic abnormalities. In these cases, the addition of supplemental insulin (written as a sliding scale) may help to correct mild hyperglycemia that might occur in the postoperative setting.

However, in many cases, the patient's home insulin regimen requires modification to appropriately suit the patient's needs in the postoperative setting. Patients that are unstable, fasting, or experiencing hyperglycemia despite the home insulin

TABLE 11.3. General Overview of Postoperative Management of Diabetes and Hyperglycemia

Patient characteristics and circumstances	Management recommendations
Stable (i.e., clinically stable after minor surgery) Without nutritional issues (i.e., able to resume a diet soon after surgery) Not experiencing significant hyperglycemia[a]	• Resume preoperative (home) diabetes regimen • Close monitoring of glycemic control perioperatively • Consider supplemental insulin

Uncertain stability (i.e., being monitored after major surgery)
With moderately complex nutritional issues (i.e., type 2 diabetes patient expected to have a significant period of fasting)
Experiencing significant hyperglycemia but not severe hyperglycemia[a]
	• Subcutaneous insulin is the agent of choice
	  ○ Consider use of the preoperative (home) insulin regimen + supplemental insulin in patients who will receive nutrition, and without significant hyperglycemia[b]
	  ○ Consider a physiologic insulin regimen (i.e., basal–nutritional–supplemental) in patients who are unable to take nutrition, or those with significant hyperglycemia[b]

Unstable (i.e., critically ill) With complex nutritional issues (i.e., type 1 diabetes patient expected to have a significant period of fasting) Experiencing severe hyperglycemia[a]	• Continuous intravenous insulin infusion

[a] Severe hyperglycemia is variably defined as blood glucose levels consistently >250–300.
[b] Significant hyperglycemia is defined as blood glucose levels consistently outside of the target range.

regimen require a customized postoperative insulin regimen. Most experts agree that the best way to provide such a regimen is via the use of an anticipatory, physiologic insulin regimen (aka basal–bolus insulin).[1,5,6] Quality improvement studies in hospitalized patients have demonstrated improvements in glycemic control when these principles were used to guide interventions.[26,27] To do this successfully, the clinician must estimate an appropriate dose of insulin, and prescribe it in a way that gives approximately one-half of the dose as basal insulin (insulin that is given even if the patient is fasting), and the other half as nutritional insulin (insulin that is given to match the carbohydrate intake of the patient, and held if the patient is fasting). Supplemental insulin (insulin that is given in small amounts in addition to basal and nutritional insulin to correct for hyperglycemia, written in a sliding-scale format) is usually also added to a physiologic regimen. Importantly, the patient's blood glucose should be carefully monitored, and the insulin regimen should be adjusted accordingly. Changes in the patient's insulin needs in the postoperative setting should be anticipated. Recovery from the stress of surgery often results in a gradual decrease in insulin resistance. A simplified approach to using insulin in the postoperative setting is shown in Figure 11.1.

The Challenge of Matching Nutritional Insulin with Nutritional Intake
Using the approach illustrated above, it is relatively easy to estimate a reasonable insulin dose, and to administer the basal portion of the regimen. However, one of

Step 1. Estimate the dose of insulin:

The **total daily dose (TDD)** of insulin is the total number of units of insulin that a patient requires over the course of a day to meet basal and nutritional needs. It can be estimated in two different ways:

- Consider the TDD of insulin that the patient required before hospitalization, and the glycemic control achieved on that regimen. Adjust dose(s) accordingly.

- Weight-based estimation: TDD (in units) = the patient's weight (in kg) × N (units/kg/day). Select multiplier based on the features listed in the table.

Dose-guiding features	N (units/kg/day)
Likely insulin sensitive (lean or malnourished patients, especially if type 1 diabetes), elderly, acute or chronic kidney disease (especially dialysis requiring)	0.3
Patients with neither features of insulin sensitivity nor insulin resistance	0.4
Likely insulin resistant (obese), or receiving high doses of corticosteroids	0.5–0.6 or higher

Step 2. Determine the patient's nutritional status, and how the TDD should be given:

- Give approximately one-half of the TDD as basal insulin.
    - Usually given regardless of the patients nutritional intake.
    - Usually given as a long-acting insulin analogue (e.g., glargine) once or twice daily, or as an intermediate-acting insulin analogue (NPH, detemir) twice daily.
- Give approximately one-half of the TDD as nutritional insulin, to match the patient's nutritional intake.
    - Usually given as boluses of regular insulin or a rapid-acting insulin analogue, at the time of nutrition intake.
    - Nutritional insulin must be matched to nutritional intake, and is held when a patient is fasting.
- Give supplemental insulin (written in a sliding-scale format) in addition to the insulin above to correct for unexpected hyperglycemic episodes.

Step 3. Frequently assess blood glucose control and nutritional circumstances, and adjust the regimen as needed.

Figure 11.1. Stepwise approach to the physiologic use of insulin in the postoperative patient.

the key challenges to effectively using subcutaneous insulin in the postoperative setting is matching a patient's nutrition to the appropriate insulin. If a patient is not getting any nutrition, this component of the insulin regimen is held. If patients are eating, but intake is sporadic, the subcutaneous bolus of a rapid-acting insulin analogue can be given *after* the patient eats a meal, *in proportion to what was eaten.*

Special Nutritional Circumstances   After surgery, not all patients resume a regular diet of three meals per day. Sometimes other nutritional strategies such as enteral or parenteral nutrition are employed. Table 11.4 shows the Society of Hospital Medicine Glycemic Control Task Force recommendations for insulin regimens for a variety of nutritional situations.[6]

The Use of Sliding-Scale Insulin   A common way of prescribing insulin in the hospital is by "sliding scale." Sliding-scale insulin refers to insulin that is administered in a dose that depends on the glucose level at the time of administration. On one hand, this seems to be a very logical way to prescribe insulin in situations where it is uncertain how much insulin the patient might need. However, the goal of diabetes management is to provide the patient with the necessary insulin *in an anticipatory manner*, with scheduled insulin (as opposed to an approach that simply reacts to hyperglycemia). The use of sliding-scale insulin, unaccompanied by scheduled insulin, is a reactive strategy that has been associated with poor glycemic control.[26,28] One randomized trial has shown that the use of sliding-scale insulin alone is inferior to a basal–bolus insulin regimen in hospitalized type 2 diabetes patients.[29]

The Postoperative Management of IV Insulin   Through experience, it has become clear that the most flexible way of delivering insulin is via an IV infusion. IV insulin acts rapidly and has a half-life that is on the order of minutes, so changes made to the infusion rate have an almost immediate effect. IV insulin infusions are especially useful in situations where a patient's clinical instability demands minute-to-minute flexibility in the insulin regimen (e.g., critically ill patients, high-complexity patients). IV insulin infusion are also indicated when it is necessary to rapidly attain control of severe hyperglycemia, or when a fasting patient is difficult to control (e.g., a fasting type 1 diabetes patient, or a poorly controlled, fasting type 2 diabetes patient). In general, dextrose should be added to the IV fluids of any fasting patient that is receiving insulin. IV infusion orders should be standardized and used only in settings that have trained personnel and protocols that allow for safe management.[18]

The Transition from an Inpatient to an Outpatient Medical Regimen   For patients that are hyperglycemic after surgery, deciding on the best medical regimen for discharge can be difficult. When approaching discharge, the postoperative patient may be receiving a diabetes regimen that is different from the home regimen, blood glucose control might be different than is usual at home, and the postoperative diet and insulin resistance may be changing as well. So, a patient may be stable for discharge from a surgical standpoint before the patient's diabetes has returned to its presurgical state. This is particularly true for patients with hyperglycemia that is

TABLE 11.4. Society of Hospital Medicine (SHM) Glycemic Control Task Force Recommendations: Preferred Insulin Regimens for Different Nutritional Situations

Nutritional situation	Necessary insulin components	Preferred regimen[a]
NPO (or clear liquids)	Basal insulin: 50% of TDD Nutritional insulin: none	*Basal insulin*: glargine given once daily *or* detemir given twice daily. *Nutritional insulin*: none *Correctional insulin*: regular insulin q 6 h *or* RAA insulin q 4 h. *Other comments*: dextrose infusion (e.g., D5-containing solution at 75–150 cc/h) recommended when nutrition is held. An IV insulin infusion is preferred for management of prolonged fasts or fasting type 1 diabetes patients.
Eating meals	Basal insulin: 50% of TDD Nutritional insulin: 50% of TDD, divided equally before each meal	*Basal insulin*: glargine given once daily *or* detemir given twice daily. *Nutritional insulin*: RAA insulin with meals. *Correctional insulin*: RAA insulin with meals and at bedtime (reduced dose at bedtime).
Bolus tube feeds	Basal insulin: 40% of TDD Nutritional insulin: 60% of the TDD, divided equally before each bolus feed	*Basal insulin*: glargine given once daily *or* detemir given twice daily. *Nutritional insulin*: RAA insulin with each bolus. *Correctional insulin*: RAA insulin with each bolus.
Continuous tube feeds	Basal insulin: 40% (conservative) of TDD Nutritional insulin: 60% of the TDD in divided doses	*Basal insulin*: glargine given once daily *or* detemir given twice daily. *Nutritional insulin*: RAA insulin q 4 h *or* regular insulin q 6 h. *Correctional insulin*: Should match nutritional insulin choice.
Parenteral nutrition	Insulin is usually given parenterally, with the nutrition.	Initially, a separate insulin drip allows for accurate dose finding. Then, 80% of the amount determined as TDD using drip is added to subsequent TPN bags as regular insulin. Use correctional subcutaneous insulin doses cautiously, in addition.

[a] Note: These are the preferred regimens for most patients in these situations by consensus of the SHM Glycemic Control Task Force. Alternate regimens may appropriately be preferred by institutions or physicians to meet the needs of their own patient population.
NPO, "nothing by mouth"; TDD, total daily dose; RAA, rapid-acting analogue insulins (which include lispro, aspart, and glulisine); TPN, total parenteral nutrition.
Taken from Wesorick et al.[6], with permission.

newly recognized in the postoperative state. It is very difficult to predict how a patient's glycemic control will change in the days to weeks after surgery, and which treatment, if any, should be given at discharge. Ultimately, close outpatient follow-up is the best way to deal with this uncertainty.

The measurement of the HbA1c level can be very helpful in further characterizing a patient's glycemic status when hyperglycemia is encountered in the postoperative setting.[30] The HbA1c is a marker of glycemic control over time and provides information about the patient's glycemic status prior to any perturbations related to the surgery. Table 11.5 shows how the HbA1c level can be used to make decisions

TABLE 11.5. Using Hemoglobin A1c[a] Data to Characterize a Hyperglycemic Patient's Baseline Glycemic Control and Guide Management Postoperatively

Type of patient	HbA1c level (recent average blood glucose represented by this HbA1c level)	Characterization of the patient's glycemic situation	Suggested management
Preoperative history of diabetes	≤7% (≤154 mg/dL)	Adequate glucose control preoperatively	HbA1c does not suggest need for intensification of diabetes medication regimen
	>7% (>154 mg/dL)	Glucose control probably not at goal preoperatively	HbA1c suggests possible opportunity for diabetes medication regimen intensification, especially for those patients with an HbA1c that is significantly >7
No preoperative history of diabetes	≤5.2% (≤103 mg/dL)	Unlikely to develop diabetes	HbA1c suggests that long-term medical management will not be needed
	5.3–6.4% (105–138 mg/dL)	Unable to diagnose diabetes, but may be at increased risk for diabetes if HbA1c >6%	HbA1c suggests that monitoring of glycemic status may be appropriate, especially if >6%
	≥6.5% (≥140 mg/dL)	Meets diagnosis of diabetes	HbA1c suggests need for initiation of diabetes treatment and follow-up
	≥8.5% (≥197 mg/dL)	Diabetes with poor preoperative glycemic control	HbA1c suggests need for more aggressive initial diabetes treatment (e.g., combination medical therapy or insulin therapy)

[a] The HbA1c is just one of many pieces of clinical data that must be considered in decisions about treatment of hyperglycemia and diabetes, and this table should only be viewed as a rough guide to these decisions.

about treatment of hyperglycemia after surgery.[31,32] Scientific investigation of the use of HbA1c in the postoperative setting is limited, and the use of the HbA1c in this setting represents an extrapolation of how this test is used in other settings. Although the HbA1c can be useful in the perioperative setting, the test does have important limitations. The HbA1c is not reliable (and will be artificially low) in settings of high red blood cell turnover such as hemolysis or bleeding (with reticulocytosis), or recent red blood cell transfusion.

Importantly, the insulin regimen that is employed in the postoperative period in the hospital may not be appropriate for discharge. Although basal–bolus insulin regimens may be advantageous for achieving good glycemic control in the hospital, they are often too complex for patients to manage themselves. Therefore, clinicians must consider the patient's preferences, goals, cognitive and functional status, and life expectancy when deciding when and how to intensify the insulin regimen. A detailed discussion of the initiation and intensification of medical treatment in diabetes is beyond the scope of this text, but can be found elsewhere.[33]

Patient Education

All patients suffering from postoperative hyperglycemia should be given specific instructions for medication use and glycemic monitoring at home after discharge. Patients given new insulin prescriptions should be taught "insulin survival skills," including how to self-administer insulin, how to check their blood glucose, how to recognize and respond to low blood glucoses, and when to call the doctor.[30]

Thyroid Disease

The physiologic effects of thyroid hormones are wide ranging, so it makes sense that active thyroid disease might influence the outcome of surgery.[4,34,35] Clinicians must be able to recognize severe thyroidal illness in the preoperative setting, so that optimal management can be assured.

Hypothyroidism

Although there are no prospective studies of the effects of hypothyroidism on surgical outcomes, observational studies offer some information. In one study, 40 patients with mild-to-moderate hypothyroidism suffered higher rates of hypotension, congestive heart failure, constipation, ileus, and neuropsychiatric complications in the perioperative period compared with 80 euthyroid control patients.[36] However, in all cases the complications were reversible, and there were no significant differences in length of stay or death. Another study found no significant difference in surgical outcomes comparing 59 mild-to-moderate hypothyroid patients to matched controls.[37] Of note, neither of these studies included significant numbers of patients with severe hypothyroidism. Many authors have concluded from these studies that mild-to-moderate hypothyroidism is not an absolute contraindication to surgery. However, rarely, surgery can precipitate myxedema coma (an extreme form of hypothyroidism that carries a high mortality rate) in hypothyroid patients.[38,39]

Thyroid hormone testing cannot be recommended as a routine part of the preoperative assessment. Furthermore, patients with known hypothyroidism, treated with chronic hormone replacement and monitored with periodic thyroid-stimulating hormone (TSH) levels, typically do not need any specific assessment in preparation for surgery. However, if patients complain of symptoms that might be caused by hypothyroidism (e.g., cognitive impairment, cold intolerance, constipation/ileus, menstrual changes, and unexplained weight gain) or they have objective findings that raise the possibility of the diagnosis (e.g., delayed relaxation phase of deep tendon reflexes, nonpitting edema [including periorbital], bradycardia, pericardial effusion, goiter, and hyponatremia), laboratory screening with a serum TSH is appropriate.

Perioperative Management For patients with known hypothyroidism who are stable on levothyroxine treatment, the oral form of the medication can be continued throughout the perioperative period. While brief interruptions in treatment are of little consequence due to the long half-life of the medication, patients who are unable to take or absorb the medication for a period of over 7 days should be treated with daily IV levothyroxine (at 80% of the usual oral dose).[34]

For patients with a new diagnosis of hypothyroidism in the preoperative setting, the treatment strategy depends on the severity of the disease, the urgency of surgery, and the presence or absence of underlying heart disease (see Table 11.6).[4,40] Patients with overt symptoms, significant clinical findings of hypothyroidism, or

TABLE 11.6. Perioperative Management of Hypothyroidism

Severity of hypothyroidism	Perioperative management
Severe hypothyroidism (overt symptoms, significant clinical findings, severely decreased hormone levels)	Elective surgery • Delay surgery to allow treatment[a] • Consider endocrinology consultation Urgent/emergent surgery • If surgery cannot be delayed, consider aggressive intravenous thyroid hormone treatment to prevent myxedema coma • Optimal medical treatment is controversial, endocrinology consultation is appropriate • If treating with thyroid hormone emergently, also treat empirically for concomitant adrenal insufficiency
Mild–moderate hypothyroidism (absence of features above)	Elective surgery • Consider delaying surgery, based on the elective nature of the surgery, to allow treatment[a] Urgent/emergent surgery • Proceed with surgery, monitoring for complications of hypothyroidism • Initiate treatment[a]

[a] Treatment in most cases is oral levothyroxine, unless the disease severity warrants intravenous treatment. A typical initial dose of oral levothyroxine is 50 μg/day but should be reduced in the elderly and in patients with known or suspected ischemic heart disease.

very low thyroid hormone levels should be considered to have severe disease,[41] and surgery should be delayed, if possible, until the patient can be made euthyroid with treatment. There is a lack of evidence to guide the treatment of these patients if they require urgent or emergent surgery, but they are often treated with aggressive hormone replacement (i.e., IV levothyroxine, IV triiodothyroxine, or both) to avoid precipitation of myxedema coma by the surgery.[38,40]

Patients with significant hypothyroidism *and* underlying ischemic cardiac disease present an interesting challenge. The administration of exogenous thyroid hormone in these patients can exacerbate symptoms of ischemia.[41] Two small reports suggest that patients with mild-to-moderate hypothyroidism may have good outcomes from cardiac surgery performed without the administration of exogenous thyroid hormone,[42,43] and some experts have recommended that these patients undergo any indicated coronary revascularization before the initiation of thyroid hormone therapy. However, this approach is based on very limited data and is controversial. In any case, patients with ischemic cardiac disease are often treated with very small initial doses of levothyroxine (e.g., 25 µg/day to start) and the dose is gradually titrated, monitoring for adverse cardiac effects.[44]

Hyperthyroidism

As is the case with hypothyroidism, routine laboratory screening for hyperthyroidism before surgery is not recommended. However, a preoperative review of systems might reveal symptoms suggestive of hyperthyroidism (e.g., heat intolerance, palpitations, anxiety, sweating, tremor, and unexplained weight loss). Other findings suggestive of hyperthyroidism include goiter, thyroid nodules, tachycardia, atrial fibrillation, rapid relaxation phase of the deep tendon reflexes, lid lag, or findings specific to Grave's disease (ophthalmopathy or dermopathy). The presence of any of these signs or symptoms should prompt testing of thyroid function with a TSH.

Perioperative Management The preferred approach to the hyperthyroid patient in the preoperative setting is to delay surgery until the patient can be rendered euthyroid by medical treatment.[35,45] Little is known about the risk of undergoing nonthyroidal surgery while suffering from untreated hyperthyroidism, but surgery in hyperthyroid patients can precipitate thyroid storm, a severe and life-threatening form of hyperthyroidism.[35,46] When hyperthyroid patients require urgent or emergent surgery, consultation with an endocrinologist can prove very helpful in guiding medical treatment.

Medications for the preoperative management of hyperthyroidism include beta-adrenergic antagonists to counter the adrenergic effects of the disease, thionamides to decrease thyroid hormone synthesis, iodine loading to inhibit the release of thyroid hormone, and corticosteroids to decrease peripheral conversion of T4 to T3. Although it may take weeks of treatment with these agents to achieve a euthyroid state, immediate use of these agents in the setting of emergent surgery may be beneficial as well.[35] A detailed discussion of the medical preparation of a hyperthyroid patient for surgery or the treatment of thyroid storm is beyond the scope of this text, but can be found elsewhere.[35,46]

REFERENCES

1. Clement S, Baithwaite SS, Magee MF, et al. Management of diabetes and hyperglycemia in hospitals. *Diabetes Care.* 2004;27:553–591.
2. Hirsch IB, McGill JB, Cryer PE, White PF. Perioperative management of surgical patients with diabetes mellitus. *Anesthesiology.* 1991;74:346–359.
3. Jacober SJ, Sowers JR. An update on perioperative management of diabetes. *Arch Intern Med.* 1999;159:2405–2411.
4. Schiff RL, Welsh GA. Perioperative evaluation and management of the patient with endocrine dysfunction. *Med Clin North Am.* 2003;87:175–192.
5. Inzucchi SE. Management of hyperglycemia in the hospital setting. *N Engl J Med.* 2006;355:1903–1911.
6. Wesorick D, O'Malley C, Rushakoff R, et al. Management of diabetes and hyperglycemia in the hospital: a practical guide to subcutaneous insulin use in the non-critically ill, adult patient. *J Hosp Med.* 2008;3(Suppl 5):s17–s28.
7. Maynard G, O'Malley CW, Kirsh SR. Perioperative care of the geriatric patient with diabetes or hyperglycemia. *Clin Geriatr Med.* 2008;24:649–665.
8. Salpeter SR, Greyber E, Pasternak GA, Salpeter EE. Risk of fatal and nonfatal lactic acidosis with metformin use in type 2 diabetes mellitus. *Cochrane Database Syst Rev.* 2009;(1):CD002967. DOI:10.1002/14651858.CD002967.pub2.
9. Misbin RI. The phantom of lactic acidosis due to metformin in patients with diabetes. *Diabetes Care.* 2004;27:1791–1793.
10. Van den Berghe G, Wouters P, Weekers F, et al. Intensive insulin therapy in critically ill patients. *N Engl J Med.* 2001;345:1359–1367.
11. Van den Berghe G, Wilmer A, Hermans G, et al. Intensive insulin therapy in the medical ICU. *N Engl J Med.* 2006;354:449–461.
12. Brunkhorst FM, Engel C, Bloos F, et al. Intensive insulin therapy and pentastarch resuscitation in severe sepsis. *N Engl J Med.* 2008;358:125–139.
13. Wiener RS, Weiner DC, Larson RJ. Benefits and risks of tight glucose control in critically ill adults: a meta-analysis. *JAMA.* 2008;300:933–944.
14. The NICE-SUGAR Study Investigators, Finfer S, Chittock DR, et al. Intensive versus conventional glucose control in critically ill patients. *N Engl J Med.* 2009;360:1283–1297.
15. Griesdale DEG, de Souza RJ, van Dam RM, et al. Intensive insulin therapy and mortality among critically ill patients: a meta-analysis including NICE-SUGAR study data. *CMAJ.* 2009;180:821–827.
16. Inzucchi SE, Siegel MD. Glucose control in the ICU—how tight is too tight? *N Engl J Med.* 2009;360:1346–1349.
17. Moghissi ES, Korytkowsk MT, DiNardo M, et al. American Association of Clinical Endocriniologists and American Diabetes Association consensus statement on inpatient glycemic control. *Diabetes Care.* 2009;32:1119–1131.
18. Ahmann AJ, Maynard G. Designing and implementing insulin infusion protocols and order sets. *J Hosp Med.* 2008;5(Suppl 5):s42–s54.
19. Umpierrez GE, Isaacs SD, Bazargan N, et al. Hyperglycemia: an independent marker of in-hospital mortality in patients with undiagnosed diabetes. *J Clin Endocrinol Metab.* 2002;87:978–982.
20. McAlister FA, Majumdar SR, Blitz S, et al. The relation between hyperglycemia and outcomes in 2471 patients admitted to the hospital with community-acquired pneumonia. *Diabetes Care.* 2005;28:810–815.
21. Yendamuri S, Fulda G, Tinkoff G. Admission hyperglycemias a prognostic indicator in trauma. *J Trauma.* 2003;55:33–38.
22. Furnary A, Zerr K, Grunkemeier G, Starr A. Continuous intravenous insulin infusion reduces the incidence of deep sternal wound infection in diabetic patients after cardiac surgical procedures. *Ann Thorac Surg.* 1999;67:352–362.
23. Furnary AP, Gao G, Grunkemeier GL, et al. Continuous insulin infusion reduces mortality in patients diabetes undergoing coronary artery bypass grafting. *J Thorac Cardiovasc Surg.* 2003;125:1007–1021.

24. Furnary A, Wu Y. Clinical effect of hyperglycemia in the cardiac surgery population: the Portland Diabetic Project. *Endocr Pract*. 2006;12:22–26.
25. Pomposelli JJ, Baxter JK, 3rd, Babineau TJ, et al. Early postoperative glucose control predicts nosocomial infection rate in diabetic patients. *JPEN J Parenter Enteral Nutr*. 1998;22:77–81.
26. Schnipper JL, Ndumele CD, Liang CL, Pendergrass ML. Effects of a subcutaneous insulin protocol, clinical education, and computerized order set on the quality of inpatient management of hyperglycemia: results of a clinical trial. *J Hosp Med*. 2009;4:16–27.
27. Maynard G, Lee J, Phillips G, et al. Improved inpatient use of basal insulin, reduced hypoglycemia, and improved glycemic control: effect of structured subcutaneous insulin orders and an insulin management algorithm. *J Hosp Med*. 2009;4:3–15.
28. Queale WS, Seidler AJ, Brancati FL. Glycemic control and sliding scale use in medical inpatients with diabetes mellitus. *Arch Intern Med*. 1997;157:545–552.
29. Umpierrez GE, Andres P, Smiley D, et al. Randomized study of basal-bolus insulin therapy in the inpatient management of patients with type 2 diabetes (Rabbit 2 trial). *Diabetes Care*. 2007;30: 2181–2186.
30. O'Malley CW, Emanuele M, Halasyamani L, Amin A. Bridge over troubled waters: safe and effective transitions of the inpatient with hyperglycemia. *J Hosp Med*. 2008;3(Suppl 5):s55–s65.
31. Greci LS, Kailasam M, Malkani S, et al. Utility of HbA1c levels for diabetes case finding in hospitalized patients with hyperglycemia. *Diabetes Care*. 2003;26:1064–1068.
32. The International Expert Committee. International Expert Committee Report on the Role of the A1c Assay in the Diagnosis of Diabetes. *Diabetes Care*. 2009;32:1327–1334.
33. Nathan DM, Buse JB, Davidson MB, et al. Management of hyperglycemia in type 2 diabetes: a consensus algorithm for the initiation and adjustment of therapy. *Diabetes Care*. 2006;8: 1963–1972.
34. Stathatos N, Wartofsky L. Perioperative management of patients with hypothyroidism. *Endocrinol Metab Clin North Am*. 2003;32:503–518.
35. Langley RW, Burch HB. Perioperative management of the thyrotoxic patient. *Endocrinol Metab Clin North Am*. 2003;32:519–534.
36. Ladenson PW, Levin AA, Ridgway EC, Daniels GH. Complications of surgery in hypothyroid patients. *Am J Med*. 1984;77:261–266.
37. Weinberg AD, Brennan MD, Gorman CA, et al. Outcome of anesthesia and surgery in hypothyroid patients. *Arch Intern Med*. 1983;143:893–897.
38. Wartofsky L. Myxedema coma. *Endocrinol Metab Clin North Am*. 2006;35:687–698.
39. Appoo JJ, Morin JF. Severe cerebral and cardiac dysfunction associated with thyroid decompensation after cardiac operations. *J Thorac Cardiovasc Surg*. 1997;114:496.
40. Bennett-Guerrero E, Kramer DC, Schwinn DA. Effects of chronic and acute thyroid hormone reduction on perioperative outcome. *Anesth Analg*. 1997;85:30–36.
41. Keating FR, Jr., Parkin TW, Selby JB, Dickenson LS. Treatment of heart disease associated with myxedema. *Prog Cardiovasc Dis*. 1960;3:364–381.
42. Myerowitz PD, Kamienski RW, Swanson DK, et al. Diagnosis and management of the hypothyroid patient with chest pain. *J Thorac Cardiovasc Surg*. 1983;86:57–60.
43. Drucker DJ, Burrow GN. Cardiovascular surgery in the hypothyroid patient. *Arch Intern Med*. 1985;145:1585–1587.
44. Woeber KA. Update in the management of hyperthyroidism and hypothroidism. *Arch Intern Med*. 2000;160:1067–1071.
45. Alderberth A, Stenstrom G, Hasselgren P. The selective β-1 blocking agent metoprolol compared with antithyroid drug and thyroxine as preoperative treatment of patients with hyperthyroidism: results from a prospective, randomized study. *Ann Surg*. 1987;205(2):182–188.
46. Burch HB, Wartofsky L. Life-threatening thyrotoxicosis: thyroid storm. *Endocrinol Metab Clin North Am*. 1993;22(2):263–277.

CHAPTER 12

ASSESSING AND MANAGING HEPATOBILIARY DISEASE

Aijaz Ahmed and Paul Martin

EPIDEMIOLOGY

The prevalence of abnormally elevated serum aminotransferases in the adult U.S. population is approximately 10%.[1-5] The role of preoperative diagnostic testing (biochemical and imaging studies) in asymptomatic and apparently healthy adults to screen for underlying liver disease is unclear.[4] Although individuals with unclear etiology for abnormally elevated serum alanine aminotransferase (ALT) levels have a higher likelihood of cardiovascular events in long-term follow-up.[3] This in turn may reflect metabolic syndrome-related obesity, diabetes mellitus, and coronary artery disease.[3] There is an ongoing debate to redefine the normal ALT level in healthy adults (<19 U/L for women and <30 U/L for men). Patients with underlying liver disease may demonstrate intermittently normal ALT levels, and some cirrhotics can present with persistently normal ALT levels.[6] Therefore, ALT alone is not a reliable screening test for underlying liver disease or to assess the state of hepatic reserve.[6]

A comprehensive preoperative clinical evaluation is the important initial step to establish surgical risk (Figure 12.1). Key components of preoperative clinical evaluation include detailed history taking and a complete physical examination. On the other hand, implementation of widespread screening for liver disease in prospective surgical patients may not be pragmatic, although subtle clues to the underlying liver disease such as a modestly reduced platelet count reflecting portal hypertension or a firm liver edge on physical examination should not be ignored. A reduction in hepatic blood supply occurs universally following administration of anesthesia in most surgical procedures and may be associated with transient liver enzyme abnormalities. These changes in hepatic perfusion are well tolerated and uneventful.

MEDICAL HISTORY

Certain ethnic groups are at increased risk for causes of chronic liver disease, for example, Asian immigrants for chronic hepatitis B based on the current Centers for

Perioperative Medicine: Medical Consultation and Co-Management, First Edition.
Edited by Amir K. Jaffer and Paul J. Grant.
© 2012 Wiley-Blackwell. Published 2012 by John Wiley & Sons, Inc.

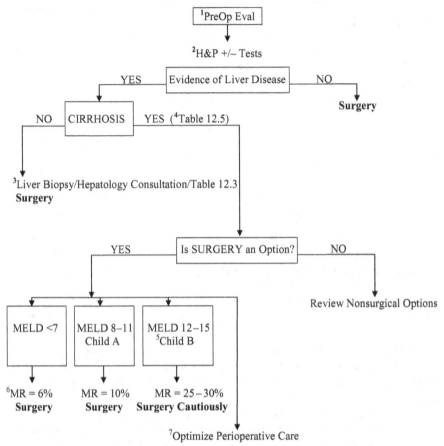

Figure 12.1. Algorithm for preoperative evaluation. [1]PreOp Eval = preoperative surgical evaluation; [2]H&P +/– Tests = history and physical examination with or without diagnostic testing for liver disease based on clinical suspicion; [3]Liver Biopsy/Hepatology Consultation/Table 12.3 = liver biopsy and hepatology consult are optional (not mandatory) and individualized, based on the complexity of surgery and presence of any contraindications to elective surgery (Table 12.3); [4]Table 12.5 = determine if surgery is contraindicated based on the number of risk factors present; [5]Child B = hepatic resection and cardiothoracic surgery is contraindicated in patients with Child class B; [6]MR = mortality rate; [7]Optimize Perioperative Care = perform surgery at a tertiary center (transplant center) with experienced team, ICU monitoring, prophylactic antibiotics, aggressive wound care, and proper nutrition. Note: Liver transplant surgery is not contraindicated in cirrhotic patients with Child class C or MELD score >20.

Disease Control (CDC) guidelines. Useful clues for underlying liver diseases include metabolic syndrome in patients with obesity, glucose intolerance, hypertension, hyperlipidemia, or history of bariatric surgery; autoimmune liver disease in patients with other autoimmune medical conditions (systemic lupus erythematosus, thyroid dysfunction, renal disease, skin disorders, rheumatoid arthritis, etc.); cholestatic liver disease, primary biliary cirrhosis (PBC), or primary sclerosing cholangitis (PSC) in patients with pruritus; PSC in patients with inflammatory bowel disease; asymptomatic mild hepatic dysfunction to advanced liver disease in patients with celiac disease; Wilson's disease in patients with visual and neuropsychiatric symptoms; hemochromatosis in patients with congestive heart disease, diabetes mellitus, and skin discoloration; viral hepatitis in patients with hemophilia, HIV infection, renal failure requiring hemodialysis and history of surgery with transfusion prior to 1992; and cirrhosis in patients with easy bruising, periodic nosebleeds, history of major gastrointestinal bleeding, jaundice (or remote history of jaundice), fluid retention, and mental status changes suspicious for hepatic encephalopathy. Allergies and active medications may help identify drug-induced hepatotoxicity. Social history should include work-related exposure to chemicals, alcohol use, injection drug use, intranasal drug use, recreational drug use, tattoos, body piercing, herbs/supplement use, over-the-counter drug use, and sexual promiscuity. If there is suspicion of excessive alcohol use, directed questioning should quantify the amount and frequency of alcohol consumption, symptoms of alcohol dependence, and alcohol-related problems such as brushes with the law for drunken driving. Family history should be obtained to rule out presence of liver disease in family members.

PHYSICAL EXAMINATION

Signs of advance liver disease may be noted during physical examination and include temporal or generalized muscle wasting, icteric sclera, Keyser–Fleisher rings, metacarpophalangeal (MCP) arthropathy, palmar erythema, spider telangiectasias, gynecomastia, testicular atrophy, firm liver edge, hepatomegaly, splenomegaly, fluid retention (ascites and peripheral edema), mental status changes suspicious for hepatic encephalopathy, and neuropsychiatric changes.

DIAGNOSTIC TESTING

If there is clinical suspicion of liver disease, further preoperative workup is crucial to establish the diagnosis and severity of liver disease.[7] Biochemical laboratory testing and imaging studies are sufficient in the majority of cases, although a liver biopsy may be needed to assess the severity of hepatic injury. Elective surgical procedure should be deferred until the completion of preoperative surgical risk assessment. Patients with features of cirrhosis on diagnostic testing (thrombocytopenia, evidence of varices, splenomegaly, shrunken and nodular liver, etc.) should be presumed to be cirrhotic. Patients with chronic liver disease without evidence of cirrhosis undergoing evaluation for a high-risk surgical procedure (e.g., a patient with chronic hepatitis C undergoing evaluation for kidney transplantation) should have a liver biopsy. In these situations, patients are at acceptable risk for surgery if they are noted to have mild-to-moderate histological damage (Stage 0, I, and II fibrosis based on Knodell Histology Activity Index criteria) and patients with evidence of bridging fibrosis or cirrhosis (Stage III and IV fibrosis based on Knodell

TABLE 12.1. CTP Scoring (Child) and Classification

	1 point	2 points	3 points
Hepatic encephalopathy	None	Grade 1–2	Grade 3–4
Ascites	Absent	Slight	Moderate
Albumin	>3.5	3.5–2.8	<2.8
Total bilirubin (for PBC or PSC)	<2	2–3	>3
	<4	4–10	>10
Prothrombin time (seconds prolonged)	<4	4–6	>6
INR	<1.7	1.7–2.3	>2.3

Total CTP scores 5–15 and Child class A to C:
CTP 5–6 = Child's class A.
CTP 7–10 = Child's class B.
CTP 11–15 = Child's class C.

TABLE 12.2. MELD Scoring Equation

MELD score for TIPSS = $0.957 \times \log_e$(creatinine mg/dL) + $0.378 \times \log_e$(bilirubin mg/dL) + 1.12
  $0 \times \log_e$(INR) + 0.643(cause of liver disease)[a]
[b]MELD score for liver transplantation = $0.957 \times \log_e$(creatinine mg/dL) + $0.378 \times \log_e$(bilirubin
  mg/dL) + $1.120 \times \log_e$(INR) + 0.643

[a] 0 if cholestatic or alcoholic liver disease, and 1 if other liver disease.
[b] Multiply by 10 and round to the nearest whole number. Laboratory values less than 1.0 are set to 1.0. The maximum serum creatinine considered in the MELD score equation is 4.0 mg/dL.

Histology Activity Index criteria) may require a more cautious approach (e.g., listing or evaluation for liver transplantation before proceeding with high-risk surgery).[8] Child–Turcotte–Pugh (CTP) score (Table 12.1) should be calculated in patients with cirrhosis to determine the CTP classification (Child class). Patients with cirrhosis are categorized as well-compensated (Child class A with a few exceptions) or decompensated cirrhosis (Child class B and C). Child class A patients with a prior history of variceal bleed, spontaneous bacterial peritonitis, and hepatocellular carcinoma should be referred to as decompensated due to poor prognosis compared with other patients with Child class A. Currently, Model for End-Stage Liver Disease (MELD) score (Table 12.2) is being increasingly utilized to predict perioperative mortality in patients with cirrhosis.

PREDICTING RISK

The key determinants of operative risk in patients with liver disease are severity of hepatic dysfunction (presence or absence of cirrhosis and severity of hepatic decompensation in patients with cirrhosis determined by Child class/MELD score), presence of comorbid medical conditions, and the planned surgical procedure (complexity

TABLE 12.3.   Absolute Contraindications to Elective Surgery in a Patient with Liver Disease

1. Acute liver failure
2. Acute viral hepatitis
3. Alcoholic hepatitis
4. Severe coagulopathy (refractory to treatment)
5. Hypoxemia
6. Cardiomyopathy
7. Unstable coronary artery disease
8. Acute renal failure
9. Multiorgan failure
10. Septicemia
11. MELD score >20 and/or Child class C in patients with cirrhosis

of surgery, elective vs. urgent/emergent, type of anesthesia, etc.). Absolute contraindications to elective surgery include acute liver failure, acute viral hepatitis, alcoholic hepatitis, severe coagulopathy (refractory to treatment), hypoxemia,
cardiomyopathy, unstable coronary artery disease, acute renal failure, multiorgan
failure, septicemia, Child class C, and MELD score >20 (Table 12.3). In the absence
of absolute contraindications to elective surgery, a comprehensive preoperative risk
assessment should be performed. In noncirrhotics, preoperative care should be individualized to optimize the outcome. In cirrhotics, surgical risk stratification should
be pursued (based on Child class and MELD score), and efficacy of nonsurgical
options should be reviewed. Although evidence-based data should be utilized to
formulate a management plan, most published data are limited by retrospective study
design.[9–14]

The risk of surgery is increased in patients with cirrhosis. Therefore, surgical
risk stratification based on Child class and MELD score are crucial in optimizing
outcomes. The perioperative mortality based on Child class in patients with cirrhosis
is as follows: Child class A 10%, Child class B 30%, and Child class C
76–82%.[9,10]Therefore, patients with Child class A are usually at acceptable risk to
undergo elective surgery, while those with Child class B are cautiously allowed with
a few exceptions (hepatic resection and cardiac surgery). Child class C is an absolute
contraindication for elective surgery (except for liver transplant surgery), and nonsurgical options are recommended. Child class influences the risk of postoperative
complications including hepatocellular failure, bleeding, hepatic encephalopathy,
refractory ascites, renal failure, hypoxia, and infection. Severe portal hypertension
is associated with increased postoperative morbidity irrespective of the Child class.
Placement of transjugular intrahepatic portosystemic shunt (TIPSS) in the preoperative period reduces the risk of morbidity.[11] The perioperative risk of mortality rises
significantly in emergency versus elective surgery (Child class A 22% vs. 10%, Child
class B 38% vs. 30%, and Child class C 100% vs. 82%).[10] However, the role of
Child classification for risk stratification is based on small retrospective studies.[9,10]
More recently, MELD score has been preferred due to its greater accuracy as a model

TABLE 12.4.   American Society of Anesthesiologists (ASA) Classification

Class	Patient
ASA class I	Healthy patient
ASA class II	Mild systemic disease without functional limitation
ASA class III	Severe systemic disease with functional limitations
ASA class IV	Severe systemic disease that is a constant threat to life
ASA class V	Moribund, not expected to survive >24 h with or without surgery
ASA class E	Emergent surgery (ASA classes I to V above)

Adapted from O'Leary et al.[4]

for postoperative mortality in patients with cirrhosis.[12] It has been estimated based on a retrospective experience that there is 1% increase in mortality rate for every 1 point increment in MELD score between 5 and 20, and a 2% increase in mortality rate for every 1 point increment in MELD score above 20.[13] Teh and colleagues defined the role of MELD score as predictor of perioperative mortality in the largest retrospective study to date.[14] In this study, 772 patients with cirrhosis who underwent major gastrointestinal (laparotomy with operative intervention on a visceral organ), orthopedic, and cardiovascular surgeries were included. Patients with laparoscopic cholecystectomy were excluded. The following mortality rates were noted based on the MELD scores: mortality rate of 5.7% for a MELD score of 7 or less; mortality rate of 10.3% for a MELD score of 8–11; and mortality rate of 25.4% for a MELD score of 12–15. The median preoperative MELD score was 8. Patients with a MELD score >15 were underrepresented (58 out of 772). In addition, Teh et al.[14] demonstrated that American Society of Anesthesiologists (ASA) class (Table 12.4) and the patient age also played a role in predicting the mortality rate. The majority of patients in this study were classified as ASA class III. Patients with ASA class IV (with ASA class III as a baseline reference group) added an equivalent of 5.5 MELD points to postoperative mortality rate. There were only 10 patients classified as ASA class V who underwent surgery and had a 100% mortality. Therefore, ASA class V is an absolute contraindication for surgery in patients with cirrhosis except for liver transplantation. ASA class was the most reliable predictor of 7-day mortality, while MELD score was the strongest predictor of 30-day, 90-day, and long-term postoperative mortality for all types of surgery. In this study, none of the patients under 30 years of age died. On the contrary, age over 70 added an equivalent of 3 MELD points to the mortality rate. This study[14] is limited by its retrospective design; results may not be generalizable to patients with MELD >15 due to underrepresentation and selection bias for patients with platelets >60,000/µL and international normalized ratio (INR) <1.5. Teh et al.[14] may have underestimated the mortality rate in patients with cardiovascular disease due to selection bias (majority of patients in this study underwent abdominal surgery) and other studies have estimated higher mortality rates for cardiothoracic surgery.[15,16] In addition, other risk factors associated with poor surgical outcomes in cirrhosis include chronic obstructive lung disease, surgery on respiratory tract, hepatic resection, open abdominal surgery (vs.

TABLE 12.5.   Risk Factors for Surgery in a Patient with Cirrhosis

1. Age (>70)
2. ASA class (classes IV and V)
3. MELD score (score >12)
4. Child class (classes B and C)
5. Complications of cirrhosis: (1) portal hypertension, (2) refractory coagulopathy (prothrombin time prolonged by >2.5 s), (3) ascites, (4) hepatic encephalopathy, (5) hepatorenal syndrome, (6) severe pulmonary hypertension, (7) hepatopulmonary syndrome, (8) hypoalbuminemia, and (9) malnutrition
6. Comorbid medical conditions: (1) anemia, (2) chronic obstructive lung disease, (3) renal failure, (4) hypoxemia, and (5) active infection
7. Surgical procedure: (1) emergency surgery, (2) cardiothoracic surgery, (3) surgery on respiratory tract, (4) hepatic resection, and (5) open abdominal surgery
8. Anesthetic agent: (1) type and (2) dose

Adapted from O'Leary et al.[4]

laparoscopic surgery), anemia, refractory coagulopathy (prothrombin time prolonged by >2.5 s), ascites, hepatic encephalopathy, renal failure, hepatorenal syndrome, hypoalbuminemia, malnutrition, hypoxemia, and active infection (Table 12.5 and Figure 12.1).[4,12,15–18]

Minor abnormalities in liver enzymes and bilirubin levels can be expected with general, spinal, and epidural anesthesia even in the absence of underlying liver disease. These fluctuations are transient and of no clinical significance in noncirrhotic patients. On the contrary, cirrhotic patients may develop overt hepatic decompensation postoperatively. The type and dose of anesthetic agent may influence the surgical outcome, while mode of anesthesia (general or spinal) is less likely to affect the outcome.[19–23] Halothane was associated with acute hepatitis in the genetically predisposed patients.[21] Halothane use has fallen out of favor. Propofol is the anesthetic of choice due to its short half-life even in decompensated liver disease.[22] In cirrhotics, the duration of action of anesthetic agents is prolonged due to ineffective hepatic metabolism and biliary excretion as a result of impaired drug–albumin binding in the setting of hypoalbuminemia. The volume of distribution of drugs may be increased in cirrhotics requiring larger doses. Suitable anesthetic agents with minimal hepatic metabolism and negligible risk of hepatitis include isoflurane, desflurane, and sevoflurane.[23] Choice of muscle relaxants include atracurium and cisatracurium as they do not require hepatic or renal clearance. Doxacurium used in longer procedures is eliminated by the kidneys. It is recommended that sedatives and narcotics be used with extreme caution in patients with underlying liver disease and in particular, cirrhotic patients with decompensated liver disease. Narcotics, which undergo first-pass hepatic breakdown, may have a prolonged effect if hypotension and poor hepatic perfusion occur. Benzodiazepines metabolized by glucuronidation (oxazepam and lorazepam) are unaffected by underlying liver disease and therefore preferred. In contrast, benzodiazepines, which undergo elimination by nonglucuronidation pathways, such as diazepam and chlordiazepoxide, may have prolonged effects. Patients with cirrhosis may develop new onset hepatic encephalopathy or worsening of existing hepatic encephalopathy with narcotics and sedatives use. Drugs with nonhepatic metabolism are preferred, such as oxazepam as a sedative and remifentanil as a narcotic.

LIVER TRANSPLANTATION

The two fundamental goals of liver transplantation are to improve survival and functional status of patients with liver failure.[24,25] Major indications for liver transplantation include acute liver failure, decompensated cirrhosis, unresectable primary hepatic malignancies, inborn metabolic disorders, and miscellaneous causes (Table 12.6).[26] First, acute liver failure accounts for approximately 6.0% of liver transplants. Candidacy for liver transplantation in patients with acute liver failure is based on selection criteria described by O'Grady et al.[27,28] at King's College Hospital and Bernuau et al.[29] at Villejuif (Table 12.7). Second, in patients with chronic liver diseases, hepatitis C-related cirrhosis is the most frequent indication for liver transplantation in the United States. Third, hepatic malignancy is now a frequent indication for liver transplantation as patients with hepatocellular carcinoma and cirrhosis are provided priority listing for liver transplantation as posttransplant survival in carefully selected cases equal that of decompensated cirrhosis without hepatocellular carcinoma. Liver transplantation provides improved survival and better cost-effectiveness compared with hepatic resection in patients with hepatocellular carcinoma in the setting of cirrhosis.[30–32] Listing criteria for patients with hepatocellular

TABLE 12.6. Indications for Liver Transplantation

Acute liver failure
   Acute hepatitis A, acute hepatitis B, and drug/toxin hepatotoxicity
Chronic liver diseases
   Chronic hepatitis B virus and chronic hepatitis C virus infection
   Alcoholic liver disease
   Autoimmune hepatitis
   Cryptogenic liver disease
   PBC and PSC
   Secondary biliary cirrhosis
α-1 antitrypsin deficiency, hereditary hemochromatosis, and Wilson's disease
   Glycogen storage disorders
   Budd–Chiari syndrome
   Polycystic liver disease
Malignancy
   Primary hepatic cancer: hepatocellular carcinoma and cholangiocarcinoma
   Metastatic: carcinoid tumors and islet cell tumors

Adapted from Ahmed and Keeffe.[26]

TABLE 12.7.   Criteria for Liver Transplantation in Fulminant Hepatic Failure

Criteria of King's College, London

Acetaminophen patients
  pH < 7.3, or
  Prothrombin time >6.5 (INR) and serum creatinine >3.4 mg/dL
Nonacetaminophen patients
  Prothrombin time >6.5 (INR), or
  Any three of the following variables:
  1. Age <10 or >40 years
  2. Etiology: non-A, non-B hepatitis; halothane hepatitis; idiosyncratic drug reaction
  3. Duration of jaundice before encephalopathy >7 days
  4. Prothrombin time >3.5 (INR)
  5. Serum bilirubin >17.5 mg/dL

Criteria of Hospital Paul-Brousse, Villejuif

Hepatic encephalopathy and Factor V level:
1. <20% in patient younger than 30 years of age, or
2. <30% in patient 30 years of age or older

INR, international normalized ratio.
Adapted from O'Grady et al.[27]

carcinoma includes solitary lesion less than 5 cm or multifocal cancer with up to three lesions, each less than 3 cm in the absence of metastatic disease.[33] The long-term tumor-free survival following liver transplantation in patients meeting the criteria is over 80%. Fourth, metabolic/genetic disorders requiring liver transplantation may include hereditary hemochromatosis, Wilson's disease, and alpha$_1$-antitrypsin deficiency. Finally, other uncommon indications for liver transplantation include polycystic liver disease and Budd–Chiari syndrome. A patient with cirrhosis can be referred for liver transplantation when the posttransplant survival rate exceeds the pretransplant life expectancy. Patients undergoing liver transplantation have a 1-year mortality rate of 10–15%. It is estimated that patients with decompensated Child class B cirrhosis have a 1-year survival rate of 85–90%. Therefore, patients with decompensated Child class B or C (CTP score 7 or higher) cirrhosis should be referred for liver transplantation. In addition, patients with Child class A cirrhosis with a history of gastrointestinal bleeding caused by portal hypertension; a single episode of systolic blood pressure (SBP); fulminant hepatic failure; and nonmetastatic, primary hepatocellular cancer are suitable candidates for liver transplantation evaluation. PBC and PSC use a different point system (Table 12.1). Other indications that may qualify patients with PBC and PSC for liver transplantation include intractable pruritus, progressive bone disease with recurrent fractures, and, in the case of PSC, recurrent bacterial cholangitis. Contraindications for liver transplantation include poor compliance, lack of adequate support system, and clinical conditions associated with poor posttransplant outcome (Table 12.8). Brain death and metastatic

TABLE 12.8.   Contraindications to Liver Transplantation

Absolute
  Brain death
  Extrahepatic malignancy
  Active uncontrolled infection
  Active substance abuse
  Acquired immunodeficiency syndrome
  Severe cardiopulmonary disease
  Inability to comply with medical regimen
Relative
  Advanced age
  Cholangiocarcinoma
  Portal vein thrombosis
  Psychological instability
  Lack of social support

Adapted from Ahmed and Keeffe.[26]

cancer are considered absolute contraindications for liver transplantation. Patients with relative contraindications should undergo preliminary discussion with the liver transplant selection committee and receive approval for pretransplant evaluation. Currently, MELD score is used for organ allocation.[34–36]

MINIMIZING RISK

It is recommended that elective procedures should be postponed to minimize the risk of surgery in the setting of absolute contraindications (Table 12.3). Patients with cirrhosis have an altered hemodynamic status at baseline (high cardiac output, arteriovenous shunting, reduced systemic vascular resistance, reduced hepatic arteriovenous perfusion, reduced portal blood flow, portal hypertension). Hepatic perfusion pressures are further compromised with induction of anesthesia during surgery. Poor baseline hepatic perfusion in the setting of cirrhosis increases the risk of hemodynamic instability following induction with anesthetic agent. It is recommended that anesthetic agents least likely to influence hepatic artery perfusion pressure (isoflurane, desflurane, and sevoflurane) be utilized. Patients with underlying liver disease should be operated by a highly skilled and experienced team (surgeons, anesthesiologists, and nursing staff). There should be a low threshold to monitor these patients in the ICU in the immediate postoperative course.

POSTOPERATIVE MANAGEMENT

Hemodynamic instability in the perioperative period can result in worsening hepatic dysfunction in patients with known liver disease. Degree and duration of intravascular volume depletion is the key determinant of severity of hepatic dysfunction. Other predictors include severity of underlying liver disease (presence or absence of cirrhosis), age of the patient, comorbid medical conditions, and complexity of the procedure performed. On the other hand, infusion of excessive fluid can result in acute hepatic congestion. Fluid overload (pulmonary edema, ascites, and peripheral edema) may lead to surgical wound complications. A careful individualized approach is needed to optimally manage a patient with underlying liver disease in the perioperative period. There should be a low threshold to use prophylactic/empiric antibiotics and monitor these patients in the ICU in the immediate postoperative course. A patient with cirrhosis should be monitored very closely for signs of hepatic decompensation in the postoperative period. An important marker of hepatic synthetic dysfunction is the prothrombin time. Other indicators of hepatic decompensation include hepatic encephalopathy, ascites, jaundice, renal failure, hypoglycemia, and worsening MELD score. The onset of renal failure is an ominous event in any cirrhotic patient. Therefore, close attention to fluid balance and avoidance of nephrotoxic drugs is crucial. Patients with coagulopathy and thrombocytopenia are at higher risk for bleeding complications. Nutritional status should be closely monitored in the postoperative period. Enteral nutritional support should be initiated in patients with complicated postoperative course. Albumin level may be misleading and is not a reliable predictor of hepatic dysfunction in the postoperative period. Hypoglycemia can result due to poor hepatic glycogen supplies and inadequate gluconeogenesis.

In conclusion, patients with evidence of liver disease should undergo a focused evaluation to determine the severity of liver injury (Figure 12.1). The role of liver biopsy is selective and not mandatory. Patients without cirrhosis should undergo risk assessment based on comorbid medical conditions and complexity of planned surgery (Tables 12.3 and 12.4). Patients with evidence of cirrhosis are at highest risk for hepatic decompensation and should be categorized based on risk factors for surgical complications (Table 12.5 and Figure 12.1). The pros and cons of nonsurgical options should be reviewed. Current recommendations are made from retrospective data, and quality indicators have not been established.

REFERENCES

1. Ioannou GN, Boyko EJ, Lee SP. The prevalence and predictors of elevated serum aminotransferase activity in the United States in 1999–2002. *Am J Gastroenterol*. 2006;101:76–82.
2. Pratt DS, Kaplan MM. Evaluation of abnormal liver-enzyme results in asymptomatic patients. *N Engl J Med*. 2000;342:1266–1271.
3. Ioannou GN, Weiss NS, Boyko EJ, et al. Elevated serum alanine aminotransferase activity and calculated risk of coronary heart disease in the United States. *Hepatology*. 2006;43:1145–1151.
4. O'Leary JG, Yachimski PS, Friedman LS. Surgery in the patient with liver disease. *Clin Liver Dis*. 2009;13:211–231.
5. Prati D, Taioli E, Zanella A, et al. Updated definitions of healthy ranges for serum alanine aminotransferase levels. *Ann Intern Med*. 2002;137:1–10.
6. Calvaruso V, Craxi A. Implication of normal liver enzymes in liver disease. *J Viral Hepat*. 2009;16:529–536.

7. Ahmed A, Keeffe EB. Liver chemistry and function tests. In *Sleisenger & Fordtran's Gastrointestinal and Liver Disease*, 8th edition, Feldman M, Friedman LS, Brandt LJ (eds.), Philadelphia: W.B. Saunders; 2006. pp. 1575–1587.
8. Fabrizi F, Messa P, Martin P. Current status of renal transplantation from HCV-positive donors. *Int J Artif Organs* 2009;32(5):251–261.
9. Garrison RN, Cryer HM, Howard DA, et al. Clarification of risk factors for abdominal operations in patients with hepatic cirrhosis. *Ann Surg.* 1984;199:648–655.
10. Mansour A, Watson W, Shayani V, et al. Abdominal operations in patients with cirrhosis: still a major surgical challenge. *Surgery.* 1997;122:730–735.
11. Gil A, Martinez-Regueira F, Hernandez-Lizoain JL, et al. The role of transjugular intrahepatic portosystemic shunt prior to abdominal tumoral surgery in cirrhotic patients with portal hypertension. *Eur J Surg Oncol.* 2004;30:46–52.
12. O'Leary JG, Friedman LS. Predicting surgical risk in patients with cirrhosis: from art to science. *Gastroenterology.* 2007;132:1609–1611.
13. Northup PG, Wanamaker RC, Lee VD, et al. Model for End-Stage Liver Disease (MELD) predicts nontransplant surgical mortality in patients with cirrhosis. *Ann Surg.* 2005;242:244–251.
14. Teh SH, Nagorney DM, Stevens SR, et al. Risk factors for mortality after surgery in patients with cirrhosis. *Gastroenterology.* 2007;132:1261–1269.
15. Friedman LS. The risk of surgery in patients with liver disease. *Hepatology.* 1999;29:1617–1623.
16. Suman A, Barnes DS, Zein NN, et al. Predicting outcome after cardiac surgery in patients with cirrhosis: a comparison of Child-Pugh and MELD scores. *Clin Gastroenterol Hepatol.* 2004;2:719–723.
17. Ziser A, Plevak DJ, Wiesner RH, et al. Morbidity and mortality in cirrhotic patients undergoing anesthesia and surgery. *Anesthesiology.* 1999;90:42–53.
18. Teh SH, Christein J, Donohue J, et al. Hepatic resection of hepatocellular carcinoma in patients with cirrhosis: Model of End-Stage Liver Disease (MELD) score predicts perioperative mortality. *J Gastrointest Surg.* 2005;9:1207–1215.
19. Gholson CF, Provenza JM, Bacon BR. Hepatologic considerations in patients with parenchymal liver disease undergoing surgery. *Am J Gastroenterol.* 1990;85:487–496.
20. Gelman S. General anesthesia and hepatic circulation. *Can J Physiol Pharmacol.* 1987;65:1762–1779.
21. Kharasch ED, Hankins D, Mautz D, et al. Identification of the enzyme responsible for oxidative halothane metabolism: implications for prevention of halothane hepatitis. *Lancet.* 1996 18; 347:1367–1371.
22. Servin F, Desmonts JM, Haberer JP, et al. Pharmacokinetics and protein binding of propofol in patients with cirrhosis. *Anesthesiology.* 1988;69:887–891.
23. Nishiyama T, Fujimoto T, Hanaoka K. A comparison of liver function after hepatectomy in cirrhotic patients between sevoflurane and isoflurane in anesthesia with nitrous oxide and epidural block. *Anesth Analg.* 2004;98:990–993.
24. Seaberg EC, Belle SH, Beringer KC, Schivins JL, Detre KM. Liver transplantation in the United States from 1987–1998: updated results from the Pitt-UNOS liver transplant registry. In *Clinical Transplants 1998*, Cecka JM, Terasaki PI (eds.), Los Angeles, CA: UCLA Tissue Typing Laboratory; 1999. pp. 17–37.
25. Bravata DM, Olkin I, Barnato AE, et al. Health-related quality of life after liver transplantation: a meta-analysis. *Liver Transpl Surg.* 1999;5:318–331.
26. Ahmed A, Keeffe EB. Liver transplantation: pretransplant evaluation and care. In *Zakim and Boyer's Hepatology: A Textbook of Liver Disease*, 5th edition, Boyer TD, Wright TL, Manns MP (eds.), Philadelphia: Elsevier; 2006. pp. 933–945.
27. O'Grady JG, Alexander GJ, Hayllar KM, et al. Early indicators of prognosis in fuminant hepatic failure. *Gastroenterology.* 1989;97:439–445.
28. Ahmed A, Keeffe EB. Acute liver failure. In *Gastrointestinal Emergencies*, 2nd edition, Tham TCK, Collins JSA, Soetikno RM (eds.), Oxford: Wiley-Blackwell; 2009. pp. 149–157.
29. Bernuau J, Samuel D, Durand F, et al. Criteria for emergency liver transplantation in patients with acute viral hepatitis and factor V (FV) below 50% of normal: a prospective study (abstract). *Hepatology.* 1991;14:49A.

30. Bismuth H, Chiche L, Adam R, et al. Liver resection versus transplantation for hepatocelular carcinoma in cirrhotic patients. *Ann Surg.* 1993;218:145–151.
31. Iwatsuki S, Starzl TE, Sheahan DG, et al. Hepatic resection versus transplantation for hepatocellular carcinoma. *Ann Surg.* 1991;214:221–228.
32. Sarasin FP, Giostra E, Mentha G, et al. Partial hepatectomy or orthotopic liver transplantation for the treatment of resectable hepatocellular carcinoma? A cost-effectiveness perspective. *Hepatology.* 1998;28:436–432.
33. Mazzaferro V, Regalia E, Doci R, et al. Liver transplantation for the treatment of small hepatocellular carcinomas in patients with cirrhosis. *N Engl J Med.* 1996;334:693–699.
34. Wiesner RH, McDiarmid SV, Kamath PS, et al. MELD and PELD: application of survival models to liver allocation. *Liver Transpl.* 2001;7:567–580.
35. Kamath PS, Wiesner RH, Malinchoc M, et al. A model to predict survival in patients with end-stage liver disease. *Hepatology.* 2001;33:464–470.
36. Wiesner R, Edwards E, Freeman R, et al. The United Network for Organ Sharing Liver Disease Severity Score Committee. Model for End-Stage Liver Disease (MELD) and allocation of donor livers. *Gastroenterology.* 2003;124:91–96.

CHAPTER 13

ASSESSING AND MANAGING HEMATOLOGIC DISORDERS

M. Chadi Alraies and Ajay Kumar

INTRODUCTION

Hematologic abnormalities are common among perioperative patients. These abnormalities can cause significant challenges in the perioperative period, and early recognition and management is important to prevent complications such as excessive bleeding and thrombosis. This chapter will focus on the risk assessment, diagnosis, and management of specific hematologic problems including anemia, hemostatic abnormalities, and thrombocytopenia. Most of the recommendations are based on clinical practice standards and expert opinion due to the paucity of evidence-based guidelines for many of these hematologic disorders.

ANEMIA

Epidemiology

Anemia is the most commonly encountered hematologic problem in perioperative patients. It is a condition defined as having less than a normal number of red blood cells (RBCs) (either from decreased production, increased loss, or destruction) or inadequate quality of hemoglobin (Hgb) in the blood. The World Health Organization defines anemia as less than 13 g/dL for men and less than 12 g/dL for nonpregnant women. Anemia is often a sign of an underlying disease or condition that could affect the surgical outcome. The major function of the RBC is to facilitate oxygen transport and a sufficient number is needed to provide adequate oxygenation to tissues. However, there are additional factors such as pulmonary gas exchange, cardiac output, blood vessel compliance, blood viscosity, and oxygen affinity for Hgb that play a role in tissue oxygenation.

Perioperative Medicine: Medical Consultation and Co-Management, First Edition.
Edited by Amir K. Jaffer and Paul J. Grant.

Anemia is frequently discovered during routine preadmission testing of patients scheduled for elective surgery. Reported frequencies range from 5% to 75% of patients going for elective surgery.[1] One study demonstrated 35% of patients going for elective orthopedic surgery have an Hgb of <13 g/dL that was not previously discovered.[2] One-third of these patients were found to have iron-deficiency anemia (IDA) and the majority were females.[3] The remainder of anemia is usually attributed to inflammation or chronic disease. Optimization of Hgb levels before surgery is an important strategy to reduce the need for allogeneic blood transfusion during and after surgery, thereby minimizing the incidence of transfusion-related blood interactions and infection.[4]

Preoperative Risk Assessment

To evaluate the risk of anemia, a few studies have evaluated patients who refuse blood transfusion for religious reasons. One retrospective cohort study involved 1958 surgical patients who refused blood transfusion.[5] The 3-day risk of mortality increased with decreased preoperative Hgb levels, especially in patients with an Hgb of <6 g/dL. Furthermore, in patients with underlying cardiovascular disease, mortality risk increased when the Hgb value was 10 g/dL or less. A subsequent study on the same population showed that there is no increased risk of death for patients with postoperative Hgb concentrations between 7 and 8 g/dL; however, there was a sharp increase in mortality in those patients with an Hgb level less than 5–6 g/dL.[6] A few other studies with small sample sizes were conducted on healthy individuals. Leung et al. showed evidence of reversible ST-segment changes suggestive of myocardial ischemia in 5 of 87 asymptomatic patients with Hgb concentrations between 5 and 7 g/dL.[7]

Elderly patients tolerate anemia differently than young patients. A study involving patients greater than 65 years of age with a history of cardiac disease showed that an Hgb of 8.8 g/dL was well tolerated.[8] However, this study had a small sample size and careful interpretation of this result is advised. A later study analyzed preoperative hematocrit levels in over 310,000 elderly veterans undergoing noncardiac surgery and concluded that even mild anemia was associated with an increased risk of 30-day morbidity and mortality, especially in patients with a hematocrit level of ≤39%.[9]

As mentioned, anemia is associated with perioperative morbidity and mortality with additional potential risks when blood product transfusion is required. Therefore, an anemia workup before elective surgery is critical and associated with better surgical outcomes and patient satisfaction.

History and Physical Examination

The evaluation of anemia should always start with a detailed history and physical examination. The history should illicit symptoms of bleeding (i.e. menstrual blood loss, hematochezia, melena, hematemesis, hemoptysis, and hematuria) and constitutional symptoms (i.e., palpitations, fatigue, anginal chest pain, and dyspnea). Questions to ask patients with a past history of anemia should include onset and duration of anemia, previous Hgb values, need for previous blood transfusions, history of blood donation, and history of splenectomy. Other important historical information should include any family history of anemia, bleeding, splenectomy, or hemolysis. The social history may elicit information on previous toxin exposure, alcohol consumption, and illicit drug use. The medication history should review prescription and nonprescription medications that include herbal and over-the-counter medications such as nonsteroidal anti-inflammatory drugs (NSAIDs).

The physical examination should assess pallor of the skin and mucus membranes, jaundice, petechiae, purpura, lymphadenopathy, organomegaly, and neurological dysfunction. Heart auscultation of a flow murmur resulting from decreased blood viscosity and increased cardiac output may be due to anemia. Pelvic and/or rectal examination (with stool guaiac testing) may be indicated to evaluate for a possible source of blood loss anemia.

Diagnostic Testing

All patients scheduled for major elective surgery should have their Hgb checked within 30 days of surgery. If anemia is discovered prior to surgery and is unrelated to the condition for which surgery is indicated, the surgery should be delayed so an anemia workup can be initiated.[9] The main etiologies of anemia are either blood loss from bleeding, underproduction of RBCs, or RBC destruction.

The initial laboratory evaluation of anemia starts with a complete blood count (CBC), peripheral blood smear, and reticulocyte count. The reticulocyte count serves to differentiate anemia caused by inadequate bone marrow production (low reticulocyte count) from anemia caused by excessive RBC loss (high reticulocyte count). However, the reticulocyte count should be corrected for differences in hematocrit and the effect of erythropoietin on the marrow. This is done by calculating a Reticulocyte Production Index (RPI) (Table 13.1). When the reticulocyte count is high, a compensatory phase of acute blood loss or hemolysis is present. In addition to obtaining a more detailed history from the patient, the next step is to order labs to assess for hemolysis (i.e., lactate dehydrogenase, haptoglobin level, and examination of a peripheral blood smear). Additional labs that may be helpful in the assessment of hemolysis include a direct and indirect Coombs test, direct and indirect bilirubin,

TABLE 13.1.   Reticulocyte Production Index (RPI)

Hematocrit (%)	Maturation correction
36–45	1.0
26–35	1.5
16–25	2.0
≤15	2.5

RPI = retic count × patient's hematocrit/normal hematocrit (45) × maturation correction.
∘ RPI <2 indicates an inappropriate/decreased marrow response to anemia.
∘ RPI >2 indicates an appropriate marrow response to anemia, usually due to blood loss or hemolysis.

and a sickle-cell preparation or Hgb electrophoresis. The peripheral smear should be reviewed for clues to the underlying process. Polychromasia, basophilic stippling, and nucleated RBCs can all be seen in hemolytic anemia. Additionally, schistocytes can be seen and are generally associated with microangiopathic hemolytic anemias, such as those resulting from disseminated intravascular coagulation (DIC), thrombotic thrombocytopenic purpura (TTP)/hemolytic uremic syndrome (HUS), and hemolysis from prosthetic heart valves. Spherocytes may be seen in hereditary spherocytosis, autoimmune hemolytic anemia, and microangiopathic hemolytic anemias.

Alternatively, a low reticulocyte count should be followed with obtaining the mean corpuscular volume (MCV) and the peripheral blood smear to determine if the anemia is microcytic, normocytic, or macrocytic:

1. Microcytic anemia is usually the result of iron deficiency or thalassemia. Further tests are required to identify the etiology.

   a) Iron (Fe), total iron-binding capacity (TIBC) or transferrin, and ferritin: Fe and TIBC are both low with anemia of chronic disease, which is due to an underlying illness. Fe is low and TIBC is high with IDA. Patients over the age of 50 usually need a gastrointestinal (GI) workup with upper and lower endoscopy as GI tract is the most common site for blood loss.

   b) Ferritin levels of <30 ng/mL in men and <10 ng/mL in women are suggestive of IDA.

   c) Determination of Hgb A2, which is elevated in β-thalassemia. Thalassemia minor is rarely the cause of Hgb values below 9 g/dL. The more severe form of thalassemia is associated with splenomegaly.

   d) Occult Hgb testing of the stool is necessary to document blood loss from the GI tract; however, false-positive and false-negative results are common with this test.

2. Normocytic anemia can result from several causes; however, acute blood loss should be excluded first. Additional causes may include underlying renal or liver disease; early iron, vitamin B_{12}, or folate deficiency; myelodysplastic/aplastic anemia; or anemia of chronic disease resulting from a chronic inflammatory or infectious disease.

3. Macrocytic anemia is most often the result of alcoholism, liver disease, hypothyroidism, vitamin B_{12} or folate deficiency, drugs (such as chemotherapy and anticonvulsants), or primary marrow dysfunction (myelodysplasia). Ovalocytes and hypersegmented neutrophils are virtually diagnostic of vitamin B_{12} or folate deficiency. Appropriate vitamin levels or bone marrow examination may be necessary to confirm the diagnosis.

Figure 13.1 summarizes the recommended evaluation for preoperative anemia.

Prior to surgery all patients should have a Type and Screen (T/S) obtained, which provides information about the patient's blood type and the presence of red cell antibodies. If the antibody screen is positive, additional testing must be performed to identify the specific antibodies present and to rule out other clinically

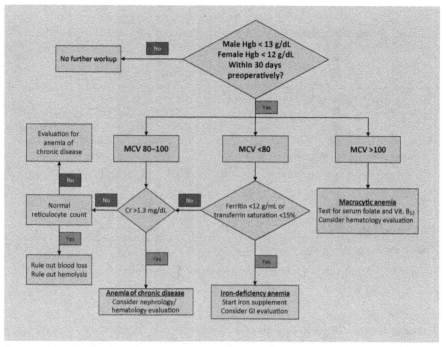

Figure 13.1.   Evaluation of preoperative anemia. See color insert.

significant antibodies to red cell antigens. Time for test completion and blood product availability depends on the number of antibodies present, antibody reactivity, and frequency of the corresponding antigen in our donor population. Once clinically significant antibodies are identified, national standards require the blood bank to provide antigen-negative, crossmatch-compatible units for transfusion.

We recommend a comprehensive multifaceted approach to blood conservation in order to achieve optimal outcomes for elective noncardiac surgery (Figure 13.2). This starts with identifying the cause of anemia and treating it before surgery. Erythropoietin alpha may be a preoperative option for anemia of chronic disease in patients with an Hgb of <13 g/dL for noncardiac, nonvascular surgery such as major joint replacement. Intraoperatively, several blood salvage techniques are also available for blood conservation.

IDA

In the case of IDA, iron (Fe) is low and TIBC is high. Ferritin levels of <30 ng/mL in men and <10 ng/mL in women suggest IDA. History and physical examination can often lead to the underlying cause, such as blood loss. Therefore, a thorough GI evaluation with colonoscopy and upper endoscopy is typically indicated. The supplementation of iron should also be initiated. Iron is most easily given in the oral form. Ferrous sulfate provides 65 mg of elemental iron per 325 mg tablet. It is recommended that adults receive 150–200 mg of elemental iron per day in

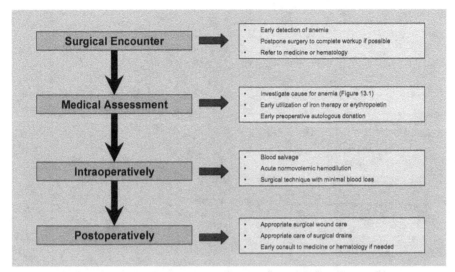

Figure 13.2. Multifaceted approach to perioperative blood conservation. See color insert.

deficiency states. Ascorbic acid should be prescribed to facilitate iron absorption. A rise in the reticulocyte count, the earliest evidence of successful treatment, takes approximately 10 days. On the other hand, Hgb levels should increase by 1 g/dL every 2–3 weeks. If patients have failed oral iron therapy or if iron loss exceeds capacity for oral iron absorption, intravenous iron therapy may be necessary. Common clinical scenarios in which this occurs include patients with inflammatory bowel disease, intestinal malabsorption from celiac disease, patients intolerant to oral iron therapy, or patients undergoing cancer chemotherapy. Of the intravenous iron preparations, ferric gluconate and iron sucrose are generally believed to have the best safety profile. Multiple studies including systematic reviews, however, suggest that low-molecular-weight iron dextran may have a comparable toxicity profile with iron sucrose.[10–13]

Vitamin B$_{12}$ and Folate-Deficiency Anemia

Anemia resulting from vitamin B$_{12}$ or folate deficiency causes a macrocytic anemia with an elevated MCV of >100 fL. This anemia is easily treated with supplementation. Folate deficiency should be treated with folic acid, 1 mg/day for up to 4 months, or until the patient's anemia is corrected. Vitamin B$_{12}$ deficiency is usually treated with intramuscular cyanocobalamin injections. The dosage of cyanocobalamin varies from 1000 mg daily for 7 days to 1000 mg every 1–4 weeks. Studies have also shown that oral cyanocobalamin supplementation of 1000–2000 mg/day for 4 months is as effective as parenteral administration, but this requires greater patient compliance.[14,15] Reticulocytosis may be expected in 3–5 days, and Hgb levels should rise within 10 days.

Anemia of Chronic Disease (AOCD)

AOCD is the second most common type of anemia after IDA. AOCD occurs in patients with acute or chronic inflammatory conditions. It is immune driven in which cytokines are stimulated to induce changes in iron hemostasis, proliferation of erythroid progenitor cells, and production of erythropoietin, and to regulate the life span of red cells. Causes of AOCD include infections (acute or chronic), underlying cancer (hematologic or solid tumors), autoimmune diseases (rheumatoid arthritis, lupus, vasculitis, sarcoidosis, and inflammatory bowel disease), chronic rejection after solid organ transplantation, and chronic kidney disease. AOCD due to chronic kidney disease has several mechanisms including decreased production of erythropoietin, uremic toxin accumulation that has an antiproliferative effect, activation of immune cells by contact with the dialysis membranes, and the tendency for recurrent infections in this patient population.[16]

The hallmark of AOCD, as mentioned above, is a disturbance in iron homeostasis. Specifically, there is an increased uptake and retention of iron within cells of the reticuloendothelial system, which leads to decreased iron in the circulation. This limits its availability for erythroid progenitor cells and subsequently causes a decrease in blood cell formation. Furthermore, the response of erythropoietin on AOCD is inadequate for the degree of anemia. And the response from erythroid progenitor cells to erythropoietin decreases and is inversely related to the severity of the underlying chronic inflammatory disease.[17–19]

AOCD is a normochromic, normocytic anemia with Hgb ranging from 8 to 9.5 g/dL. Reticulocyte count is also low indicating underproduction of RBCs. The workup of ACOD should start by assessing the iron stores since treatment will most likely fail if IDA is also present. The main difference between IDA and AOCD is that in IDA, there is an absolute iron deficiency, while in the latter, hypoferremia is due to acquisition of iron by the reticuloendothelial system causing decreased availability for the bone marrow. In both IDA and AOCD, transferrin saturation is decreased. However, transferrin is increased in IDA and normal or reduced in AOCD.[17,19–21] Because iron stores are full in AOCD due to decreased utilization, the ferritin level is normal or high. Increased ferritin levels seen in AOCD can also be due to immune activation.[22] Ferritin level is decreased in IDA. Soluble transferrin receptor levels can be determined by commercially available assays and is helpful for differentiation between AOCD alone (with normal or high ferritin and low levels of soluble transferrin receptors) and patients with AOCD and IDA (with low ferritin levels and high levels of soluble transferrin receptors). The ratio of the concentration of soluble transferrin receptors to the log of the ferritin level may also be helpful. A ratio of <1 suggests AOCD, whereas a ratio of >2 suggests absolute iron deficiency coexisting with AOCD.[23,24] See Table 13.2.

Erythropoietin levels can be used to assess the response from erythropoietin treatment. It is useful only for patients with an Hgb less than 10 g/dL.[25] After 2 weeks of erythropoietin treatment, either a serum erythropoietin level of more than 100 U/L, or a ferritin level of >400 ng/mL predicts a lack of treatment response in 88% of patients with cancer who are not receiving chemotherapy.[26]

TABLE 13.2.   Laboratory Testing to Differentiate Anemia of Chronic Disease and Iron-Deficiency Anemia

Variable	Anemia of chronic disease	Iron-deficiency anemia	Both conditions
Iron	Reduced	Reduced	Reduced
Transferrin	Reduced or normal	Increased	Reduced
Transferrin saturation	Reduced	Reduced	Reduced
Ferritin	Normal to increased	Reduced	Reduced to normal
Soluble transferrin receptor	Normal	Increased	Normal to increased

Adapted from Weiss and Goodnough.[79]

Erythropoietin has been proven to raise the Hgb concentration and reduce the need for allogeneic blood transfusion after surgery.[27,28] In patients with chronic renal failure not receiving hemodialysis, the use of erythropoietin is becoming more common with a target Hgb no greater than 12 g/dL. The usual dose is 50 units/kg three times weekly, or 10,000 units weekly. The initial response to erythropoietin therapy takes a few weeks and subsequent iron replacement therapy should be used in all patients with AOCD. Erythropoietin therapy should be limited when possible to avoid the potential risks associated with this medication (i.e., thromboembolism,[29,30] serious cardiovascular events,[31,32] and mortality[29]). Furthermore, a few studies have demonstrated an increased risk for tumor progression or recurrence.[33–35]

Sickle-Cell Disease (SCD)

SCD is the most common hemoglobinopathy that affects approximately 1 in 650 African–American infants in the United States. Sickle-cell anemia is usually a chronic, well-compensated hemolytic anemia with an appropriate reticulocytosis that leads to accelerated clearance of RBCs from the circulation. Exposure of these patients to precipitating factors (i.e., hypoxia, hypothermia, dehydration, hypoperfusion, and acidosis) produces irreversible RBC membrane damage, sludging of blood in capillaries, organ ischemia, and hemolysis. The clinical consequences of these events are recurrent painful crises and dysfunction of the nervous, cardiac, pulmonary, renal, and immune systems. Individuals with this illness are more likely to undergo surgery than persons in the general population during their lifetime. Yet with meticulous care, approximately 25–30% of patients will have a postoperative complication, even without a known history of cardiopulmonary disease.[36,37] Individuals with sickle-cell anemia (HgbSS) are at greatest risk. Patients who are compound heterozygotes for HgbS and HgbC (HgbSC) or HgbS and β-thalassemia (HgbSβ-thal) may be at increased risk, but this is not well defined. Generally, individuals with sickle-cell trait (heterozygosity for HgbS) are not at increased perioperative risk.

Cholecystectomy (as a result of cholelithiasis due to chronic hemolytic anemia) and splenectomy (usually performed in children following sequestration events)[38]

are the most common type of surgery in patients with SCD. Laparoscopic cholecystectomy has been widely used in patients with SCD. Although it is associated with longer anesthesia time,[39] it has a shorter recovery time after the surgery. This approach, however, has not been shown to reduce the rate of postoperative acute chest syndrome.[39,40]

Another common surgery in this patient population is hip arthroplasty secondary to osteonecrosis of the hip joint that occurs in 50% of adults with SCD.[41] The use of a tourniquet during orthopedic procedures should be used with caution because of the increased circulatory stasis, acidosis, and hypoxia underneath the cuff. Several factors have been shown to decrease the risk of sickling during and after the period of tourniquet application: HgbS <50%, optimal hydration, mild hyperventilation to keep pCO_2 at 30 mm Hg, and minimizing duration of surgery.[42]

The perioperative management of individuals with SCD is complicated and consideration should be given to multiple factors. The surgical stress by itself is a risk for triggering sickling and vaso-occlusive crisis.

Blood Transfusion   It is generally agreed that the Hgb should be corrected by transfusion of packed red cells to an Hgb level of 9–10 g/dL for moderate and high-risk procedures. Koshy et al. concluded in his Cooperative Study of Sickle Cell Disease, that surgery was safe in patients with SCD and preoperative transfusion was beneficial for all surgical risk levels; however, complication rates were low in most patients who had low risk surgery and did not receive blood transfusions.[38] When aggressive and conservative regimens were compared in 604 surgical procedures in patients with SCD, the conservative transfusion (correcting Hgb to 10 g/dL) was as effective as the aggressive regimen (reducing HgbS to ≤30%) in reducing the complications of surgery and anesthesia. The incidence of serious complications (31% and 35%) and acute chest syndrome (10%) were not significantly different in the two groups, although the aggressive transfusion group had a higher rate of transfusion-related complications (14% vs. 7%).[36] Other studies have confirmed equivalent outcomes in the two groups as well.[43–45] Simple transfusion to raise Hgb levels above 10 g/dL is not recommended because of the increased viscosity of the sickle blood.

Hydration   Due to an inability to concentrate urine, these patients are prone to dehydration, increased viscosity, cellular dehydration, and acidosis. For this reason, patients are advised to drink clear liquids prior to surgery at which time intravenous fluids are started and continued until they can tolerate adequate oral fluids postoperatively.

Oxygenation   Acute chest syndrome is the most common cause of death in young patients with SCD.[46] Hypoxia and ventilation–perfusion mismatch can increase the risk of pulmonary infarction and/or infections in patients with SCD. Adequate oxygenation should be maintained with careful anesthesia and postoperative respiratory management with hyperoxygenation administered at the induction of anesthesia. Postoperative hypoxia should be assessed carefully to rule out mucus plugging, pneumonia, pulmonary embolism (PE), or acute chest syndrome.

Hypothermia   A decrease in body temperature can increase peripheral resistance, reduce local blood flow, increase capillary transit time, and trigger vaso-occlusion.[47] Appropriate body temperature should be maintained during and after the surgery.

Infection Control   Patients with SCD are more prone to infection than the general population, especially patients with functional asplenia.[48] Furthermore, infections are a precipitating factor for sickle-cell crisis and vaso-occlusive attacks. It is extremely important to institute infection prevention measures, such as frequent hand washing, early mobilization after surgery, and incentive spirometry, and to carefully assess any postoperative fever.

Thalassemia

Thalassemia is characterized by ineffective production of Hgb and intramedullary destruction of RBCs. Individuals with severe thalassemia disease often have a history of long-term transfusion therapy and may suffer from multiorgan dysfunction caused by iron overload. These patients need a thorough evaluation of renal, hepatic, cardiac, and pulmonary function before surgery. Milder and less severe thalassemia syndromes usually have mild-to-moderate anemia that do not require blood transfusion. These patients are at no increased perioperative risk beyond that of the anemia itself. Treatment, although seldom indicated, is usually blood transfusion.

Autoimmune Hemolytic Anemia (AIHA)

One of the most common causes of acquired hemolytic anemia is immunologic destruction of RBCs mediated by autoantibodies directed against antigens on the patient's RBCs. The clinical manifestations of this group of diseases, called AIHA, depend greatly on the type of antibody that is produced by the abnormal immune reaction. AIHA is one of the most difficult problems to manage in the perioperative period.

Broadly speaking, there are two types of antibodies involved with AIHA, warm and cold antibodies. Most immune hemolytic anemias are of the warm antibody type and mediated by immunoglobulin G (IgG), which occurs at physiologic temperature. These are most often idiopathic or associated with other autoimmune or lymphoproliferative disorders such as lymphomas, chronic lymphocytic leukemia, HIV disease, and multiple myeloma. It is associated with positive direct Coombs test for IgG, complement, or both. Less common is the cold antibody type, mediated mainly by immunoglobulin M (IgM) and most often seen in association with infectious diseases such as mycoplasma pneumonia, mononucleosis, syphilis, viruses, or lymphoproliferative diseases. This type is associated with positive direct Coombs for complement and high titer cold agglutinin levels.

In general, patients should be treated and the AIHA controlled before surgery is undertaken. However, the management is challenging for two reasons. First, if transfusion is indicated, the transfused RBCs are as sensitive to the hemolytic process as the native cells. Second, the autoantibody makes it difficult to find compatible blood in the event that transfusion is needed. These autoantibodies can prevent the detection of alloantibodies that may precipitate immediate or delayed transfusion reactions and increase hemolysis caused by the autoimmune process. Management of this type of anemia should be coordinated by experienced teams of hematologists, clinical pathologists, and anesthesiologists. Elective surgeries should be delayed until the hemolysis process is controlled.

Warm antibody hemolytic anemia generally responds to corticosteroids at a usual starting dose of 1–2 mg/kg of prednisone. Improvement typically occurs in several days. In patients with poorly controlled hemolysis, some advocate administering intravenous immunoglobulin before transfusion. If transfusion is necessary, it should be administered with close monitoring for any signs or symptoms of hemolysis. Transfusion should be done while the patient is awake to report any reaction to the transfusion.

Patients with cold antibodies should be kept warm so the blood temperature exceeds 37 degrees. All blood products and fluids must be warmed to 37 degrees before infusion. This type of hemolytic anemia has a poor response to steroids. In rare circumstances, plasmapheresis may be helpful to limit hemolysis, especially in patients who have demonstrated a significant degree of hemolysis.

BLEEDING DISORDERS

Bleeding Risk Assessment and Preoperative Evaluation

The most important component of the evaluation for hemostatic function is a careful history.[49] Nearly all potential hemostatic problems can be uncovered through a careful history and physical examination. A positive response to any of the following questions has the potential to lead to perioperative bleeding problems:

- excessive bruising;
- bleeding gums after brushing teeth;
- nosebleeds;
- prolonged bleeding after cuts;
- heavy, prolonged menstrual periods;
- history of occult or frank blood loss through the GI or genitourinary tract;
- excessive bleeding after dental extraction, surgery, or childbirth;
- history of hemophilia or a co-inherited familial hematologic disorder;
- personal history of liver disease, renal failure, hypersplenism, hematologic disorder, or collagen vascular disease;
- current or recent use of medications that may interfere with hemostasis.

Moreover, if unexpected bleeding occurs during any surgery that is not explained by a local lesion or to the specific type of surgery being performed, an undiscovered hemostatic defect should be considered followed by an expeditious evaluation. The physical examination focuses on signs of petechiae, purpura, hematomas, jaundice, and cirrhosis, which alert the clinician that postoperative bleeding may be an issue.

Prothrombin Time (PT) and Activated Partial Thromboplastin Time (aPTT) Preoperative Testing

Rarely is a previously unsuspected bleeding disorder identified by laboratory screening if the history and physical examination are normal. The PT and aPTT are highly reproducible and automated. These tests were not designed to determine the risk of perioperative bleeding, but rather to detect factor deficiencies. Most studies have shown that these tests have poor predictive value with respect to perioperative bleeding complications.[50] The bleeding time is another laboratory test that has not been shown to be predicative of postsurgical bleeding complications upon extensive review. Thus, this test should not be performed. Given the poor predictive value provided by these labs, it underscores that there is no substitute for a good patient history to evaluate perioperative bleeding risk.

Genetic Coagulation Abnormalities

Glucose-6-Phosphate Dehydrogenase (G6PD) Deficiency G6PD deficiency is an X-linked inherited disease that causes hemolysis after exposure to infections, drugs, and certain substances including antipyretics, sulfonamides, nitrates, and antimalarials. The severity of hemolysis depends on the exposure to the offending agent and the enzymatic activity in the patient.

During surgery, hypoxia, sustained mechanical ventilation, and the need for blood products increases the risk for hemolysis. Autoantibody-coated erythrocytes rapidly undergo destruction in the reticuloendothelial system in AIHA leading to severe hemolysis. This disease responds well to steroids, which should be instituted and continued until signs of hemolysis disappear. In patients with sustained hemolysis despite steroid therapy, splenectomy is advocated. Normothermia is maintained because hypothermia is a known trigger for hemolysis. In the postoperative period, patients are monitored for hemolysis with regular Hgb and haptoglobin levels.[51]

Von Willebrand Disease (vWD) vWD is the most common inherited bleeding disorder in humans, with a prevalence of approximately 1%.[52] In vWD, there is a deficiency of von Willebrand factor (vWF), which causes platelet dysfunction. There are several subtypes of vWD, the most common subtype being type 1 (70%), which is characterized by a partial quantitative defect of normal vWF. Inheritance is autosomal dominant, with incomplete penetrance.[53] Most of the remaining cases (20–30%) are type 2 and are characterized by both qualitative and quantitative defects of vWF. Type 2 has three variants of approximately equal prevalence.[52] Type 2A has autosomal dominant inheritance and patients lack high-molecular-weight vWF multimers. Type 2B is also an autosomal dominant disease and is associated with both thrombocytopenia and loss of high-molecular-weight multimers.[54] Type 2N, an uncommon form of vWD, is an X-linked recessive disorder associated with decreased binding of Factor VIII to vWF. This decreased binding leads to a rapid clearance of Factor VIII from the plasma and resembles hemophilia A.[55] A much rarer form, type 2M, is associated with decreased vWF binding to platelet GPIb. Approximately 5% of patients with vWD have the type 3 variant. It is autosomal recessive and associated with little to no production of vWF. In addition to the inherited forms, an acquired form also exists and is associated most commonly with lymphoproliferative disorders, cardiac disease, and cancer.

Treatment of vWD depends on the subtype. Approximately 75% of patients with types 1, 2A, and 2M will respond to desmopressin, which releases vWF and Factor VIII from endothelial cells.[53] The dose is 0.3 mg/kg (maximum 20 mg) by intravenous infusion administered over approximately 30 min. vWF levels increase by a factor of 3–5 within 1 h and stay elevated for approximately 8–10 h.[56] During preparation of a patient for elective surgery, a desmopressin challenge followed by verification of an increase in vWF levels is useful. The addition of an antifibrinolytic agent also improves clot stability. Of note is that desmopressin is contraindicated in type 2B vWD because it may worsen thrombocytopenia. Also, desmopressin may cause hyponatremia; therefore, electrolytes should be monitored with repeated dosing. Patients who do not respond favorably to desmopressin will need exogenous vWF. Although vWF is present in cryoprecipitated anithemophilic factor (or simply called cryoprecipitate), the use of this blood product carries the risk of viral disease transmission and is not recommended. Purified plasma factor concentrates are the recommended therapy, and expert consultation is advised to assist with dosing. For surgery, patients should receive approximately 60–80 units of ristocetin cofactor activity per kilogram every 8–12 h, and this should continue for 7–10 days after major surgery and 3–5 days after minor surgery.[53]

Factor II Deficiency   Factor II deficiency is a rare, autosomal recessive disorder characterized by either low or dysfunctional prothrombin.[53,57] Prothrombin levels may vary from <1% to 75%, although levels from 5% to 50% are usually well tolerated except when challenged with trauma or surgery.[57] It is important to rule out vitamin K deficiency when diagnosing this disease. Prothrombin complex concentrates (PCCs) can be used to treat this deficiency. Prothrombin has a long serum half-life of about 60 h, which simplifies maintenance therapy. The loading dose is 20 units/kg, with a maintenance dose of 5 units/kg daily. Fresh frozen plasma (FFP) is an alternative, although it has an increased risk of viral disease transmission and fluid overload.[58] The loading dose of FFP is 20 mL/kg, with maintenance doses of 5 mL/kg daily.[57]

Factor V Deficiency   Factor V deficiency is an extremely rare, autosomal recessive disorder, with approximately 200 reported cases.[59] Signs and symptoms include ecchymosis, epistaxis, gingival bleeding, menorrhagia, and excess bleeding associated with surgery or trauma. Factor V is synthesized by the liver and has a serum half-life of 12–36 h. Surgical hemostasis is achieved when levels are approximately 30% of normal. Replacement therapy is FFP with a loading dose of 20 mL/kg and maintenance doses of 5–10 mL/kg daily for 7 days.

Factor VII Deficiency   Factor VII is an autosomal recessive disorder and the only hereditary clotting factor deficiency with a prolonged PT and a normal partial thromboplastin time (PTT). Diagnosis requires a specific Factor VII assay. Heterozygotes are usually asymptomatic, but the bleeding in homozygotes does not always correlate with Factor VII levels. Replacement therapies have included PCCs or FFP; however, the newer recombinant Factor VIIa has advantages because it removes the risk of both viral disease transmission and fluid overload. Dosing regimens are still anecdotal. Surgical hemostasis may be achieved with Factor VII levels approximately 25% of normal, but this is not certain.[57] A higher Factor VII level may be required when small amounts of bleeding would be poorly tolerated. For example, in neurosurgery, a loading dose of 50 mg/kg followed by 20 mg/kg every 12 h has been successful.[60] Frequent dosing or continuous infusion may be required perioperatively because of Factor VII's short half-life of about 5 h. A case report of a patient with Factor VII deficiency (native level 5% of normal) who underwent a caesarean section described no excessive bleeding after administration of a 13.3 mg/kg bolus followed by 96 h of continuous infusion.[61] Expert hematology consultation is recommended when using this expensive therapy.

HEMOPHILIA

Hemophilia A is an X-linked recessive disorder caused by a deficiency of Factor VIII. This defect occurs in approximately 1/10,000 males and is diagnosed definitively with a Factor VIII assay. Carriers have Factor VIII levels >50% of normal and are usually asymptomatic. Symptomatic patients are classified as mild, moderate, or severe. Mildly affected patients (Factor VIII levels 6–30% of normal) rarely suffer spontaneous hemorrhaging, although surgery or trauma may lead to excess bleeding. Moderately affected patients (Factor VIII levels 1–5% of normal) have occasional spontaneous hemorrhages, while severely afflicted patients (Factor VIII levels <1% of normal) experience frequent, spontaneous hemorrhages from early infancy.

Treatment varies with disease severity and should be coordinated through the patient's hematologist. Mildly affected patients may respond to desmopressin (either 0.3 mg/kg intravenously or 300 mg intranasally) and antifibrinolytic therapy with aminocaproic acid or tranexamic acid.[62,63] Despite this, patients may still require Factor VIII replacement with recombinant Factor VIII. Although patients with a history of moderate hemorrhages who are undergoing minor surgical procedures may respond adequately when Factor VIII activity is increased to 30–60%, patients with a history of life-threatening hemorrhages undergoing major surgery will need 100% of normal Factor VIII activity. Dosing is based on the empiric observation that 1 unit/kg will generally increase Factor VIII activity by 2%. The initial preoperative dose is 50 units/kg, and verification of 100% activity is needed to document benefit. This dose will need to be repeated every 6–12 h to bring the level back up from 50% to 100%.[64] Maintenance of 100% Factor VIII activity will be required for 10–14 days or until healing is complete.

Despite the advantages of recombinant Factor VIII therapy, the incidence of inhibitor formation to Factor VIII is approximately 30% and most inhibitor patients have severe hemophilia.[65] Patients with inhibitors are classified as high responders (high inhibitor titers) or low responders (low inhibitor titers). Patients with low antibody titers may respond favorably to high doses of Factor VIII concentrates.

Patients with high antibody titers generally do not respond favorably to Factor VIII concentrates and should be treated with recombinant Factor VIIa. Before major surgery, the dose of recombinant Factor VIIa is 90 mg/kg intravenously, with repeat dosing every 2–3 h to maintain hemostasis.[66] Hematology consultation is recommended.

Hemophilia B (Factor IX deficiency) is an X-linked recessive disorder with an incidence of 1/25,000 males and is clinically identical to hemophilia A. Similarly, mildly affected patients have Factor IX levels 5–40% of normal, moderately affected patients have levels in the 1–5% range, and severely afflicted patients have levels below 1%. Definitive diagnosis is based on measuring Factor IX levels.

Although PCCs have been used in the past, they are no longer the first-line therapy because of the risks of thromboembolic complications. The preferred agent is recombinant Factor IX. Dosing is based on the empiric observation that 1.3 units/kg of recombinant Factor IX will increase Factor IX activity by 1%. Recombinant Factor IX has a half-life of 18–20 h and maintenance doses should be repeated at 12- to 18-h intervals until healing is complete. Therapy should be guided by measuring Factor IX levels.[53,64] In contrast to hemophilia A, only about 3% of hemophilia B patients will develop inhibitors to Factor IX.[67] Also unique in hemophilia B patients with inhibitors is reported cases of anaphylaxis and nephrotic syndrome upon exposure to Factor IX.[68] In patients with Factor IX inhibitors, recombinant Factor VIIa can be used and is dosed as described for hemophilia A patients with inhibitors. Once again, it is important to coordinate therapy with the patient's hematologist.

Factor XI Deficiency

Factor XI deficiency is an autosomal recessive disorder that occurs with a frequency of 1/450 among Ashkenazi Jews but occurs about 1/1,000,000 outside that population.[69] Spontaneous bleeding is rare, but hemorrhaging often occurs with surgery or trauma.[53,69] Bleeding does not always correlate with Factor XI levels and can be associated with vWD.[70] Treatment with antifibrinolytic agents is often sufficient (especially for dental surgery) and fibrin sealant has also been used successfully.[71] The preferred therapy for Factor XI deficiency is FFP or Factor XI concentrate; however, FFP is associated with fluid overload and viral disease transmission, and Factor XI concentrate is not available in the United States. Recombinant Factor VIIa (major surgery: 90 mg/kg every 2 h for 24 h, followed by 90 mg/kg every 4 h for 24 h) in combination with tranexamic acid (15 mg/kg given orally every 6 h for 7 days) was used successfully in a pilot study involving 14 patients, although one patient suffered a fatal cerebrovascular accident.[69]

Hageman Factor (Factor XII) Deficiency

Factor XII deficiency is a rare, autosomal recessive disorder that is not associated with a bleeding diathesis despite an elevated PTT. Paradoxically, it has been associated with thromboembolic complications. It is uncertain if this is related to Factor

XII levels or some other abnormality, such as antiphospholipid antibody syndrome or lupus anticoagulant.[72]

Thrombocytopenia

Thrombocytopenia is defined as a platelet count of less than 150,000 per cubic millimeter (mm^3). Unlike most other coagulation laboratory testing, the platelet count can be useful in assessing perioperative bleeding risk. Platelets can be low in certain diseases, such as cirrhosis, or be normal but dysfunctional in patients with end-stage renal disease (ESRD). The causes of thrombocytopenia include decreased production, sequestration, or increased destruction of platelets (Table 13.3). Patients who are otherwise healthy should always first be assessed for pseudothrombocytopenia, which occurs due to platelet agglutination caused by ethylenediaminetetraacetic acid (EDTA). EDTA is a chelating agent that is widely used to sequester di- and trivalent metal ions and used in blood collection tubes for CBC determination. The workup

TABLE 13.3. Causes of Thrombocytopenia

Decreased production	
Congenital	Acquired
1. Bernard–Soulier syndrome (loss of glycoprotein 1b)	1. Bone marrow infiltration Metastatic cancers Myelofibrosis
2. Alport's syndrome	
3. May–Hegglin anomaly	2. Ineffective thrombopoiesis Folate, B_{12}, or iron deficiency Myelodysplastic syndrome
4. Wiskott–Aldrich syndrome	

Increased destruction	
Idiopathic	
Drugs	

1. Immune mechanism: that is, penicillin, digitalis derivatives, sulfa compounds, quinine, quinidine, phenytoin, heparin, ampicillin
2. Nonimmune mechanism: that is, ticlopidine, mitomycin, cisplatin, cyclosporine
3. Altered function: that is, nonsteroidal anti-inflammatory agents, β-lactam antibiotics, heparin, isoniazid, penicillin, aminoglycosides

Autoimmune	Nonimmune
1. Chronic lymphocytic leukemia	1. Preeclampsia
2. Systemic lupus erythematosus	2. Hemolytic–uremic syndrome
3. Thyroid disease	3. Thrombotic thrombocytopenic purpura
4. Hypogammaglobulinemia	4. Cardiopulmonary bypass
5. Antiphospholipid syndrome	5. Disseminated intravascular coagulation
6. Posttransfusion purpura	
7. Sepsis	

for thrombocytopenia should also include a peripheral smear examination to esti-mate platelet numbers, morphology, and to evaluate red and white blood cell abnormalities.

A preoperative finding of thrombocytopenia needs to be investigated and cor-rected because thrombocytopenia poses a risk of bleeding that is inversely related to the platelet count. Surgery can generally proceed at levels above 50,000/mm^3 as long as the patient is supplemented with platelets on call to the operating room. In general, anesthesia via neuraxial blockade is contraindicated at levels below 100,000/mm^3. For any given platelet count, the risk of bleeding increases when anemia, fever, infection, or a platelet function defect (i.e., use of aspirin or NSAIDs) coexist. In consumptive disorders caused by drugs, discontinuation of the offending agent should lead to a normal platelet count within 5–10 days. If thrombocytopenia is caused by DIC, treatment should be directed at the underlying disease.[73]

Idiopathic thrombocytopenic purpura (ITP) in adults is a chronic autoimmune condition usually with an insidious onset. It is characterized by a reduced platelet count, increased peripheral destruction of platelets, and augmented platelet produc-tion. Autoantibodies are produced against platelets and possibly against megakaryo-cytes, which leads to the phagocytic destruction of these cells. The diagnosis of ITP is based solely on clinical criteria because platelet antibody studies and bone marrow aspiration are of uncertain diagnostic value. The history, physical examination, and peripheral blood smear can exclude most alternative diagnoses.[73]

The treatment of chronic ITP is supportive, not curative, and is directed toward the inactivation or removal of the major site of platelet destruction and antiplatelet antibody production, the spleen. Corticosteroids prevent sequestration of antibody-coated platelets by the spleen and probably impair antibody production. Gamma globulin or platelet transfusions are used in urgent situations.

Thrombocytopenia in the presence of heparin should raise concerns for heparin-induced thrombocytopenia (HIT). It usually occurs within 5–10 days after initiation of heparin; however, 30% of cases occur within 24 h after initiation of heparin. This condition is often referred to as rapid-onset HIT, and these patients usually have had a prior exposure to heparin within the past 30 days. Some of the associated complications include arterial thromboses, deep venous thrombosis (DVT), PE, cerebral sinus thrombosis, and thromboses of arterial venous (AV) fis-tulas. The overall risk of HIT depends on the type of heparin and patient character-istics. This diagnosis can be catastrophic if undiagnosed or untreated as up to 30% of patients die. An additional 10–20% of patients will require an amputation. Half of all patients with HIT will have a thrombosis in 30 days. Treatment of HIT starts with the immediate discontinuation of all heparin products followed by initiation of an alternative anticoagulant. The direct thrombin inhibitors are considered first-line agents and include lepirudin, bivalirudin, and argatroban. The Factor Xa inhibitor fondaparinux has also been used for the treatment of HIT; however, this drug does not have a formal indication for this use. The heparinoid drug, danaparoid sodium, is another treatment option but is not available in the United States. It is important to note that low-molecular-weight heparin (LMWH) use is contraindicated if HIT is suspected.[74,75]

Thrombocytosis

Thrombocytosis, defined as a platelet count of more than $500,000/mm^3$, may be physiologic (exercise, parturition, acute blood loss), primary (a myeloproliferative disorder with increased platelet production independent of normal regulatory control), or secondary (associated with iron deficiency, malignancy, infection, chronic inflammatory states, and postoperative states). The platelet count usually returns to normal with treatment of the underlying disorder. Patients with polycythemia vera and essential thrombocythemia (primary thrombocytosis) have an increased risk of thrombotic or bleeding events, respectively. The risk of thrombosis and hemorrhage seems to be increased in older patients and those with prior thrombotic or hemorrhagic events. Aspirin use may worsen the hemorrhagic tendency in these patients. No specific platelet count is predictive of hemorrhage or thrombosis. The most common sites of hemorrhage are mucosal surfaces; the most common thrombotic events are mesenteric, DVT, PE, and cerebral, coronary, and peripheral arterial occlusions.

Secondary thrombocytosis rarely leads to platelet counts $>1,000,000/mm^3$, and the cause may be obvious from the history, physical examination, radiologic, or blood testing. Treatment of the underlying disorder usually returns the platelet count to normal. Thromboembolic events are rare in patients with secondary thrombocytosis or chronic myelogenous leukemia. Platelet pheresis has been used (i.e., in serious hemorrhage or thrombosis; before an emergent operation); however, it is rarely necessary. Due to the long half-life of platelets (7 days), medical therapy with agents such as hydroxyurea and anagrelide does not provide an immediate effect.

Thrombophilias

Pathogenesis for venous thromboembolism (VTE) is multifactorial often involving acquired or environmental risk factors as well as genetic predisposition. These risk factors can be placed into one or more of the following categories, namely, circulatory stasis, endothelial (vessel wall) injury, and changes in composition of blood (hypercoagulable state). Hypercoagulability can be inherited or acquired and is now termed thrombophilia. There is little role for routine preoperative screening for thrombophilias in the asymptomatic individual[76]; however, in the setting of a patient who has experienced a prior VTE and has a known thrombophilia (such as Factor V Leiden, prothrombin gene mutation, protein C or protein S deficiency), they should receive aggressive pharmacologic prophylaxis with either unfractionated heparin 5000 units subcutaneously (sc) three times daily, LMWH (such as enoxaparin 40 mg sc daily or dalteparin 5000 units sc daily), or fondaparinux 2.5 mg sc daily.[77] In situations where patients are undergoing major surgery, extended prophylaxis beyond hospital discharge can be considered in the presence of a known thrombophilia.

Special Considerations with Neuraxial Blockade

The American Society of Regional Anesthesia (ASRA) has published the following recommendations[78] to reduce the risk of paraspinal hematomas, a potentially catastrophic complication. Full recommendations are available online at http://www.asra.com:

1. Coadministration of antiplatelet and anticoagulant medications is contraindicated with indwelling epidural catheters. Clopidogrel must be held for 7 days before neuraxial blockade.

2. Spinal or epidural anesthesia should occur at least 12 h after the last thromboprophylaxis dose of LMWH and at least 24 h after the last full (weight-based) dose of LMWH.

3. In general, an epidural catheter should not be removed until 12 h after the last prophylaxis dose of LMWH.

4. The first dose of LMWH should be administered no sooner than 2 h after catheter removal.

5. Delay LMWH use for 24 h if the patient experienced excessive trauma during attempted epidural or spinal anesthesia.

CONCLUSIONS

The preoperative management of the patient with anemia, platelet disorders, or a defect affecting thrombosis or hemostasis can be complicated. This chapter provides an evidence-based overview with recommendations to manage these commonly encountered hematologic conditions in the perioperative setting.

REFERENCES

1. Bierbaum BE, et al. An analysis of blood management in patients having a total hip or knee arthroplasty. *J Bone Joint Surg Am.* 1999;81(1):2–10.
2. Wilson A, et al. Prevalence and outcomes of anemia in rheumatoid arthritis: a systematic review of the literature. *Am J Med.* 2004;116(Suppl 7A): 50S–57S.
3. Goodnough LT, et al. Prevalence and classification of anemia in elective orthopedic surgery patients: implications for blood conservation programs. *Vox Sang.* 1992;63(2):90–95.
4. Goodnough LT, Shander A, Spence R. Bloodless medicine: clinical care without allogeneic blood transfusion. *Transfusion.* 2003;43(5):668–676.
5. Carson JL, et al. Effect of anaemia and cardiovascular disease on surgical mortality and morbidity. *Lancet.* 1996;348(9034):1055–1060.
6. Carson JL, et al. Mortality and morbidity in patients with very low postoperative Hb levels who decline blood transfusion. *Transfusion.* 2002;42(7):812–818.
7. Leung JM, et al. Electrocardiographic ST-segment changes during acute, severe isovolemic hemodilution in humans. *Anesthesiology.* 2000;93(4):1004–1010.
8. Spahn DR, et al. Hemodilution tolerance in elderly patients without known cardiac disease. *Anesth Analg.* 1996;82(4):681–686.
9. Wu WC, et al. Preoperative hematocrit levels and postoperative outcomes in older patients undergoing noncardiac surgery. *JAMA.* 2007;297(22):2481–2488.
10. Auerbach M, et al. The role of intravenous iron in anemia management and transfusion avoidance. *Transfusion.* 2008;48(5):988–1000.
11. Critchley J, Dundar Y. Adverse events associated with intravenous iron infusion (low-molecular-weight iron dextran and iron sucrose): a systematic review. *Transfus Altern Transfus Med.* 2007;9(1): 8–36.

12. Moniem KA, Bhandari S. Tolerability and efficacy of parenteral iron therapy in hemodialysis patients, a comparison of preparations. *Transfus Altern Transfus Med.* 2007;9(1):37–42.
13. Sav T, et al. Is there a difference between the allergic potencies of the iron sucrose and low molecular weight iron dextran? *Ren Fail.* 2007;29(4):423–426.
14. Eussen SJ, et al. Oral cyanocobalamin supplementation in older people with vitamin B12 deficiency: a dose-finding trial. *Arch Intern Med.* 2005;165(10):1167–1172.
15. Kuzminski AM, et al. Effective treatment of cobalamin deficiency with oral cobalamin. *Blood.* 1998;92(4):1191–1198.
16. Eschbach JW. Anemia management in chronic kidney disease: role of factors affecting epoetin responsiveness. *J Am Soc Nephrol.* 2002;13(5):1412–1414.
17. Means RT, Jr. Recent developments in the anemia of chronic disease. *Curr Hematol Rep.* 2003;2(2):116–121.
18. Sullivan PS, et al. Epidemiology of anemia in human immunodeficiency virus (HIV)-infected persons: results from the multistate adult and adolescent spectrum of HIV disease surveillance project. *Blood.* 1998;91(1):301–308.
19. Weiss G. Pathogenesis and treatment of anaemia of chronic disease. *Blood Rev.* 2002;16(2):87–96.
20. Matzner Y, et al. Prevalence and causes of anemia in elderly hospitalized patients. *Gerontology.* 1979;25(2):113–119.
21. Spivak JL. Iron and the anemia of chronic disease. *Oncology (Williston Park).* 2002;16(9 Suppl 10):25–33.
22. Torti FM, Torti SV. Regulation of ferritin genes and protein. *Blood.* 2002;99(10):3505–3516.
23. Brugnara C. Iron deficiency and erythropoiesis: new diagnostic approaches. *Clin Chem.* 2003;49(10):1573–1578.
24. Punnonen K, Irjala K, Rajamaki A. Serum transferrin receptor and its ratio to serum ferritin in the diagnosis of iron deficiency. *Blood.* 1997;89(3):1052–1057.
25. Miller CB, et al. Decreased erythropoietin response in patients with the anemia of cancer. *N Engl J Med.* 1990;322(24):1689–1692.
26. Ludwig H, et al. Prediction of response to erythropoietin treatment in chronic anemia of cancer. *Blood.* 1994;84(4):1056–1063.
27. Faris PM, Ritter MA, Abels RI. The effects of recombinant human erythropoietin on perioperative transfusion requirements in patients having a major orthopaedic operation. The American Erythropoietin Study Group. *J Bone Joint Surg Am.* 1996;78(1):62–72.
28. Laupacis A, Feagan B, Wong C. Effectiveness of perioperative recombinant human erythropoietin in elective hip replacement. COPES Study Group. *Lancet.* 1993;342(8867):378.
29. Phrommintikul A, et al. Mortality and target haemoglobin concentrations in anaemic patients with chronic kidney disease treated with erythropoietin: a meta-analysis. *Lancet.* 2007;369(9559):381–388.
30. Bennett CL, et al. Venous thromboembolism and mortality associated with recombinant erythropoietin and darbepoetin administration for the treatment of cancer-associated anemia. *JAMA.* 2008;299(8):914–924.
31. Drueke TB, et al. Normalization of hemoglobin level in patients with chronic kidney disease and anemia. *N Engl J Med.* 2006;355(20):2071–2084.
32. Singh AK, et al. Correction of anemia with epoetin alfa in chronic kidney disease. *N Engl J Med.* 2006;355(20):2085–2098.
33. Henke M, et al. Erythropoietin to treat head and neck cancer patients with anaemia undergoing radiotherapy: randomised, double-blind, placebo-controlled trial. *Lancet.* 2003;362(9392):1255–1260.
34. Henke M, et al. Do erythropoietin receptors on cancer cells explain unexpected clinical findings? *J Clin Oncol.* 2006;24(29):4708–4713.
35. Longmore GD. Do cancer cells express functional erythropoietin receptors? *N Engl J Med.* 2007;356(24):2447.
36. Vichinsky EP, et al. A comparison of conservative and aggressive transfusion regimens in the perioperative management of sickle cell disease. The Preoperative Transfusion in Sickle Cell Disease Study Group. *N Engl J Med.* 1995;333(4):206–213.

37. Wali YA, Al Okbi H, Al Abri R. A comparison of two transfusion regimens in the perioperative management of children with sickle cell disease undergoing adenotonsillectomy. *Pediatr Hematol Oncol.* 2003;20(1):7–13.

38. Koshy M, et al. Surgery and anesthesia in sickle cell disease. Cooperative Study of Sickle Cell Diseases. *Blood.* 1995;86(10):3676–3684.

39. Wales PW, et al. Acute chest syndrome after abdominal surgery in children with sickle cell disease: is a laparoscopic approach better? *J Pediatr Surg.* 2001;36(5):718–721.

40. Delatte SJ, et al. Acute chest syndrome in the postoperative sickle cell patient. *J Pediatr Surg.* 1999;34(1):188–191; discussion 191–192.

41. Firth PG, Head CA. Sickle cell disease and anesthesia. *Anesthesiology.* 2004;101(3):766–785.

42. Abdulla Al-Ghamdi A. Bilateral total knee replacement with tourniquets in a homozygous sickle cell patient. *Anesth Analg.* 2004;98(2):543–544, table of contents.

43. Haberkern CM, et al. Cholecystectomy in sickle cell anemia patients: perioperative outcome of 364 cases from the National Preoperative Transfusion Study. Preoperative Transfusion in Sickle Cell Disease Study Group. *Blood.* 1997;89(5):1533–1542.

44. Vichinsky EP, et al. The perioperative complication rate of orthopedic surgery in sickle cell disease: report of the National Sickle Cell Surgery Study Group. *Am J Hematol.* 1999;62(3):129–138.

45. Waldron P, et al. Tonsillectomy, adenoidectomy, and myringotomy in sickle cell disease: perioperative morbidity. Preoperative Transfusion in Sickle Cell Disease Study Group. *J Pediatr Hematol Oncol.* 1999;21(2):129–135.

46. Platt OS, et al. Mortality in sickle cell disease. Life expectancy and risk factors for early death. *N Engl J Med.* 1994;330(23):1639–1644.

47. Marchant WA, Walker I. Anaesthetic management of the child with sickle cell disease. *Paediatr Anaesth.* 2003;13(6):473–489.

48. Tobin JR, Butterworth J. Sickle cell disease: dogma, science, and clinical care. *Anesth Analg.* 2004;98(2):283–284.

49. Chee YL, et al. Guidelines on the assessment of bleeding risk prior to surgery or invasive procedures. British Committee for Standards in Haematology. *Br J Haematol.* 2008;140(5):496–504.

50. Munro J, Booth A, Nicholl J. Routine preoperative testing: a systematic review of the evidence. *Health Technol Assess.* 1997;1(12):i–iv. 1–62.

51. Gayyed NL, Bouboulis N, Holden M. Open heart operation in patients suffering from hereditary spherocytosis. *Ann Thorac Surg.* 1993;55(6):1497–1500.

52. Ramasamy I. Inherited bleeding disorders: disorders of platelet adhesion and aggregation. *Crit Rev Oncol Hematol.* 2004;49(1):1–35.

53. Lee JW. Von Willebrand disease, hemophilia A and B, and other factor deficiencies. *Int Anesthesiol Clin.* 2004;42(3):59–76.

54. Fausett B, Silver RM. Congenital disorders of platelet function. *Clin Obstet Gynecol.* 1999;42(2):390–405.

55. Nichols WC, Ginsburg D. Von Willebrand disease. *Medicine (Baltimore).* 1997;76(1):1–20.

56. Mannucci PM, et al. Response of factor VIII/von Willebrand factor to DDAVP in healthy subjects and patients with haemophilia A and von Willebrand's disease. *Br J Haematol.* 1981;47(2): 283–293.

57. Lechler E. Use of prothrombin complex concentrates for prophylaxis and treatment of bleeding episodes in patients with hereditary deficiency of prothrombin, factor VII, factor X, protein C protein S, or protein Z. *Thromb Res.* 1999;95(4 Suppl 1):S39–S50.

58. Preiss DU, et al. Safety of vapour heated prothrombin complex concentrate (PCC) Prothromplex S-TIM 4. *Thromb Res.* 1991;63(6):651–659.

59. Girolami A, et al. Hemorrhagic and thrombotic disorders due to factor V deficiencies and abnormalities: an updated classification. *Blood Rev.* 1998;12(1):45–51.

60. Cohen LJ, et al. Prophylaxis and therapy with factor VII concentrate (human) immuno, vapor heated in patients with congenital factor VII deficiency: a summary of case reports. *Am J Hematol.* 1995;50(4):269–276.

61. Jimenez-Yuste V, et al. Continuous infusion of recombinant activated factor VII during caesarean section delivery in a patient with congenital factor VII deficiency. *Haemophilia.* 2000;6(5): 588–590.

62. Tischkowitz M, Dokal I. Fanconi anaemia and leukaemia—clinical and molecular aspects. *Br J Haematol*. 2004;126(2):176–191.
63. Djulbegovic B, et al. Safety and efficacy of purified factor IX concentrate and antifibrinolytic agents for dental extractions in hemophilia B. *Am J Hematol*. 1996;51(2):168–170.
64. Berntorp E, Bjorkman S. The pharmacokinetics of clotting factor therapy. *Haemophilia*. 2003;9(4):353–359.
65. Scharrer I, Bray GL, Neutzling O. Incidence of inhibitors in haemophilia A patients—a review of recent studies of recombinant and plasma-derived factor VIII concentrates. *Haemophilia*. 1999;5(3):145–154.
66. Goodnough LT, et al. Transfusion medicine service policies for recombinant factor VIIa administration. *Transfusion*. 2004;44(9):1325–1331.
67. Shapiro AD, et al. The safety and efficacy of recombinant human blood coagulation factor IX in previously untreated patients with severe or moderately severe hemophilia B. *Blood*. 2005; 105(2):518–525.
68. Warrier I, et al. Factor IX inhibitors and anaphylaxis in hemophilia B. *J Pediatr Hematol Oncol*. 1997;19(1):23–27.
69. O'Connell NM. Factor XI deficiency. *Semin Hematol*. 2004;41(1 Suppl 1):76–81.
70. Tavori S, Brenner B, Tatarsky I. The effect of combined factor XI deficiency with von Willebrand factor abnormalities on haemorrhagic diathesis. *Thromb Haemost*. 1990;63(1):36–38.
71. Rakocz M, et al. Dental extractions in patients with bleeding disorders. The use of fibrin glue. *Oral Surg Oral Med Oral Pathol*. 1993;75(3):280–282.
72. Kitchens CS. The contact system. *Arch Pathol Lab Med*. 2002;126(11):1382–1386.
73. Cines DB, Blanchette VS. Immune thrombocytopenic purpura. *N Engl J Med*. 2002; 346(13):995–1008.
74. Bartholomew JR, Begelman SM, Almahameed A. Heparin-induced thrombocytopenia: principles for early recognition and management. *Cleve Clin J Med*. 2005;72(Suppl 1):S31–S36.
75. Warkentin TE, Kelton JG. Temporal aspects of heparin-induced thrombocytopenia. *N Engl J Med*. 2001;344(17):1286–1292.
76. Eckman MH, et al. Screening for the risk for bleeding or thrombosis. *Ann Intern Med*. 2003; 138(3):W15–W24.
77. Geerts WH, et al. Prevention of venous thromboembolism: the Seventh ACCP Conference on Antithrombotic and Thrombolytic Therapy. *Chest*. 2004;126(3 Suppl):338S–400S.
78. Horlocker TT, et al. Regional anesthesia in the anticoagulated patient: defining the risks (the second ASRA Consensus Conference on Neuraxial Anesthesia and Anticoagulation). *Reg Anesth Pain Med*. 2003;28(3):172–197.
79. Weiss G, Goodnough LT. Anemia of chronic disease. *N Engl J Med*. 2005;352(10):1011–1023.

CHAPTER 14

RENAL DISEASE AND ELECTROLYTE MANAGEMENT

Maninder S. Kohli

The spectrum of perioperative renal disease encompasses several types of patient populations in a variety of surgical settings. The significant increase in perioperative morbidity and mortality in such patients depends on a number of preexisting risk factors and comorbidities, the nature and timing of the operation, and anesthesia. Patients with chronic kidney disease (CKD) and dialysis patients are at significant risk for excessive morbidity and mortality from major surgery. Preoperative renal insufficiency is the most important risk factor for developing acute on chronic renal failure after a major surgical procedure and is associated with a high mortality.[1] The presence of preoperative renal insufficiency is also an important predictor of postoperative cardiac complications in patients undergoing a major operation. Cardiac dysfunction and sepsis are significant causes of death after a major surgery in patients with CKD. Other serious complications include volume overload, hypertension, bleeding, acidosis, and electrolyte disturbances such as hyperkalemia. Patients on dialysis present unique management challenges in the perioperative period. This chapter will focus on the risk factors, diagnosis, and assessment and management of perioperative renal disease in addition to common electrolyte abnormalities.

EPIDEMIOLOGY

It is clear from national data that the prevalence of CKD is steadily rising. Recent data from the U.S. Renal Data System show that the number of patients on dialysis has risen 12% in the previous decade.[2] New cases of acute renal failure (ARF) in the perioperative setting account for 25% of all episodes of hospital-acquired renal insufficiency and for a substantial number of patients requiring urgent renal replacement therapy (RRT).[3] Postoperative acute kidney injury (AKI) is defined as an acute decline in renal function resulting in a rise of serum creatinine and accumulation of

Perioperative Medicine: Medical Consultation and Co-Management, First Edition.
Edited by Amir K. Jaffer and Paul J. Grant.

nitrogenous wastes. Although earlier studies used absolute values of serum creatinine elevation, more recent studies have used estimation of creatinine clearance. A decline of 50% or more in the glomerular filtration rate (GFR) or the need for RRT are better descriptions of postoperative AKI. The mortality of postoperative AKI ranges from 25% to 90% despite vast improvements in intensive care support and RRT.[4] This topic is covered in more detail in Chapter 34.

PREDICTION OF RISK: PATIENT- AND SURGERY-RELATED RISK FACTORS

Patients with GFR or >60 mL/min without additional risk factors are unlikely to experience serious postoperative complications and as such no specific precautions are necessary. In a recent cohort of patients with normal renal function undergoing noncardiac surgery, there was a low (0.8%) risk of postoperative AKI and an even lower (0.1%) risk of requiring RRT.[5] Preoperative predictors of increased risk were age ≥60, body mass index (BMI) ≥32, peripheral vascular disease, liver disease, chronic obstructive pulmonary disease, high-risk surgery, and emergent surgery. Among those with three or more risk factors, 4.3% developed AKI and had a sixfold increase in 30-day mortality.

However, patients with preexisting CKD are at high risk for postoperative AKI and a low GFR predicts the need for RRT. Diabetics with established nephropathy and patients with immunologic glomerular disease are at elevated risk of postoperative renal dysfunction. Those with a severely reduced GFR (<20 mL/min) are quite likely to experience postoperative volume overload, acidosis, hyperkalemia, and the need to initiate immediate RRT after surgery. A recent systematic review of 31 studies found the presence of CKD to be an independent risk factor for postoperative cardiovascular death after elective noncardiac surgery.[6] Moreover, the severity of kidney disease predicted the increased perioperative risk of death.

Patients with advanced CKD on dialysis have an overall increased risk of surgical morbidity and mortality. An earlier review of dialysis patients undergoing general surgery had a morbidity rate of 54%.[1] The overall mortality rate was 4%, with a disturbing 47% mortality in the subset requiring emergency surgery.

Increases in perioperative risk are also noted in several studies of patients with an estimated GFR below 60 mL/min undergoing major aortic and lower-extremity vascular surgery. Analysis of operative outcomes and long-term follow-up of patients undergoing thoraco-abdominal aneurysm surgery with cross-clamping showed that advanced age and preoperative CKD were risk factors for postoperative dialysis.[7] Other factors that increase the risk for postoperative renal failure include complicated aneurysms (i.e., ruptured aneurysms, suprarenal aneurysms, and those that require renal artery bypass), intraoperative blood loss and hypotension, prolonged cardiopulmonary bypass, and cholesterol embolization.[1]

In a large cohort of patients requiring infrainguinal vascular surgery, preoperative renal disease was independently associated with postoperative death, cardiac arrest, myocardial infarction, and re-intubation.[8] In another study of 57 infrainguinal bypass procedures in 44 patients requiring maintenance dialysis (33 of which were diabetics), the perioperative mortality rate was 9%.[9] The 30-day surgical morbidity rate was 39%, and the major complications were wound breakdown (19%), graft thrombosis (9%), and major limb amputation (4%). Patient survival was only 52% at 2 years.

Of all the surgical procedures, AKI in the cardiac surgery patient by far carries the highest rates of perioperative morbidity and mortality. In a review of 13 studies of patients with end-stage renal disease undergoing cardiac surgery, a morbidity rate of 46% and a mortality rate of 10% was reported.[1] The mortality of valve repair was twice that of coronary artery bypass grafting (CABG). A more recent trial studied outcomes in a cohort of 7152 patients on dialysis undergoing coronary artery bypass surgery.[10] Patients on dialysis carried a greater than sixfold increase in operative mortality and a greater than threefold increase in the frequency of stroke, septicemia, prolonged ventilation, and prolonged postoperative stay compared with patients with a normal GFR. In the same study, patients with severe renal dysfunction (GFR < 30 mL/min) experienced longer pump times (cross-clamp and perfusion times) and more frequent balloon pump usage compared with patients who had a normal GFR. A large cohort of patients at the Cleveland Clinic who underwent open heart surgery were assessed for the frequency of postoperative AKI requiring RRT or a >50% decline from preoperative GFR.[11] Combined outcomes were seen in 3.8% of patients undergoing CABG, 4.5% in those undergoing valve surgery, and 7.9% among patients requiring combined CABG and valve procedures.

Although the literature is sparse, patients undergoing surgery for obstructive jaundice appear to have a high incidence of postoperative renal failure. Severity of preoperative jaundice, CKD, and perioperative hypotension predict postoperative AKI. Patients with obstructive jaundice appear to have significant postoperative reductions in the GFR. This effect may be explained by the fact that absorption of endotoxins is limited due to the decreased excretion of bile salts in deeply jaundiced patients.[12] The result of the endotoxinemia is enhanced renal vasoconstriction, which in the presence of systemic hypotension or preexisting renal disease can lead to worsening of renal function in the postoperative period.

AGE

Earlier studies have determined advanced age to be an independent predictor of developing postoperative renal failure. One study found age >65 to be a multivariate predictor for developing postoperative ARF after cardiac surgery; however, advanced age did not predict the need for dialysis.[13] Advanced age was not predictive of postoperative renal failure requiring dialysis in a large prospective study of 4315 patients undergoing noncardiac surgery.[14] More recently, a large prospective study found that patients ≥59 years of age with normal preoperative renal function were more likely to develop postoperative ARF than younger patients.[15] It is likely that age-related reductions in GFR and the presence of comorbid conditions can lead to renal dysfunction after surgery. Important variables that predict mortality in the elderly with postoperative renal failure include sustained perioperative hypotension, the need for mechanical ventilation, and multiorgan failure.

PREDICTION OF RISK: RISK INDICES

Several indices exist for the preoperative cardiovascular risk stratification of patients undergoing major surgery. The Revised Cardiac Risk Index (RCRI) is the most commonly used index to predict cardiac complications in patients undergoing non-cardiac surgery and includes CKD (defined as serum creatinine of >2.0 mg/dL) as one of the indices.[16]

A recent study using similar methodology prospectively developed and validated a risk index to predict AKI for patients undergoing general surgery from a large national data set.[15] Patients with the highest weighted score for increased risk were those undergoing intraperitoneal surgery, the presence of mild–moderate CKD, ascites, congestive heart failure (CHF), and emergency surgery (Table 14.1). The incidence of AKI increased with risk class and demonstrated consistency across the derivation and validation cohorts. In addition, patients without postoperative AKI had a morbidity of 19% and a 30-day mortality of 8.6%. Patients who did develop postoperative AKI had a corresponding morbidity of 66% and a mortality of 42%.

Multiple studies have attempted to produce predictive indices with moderate accuracy (areas under the receiver operating characteristic [ROC] curve of 0.75–0.81 in external validation) to predict postoperative AKI and need for RRT after cardiac surgery. A recent study by Wijeysundera et al. developed and validated a simplified risk index in 20,131 patients to predict RRT after cardiac surgery.[17] Multivariate analysis identified eight variables of increased risk (Table 14.2). The predictive index was scored from 0 to 8 points. The presence of severe preoperative CKD again carried the highest risk of postoperative RRT. Among half of the cohort with low risk scores (≤1 point), the risk of RRT was 0.4%. In contrast, patients with the highest risk (≥4 points) had a 10% risk of requiring postoperative RRT.

TABLE 14.1. Acute Kidney Injury (AKI) Risk Index for Patients Undergoing General Surgery

Preoperative risk class	AKI incidence (%) Derivation cohort	AKI incidence (%) Validation cohort
Class I (0–2 risk factors)	0.2	0.2
Class II (3–4 risk factors)	0.8	0.8
Class III (4 risk factors)	1.8	2.0
Class IV (5 risk factors)	3.3	3.6
Class V (≥6 risk factors)	8.9	9.5

Risk factors to predict risk: age ≥56 years, male sex, active congestive heart failure, ascites, hypertension, emergency surgery, intraperitoneal surgery, renal insufficiency (mild or moderate; preoperative serum creatinine >1.2 mg/dL), and diabetes mellitus on oral or insulin therapy.
Adapted from Kheteral et al.[15]

TABLE 14.2.   Risk Index to Predict Renal Replacement Therapy (RRT) in Cardiac Surgery

Risk variable	Points assigned	Risk class	Complication rate
Estimated GFR ≤30 mL/min	2	Low risk (0–1 points)	<1%
Estimated GFR 31–60 mL/min	1	Intermediate risk (2–3 points)	2–5%
Diabetes mellitus (on therapy)	1	High risk (≥4 points)	10%
LVEF ≤40%	1		
Previous cardiac surgery	1		
Surgery other than CABG/ASD repair	1		
Urgent/emergent procedure	1		
Preoperative intra-aortic balloon pump	1		

GFR, glomerular filtration rate; LVEF, left ventricular ejection fraction; CABG, coronary artery bypass grafting; ASD, atrial septal defect.
Adapted from Wijeysundera et al.[17]

The significance of a preoperative risk index to a clinician is to classify patients into various categories of risk. A valuable risk index can adequately identify low-risk patients who may not need further evaluation or specific perioperative precautions. More importantly, it can classify patients at increased risk of serious postoperative complications who may require additional preoperative testing or focused perioperative management (discussed below).

PREOPERATIVE EVALUATION

A basic evaluation of patients with CKD consists of a careful history and physical examination; a panel of laboratory tests including serum chemistry, calcium, and phosphate levels; a complete blood count; a coagulation profile; and an electrocardiogram. Specific risk factors requiring preoperative evaluation and possible intervention include the presence of preoperative CKD (serum creatinine >2 mg/dL, estimated GFR <60 mL/min, and especially <30 mL/min), hyperkalemia, metabolic acidosis, significant anemia, and presence of cardiac disease.

Patients with unexplained CKD discovered during the preoperative evaluation should have elective surgery postponed to determine the etiology of the renal disease.

Cardiovascular Evaluation

Cardiac disease is the most serious comorbidity in patients with CKD. It is estimated that 50% of all deaths in this patient population are from underlying cardiac disease. Coronary atherosclerosis is the key factor in the development of significant cardiac disease in patients with CKD with a prevalence of about 40%.[18] In patients with advanced CKD on hemodialysis or peritoneal dialysis, the prevalence of heart failure is approximately 40%. Both coronary artery disease and left ventricular hypertrophy are risk factors for developing CHF.

Cardiovascular mortality approaches 9% per year in patients with CKD. In dialysis patients, the annual mortality is 10–20 times higher than the general population.[18] Preexisting renal disease (serum creatinine >2 mg/dL) has been shown to be an independent predictor of increased cardiac risk in patients undergoing major noncardiac surgery.[16] Given the high prevalence of cardiac disease, a careful cardiac risk assessment is mandated in CKD patients undergoing major surgery. Many patients with CKD are asymptomatic of the typical manifestations of coronary disease and heart failure. Therefore, further preoperative evaluation is often necessary, particularly in dialysis recipients.

Additional testing for significant coronary artery disease may need to be performed in select patients with CKD. One study of cardiac risk stratification in patients undergoing renal transplantation found that patients who had no risk factors (age >50, angina, CHF, insulin-dependent diabetes, abnormal electrocardiogram) were at low risk for cardiac events with an overall cardiac mortality of 1%. Those with one or more risk factors had a 17% overall mortality.[19] A number of trials have explored the role of noninvasive evaluation in the preoperative assessment of cardiac risk in patients with CKD undergoing surgery. The majority of the patients were renal transplant candidates and thus represented a relatively healthy dialysis population. Many trials have noted limitations of exercise stress testing and dipyridamole thallium scanning in patients with CKD, reporting lower sensitivities and specificities for the detection of significant coronary disease.[18]

Studies of combined dipyridamole and exercise thallium scanning as well as the use of dobutamine echocardiography have shown favorable results in identifying significant coronary disease in patients undergoing renal transplantation. Dipyridamole-exercise thallium imaging and coronary angiography were both performed prospectively in a study of 60 asymptomatic hemodialysis patients who were followed for major coronary events. After follow-up of almost 3 years, 47% of patients with abnormal thallium uptake experienced a coronary event, as compared with 9% of patients with a normal thallium uptake.[20] In a study of 53 patients with insulin-dependent diabetes mellitus being considered for kidney and/or pancreas transplantation, cardiac event rates were 45% among those with an abnormal, compared with 6% among those with a normal dobutamine stress echocardiogram.[21]

Given the high prevalence of significant cardiac disease in dialysis patients, some authors have questioned the use of noninvasive testing before renal transplantation. One study examined 126 renal transplant candidates who were classified as moderate (≥50 years) or high coronary risk (diabetes, peripheral atherosclerosis, or clinical coronary artery disease), and underwent myocardial scintigraphy (SPECT), dobutamine stress echocardiography, and angiography.[22] The prevalence of CAD was 42%, and the sensitivities and negative predictive values for the two noninvasive tests and risk stratification were <75%. The probability of event-free survival at 48 months was 94% in patients with <70% stenosis on coronary angiography, and 54% in patients with >70% stenosis. Multivariate analysis showed that the presence of critical coronary lesions was the sole predictor of cardiac events.

Patients with evidence of valvular heart disease or CHF by history and physical examination should undergo a preoperative echocardiogram to determine the magnitude of left ventricular dysfunction.

Many trials of medical therapy (largely beta-blockers) have shown favorable immediate- and long-term outcomes in patients with established CAD or risk factors for CAD. Although the published trials were not specific to patients with CKD, the results indicate that barring contraindications, patients with CKD in addition to significant CAD risk, may be justified in receiving perioperative beta-blockers. Ideally, these agents should be initiated several days or weeks before the surgery and titrated to a resting heart rate of 55–65 beats per minute. Immediate preoperative initiation of beta-blockers in high doses is not recommended due the elevated risk of stroke and overall mortality reported in a recent large, randomized controlled trial.[23]

ANESTHETIC CONSIDERATIONS

Important considerations in the patient with CKD are the use of anesthetic agents and sedatives in the perioperative period.[24] The choice of inhalational anesthetic agents is best left to the anesthesiology team. General anesthesia, and particularly spinal anesthesia, can cause hypotension and reduce effective renal blood flow. This effect is probably proportional to the depth of the anesthesia achieved.[25] Propofol and isoflurane are well tolerated and widely used anesthetic agents, although induction doses may need to be reduced in a patient with CKD. The potential for hyperkalemia in patients with CKD who are given succinylcholine is well recognized; however, if the preoperative potassium level is less than 5.5 mEq/L, then it may be safely administered. Long-acting muscle relaxants such as pancuronium are best avoided. Vecuronium may be safe for induction, but the preferred agent is atracurium since it does not accumulate in patients with preexisting renal disease. Local and regional anesthetic agents are usually well tolerated.

Extreme caution must be exercised with the use of perioperative sedatives and opiates.

Dialysis patients are particularly sensitive to the effects of benzodiazepines. The free fraction of these protein-bound drugs is increased in such patients. Midazolam is excreted as its active metabolite and can rapidly accumulate in renal failure.[25] Morphine may be used in renal failure patients, but with caution. Although the half-life of morphine is essentially unchanged, its metabolites can accumulate and are pharmacologically active. Meperidine must be avoided in patients with advanced kidney disease since its active metabolite normeperdine accumulates in toxic levels and can lead to seizures.

PERIOPERATIVE MANAGEMENT

Perioperative management of CKD patients undergoing major surgery requires aggressive metabolic, cardiovascular, hematologic, and pharmaceutical management.

Fluid Management

Euvolemia is mandated in patients with CKD in preparation for surgery as the ability to respond to volume expansion and depletion as well as other homeostatic changes is limited in these patients. Patients with mild-to-moderate reductions in the GFR may have impaired excretion of a large and rapid sodium load in the perioperative period. This may occur in circumstances where other comorbidities also inhibit sodium excretion, such as CHF, cirrhosis, and nephrotic syndrome.

In patients with a GFR of <10 mL/min, administration of large quantities of intravenous fluids can quickly lead to volume overload. The presence of volume overload preoperatively can be managed with aggressive sodium restriction and the use of diuretics. Large doses of loop diuretics such as furosemide or bumetanide are often required in patients not already receiving dialysis. At times, the judicious use of metolazone can enhance the effect of the loop diuretics. Maintenance infusions of furosemide are not recommended. The use of mannitol, low-dose dopamine, or calcium channel blockers has not been proven to prevent postoperative renal failure in patients with normal renal function or with preexisting renal disease.[26,27] With careful preoperative resuscitation and control of fluid and electrolyte balance, the incidence of postoperative renal dysfunction can be minimized. The role of prophylactic dialysis in patients with severe renal dysfunction not previously on RRT is controversial. A small study of 44 adult patients with a serum creatinine of >2.5 mg/dL undergoing cardiac surgery noted decreased morbidity and mortality in those receiving perioperative prophylactic RRT.[28]

Dialysis Patients

Ideally, dialysis patients should be at or close to their "dry weight" by the time of surgery.

Preoperative consultation with the surgeon and anesthetist is useful to estimate the amount of fluids likely to be administered in the perioperative period. Besides the type of fluid to be given (preferably isotonic saline and not lactated ringers), the timing and intensity of preoperative dialysis can help to ensure a safe outcome.

In general, dialysis should be provided on the day before the procedure. Care must be taken to avoid volume depletion in patients with some preservation of renal function. Worsening renal function is common in those with preoperative volume depletion who then experience sustained hypotension. Dialysis patients who undergo intensive preoperative dialysis are at risk for anesthesia-induced vasodilatation that can lead to thrombosis of the vascular access graft.[25]

The timing of postoperative dialysis depends on the amount of fluids administered perioperatively. Critically ill patients and those who have received excessive fluids may need immediate postoperative dialysis. Ultrafiltration provides a means to preferentially remove fluid in volume-overloaded patients. This must be balanced with the risk of hypotension, especially in patients with postoperative cardiac dysfunction or sepsis. In stable patients, dialysis can be safely resumed 24 h after the surgery. The decision to use heparin with dialysis should be made in consultation with the surgical team.

Dialysis patients needing emergency surgery are at particular risk for serious morbidity and higher mortality. When possible, a "no heparin" dialysis should be performed for 2–3 h before surgery. However, dialysis can be continued through the surgical procedure if necessary. Hypotension, hyperkalemia, and wound complications are common in the postoperative setting.

Peritoneal dialysis patients present unique management challenges in the perioperative period. Dwells must be individualized and based on the preoperative assessment of fluid status, type of surgery, and expected fluid administration. The dialysate fluid should be exchanged before the start of surgery and the dwell maintained through the course of a short procedure. For a longer procedure, an intraoperative exchange may be necessary. Dialysate concentrations can be adjusted to manage excess fluid administration during surgery. Postoperatively, dwells should be resumed on a scheduled basis, with modifications to the dialysate fluid based on volume status and serum electrolyte measurements. Patients on peritoneal dialysis undergoing abdominal surgery are at an increased risk for anastomotic leaks, poor wound healing, and incisional hernia formation. For such patients, the peritoneal fluid should be drained completely just before the surgery. Alternative dialysis modes such as hemodialysis or continuous arteriovenous hemodialysis may be undertaken in the perioperative period. Peritoneal dialysis can be resumed after a few weeks beginning with small volumes and short dwell times.

POSTOPERATIVE AKI

The early diagnosis of postoperative renal insufficiency is frequently not apparent. A decrease in urine output may be the first sign of ARF; although many patients have nonoliguric renal insufficiency.

Symptoms and signs of AKI include reduced oral intake, vomiting, flank pain, mental status changes, hypertension, and volume overload. However, symptoms manifest only after the occurrence of significant renal dysfunction. Variations in serum sodium levels can lead to alterations in mentation. Acidosis and hyperkalemia can lead to significant cardiovascular instability.

Measurements of serum chemistry, urine osmolality, and electrolytes, and examination of the urine sediment are crucial in the evaluation of postoperative renal failure. Estimating the creatinine clearance using the Cockroft–Gault equation (Appendix) provides a reasonable estimate of the GFR. Determining the fractional excretion of sodium can distinguish between acute tubular necrosis (ATN) and prerenal causes of postoperative AKI (Table 14.3 and Appendix). Hyaline casts (concentrated Tamm–Horsfall mucoproteins) are nonspecific and may indicate hypoperfusion. Often, the presence of brown granular casts suggests ATN. The presence of white blood cells can indicate urinary tract infection, and eosinophiluria suggests interstitial nephritis or cholesterol embolization.[24]

Impaired renal concentrating ability, salt-wasting, hypotonic fluids, and postoperative syndrome of inappropriate antidiuretic hormone secretion (SIADH) can lead to hyponatremia. However, hypernatremia can develop from the inability to replace free water losses during the polyuria phase of renal function recovery.

TABLE 14.3. Differentiating Prerenal and Renal Azotemia

	Prerenal	Renal
Urine osmolality (mOsm/kg)	>50	<350
Urine/plasma osmolality	>1.3	<1.1
Urine sodium (mEq/L)	<20	>40
Urine/plasma creatinine	>40	<20
Fractional excretion of sodium (FENa)	<1%	>1%

TABLE 14.4. Major Causes of Postoperative Renal Failure

Prerenal causes:
- Intraoperative hypotension
- Volume depletion
- Sepsis
- Congestive heart failure

Renal causes:
- Acute tubular necrosis
- Drugs-induced nephritis
- Radiocontrast dye
- Hemoglobinuria
- Myoglobinuria

Postrenal causes:
- Tubular obstruction
- Bladder dysfunction
- Pelvic/ureteral obstruction
- Retroperitoneal hematoma

A renal ultrasound should be ordered early if there is a strong suspicion for urinary tract obstruction. Older men with benign prostatic hyperplasia (BPH) and patients who have undergone urological or gynecological procedures are at a higher risk for developing postrenal causes of postoperative AKI.[24]

The highly vascular kidneys are particularly at risk for a variety of insults that can compromise renal function. The pathophysiology of postoperative AKI mirrors the causes usually found in the medical patient with compromised renal function. Table 14.4 lists the major causes and differential diagnosis of AKI.[24] Of note, a major cause is sustained hypotension from the following causes:

- perioperative blood and fluid losses,

- prolonged anesthetic time,

- aorta cross-clamp time,

– cardiopulmonary bypass,

– positive-pressure ventilation.

Prolonged renal ischemia from the above causes or vasoactive inflammatory mediators due to sepsis can lead to rapid postoperative ATN.[29] Other mechanisms of kidney injury are cholesterol embolization from cardiopulmonary bypass and aortic surgery.

There is a risk of significant morbidity in the postoperative period. In a study of 312 dialysis patients, 64% of patients experienced a major complication, with the most frequent one being hyperkalemia.[30] Other serious complications were hemodynamic instability, fluid overload, infections, arrhythmias, and bleeding. Cardiovascular complications included postoperative myocardial infarction, CHF, and arrhythmias. Hemodynamic derangements with hypertension and hypotension in the perioperative period are not infrequent in the dialysis patient. Failure to metabolize and excrete anesthetics and analgesics can lead to toxic accumulation of these agents.[25] Anemia, pericarditis, and clotting of vascular access ports can further complicate the day-to-day management of patients with CKD. Finally, dialysis patients frequently require intensive care support including the need for prolonged mechanical ventilation, vasopressor use, and a protracted length of stay.[25] The management of postoperative AKI and role of perioperative RRT is discussed in Chapter 34.

Electrolyte Management

Hyperkalemia   Hyperkalemia is one of the most important morbid complications in the perioperative period.

A preoperative electrocardiogram should be ordered to assess the physiologic effect of hyperkalemia although electrocardiographic changes may be seen only when the potassium concentration exceeds 6.0–6.5 mEq/L.[25] Patients with CKD usually tolerate a modest elevation in the serum level of potassium, but abrupt increases in levels are poorly tolerated in dialysis patients. In patients undergoing elective surgery, the preoperative potassium should be reduced to less than 5.0 mEq/L. Based on the preoperative serum potassium level, the dialysis flow rate, type of dialyzer, and the potassium concentration of the bath, hemodialysis can adequately remove an appropriate amount of potassium. In cases of emergency surgery where time does not permit an adequate preoperative dialysis, other measures must be taken to stabilize the cardiac membrane. Patients with electrocardiographic evidence of hyperkalemia (i.e., peaked T-waves, prolongation of the QRS, or arrhythmias) should be given an intravenous infusion of 1 ampule of calcium gluconate (10 mL of a 10% solution). This intervention can provide cardioprotection while attempts are under way to reduce the serum potassium.

Medical management of severe hyperkalemia before surgery can reduce potassium by varying degrees and include insulin, administered together with glucose to avoid hypoglycemia, which causes a rapid shift of potassium to the intracellular space. The expected reduction in serum potassium is 0.9 mEq/L. Other options include epinephrine and albuterol, which can be expected to reduce potassium by

0.3 mEq/L; however, the beta-2 agonists can lead to arrhythmias. Sodium bicarbonate has no effect on serum potassium in the absence of metabolic acidosis. Cation exchange resins are effective in removing excess potassium, but take several hours to take effect. The usual oral dose is 15–30 g, which can be repeated. If patients are unable to take anything by mouth, 50–100 g in 200 mL of water can be administered as a rectal enema. Of note, one complication of cation exchange resins is the risk of intestinal necrosis when administered within 1 week after abdominal surgery.[25]

Calcium and Phosphate   Severe hypocalcemia (less than 6 mg/dL) must be treated and should begin with control of the serum phosphate level. The use of phosphate binders should be initiated early to aim for a level less than 5.5 mg/dL. In emergency situations, preoperative dialysis can also lower serum phosphate. Calcium can be replaced orally with 1.5 g of oral elemental calcium per day. Coadministration of the rapidly acting vitamin D derivative 1,25-dihydroxycholcalciferol is recommended in a dose of 0.25–0.75 μg/day. Intravenous calcium can be infused rapidly in patients with signs and symptoms of severe hypocalcemia.

Acidosis   Patients with CKD are prone to metabolic acidosis. Although there is respiratory compensation, patients may be prone to severe acidemia due to perioperative ischemia. The impairment of renal function makes it difficult to buffer a large acid load. The preoperative bicarbonate level should be greater than 18 mEq/L. Bicarbonate administration with either oral replacement or intravenous infusion can raise the level without leading to significant volume expansion from the sodium load.

Hypertension and Hypotension   The incidence of hypertension is high in patients with CKD. Excessive fluid retention and exaggerated catecholamine surges are primary mechanisms that can explain hypertension in dialysis patients. Preoperative optimization can be accomplished by dialysis and ultrafiltration. Management of anxiety and continuation of most antihypertensive agents through the operative day can help control blood pressure. For refractory hypertension that does not respond to preoperative dialysis and oral medications, intravenous labetalol, enalapril, or hydralazine can immediately lower the blood pressure. The use of intravenous nitroprusside should be limited to 1–2 days since thiocyanate, a metabolite of nitroprusside, can accumulate in patients with advanced kidney disease leading to anorexia, confusion, and psychosis.

Hypotension in the dialysis patient is multifactorial and problematic as the need for pre- and postoperative dialysis arises in the surgical patient. Preoperative excessive fluid removal, CHF, autonomic dysfunction, operative blood loss, and the perioperative use of anesthetics and antihypertensive agents are important causes of hypotension.[24] Corrective measures to reduce and treat perioperative hypotension include adjusting the patient's dry weight, increasing the dialysate sodium concentration, and the use of steady ultrafiltration. Use of erythropoietin to treat underlying anemia, a higher calcium concentration in the dialysate, and cool temperature dialysis can also favorably affect cardiovascular performance.

The use of a pulmonary-artery catheter in the perioperative period is theoretically advantageous in patients with CKD. However, several studies have failed to demonstrate improved outcomes (although some excluded patients with renal failure).

At present, the use of pulmonary-artery catheters is probably justified only in CKD patients undergoing major operations who have perioperative volume or hemodynamic derangements, significant left ventricular dysfunction, and in dialysis patients undergoing emergency surgery.

Anemia and Bleeding Diathesis   Anemia is universally present in patients with significant CKD. Since the anemia is chronic, it is usually well tolerated, and most patients with hematocrit levels of 20–24% tolerate even major procedures without the need for preoperative transfusions. Patients with advanced CKD have defects in platelet aggregation and thus are at risk for postoperative bleeding. Preoperative bleeding times are not routinely recommended; however, one may be obtained in patients with CKD who have a prior history of excessive bleeding. Intensive preoperative dialysis is likely beneficial in patients with a prolonged bleeding time who require surgical procedures that are associated with excessive blood loss. Intravenous desmopressin is recommended for urgent surgery. The duration of action is 8 h, although tachyphylaxis can develop after repeated doses. Postoperative dialysis without heparin can be performed if the anticipated risk of perioperative bleeding is high.

Nutrition   Poor nutritional status is common in patients with advanced CKD. Poor wound healing and infections can complicate the postoperative course in malnourished patients. Diabetics with advanced CKD disease are also predisposed to hypoglycemic events. Earlier evidence suggests that patients with CKD who receive perioperative nutritional support have a lower mortality.[25]

Patients with CKD undergoing major surgery should receive enteral or parenteral nutrition if oral intake cannot be resumed soon after major surgery. Since azotemia and fluid overload are common issues in patients with advanced CKD, administration of essential amino acids and concentrated carbohydrates and lipids can minimize nitrogen and fluid excess. Frequent measurements of serum electrolytes are essential to avoid derangements in potassium, calcium, phosphate, and sodium.

CONCLUSION

The surgical risk in patients with CKD depends on the severity of the underlying kidney disease, presence of comorbid medical conditions, type of surgical procedure, and whether the surgery is elective or emergent. A careful preoperative assessment of patients with preexisting renal disease is imperative in predicting adverse postoperative events and implementing strategies to reduce operative morbidity and mortality.

REFERENCES

1. Kellerman PS. Perioperative care of the renal patient. *Arch Intern Med.* 1994;154:1674–1688.
2. United States Renal Data System. 2009 Annual Data Report: Atlas of End-Stage Renal Disease. Bethesda, MD: NIH, NIDDK; 2009.
3. Liano F, Pascual J. Epidemiology of acute renal failure: a prospective, multicenter community-based study. *Kidney Int.* 1996;50(3):811–818.
4. Carmichael P, Carmichael AR. Acute renal failure in the surgical setting. *ANZ J Surg.* 2003;73(3):144–153.
5. Kheterpal S, Tremper KK, Englesbe MJ, et al. Predictors of acute renal failure after noncardiac surgery in patients with previously normal renal function. *Anesthesiology.* 2007;107:892–902.
6. Mathew A, Devereaux PJ, O'Hare A, et al. Chronic kidney disease and postoperative mortality: a systematic review and meta-analysis. *Kidney Int.* 2008;73:1069–1081.
7. Schepens MA, Defauw JJ, Hamerlijnck RP, et al. Surgical treatment of thoraco-abdominal aortic aneurysms by simple cross-clamping. Risk factors and late results. *J Thorac Cardiovasc Surg.* 1994;107(1):134–142.
8. O'Hare AM, Feinglass J, Sidawy AN, et al. Impact of renal insufficiency on short-term morbidity and mortality after lower extremity revascularization: data from the Department of Veterans Affairs' National Surgical Quality Improvement Program. *J Am Soc Nephrol.* 2003;14:1287–1295.
9. Baele HR, Piotrowski JJ, Yuhas J, et al. Infrainguinal bypass in patients with end-stage renal disease. *Surgery.* 1995;117(3):319–324.
10. Cooper WA, O'Brien SM, Thourani VH, et al. Impact of renal dysfunction on outcomes of coronary artery bypass surgery: results from the Society of Thoracic Surgeons National Adult Cardiac Database. *Circulation.* 2006;113:1063–1070.
11. Thaker CV, Liangos O, Yared JP, et al. Acute renal failure after open-heart surgery: influence of gender and race. *Am J Kidney Dis.* 2005;45:742–751.
12. Pain JA, Cahill CJ, Gilbert JM, et al. Prevention of postoperative renal dysfunction in patients with obstructive jaundice: a multicentre study of bile salts and lactulose. *Br J Surg.* 1991;78(4):467–469.
13. Conlon PJ, Stafford-Smith M, White WD, et al. Acute renal failure following cardiac surgery. *Nephrol Dial Transplant.* 1999;14:1158.
14. Polanczyk CA, Marcantonio E, Goldman L, et al. Impact of age on perioperative complications and length of stay in patients undergoing noncardiac surgery. *Ann Intern Med.* 2001;134:637–643.
15. Kheteral S, Tremper KK, Heung M, et al. Development and validation of an acute kidney injury risk index for patients undergoing general surgery. *Anesthesiology.* 2009;110:505–515.
16. Lee TH, Marcantonio ER, Mangione CM, et al. Derivation and prospective validation of a simple index for prediction of cardiac risk for noncardiac surgery. *Circulation.* 1999;100:1043–1049.
17. Wijeysundera DN, Karkouti K, Dupuid JY, et al. Derivation and validation of a simplified predictive index for renal replacement therapy after cardiac surgery. *JAMA.* 2007;297:1801–1809.
18. Joseph AJ, Cohn SL. Perioperative care of the patient with renal failure. *Med Clin North Am.* 2003;87:193–210.
19. Le A, Wilson R, Douek K, Pulliam L, et al. Prospective risk stratification in renal transplant candidates for cardiac death. *Am J Kidney Dis.* 1994;24(1):65–71.
20. Dahan M, Viron BM, Faraggi M, et al. Diagnostic accuracy and prognostic value of combined dipyridamole-exercise thallium imaging in hemodialysis patients. *Kidney Int.* 1998;54(1):255–262.
21. Bates JR, Sawada SG, Segar DS, et al. Evaluation using dobutamine stress echocardiography in patients with insulin-dependent diabetes mellitus before kidney and/or pancreas transplantation. *Am J Cardiol.* 1996;77(2):175–179.
22. De Lima JJ, Sabbaga E, Vieira ML, et al. Coronary angiography is the best predictor of events in renal transplant candidates compared with noninvasive testing. *Hypertension.* 2003;42(3):263–268.
23. Devereaux PJ, Yang H, Yusuf S, et al. Effects of extended-release metoprolol succinate in patients undergoing non-cardiac surgery (POISE trial): a randomised controlled trial. *Lancet.* 2008;371(9627):1839–1847.
24. Kohli MS, Kerns JC. Postoperative renal failure. In: *Just the Facts: Perioperative Medicine*, Cohn SL, Smetana G, Weed H (eds.), pp. 317–319. New York: McGraw-Hill; 2006.

25. Shusterman N. Surgery in the patient with chronic renal failure. In: *Perioperative Medicine*, 2nd edition, Goldmann DT, Brown FH, Guarnieri DM (eds.), pp. 309–317. New York: McGraw-Hill; 1994.
26. Bellomo R, Chapman M, Finfer S, et al. Low-dose dopamine in patients with early renal dysfunction: a placebo-controlled randomized trial. *Lancet.* 2000;356:2139.
27. Brown CV, Rhee P, Chan L, et al. Preventing renal failure in patients with rhabdomyolysis: do bicarbonate and mannitol make a difference? *J Trauma.* 2004;56(6):1191–1196.
28. Durmaz I, Yagdi T, Calkavur T, et al. Prophylactic dialysis in patients with renal dysfunction undergoing on-pump coronary artery bypass surgery. *Ann Thorac Surg.* 2003;75:859–864.
29. Edwards BF. Postoperative renal insufficiency. *Med Clin North Am.* 2001;85:1241–1254.
30. Pinson CW, Schuman ES, Gross EF, et al. Surgery in long-term dialysis patients. Experience with more than 300 cases. *Am J Surg.* 1986;151(5):567–571.

APPENDIX

Cockroft–Gault Equation

$$\frac{(140 - \text{age}) \times \text{weight (kg)}}{72 \times \text{serum creatinine (mg/dL)}} \times 0.85 \text{ (for women)} = \text{creatinine clearance (mL/min)}$$

Fractional Excretion of Sodium (Na)

$$\frac{\text{Urine Na} \times \text{serum creatinine}}{\text{Serum Na} \times \text{urine creatinine}} \times 100 = \text{FENa}$$

ASSESSING AND MANAGING NEUROVASCULAR, NEURODEGENERATIVE, AND NEUROMUSCULAR DISORDERS

Peter G. Kallas

The perioperative assessment and management of patients with neurovascular, neurodegenerative, or neuromuscular disease is a topic that lacks evidence to a great degree and is mostly devoid of formal clinical guidelines. This chapter will identify the existing evidence, apply recommendations from the available literature, and distill this information to create helpful guideposts for the clinician caring for patients in the perioperative setting.

NEUROVASCULAR DISEASE

Perioperative Stroke

The incidence of perioperative stroke is relatively low in the noncardiac surgery population (0.2%)[1] but occurs at a rate of 1.7% in the coronary bypass population.[2] In-hospital mortality rates associated with perioperative stroke have shown to be 31.1% for hemicolectomy, 12.0% for total hip replacement, 32.6% for segmental lung resection,[3] and can be as high as 23.1% in patients after coronary bypass.[2] Higher stroke rates have also been associated with urgent surgery as compared with elective surgery.[4] The age of the patient also plays an important role as perioperative strokes can be as low as 1–1.5% in 50- to 60-year-old coronary bypass patients and as high as 8–9% in those over age 80.[2] For strokes related to noncardiac surgery, 16.4% occur in the first 24 h[5] as opposed to 38–45% in the cardiac surgery population.[4]

Perioperative Medicine: Medical Consultation and Co-Management, First Edition.
Edited by Amir K. Jaffer and Paul J. Grant.
© 2012 Wiley-Blackwell. Published 2012 by John Wiley & Sons, Inc.

The theoretical mechanisms of perioperative strokes are many, and the true cascade that leads to a stroke in this setting likely involves a combination of factors. Hypotension and carotid stenosis resulting in watershed infarcts have implicitly been the most quoted etiologies of strokes in common practice, yet the literature does not support these. In one study, only 11.5% of strokes in a noncardiac surgery population were due to watershed or border zone infarcts. This study also showed no association between mean arterial pressure and stroke, and concluded that hypotension "rarely" accounts for perioperative strokes.[5] Similarly, in a cardiac surgery population, the incidence of watershed infarcts was 5%.[2] Likewise, a focal area of carotid stenosis does not necessarily lead to a perioperative stroke occurring in the territory supplied by that artery. A systematic review showed that 59% of strokes after cardiac surgery were not related to carotid thromboembolic disease alone. Stated in a different way, this study revealed that 48% of patients with strokes related to cardiac surgery had normal carotid arteries or stenoses less than 50%. Further analysis within this publication found that 86% of all observed cerebral events ($n = 108$) occurred ipsilateral to a hemisphere without a 50–99% stenosis or occlusion and only 7% of strokes or transient ischemic attacks occurred ipsilateral to a surgically amenable lesion.[2] Finally, in a retrospective study of patients ($n = 284$) who suffered a perioperative stroke in proximity to noncardiac surgery who also had a documented carotid ultrasound prior to surgery, the incidence of a perioperative stroke in those with less than 50% stenosis was not significantly different from the incidence in those with stenoses of 70% or greater (3.3% vs. 3.7%, respectively). Of note, 88% of these patients had a documented finding of a carotid bruit, a previous transient ischemic attack or stroke, or both.[6] For asymptomatic carotid stenosis, it is more appropriate to view this as a marker of generalized cerebrovascular disease rather than a focal problem that should be surgically corrected prior to noncardiac surgery.

Alternative mechanisms of perioperative stroke that have been proposed involve thromboembolic and hematologic mechanisms. Cardiac sources of emboli accounted for 29.5% of perioperative strokes in one study.[5] In another study, atrial fibrillation was the most common comorbid diagnosis found in perioperative stroke patients occurring at a rate of 27.6%.[3] In a large retrospective study using over 2.5 million patients in an administrative database, the risk-adjusted odds ratio (OR) of a postoperative stroke within 30 days in patients with chronic atrial fibrillation was 2.1 (confidence interval [CI]: 2.0–2.3).[7] Other cardioembolic sources include paradoxical cerebral embolism via a patent foramen ovale from clots in the lower extremity or pelvic veins and from fat emboli associated with orthopedic surgery. Postoperative myocardial infarctions could be a source as well as aortic atherosclerotic disease, especially in surgeries that require manipulation of the ascending aorta. It is well recognized that the perioperative period is a time of hypercoagulability, which may include activation of the hemostatic system and reduced fibrinolysis.[8–10] Neck extension for endotracheal intubation is another proposed mechanism. Compression of basilar artery flow in the presence of vertebral artery stenosis or stretching of diseased carotid arteries in the drowsy perioperative patient may result in thrombus formation and embolization.[11] Manipulation of extracranial carotid arteries or vertebral arteries during neck surgeries has also been implicated through similar mechanisms. Others have mentioned general anesthesia, dehydration, bed rest, and

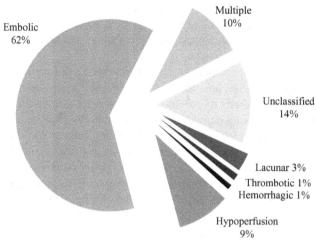

Figure 15.1. Proposed mechanisms for perioperative stroke. Data from Likosky DS, Caplan LR, Weintraub RM, et al. Heart Surg Forum 2004;7:E271–E276. Reproduced with permission from Selim,[12] figure 1. See color insert.

stasis in the postoperative period as potentially causative.[12] Lastly, and possibly most importantly, the withholding of antiplatelet and anticoagulant medications in the perioperative period may play a major role in causation (Figure 15.1).

Numerous attempts have been made to identify and risk-stratify patients at risk for a perioperative cerebrovascular event. One such study found that atrial fibrillation, history of stroke, cardiac valvular disease, and renal disease all carried an OR greater than 1.5 in the noncardiac surgery population.[3] Another study found an association with previous cerebrovascular disease, chronic obstructive pulmonary disease, higher blood pressure on admission, and a higher blood urea nitrogen at the time of stroke.[5] Of note, the rate of perioperative stroke in patients with a prior stroke going for noncardiac surgery is 2.9% and is probably the most important risk factor. Interestingly, an incidental carotid bruit found preoperatively on the day of noncardiac surgery was found to only carry a perioperative stroke incidence of 0.7%. As noted earlier, carotid stenosis found on a preoperative carotid ultrasound carried a perioperative stroke risk between 3% and 4%[6]; however, a number of these patients had a history of a cerebrovascular event, which is consistent with the 2.9% perioperative stroke rate in those with prior cerebrovascular events.

Risk assessment for patients undergoing cardiac surgery has been more closely analyzed in the literature and involves procedure-specific risks; therefore, it deserves to be handled separately from noncardiac surgery. Charlesworth et al. created a model for predicting the risk of stroke among patients undergoing coronary bypass surgery.[13] The risk factors are additive, producing an aggregate estimate of the risk of perioperative stroke. These risk factors in this model include age, urgency of surgery, female sex, left ventricular ejection fraction, vascular disease, diabetes mellitus, and renal disease. Risk assessment in the noncardiac surgery population is less formalized, but it seems prudent to be wary of those patients with known history of stroke or transient ischemic attack, atrial fibrillation, severe valvular disease, or documented carotid artery disease.

In preoperative patients thought to be at increased risk for stroke, there are no formal guidelines to suggest how these patients should be evaluated or optimized. A thorough history in search of stroke-like symptoms and a complete neurologic examination looking for stroke findings are appropriate. Asymptomatic carotid bruits found on the preoperative evaluation should not delay surgery, but if time allows, a carotid ultrasound to assess degree of stenosis and the need for follow-up seems reasonable. When a stenotic lesion is known or newly discovered, some experts recommend brain imaging with computed tomography (CT) or magnetic resonance imaging (MRI) to capture those patients with silent ipsilateral infarcts, which would prompt surgical correction prior to other procedures.[12] For cardiac surgery patients, identifying the extent and location of aortic atherosclerosis prior to surgery using transesophageal echocardiography or intraoperative epiaortic ultrasound is important to modify surgical technique and determine the location for aortic cannulation or clamping.

The management of a patient with perioperative risk for stroke starts with determining if antiplatelet or anticoagulant therapy should be continued up until surgery, as most of these patients are typically taking aspirin, clopidogrel, dipyridamole, warfarin, or a combination of these agents. Studies that have investigated the time relationship between cessation of antiplatelet therapy and stroke have found the average time interval to be 7.4–14.3 days.[14-16] Evidence suggests that the etiology of an increased stroke risk at 7–10 days may not only result from the removal of the antiplatelet agent or from the hypercoagulable state associated with surgery, but that a possible "rebound" effect associated with the withdrawal of these drugs could also be contributory. For instance, a study using a single dose of aspirin in rats followed by laser injury to a vessel measured the presence of embolization. Compared with day 2 after aspirin administration, day 8 had significantly more emboli and a longer duration of embolization, suggesting a late prothrombotic effect.[17] One theoretical mechanism involves the possibility that ultralow doses of aspirin seen at the 7- to 10-day mark after cessation may actually induce prothrombotic effects by endothelial cells, such as the release of the platelet-activating factor.[18]

Hence, continuation of antiplatelet or anticoagulant agents through surgery would be ideal from a stroke prevention perspective, but potentially hazardous from a surgical bleeding standpoint. In a meta-analysis investigating the bleeding risk associated with various surgeries from 41 studies, the authors found that aspirin multiplied the bleeding rate by a factor of 1.5. Bleeding risk ranged from 0% in some skin and eye surgeries to 75% for transrectal prostate biopsy. Mortality possibly related to bleeding occurred only after transurethral prostatectomy.[16] The continuation of aspirin through surgery is finding more and more acceptance among surgeons. It is advisable to discuss with the surgeon the need for perioperative aspirin dosing in patients at risk for stroke. The following surgeries, however, likely carry unacceptable risk for hemorrhage while under the effects of aspirin: craniotomies or procedures entering the brain, spine surgeries in which the spinal cord is at risk, urologic procedures, and some liver surgeries.

Warfarin has been used safely through procedures such as cutaneous dermatologic surgeries,[19] dental extractions,[20] diagnostic endoscopies, and cataract extractions.[21] Seventy-five percent of ophthalmologists in one survey responded that they now continue warfarin through cataract surgery.[22] Adenosine diphosphate inhibitors, such as clopidogrel, have been studied mainly in the coronary bypass population. The CURE trial showed an elevated risk of postoperative bleeding in those patients who received a dose of clopidogrel within 5 days of surgery.[23] Another study found that the risk of reexploration due to bleeding after coronary bypass surgery was independently associated with clopidogrel use at the time of surgery and carried an OR of 6.9. There was no association with aspirin use alone for reexploration secondary to bleeding in this study.[24] The continuation of the combination of dipyridamole and aspirin through surgery has not been studied. It is a reasonable strategy to substitute low-dose aspirin for clopidogrel or warfarin in high-risk patients when the latter two agents are contraindicated. Though aspirin used for primary prevention is often reflexively discontinued by surgeons' offices prior to surgery, the medical doctor must actively guard those patients who take antiplatelet and anticoagulant medications for secondary prevention of conditions such as stroke. A firm grasp of the safety profile of these agents through various types of surgeries will enhance the conversation with the surgeon, which is of utmost importance before recommendations are made.[25,26]

Recent evidence supports the positive effects of HMG CoA reductase inhibitors, or statins, in reducing perioperative stroke risk. Among 1566 patients undergoing carotid endarterectomy in a retrospective study, those receiving statin therapy for at least 1 week had a threefold decrease in stroke rates and a fivefold decrease in all-cause mortality using multivariate analysis.[27] A prospective observational study of 810 consecutive patients going for coronary bypass surgeries found a fourfold lower risk of perioperative stroke in those patients who were on statin therapy prior to surgery.[28] In a prospective, randomized control study, atorvastatin was started an average of 31 days prior to major vascular surgery ($n = 100$). The composite end point of death from cardiac causes, nonfatal acute myocardial infarction, ischemic stroke, and unstable angina was significantly reduced in the treatment group. With respect to stroke, the placebo group had two strokes versus none in the atorvastatin group, which was not statistically significant.[29] In DECREASE IV, a randomized controlled trial, noncardiac surgery patients assigned to fluvastatin 80 mg starting 21–53 days prior to surgery did not show a significant decrease in perioperative stroke rate compared with placebo.[30] Plaque stabilization through multiple mechanisms is thought to drive the favorable effects of statins on stroke prevention. Statins have been shown to have a beneficial effect on inflammation, vasomotor function, fibrinolysis, and platelet reactivity. In patients who received pravastatin 40 mg for 3 months prior to carotid endarterectomy, carotid plaque composition had significantly less lipid content, fewer macrophages, fewer T cells, and a significantly higher collagen content than placebo.[31] The minimum time to achieve treatment effect for statins prior to surgery has not been determined.

The safety profile of statin use throughout the perioperative period has been excellent.

The initiation of beta-blocking agents within 24 h of surgery has been associated with a higher incidence of perioperative stroke in the noncardiac surgery population making this practice unadvisable.[32] A possible exception may be in patients with the highest risk for perioperative cardiac complications. However, studies that have titrated the beta-blocking agent weeks in advance of surgery have not found the same elevation in stroke risk.[30,33] In one retrospective study of coronary bypass patients, those receiving a perioperative beta-blocker prior to surgery as well as those who had initiation of the drug intraoperatively ($n = 2296$) actually had a reduction in severe neurologic outcomes (stroke and coma) compared with those who were not receiving this drug class ($n = 279$), OR 0.45, 95% CI 0.23–0.83.[34] Though the influence of preoperative beta-blocker initiation on stroke rates remains controversial, studies have shown that beta-blockers can be initiated safely in the perioperative period if titrated over a safe time interval. A minimum time interval has yet to be defined.

Surgical intervention or stenting of an asymptomatic stenotic carotid artery lesion prior to major surgery is often contemplated in the preoperative patient. For stenotic lesions ranging from less than 50% to critical stenosis and complete occlusion, one study found that the incidence of perioperative stroke in the noncardiac surgery population did not differ significantly from low-grade to high-grade stenosis (stroke incidence was 3–4%).[6] Since the incidence of perioperative stroke associated with carotid endarterectomy in asymptomatic patients is at best 2.5%,[35] experts have recommended against prophylactic endarterectomy in the asymptomatic noncardiac surgery population.[11] Coronary artery bypass surgery in the presence of known carotid disease is associated with a stroke rate of 3.0% with unilateral carotid stenosis, 5.0% with bilateral disease, and 7.0% when there is carotid occlusion. Despite the common occurrence of simultaneous coronary and carotid artery disease, there is no clear consensus regarding the management of such patients other than the suggestion that the symptomatic stenosis be addressed first.[11] A staged approach, a combined approach, and a sequential carotid stent followed by coronary bypass strategy[36] are all options that are best vetted by the cardiovascular surgeon.

In the event of a perioperative stroke, systemic tissue plasminogen activator (tPA) is contraindicated due to the high surgical bleeding risk. However, catheter-guided intra-arterial thrombolysis has been used successfully. A retrospective case series showed that among 36 patients with postoperative stroke, 38% of patients achieved a good outcome (Rankin score less than or equal to 2) with intra-arterial thrombolysis.[37] Twenty-five percent of the total population had surgical site bleeding related to thrombolysis, most notably in two of the three craniotomies, both of whom died. Another case series of 13 coronary bypass patients with postoperative stroke who underwent intra-arterial thrombolysis demonstrated that, again, 38% of patients showed improvement in their stroke scores, and notably there was no bleeding that required reoperation.[38] Both of these studies showed a 25% mortality rate. The range of time to angiogram from stroke symptom onset was 10 min to 5.5 h in these trials. Hence, it seems reasonable to consider urgent angiogram and intra-arterial thrombolysis in the postoperative stroke patient who meets the criteria from a stroke perspective. However, from the limited data that is available, it seems that postcraniotomy patients carry too much risk of intracranial bleeding to consider this an option.

Finally, the recommended timing to perform noncarotid artery surgery after the patient has suffered a stroke is generally thought to be 30 days.[11] This recommendation is based more on the pathophysiology of a healing stroke rather than actual data. It is thought that the autoregulatory mechanisms of cerebral blood flow take approximately 1–2 weeks to return to baseline after a stroke. Also, the area of infarct undergoes a series of changes over the first 30 days that are mediated by inflammation and are thought to "soften" the tissue, making it potentially more vulnerable to hemorrhagic transformation or ischemia.

Cerebral Aneurysms and Arterial Venous Malformations (AVMs)

Unruptured intracranial aneurysms and AVMs are as prevalent as 6% and 0.01% of the population, respectively.[39] A basic understanding of these diseases and their treatment options is helpful when the perioperative physician encounters a patient with a stated history of these vascular abnormalities or a history of cerebral hemorrhage who now needs a non-neurosurgical procedure. One should obtain the most recent reports of imaging of the brain and, ideally, a report of the cerebral angiogram. It is safe to say that aneurysms less than 13 mm in the cavernous carotid artery are at low risk for bleeding and do not require further investigation preoperatively.[40] Intracranial aneurysms in the posterior circulation, however, carry significant risk for bleeding, even if they are small in size. Bleed rates of intracranial aneurysms at the other locations depend heavily on a patient's history or image findings of a prior bleed or leak. For those patients with an aneurysm in the anterior, middle, and noncavernous internal carotid artery systems and with no evidence of bleeding, bleed rates have been found to be 0% in those with an aneurysm less than 7 mm. Those patients with evidence of an aneurysm in these locations and a prior bleed, however, carry significant risk of another bleed no matter how small the aneurysm size.

Since surveillance CT scans of aneurysms less than 5 mm have not been found to be useful, reimaging prior to nonaneurismal surgery may not be necessary.[41] Whether or not to treat risky intracranial aneurysms prior to nonaneurismal surgery is dependent on the nature of the planned surgery and the need for anticoagulant and antiplatelet therapy. Surgeries that may pose higher risk for aneurismal bleed include cardiopulmonary bypass surgeries and carotid artery surgery since there is direct manipulation of the major feeder arteries; sinus surgery due to the common use of strong decongestants; and finally, total joint replacements that often require full anticoagulation with warfarin postoperatively. In this last scenario, the use of low–molecular-weight heparin at prophylaxis dosing is advisable.

AVMs pose similar challenges to the perioperative physician though they are far less common. Worrisome AVM characteristics include previous hemorrhage, younger age of the patient, deep location in the brain, and exclusive deep venous drainage.[42]

NEURODEGENERATIVE, NEUROMUSCULAR, AND MUSCULAR DYSTROPHY DISORDERS

Parkinson's Disease

Parkinson's disease is one of the more common neurodegenerative diseases that clinicians encounter in the perioperative period. It is associated with a reduction in respiratory reserve capacity predisposing postoperative patients to atelectasis. This together with risk of levodopa withdrawal during prolonged surgeries and the resulting chest wall rigidity places the Parkinson's patient at risk for respiratory failure. Upper airway obstruction may also occur as the result of upper airway muscle discoordination. Aspiration is a common respiratory complication. Evaluating the patient with preoperative pulmonary function testing may be appropriate for those patients undergoing intrathoracic surgery, upper abdominal surgery, and thoracic spine surgery as a way to gauge risk of postoperative respiratory failure, especially in patients with advanced disease. For surgeries lasting 6 h or longer, it may be prudent to initiate longer-acting Parkinson's disease agents preoperatively and to formulate a strategy for patients who cannot take their oral medication postoperatively. Discussion with the patient's neurologist would be appropriate in these cases. Elevation of the head of the bed to 30 degrees at all times seems prudent. Maintaining the patients' usual dosing schedule postoperatively is crucial, via nasogastric tube or intravenously, if necessary. Avoidance of common antidopaminergic perioperative medications such as metoclopramide, droperidol, and phenothiazines is recommended.

The experienced perioperative physician expects to encounter some degree of delirium in most Parkinson's patients postoperatively. Whether these patients are more susceptible to perioperative medication side effects, are prone to delirium due to the dopaminergic effects of their drugs, or have poorer brain homeostasis mechanisms is not known. Preventative measures for delirium are identical to non-Parkinson's patients at risk (see Chapter 30, "Delirium"), but treatment options in the Parkinson's population differ. Haloperidol, the treatment of choice for many physicians, is relatively contraindicated due to its strong antidopaminergic properties. Newer antipsychotics such as olanzapine, risperidone, or quetiapine have less antidopaminergic activity and may be better choices. Finally, the postoperative nurse and physical therapists must be made aware of the common and sometimes severe cases of orthostatic hypotension that is associated with Parkinson's disease.

Multiple Sclerosis

There are approximately 250,000–350,000 people with multiple sclerosis in the United States with varying degrees of disability.[43] It is known that surgery can induce an exacerbation of this disease, and multiple mechanisms for inducing an exacerbation have been proposed. Demyelinated nerve fibers are sensitive to elevated temperatures, so perioperative pyrexia should be avoided. Hence, the perioperative physician should warn against the use of warming devices in the recovery room and possibly suggest acetaminophen or nonsteroidal anti-inflammatory agents around the clock if fevers become an issue. Infections pose another risk for multiple sclerosis exacerbation; therefore, Foley catheters and intravenous catheters should be promptly removed when no longer indicated.

Spinal and general anesthesias have been implicated in causing exacerbations as well. It has been theorized that local anesthetic agents may have a neurotoxic effect in these patients; however, it has been proposed that lower-dose bupivacaine, for instance, can be safely used for epidural anesthesia.[43] For general anesthesia, there is no evidence indicating that one intravenous or inhalational anesthetic is superior to another in multiple sclerosis patients. An introduction to this issue should be given to the patient by the perioperative physician, setting up the more detailed conversation the patient will have with the anesthesiologist. Patients with evidence of significant muscle denervation, such as flaccidity, spasticity, or hyperreflexia, should have their findings documented and highlighted for the anesthesiologist as these patients are prone to severe hyperkalemia when depolarizing neuromuscular blocking agents are employed.

Patients with cervical or thoracic lesions can have respiratory muscle dysfunction including diaphragmatic paralysis. Central control of carbon dioxide levels can also be affected by this disease, making them prone to hypercarbia. Additionally, the ability to clear secretions and swallow normally can be affected. One should consider a chest X-ray, arterial blood gas, or pulmonary function testing in multiple sclerosis patients who have worrisome findings on their history or physical exam. Consultation with an anesthesiologist for severely debilitated patients is recommended.

Postoperatively, the clinician should anticipate the many possible complications in patients with multiple sclerosis. These include blood pressure instability and orthostatic hypotension due to autonomic dysfunction, hypoventilation and atelectasis, residual neuromuscular blockade, and bladder and bowel dysfunction. Since many of these patients are on centrally acting muscle relaxants, such as baclofen, and since there is not an intravenous form of this drug, a gradual transition to diazepam can be considered perioperatively. Abrupt baclofen withdrawal can lead to seizures, hallucinations, and death. Finally, the postoperative physician should closely monitor the patient's neurologic exam for evidence of an acute exacerbation.

Myasthenia Gravis

Myasthenia gravis occurs at an incidence of 1 in 20,000 adults.[44] The medicine consultant must be wary of the potential for postoperative respiratory failure and understand the special challenge these patients pose to the anesthesiologist. Though authors have proposed strategies to risk-stratify patients with myasthenia gravis for postoperative respiratory failure,[43] no consensus currently exists. It seems reasonable to focus efforts on patients with advanced disease, disease of longer duration, or a history of respiratory failure. For these higher-risk patients, one should consider pulmonary function testing to determine forced vital capacity (FVC), and an arterial blood gas to determine carbon dioxide levels. Referral to a myasthenia gravis specialist for consideration of preoperative steroids, intravenous gamma globulin, or plasmapheresis in an attempt to optimize the disease is recommended in select patients.

For major surgery, it is prudent to consult the anesthesiologist prior to the day of surgery to allow discussion of the anesthesia plan and associated risks with the patient. Due to the nature of this disease, myasthenia gravis patients are highly resistant to the depolarizing muscle relaxants and highly sensitive to the nondepolarizing agents. Anesthesiologists who plan to use muscle relaxants with surgery may prefer to hold the anticholinesterase drugs on the day prior to surgery, or the day of surgery. Furthermore, the need for anticholinesterase drugs is decreased in the first 48 h after surgery since the patient is typically less mobile. These agents need to be restarted and titrated to avoid the risk of cholinergic crisis.[45] Drugs that affect the neuromuscular junction should be used with caution perioperatively. These include aminoglycosides, polymyxins, beta-blockers, calcium channel blockers, procainamide, and phenytoin. Lastly, patients with myasthenia gravis are particularly sensitive to the respiratory depressant effects of barbiturates, benzodiazepines, opioids, and propofol; thus, cautious administration and dosing of these drugs are recommended.

Duchenne Muscular Dystrophy

Duchenne muscular dystrophy is an inherited progressive myopathic disorder that occurs in 1 of every 3500 live male births.[46] It affects skeletal muscles, most ominously the muscles of respiration. It is also associated with dilated cardiomyopathy, making these patients especially vulnerable to the effects of general anesthesia and muscle relaxants. Mean survival of these patients is now reaching age 25, many of whom will require corrective scoliosis surgery.

A consensus statement on Duchenne muscular dystrophy patients undergoing anesthesia or sedation was published by the American College of Chest Physicians in 2007 and was primarily based on expert opinion.[46] This document recommends that patients with Duchenne muscular dystrophy obtain pulmonary function testing that includes FVC, maximum inspiratory pressure (MIP), maximum expiratory pressure (MEP), peak cough flow (PCF), and arterial blood gas measurement prior to major surgery. Those with an FVC less than 30% are considered especially high risk for respiratory failure and should be considered for preoperative noninvasive positive pressure ventilation (NPPV) training. Preoperative malnutrition is often associated with the increased work of breathing in advanced disease; hence, preoperative use of NPPV in addition to nutritional supplementation may be of benefit. For PCF less than 270 L/min or MEP less than 60 cm H_2O, consideration should be made for preoperative manual and mechanically assisted cough, such as a mechanical insufflation–exsufflation device.

Loss of cardiac muscle can sometimes be more advanced than that of skeletal muscle in patients with Duchenne muscular dystrophy. This is suggestive when progressive loss of the R-wave is noted on electrocardiogram, and with left ventricular dysfunction on serial echocardiograms. Both of these tests are important in the preoperative evaluation, even in early disease. Rhabdomyolysis and hyperkalemia have occurred with volatile anesthetics alone or in combination with succinylcholine. These patients may also be susceptible to a malignant hyperthermia-like syndrome. Hence, a total intravenous anesthetic technique for induction and maintenance of general anesthesia, such as propofol and a short-acting opioid, is recommended. Again, consultation with an anesthesiologist prior to the day of surgery is recommended.

CONCLUSION

The perioperative assessment and management of patients with neurologic disease can be challenging. A basic understanding of how these disease processes behave as well as how to manage their medications perioperatively is important, in addition to knowing when to involve the anesthesiologist or neurologist. This knowledge will allow the physician to safely guide the patient with a neurologic disease through the perioperative period.

REFERENCES

1. Larsen SF, Zaric D, Boysen G, et al. Postoperative cerebrovascular accidents in general surgery. *Acta Anaesthesiol Scand.* 1988;32:698–701.
2. Naylor AR, Mehta Z, Rothwell PM, Bell PR. Carotid artery disease and stroke during coronary artery bypass: a critical review of the literature. *Eur J Vasc Endovasc Surg.* 2002;23:283–294.
3. Bateman BT, Schumacher C, Wang S, Shaefi S, Berman M. Perioperative acute ischemic stroke in noncardiac and nonvascular surgery. *Anesthesiology.* 2009;110:231–238.
4. Bucerius J, Gummert JF, Borger MA, et al. Stroke after cardiac surgery: a risk factor analysis of 16,184 consecutive adult patients. *Ann Thorac Surg.* 2003;75:472–478.
5. Limburg M, Widjdicks E, Li H. Ischemic stroke after surgical procedures. *Neurology.* 1998;50:895–901.
6. Evans B, Wijdicks E. High grade carotid stenosis detected before general surgery: is endarterectomy indicated? *Neurology.* 2001;57:1328–1330.
7. Kaatz S, Douketis J, Zhou H, Gage BF, White RH. Risk of stroke after surgery in patients with and without chronic atrial fibrillation. *J Thromb Haemost.* 2010;8(5):884–890.
8. Dixon B, Santamaria J, Campbell D. Coagulation activation and organ dysfunction following cardiac surgery. *Chest.* 2005;128:229–236.
9. Paramo JA, Rifon J, Llorens R, Cesares J, Paloma MJ, Rocha E. Intra- and postoperative fibrinolysis in patients undergoing cardiopulmonary bypass surgery. *Haemostasis.* 1991;21:58–64.
10. Hinterhuber G, Bohler K, Kittler H. Extending monitoring of hemostatic activation after varicose vein surgery under general anesthesia. *Dermatol Surg.* 2006;32:632–639.
11. Blacker D, Flemming K, Link M, Brown RD. The preoperative cerebrovascular consultation: common cerebrovascular questions before general or cardiac surgery. *Mayo Clin Proc.* 2004;79:223–229.
12. Selim M. Perioperative stroke. *N Engl J Med.* 2007;356:706–713.
13. Charlesworth DC, Likosky DS, Marrin CA, et al. Development and validation of a predictive model for strokes after coronary bypass grafting. *Ann Thorac Surg.* 2003;76:436–443.
14. Sibon I, Orgogozo J. Antiplatelet drug discontinuation is a risk factor for ischemic stroke. *Neurology.* 2004;62:1187–1189.
15. Maulaz AB, Bezerra D, Michel P, Bogousslavsky J. Effect of discontinuing aspirin therapy on the risk of brain ischemic stroke. *Arch Neurol.* 2005;62:1217–1220.

16. Burger W, Chemnitius JM, Kneissl GD, Rucker G. Low-dose aspirin for secondary cardiovascular prevention—cardiovascular risks after its perioperative withdrawal versus bleeding risks with its continuation—review and meta-analysis. *J Intern Med.* 2005;257:399–414.

17. Aguejouf O, Belougne-Malfatti E, Doutremepuich F, Belon P, Doutremepuich C. Thromboembolic complications several days after a single-dose administration of aspirin. *Thromb Res.* 1998;89:123–127.

18. Aguejouf O, Malfatti E, Belon P, Doutremepuich C. Time related neutralization of two doses of acetyl salicylic acid. *Thromb Res.* 2000;100:317–323.

19. Kargi E, Babuccu O, Hosnuter M, Babuccu B, Altinyazar C. Complications of minor cutaneous surgery in patients under anticoagulant treatment. *Aesthetic Plast Surg.* 2002;26:483–485.

20. Wahl MJ. Dental surgery in anticoagulated patients. *Arch Intern Med.* 1998;158:1610–1616.

21. Katz J, Feldman M, Bass E, et al. Risks and benefits of anticoagulant and antiplatelet medication use before cataract surgery. *Ophthalmology.* 2003;110:1784–1788.

22. Ong-Tone L, Paluck EC, Hart-Mitchell RD. Perioperative use of warfarin and aspirin in cataract surgery by Canadian society of cataract and refractive surgery members: survey. *J Cataract Refract Surg.* 2005;31:991–996.

23. The Clopidogrel in Unstable Angina to Prevent Recurrent Events Trial Investigators. Effects of clopidogrel in addition to aspirin in patients with acute coronary syndromes without ST-segment elevation. *N Engl J Med.* 2001;345(7):494–502.

24. Yende S, Wunderink RG. Effect of clopidogrel on bleeding after coronary bypass surgery. *Crit Care Med.* 2001;29:2271–2275.

25. American Academy of Ophthalmology. Basic and Clinical Science Course, 2010. Available at http://one.aao.org/CE/EducationalProducts/snippet.aspx?F=bcsccontent\bcscsection1\bcsc2007 section1_2007-03-21_010314\perioperativemanagementinocularsurgery\bcsc-2006-s1-2933.xml. Accessed September 27 2010.

26. Eisenberg MJ, Richard PR, Libersan D, Filion KB. Safety of short-term discontinuation of antiplatelet therapy in patients with drug-eluting stents. *Circulation.* 2009;119(12):1634–1642.

27. Mcgirt MJ, Perler BA, Brooke BS, et al. 3-Hydroxy-3-methylglutaryl coenzyme a reductase inhibitors reduce the risk of perioperative stroke and mortality after carotid endarterectomy. *J Vasc Surg.* 2005;42(5):829–835.

28. Aboyans V, Labrousse L, Lacroix P, et al. Predictive factors of stroke in patients undergoing coronary bypass grafting: statins are protective. *Eur J Cardiothorac Surg.* 2006;30:300–304.

29. Durazzo A, Machado FS, Ikeoka DT, et al. Reduction in cardiovascular events after vascular surgery with atorvastatin: a randomized trial. *J Vasc Surg.* 2004;39(5):967–975.

30. Dunkelgrun M, Boersma E, Shouten O, et al. Bisoprolol and fluvastatin for the reduction of perioperative cardiac mortality and myocardial infarction in intermediate-risk patients undergoing noncardiovascular surgery (Decrease IV). *Ann Surg.* 2009;249(6):921–926.

31. Crisby M, Nordin-Fredriksson G, Shah KS, Yano J, Zhu J, Nilsson J. Pravastatin treatment increases collagen content and decreases lipid content, inflammation, metalloproteinases, and cell death in human carotid plaque. *Circulation.* 2001;103:926–933.

32. Devereux PJ, Yang H, Yusuf S, et al. Effects of extended release metoprolol succinate in patients undergoing non-cardiac surgery (POISE trial). *Lancet.* 2008;371(9627):1839–1847.

33. Poldermans D, Boersma E, Bax JJ, et al. The effect of bisoprolol on perioperative mortality and myocardial infarction in high-risk patients undergoing vascular surgery. Dutch Echocardiographic Cardiac Risk Evaluation Applying Stress Echocardiography Study Group. *N Engl J Med.* 1999;341(24):1789–1794.

34. Amory DW, Grigore JK, Ma G, et al. Neuroprotection is associated with beta-adrenergic receptor antagonist during cardiac surgery: evidence from 2575 patients. *J Cardiothorac Vasc Anesth.* 2002;16(3):270–277.

35. Executive Committee for the Asymptomatic Carotid Atherosclerosis Study. Endarterectomy for asymptomatic carotid artery stenosis. *JAMA.* 1995;273:1421–1428.

36. Versaci F, Del Giudice C, Scafuri A et al. Sequential hybrid carotid and coronary artery revascularization: immediate and mid-term results. *Ann Thorac Surg.* 2007;84:1508–1514.

37. Chalela JA, Katzan I, Liebeskind DS, et al. Safety of intra-arterial thrombolysis in the postoperative period. *Stroke.* 2001;32:1365–1369.

38. Moazami N, Smedira NG, McCarthy PM, et al. Safety and efficacy of intraarterial thrombolysis for perioperative stroke after cardiac operation. *Ann Thorac Surg.* 2001;72:1933–1939.

39. Stapf C, Mast H, Sciacca RR, et al. The New York islands AVM study. *Stroke.* 2003;34:e29–e33.

40. International Study of Unruptured Intracranial Aneurysms Investigators. Unruptured intracranial aneurysms: natural history, clinical outcome, and risks of surgical and endovascular treatment. *Lancet.* 2003;362:103–110.

41. Wermer M, van der Schaaf I, Velthuis B, Majoie CB, Albrecht KW, Rinkel GJ. Yield of short-term CT/MR angiography for small aneurysms detected at screening. *Stroke.* 2006;37:414–418.

42. Stapf C, Mast H, Sciacca RR et al. Predictors of hemorrhage in patients with untreated brain arteriovenous malformation. *Neurology.* 2006;66:1350–1355.

43. Dorotta IR, Schubert A. Multiple sclerosis and anesthetic implications. *Curr Opin Anaesthesiol.* 2002;15:365–370.

44. Baraka A. Anesthesia and myasthenia gravis. *Can J Anaesth.* 1992;39:476–486.

45. Lieb K, Selim M. Preoperative evaluation of patients with neurological disease. *Semin Neurol.* 2008;28(5):603–610.

46. Birkrant DJ, Panitch HB, Benditt JO, et al. American College of Chest Physicians consensus statement on the respiratory and related management of patients with Duchenne muscular dystrophy undergoing anesthesia or sedation. *Chest.* 2007;132:1977–1986.

CHAPTER 16

ASSESSING AND MANAGING RHEUMATOLOGIC DISORDERS

Gregory C. Gardner and Brian F. Mandell

INTRODUCTION

Orthopedic surgery has enhanced the care of patients with advanced arthritis. The rheumatologic diseases pose a unique set of challenges that can impact perioperative patient outcomes. Rheumatologists, surgeons, anesthesiologists, internists, and hospitalists should be aware of these issues to minimize patient risk and maximize favorable outcome.

RHEUMATOID ARTHRITIS (RA)

Epidemiology

Prevalence of RA in the United States is estimated at 0.6–0.8% of the population or approximately 2 million people.[1] Common surgical procedures in RA patients include synovectomies, total joint arthroplasties, and tendon rupture repairs. In a 12-year cohort study of 105 RA patients enrolled early in their disease course, 14% ultimately required surgery for joint replacement.[2] After 30 years, 33% of RA patients required at least one orthopedic procedure.[3] Weiss et al. in a 15-year retrospective study using the Swedish National Hospital Discharge Registry,[4] reported that 50,478 RA patients were admitted for surgical procedures including placement of 13,895 joint prostheses and a 42% decline in RA patients hospitalized between 1987 and 2001. Similar data were reported by da Silva et al. and Ward.[3,5] Ward reported lower cumulative rates of orthopedic surgery for RA patients diagnosed after 1985 and followed at least 10 years compared with earlier cohorts likely reflecting use of newer effective therapies.

History

Important historical features include length of disease (disease duration is associated with more joint damage, particularly neck involvement), current functional status

Perioperative Medicine: Medical Consultation and Co-Management, First Edition.
Edited by Amir K. Jaffer and Paul J. Grant.

(use of ambulatory aids and ability to perform activities of daily living independently impact rehabilitation and predict cardiac risk), problem joints, current medications, previous use of corticosteroids, extra-articular manifestations, and previous experience with surgery.

Postoperative myocardial infarction (MI) is the predominant cause of morbidity and mortality in patients undergoing noncardiac surgery.[6] Patients with chronic inflammation, like RA, are at greater risk to develop atherosclerosis. The standardized mortality ratio (SMR) for RA patients is twice the general population, similar to that of people with diabetes mellitus and excess mortality is due mostly to cardiovascular (CV) events.[7] The preoperative assessor should query the patient regarding traditional risk factors, CV symptoms, and recognize that long-standing, incompletely controlled RA increases CV risk.[6]

Metafratzi and colleagues reported mild pulmonary abnormalities in up to 69% of RA patients with early disease.[8] Lung involvement may advance to frank pulmonary fibrosis, bronchiectasis, and obliterative bronchiolitis.[9] A history of dyspnea on exertion, crackles on examination, or recurrent pulmonary infections all warrant further investigation.

Three joint areas have special perioperative implications in RA: cervical spine, cricoarytenoid articulation, and temporomandibular joints (TMJs). Cervical spine subluxation abnormalities include anterior atlantoaxial subluxation, atlantoaxial impaction, and subaxial subluxation.[10] In 154 patients awaiting orthopedic surgery in Finland, 38% had cervical spine subluxation and eight (5%) had previous surgery for cervical disease.[10] Longer duration of disease and more active disease predicted cervical subluxation. Cervical spine instability is usually clinically silent and may lead to brain stem or spinal cord compression, while affected patients are manipulated while under sedation.

The cricoarytenoid joints are joints that move with the vocal cords to vary pitch and tone of the voice.[11] Arthritis or ankylosis of these joints has been reported in up to 75% of RA patients by fiber-optic laryngoscopy and in 72% using computed tomography (CT) scan.[12] Arthritis may lead to difficulties with intubation or postoperative airway obstruction due to irritation from the endotracheal tube. A history of hoarseness, sore throat, or difficulty with inspiration may be a clue to its presence. This is an "always remember" issue in the immediate postoperative period. Bandi et al. have extensively reviewed upper airway problems in rheumatologic disorders.[13]

Temporomandibular involvement in RA may impair full opening of the mouth for intubation. Jaw pain during meals may be an indication of abnormalities.

Physical Examination

Examination of the RA patient includes special attention to the heart, lungs, neurologic findings, and joints. Joint examination includes the assessment of active and passive range of motion of the cervical spine and listening to breathing and voice sounds for any clues to cricoarytenoid impairment. Palpation of the TMJs and assessment of oral excursion should be done. Range of motion, gait assessment, and evidence of synovitis of the peripheral joints should be noted to plan rehabilitation. A skin evaluation for breakdown or infection should be made. Look between the toes and balls of the feet and over rheumatoid nodules; these areas might be sources of skin infection. The neurologic examination should focus on evidence of muscle weakness, hyperreflexia, sensation, and long-track signs suggestive of cervical spine disease. Ocular dryness should be addressed by perioperative eye lubricating ointment.

Laboratory Testing and Imaging

Patients should have a complete blood count (CBC) looking for evidence of leuko-penia or anemia. Liver and kidney status should be assessed in everyone on chronic, potentially hepatotoxic, or nephrotoxic therapy. Room air O_2 saturation at rest and after a short walk is easy to perform and potentially reveal underlying interstitial lung disease.

Neva et al. documented that 6.8% of RA patients had films showing cervical subluxation after 2 years of disease, and by 5 years, this had increased to 11%.[14,15] For patients undergoing an orthopedic procedure, the prevalence of cervical spine subluxation has been reported as 44%.[10] These numbers will likely be lower with current therapies. Cervical spine films with flexion and extension views should be obtained in all RA patients going to orthopedic surgery for a complication of their disease, in patients with any neurologic abnormality on examination, after 5 years of RA, or less than 5 years with poorly controlled disease. Cervical spine protection is necessary during patient transportation and transfers.

A cervical magnetic resonance imaging (MRI) should be obtained in patients when a neurologic abnormality is identified, those with radiographic evidence of superior migration of the odontoid, a posterior atlanto-dental interval of 14 mm or less, or a subaxial sagittal canal diameter of 13 mm or less.[16] Radiographically "silent" pannus may be present compromising the spinal cord compartment. Patients with significant abnormalities on plain films or MRI should have neurosurgical or orthopedic spine consultation. Options for the anesthesiologist in a patient with a potentially unstable spine who is felt not to need surgical stabilization prior to surgery include regional anesthesia, intubation with fixed neck positioning, fiber-optic intubation, or laryngeal mask.

JUVENILE IDIOPATHIC ARTHRITIS (JIA)

JIA is a term covering a broad range of inflammatory childhood arthritides. Periop-erative considerations are similar to RA but particularly common problems include TMJ dysfunction, cervical spine disease, with fusion, and cricoarytenoid arthritis leading to difficulty with intubation and possible airway obstruction postextubation.

Cardiac and pulmonary considerations are less of an issue in JIA. Laboratory testing and imaging suggestions are similar for JIA as for RA.

ANKYLOSING SPONDYLITIS (AS)/PSORIATIC ARTHRITIS (PsA)

Epidemiology

AS affects 350,000 people in the United States and 600,000 in Europe. HLA B27 is found in 80–95% of AS patients[17] but is not required for diagnosis. Surgical procedures in patients with AS are predominately total joint arthroplasties, especially hips followed by shoulders and knees. Less common surgeries include vertebral osteotomies to correct flexion deformities in the cervical or thoracolumbar spine and stabilization of posttraumatic hyperextension fractures in the mid to lower cervical region. Another rare operative procedure related to AS is repair of the aortic valve due to damage from aortitis.

Sixteen percent of AS patients with early-onset disease undergo hip arthroplasty within 20 years and 90% with hip involvement ultimately have bilateral disease.[17] AS patients undergo arthroplasties at a mean age of 38 years old; thus, revision arthroplasties are common.

Patients with PsA can have one, few, or many joints involved and, in addition, may have spondylitis similar to AS. Surgery related to PsA includes large joint arthroplasties and synovectomies. In a review of orthopaedic surgery in patients with PsA, Lofin et al. noted fewer procedures performed in PsA than in RA patients. Approximately 7% of PsA patients will require a surgical procedure an average of 13.9 years after diagnosis.[18] The most common orthopedic procedures performed are hip followed by knee arthroplasties followed by procedures on the hands and feet.[19]

History

The preoperative history should focus on length of disease, peripheral joint involvement, spine and neck symptoms, the TMJ, and pulmonary and cardiac symptoms as well as overall functional capacity. It is important to know the outcome of any previous joint surgery with regard to the development of postoperative heterotopic ossification.

AS has a higher mortality rate than the general population due to an excess of CV disease.[20] Patients with AS are prone to develop conduction abnormalities, atrial fibrillation and aortitis. Dik et al. reported that 28.2% of 131 AS patients had a prolonged QRS interval, first-degree atrioventricular block was seen in 4.6%, complete right bundle branch block in 0.8%, and left anterior hemiblock in 0.8%.[21] Disease duration correlates with the presence of conduction abnormalities and aortitis.[22]

Long-standing AS may result in restrictive lung disease from chest wall rigidity.[23] This does not usually lead to major ventilation problems as increased diaphragmatic excursion can make up for the chest wall stiffness, but may be an issue postoperatively and with ventilator management.

AS patients are at moderate risk for heterotopic ossification.[24] The following circumstances increase the risk and warrant consideration for prophylactic therapy to prevent clinically significant heterotopic bone formation: previous post-arthroplasty heterotopic ossification, undergoing bilateral procedures, prior arthroplasty on the opposite side, or significant bone proliferation around the native diseased joint.[24] An elevated C-reactive protein (CRP) preoperatively may also predict postoperative heterotopic ossification.[25] Prophylaxis against heterotopic ossification can include a preoperative local radiation dose of 800 Gy to the operative site or a 7- to 10-day course of a nonsteroidal anti-inflammatory drug (NSAID) started 24–48 h after surgery. Indomethacin 25 mg TID has been used but increases the risk of postoperative bleeding from 1.5% to 3.2%.[24,26] Celecoxib (which does not affect platelet function) is effective with fewer side effects.[26]

Patients with PsA have an increased prevalence of hypertension, angina, and MI.[27] The presence of more extensive skin disease increases the CV risk. PsA patients undergoing perioperative assessment should have CV risk factors addressed.

Patients with PsA may also have in increased risk of postoperative infection. Data from the 1980s suggested up to a 17% deep infection rate post-arthroplasty in patients with PsA even with the use of perioperative antibiotics.[18] Common organisms included *Staphylococcus aureus* and beta-hemolytic streptococci. A series from the early 1990s reported a less concerning 2% deep infection rate. Meticulous skin care is suggested as is avoiding incision through involved skin.[18] Heterotopic ossification can also occur in PsA patients undergoing arthroplasty, and psoriasis may occur at the site of the surgical scar.[19]

Examination

Examination should include an assessment of TMJs and cervical spine motion. Limitation of range in these joints may affect anesthesia management. Patients with severe deformities can be successfully treated with nasotracheal fiber-optic intubation if necessary.[28] Spine and hip involvement may affect positioning for epidural anesthesia. Cardiopulmonary examination includes auscultation for evidence of pulmonary fibrosis and for aortic regurgitation.

Laboratory Testing

Laboratory tests should include a CBC and comprehensive chemistry panel looking for anemia or renal abnormalities from long-term treatment with NSAIDs. A chest radiograph (CXR) is recommended in the presence of any pulmonary symptoms, and pulmonary function testings (PFTs) should be considered if abdominal laparoscopic surgery is being considered in patients with spondylitis, since this may affect diaphragm excursion. An electrocardiogram (ECG) should be done to assess cardiac conduction. Cervical spine imaging with plain films may alert the anesthesiologist to large anterior syndesmophytes that might impede intubation in patients with neck involvement. Cervical instability is less of a problem in AS/PsA than fusion with decreased mobility.

SYSTEMIC AUTOIMMUNE DISEASES

Systemic Lupus Erythematosus (SLE)

Epidemiology Surgery may be required emergently for gastrointestinal (GI) complications of SLE such as ischemic bowel disease, or electively for problems as diverse as splenectomy or arthroplasty for joints damaged by osteonecrosis. SLE patients are at higher risk for coronary artery disease (CAD) and MI at a relatively young age and may require bypass surgery. Patients with SLE and antiphospholipid antibodies (aPLAs) are at increased risk for heart valve disease (as well as thrombosis) and may need valve surgery. Domsic et al. reported a two- to sevenfold higher mortality rate for SLE patients undergoing both nonelective and elective hip and knee surgery compared with RA patients and controls.[29] The excess risk was independent of major medical comorbidities. Esdaile et al. found the relative risk of patients with SLE of nonfatal MI was 10.1, fatal MI was 17.0, coronary heart disease was 7.5, and stroke was 7.9 when controlling for Framingham Heart Study risk factors.[30]

History Issues in SLE include medication management (discussed below) hematologic abnormalities, blatant or occult renal disease, immune dysfunction, increased risk of CAD, and thromboembolic disease.

Assessment needs to include evaluation of thrombosis risk. A history of arterial or venous thrombosis, pulmonary emboli, a history of fetal loss at or beyond the 10 weeks of gestation, three of more early pregnancy losses, persistent thrombocytopenia, an elevated partial thromboplastin time (PTT), or the presence of livedo on skin examination may all be clues to the presence of aPLAs or lupus anticoagulant (LAC). Approximately 39% of SLE patients have aPLAs and 22% have LAC; however, not all of these patients will develop thromboembolic disease.[31] A recent study suggests that asymptomatic SLE patients who have an elevated D-dimer have an increased risk of near future thrombosis while those with low levels do not[31]; 42% of those with an elevated D-dimer experienced a thromboembolic event during follow-up. Seventy-six percent of these patients were aPLA positive. The negative predictive value of a low-level D-dimer was 100%. Whether this can be used to stratify perioperative risk is unclear and unknown. Patients with asymptomatic aPLA may have a higher risk for thromboembolic disease and should at least receive the usual prophylactic antithrombotic therapy, as well as compressive stockings when hospitalized for surgery.[32]

Patients with established thromboembolic disease associated with aPLA/LAC have the antiphospholipid syndrome (APS) and are at high risk for perioperative morbidity and mortality. A retrospective review involving five patients with APS undergoing cardiac surgery had a perioperative mortality rate of 60% with a 1-year mortality rate of 80%.[33] Much of the morbidity occurs around transitions between anticoagulant regimens in the immediate pre- and postoperative periods; in these patients, "bridging" anticoagulation therapy should be considered (similar to that provided to high-risk prosthetic heart valve patients).

The first step in reducing the chance of perioperative MI and thrombosis is to preoperatively address traditional risk factor such as smoking or the use of birth control pills.[34] Blood pressure should be controlled and hyperlipidemia addressed. Arthroplasty poses a high risk for thrombosis and guidelines for post-arthroplasty anticoagulation have been developed and are discussed in Chapters 22 and 32.[35] The method chosen and the length of postoperative anticoagulation needs to be individualized for each SLE patient based on the surgery, bleeding risk, and associated comorbidities (i.e., thrombocytopenia, renal disease). Patients with a history of thrombosis due to aPLA need to have their anticoagulant transitions coordinated to minimize time without therapy, a challenge when neuraxial pain control is used.

If an SLE patient has Raynaud's phenomenon, central and peripheral cooling perioperatively should be limited to limit digital ischemia. Arterial lines should be minimized. Postoperative fever/inflammatory symptoms may have several causes including SLE flare.

Laboratory Testing   Important tests include CBC, complete chemistry panel, urinalysis (assess nephritis), an assessment of coagulation profile if not already known, and, depending on history and recent labs, perhaps testing to monitor SLE activity (Ds-DNA, C_3) to assess level of preoperative disease activity. The patient's rheumatologist should have baseline labs for comparison as changes postoperatively may be useful to determine causes of fever or new symptoms. Patients with SLE may have leukopenia/lymphopenia (while infection will generally elevate the white blood cells [WBCs]); however, leukopenia does not always indicate *active* SLE. Thrombocytopenia is common and should be looked for preoperatively; intravenous immunoglobulin and steroids may be useful if the platelet count needs to be raised quickly prior to surgery.

Polymyositis/Dermatomyositis

Patients with inflammatory muscle disease who undergo surgery need attention to their cardiac and pulmonary systems. Cardiac muscle involvement and arrythmias contribute to morbidity and the mortality. Patients with active skeletal muscle disease will typically have an elevated creatine phosphokinase (CPK) (including creatine phosphokinase-MB [CPK-MB]) and troponin T levels, making detection of cardiac injury more challenging. Interstitial lung disease and thoracic muscle weakness may affect ventilation and the latter also contributes to an increased risk of aspiration. Patients often have Raynaud's, and protecting patients from excessive cold during surgery is important.

Preoperative assessment should include routine CBC, chemistry panel and baseline CPK, troponins, ECG, and PFTs looking at both ventilatory effort and diffusion capacity. Cardiac troponins are fairly specific to myocardium but can be elevated in a variety of other settings including tachyarrhythmias, pulmonary embolus, sepsis, and other noncoronary ischemia situations where myocardial workload is abnormally increased.[36] Regenerating skeletal muscle releases troponin T and CPK-MB complicating the diagnosis of acute MI.

Scleroderma

Scleroderma spectrum diseases include diffuse scleroderma and limited scleroderma, also known as the CREST syndrome. Reasons for surgery in scleroderma include digital gangrene and amputations, periarterial sympathectomies for improvement of digital blood flow, surgical exploration for intestinal pseudo-obstruction, and rarely lung transplantation. Perioperative pulmonary and CV issues include interstitial lung disease, myocardial fibrosis from the disease, and pulmonary hypertension. There is often difficulty in obtaining vascular access due to thickened skin, and there must be great caution with placing arterial monitoring lines at the wrist due to an increased incidence of baseline ulnar occlusion.[37] Pulse oximetry may be unreliable when used on fingers; alternative locations such as an earlobe may be a preferred site. Raynaud's phenomenon can be severe in scleroderma, and attention to maintaining central and peripheral warmth is critical. GI reflux can also be severe, and postoperatively, aspiration precautions are important. Enteral absorption of medications may be delayed due to dysmotility. Patients with scleroderma can have a mild myopathy or an overlap with polymyositis; baseline muscle enzymes may be elevated.

Preoperative assessment should include CBC, ECG (looking for conduction on disease or a pseudo-infarct pattern), chemistry panel, troponins, and echocardiogram (looking for pulmonary hypertension).

Postoperative Gout

Gout or pseudogout can elicit postoperative fever as well as delay post-op rehabilitation. Craig et al. described 52 patients with postoperative gout ranging in age from 20 to 82, and 7 of the 52 had their first gouty attack following surgery.[38] Most of the affected joints were in the lower extremities, and podagra was present in only 8 of the 52 cases. Seven of the 52 had polyarticular gout. Attacks occurred a mean of 4 days after surgery but ranged from 1 to 18 days. Uric acid levels may be increased or decreased at the time of an attack, and should not be used to diagnose (or exclude) gout. Clinical symptoms, findings, and lab tests other than synovial fluid analysis will not distinguish gout from joint infection. Gout and septic arthritis can rarely occur simultaneously.[39] A history of gout or hyperuricemia, bariatric surgery (obesity is a risk factor for hyperuricemia), chronic use of diuretics, posttransplant surgery (patients may have been on chronic diuretic therapy, and the calcineurin inhibitors are a notorious cause of hyperuricemia), or in the setting of chronic kidney disease (CKD) increase the possibility of postoperative gout.

Pyrophosphate gout or "pseudogout" occurs in the postoperative setting. Target joints include knee, wrist, elbow, and hip. Symptoms are similar to urate gout and fever and leukocytosis can also occur.

If gout or pseudogout is suspected, joint aspiration is indicated and the fluid sent for cell count, crystal analysis, Gram stain, and culture. Anti-inflammatory therapy can be started at once if not contraindicated. NSAIDs are a mainstay, but are often problematic in the postoperative period. Parenteral NSAIDs such as ketorolac have the same (or greater) GI/renal toxicities as the oral agents. If started within 12 h, colchicine 1.2 mg initially followed by 0.6 mg 1 h later will significantly improve symptoms, and signs of inflammation in perhaps 50% of patients[40] but can cause GI upset and diarrhea. Once possible infection has been addressed, daily oral prednisone at 30–40 mg can be started and tapered over 5–7 days or the affected joint can be injected with steroids. Anakinra, an IL-1 inhibitor, can be injected subcutaneously daily at a dose of 100 mg or every other day in patients with moderate–severe CKD.[41] Patients may respond to as few as one injection or may need as many as four. Use of anakinra usually results in prompt improvement in symptoms, but use is currently not approved by the U.S. Food and Drug Administration (FDA).

PERIOPERATIVE MEDICATION MANAGEMENT

NSAIDs

NSAIDs are commonly used in patients with rheumatologic disease. Potential side effects in the perioperative period include an increase a risk of bleeding due to their effects on platelets and GI mucosa, a decline in glomerular filtration rate (GFR), fluid retention, hypertension, masking fever, and concern about NSAIDs affecting bone healing. Perioperative use of NSAIDs increases blood loss and transfusion requirements, and unless NSAIDs are felt critical for care or for prevention of heterotopic ossification, pain control can be accomplished without their use.[42,43] It is important to remember that ketorolac, a parenteral NSAID, has the same concerns as oral NSAID.

NSAIDs should be stopped 5 half-lives before surgery to assure their elimination (Table 16.1). Thus, ibuprofen with a half-life of 1.6 h can be stopped a day before surgery, while piroxicam with a half-life of 20 h should be withdrawn 4–5 days before surgery.

Aspirin uniquely irreversibly inactivates platelet cyclooxygenase, inhibiting platelet function for the life of the platelet; thus, it should be stopped 7–10 days before surgery, to allow new platelets to accumulate before the procedure.

TABLE 16.1. Nonsteroidal Anti-Inflammatory Drugs (NSAIDs) and Half-Lives

NSAID	Brand names	Half-life (h)
Ibuprofen	Motrin, Advil	1.6–1.9
Naproxen	Aleve, Naprosyn	12–15
Diclofenac	Voltaren, Arthrotec	2
Indomethacin	Indocin	4.5
Piroxicam	Feldene	30
Etodolac	Lodine	6–7
Nabumatone	Relafen	24–29
Celecoxib	Celebrex	11

NSAIDs are generally cleared within 5 half-lives. Information obtained from Micromedex.

For patients who need an NSAID for pain control, alternatives include stopping a long-acting drug 5 half-lives before surgery and replacing it with a short half-life agent, which is then stopped the day before surgery. Celecoxib, the only cyclooxygenase-2 (COX-2) available, has been shown to neither increase perioperative blood loss nor affect the stability of the joint prosthesis.[44,45] As noted previously, celecoxib is probably effective for prevention of heterotopic ossification.[26] Celecoxib can adversely affect renal function in those with CKD.

Corticosteroids (CSs)

Many patients with rheumatologic disease take CSs. In general, patients with inflammatory arthritis are given low-dose CSs, while those with diseases like SLE or vasculitis may require high-dose CSs, which are tapered when the disease comes under control. Use of CSs impairs endogenous production of cortisol, but clinically significant perioperative adrenal insufficiency is rare, being reported in only 0.7% of patients who have been on CSs. Historically, large "stress" doses of CSs were routinely used in the perioperative period, but two thoughtful reviews on the topic of perioperative CSs provide more rational guidelines.[46,47]

Patients who have been on 20 mg of prednisone for as little as 5 days may demonstrate hypothalamic–pituitary–adrenal (HPA) suppression. Suppression is not common in patients on 5 mg a day in the morning, even for prolonged periods. Patients who have been on prolonged supraphysiologic doses of CSs may take up to 1 year to restore full HPA axis responsiveness. Exogenous CSs do not affect mineralocorticoid (aldosterone) levels.

Symptoms of glucocorticoid insufficiency may include hypotension, hyponatremia, confusion or agitation, hypoglycemia, fatigue, myalgias, and fever. Under normal circumstances, the body produces approximately 10–12 mg of cortisol per day. With moderate stress, cortisol production increases to 25–50 mg/day, and with major stress, 75–150 mg may be released into the circulation.[48] The elevated levels of cortisol return to baseline within 24–48 h following the stressor.

Salem et al. have suggested that CS replacement in patients who are thought to need stress dose steroids should be based on the surgical stress and the patient's typical steroid dose[46]:

Minor Stress Procedures   (i.e., inguinal hernia repair, knee arthroscopy, carpal tunnel release, first metacarpophalangeal joint fusion). The patient should receive 25 mg of hydrocortisone or equivalent preoperatively and return to baseline dosing (even if zero) the following day.

Moderate Stress Procedures   (i.e., joint arthroplasty, anterior curciate ligament repair, abdominal hysterectomy, partial colectomy). The patient should receive their usual CS dose or parental equivalent preoperatively and 50 mg of hydrocortisone intra-operatively. On postoperative day 1, 20 mg of hydrocortisone every 8 h is then given with resumption of the usual CS dose on postoperative day 2.

Major Stress Procedures   (i.e., coronary artery bypass grafting [CABG], bilateral knee arthroplasty, multiple trauma surgery, revision arthroplasty). Again the patient's usual daily dose of CS is given preoperatively, and 25–50 mg of hydrocortisone or equivalent is given every 8 h for 48–72 h followed by prompt return to preoperative CS dosing.

The patient who is receiving a maintenance dose CS therapy that is more than the estimated stress requirement will not need more CS coverage during the stress period.[46] There is *no* documented necessity for extended tapering of stress dose steroids, which may blunt signs of infection, cause leukocytosis, increase glucose, and so on.

Methotrexate

A 2008 review of the eight studies of methotrexate in the orthopedic perioperative period concluded that this agent can be continued through surgery.[49] Two of the eight articles concluded that methotrexate posed an infection risk postoperatively while the other six did not. The largest and best designed trial by Grennan et al. found that if methotrexate was continued, the flare rate was significantly lower, and there was no increased risk of infection compared with those that held methotrexate 2 weeks before and 2 weeks after surgery.[50]

There are little data available for nonorthopedic procedures. We suggest it be continued for most surgeries unless the surgery was done to treat serious infection, that is, colonic perforation with associated peritonitis. Methotrexate is rapidly eliminated from the blood via the kidney. Not giving methotrexate within 48 h preoperatively may be reasonable in patients at high risk for acute renal injury or other specific concerns. Important perioperative drug interactions include penicillin antibiotics (increases methotrexate levels) and full-dose bactrim (also a folate inhibitor).[51] Methotrexate toxicity includes bone marrow suppression/neutropenia that should be treated with folinic acid supplementation.

Leflunomide

The data regarding leflunomide are scant but of some concern. Fuerst and colleagues reported that 40% of 32 patients using leflunomide developed wound complications postoperatively following orthopedic procedures compared with 13% of 59 patients using methotrexate or methotrexate plus corticosteroids ($P = 0.001$).[52] Infection rate was 9.3% in the leflunomide group. The authors strongly recommended interrupting leflunomide therapy before orthopedic surgery.

In a prospective study, Tanaka et al. did not find a difference in postoperative wound infections rates for patients who had had interruption of leflunomide therapy (stopped 2 weeks before and restarted 2 weeks after surgery) versus those who had continuous therapy.[53]

For low-intensity procedures, leflunomide can be continued. For elective procedures where there will be large postoperative wounds, one should consider holding the drug 2 half-lives, that is, 4 weeks or using a cholestyramine protocol for rapid removal. Cholestyramine given orally at a dose of 8 g three times a day for 24 h to three healthy volunteers decreased plasma levels by approximately 40% in 24 h and by 49–65% in 48 h. Leflunomide can elevate levels of warfarin if used together.

Other Nonbiologic Disease-Modifying Agents

Hydroxychloroquine was at one time used as a postoperative anticoagulant.[54] It can be continued uninterrupted through surgery. Sulfasalazine can also in general be continued or interrupted 1 day before and restarted a few days after surgery. It is a folate antagonist, and folate depletion may lead to toxicity. It can also increase the international normalized ratio (INR) in patients on warfarin. Azathioprine and mycophenololate can in general be continued for minor procedures and held briefly for more intense surgeries, though there are no data indicating that this is necessary.

Biologic Agents

The use of biologics, in particular the anti-tumor necrosis factor (TNF) agents, in the perioperative period has been reviewed.[55,56] The data for the TNF agents are mixed in regard to both wound healing and postoperative infection, but it is felt by the authors and by various international rheumatology societies that holding the medication preoperatively prevent course of action, when feasible. The recommendations are to hold the TNF agents at least 2 half-lives before major elective procedures and waiting 10–14 days or until wound healing is satisfactory to restart these agents. Thus, for infliximab 3 weeks, adalimumab 4 weeks, etanercept 7–10 days, golimumab 4 weeks, and certolizumab 4 weeks. TNF agents probably do not need to be held for minor procedures. There are no major drug interactions for the TNF medications (Table 16.2).

Rituximab, a chimeric anti-CD20 agent, affects B lymphocytes and can lead to selective immunosuppression for 6–12 months following dosing. Significant bac-

TABLE 16.2. Biologic Agents and Half-Lives

Generic name	Brand names	Type	Half-life (days)
Etanercept	Enbrel	TNF inhibitor	3.5–5.5
Adalumimab	Humira	TNF inhibitor	10–20
Infliximab	Rituximab	TNF inhibitor	9.5
Certoluzimab	Cimzia	TNF inhibitor	14
Golumimab	Simponi	TNF inhibitor	14
Abatacept	Orencia	T-cell inhibitor	13
Rituximab	Rituxan	B-cell inhibitor	18
			Effects on B cells may be 6 months or more
Tocilizumab	Actemra	IL-6 receptor antagonist	11–13
Anakinra	Kineret	IL-1 receptor antagonist	4–6 h

Biologics are suggested to be held at least 2 half-lives prior to elective surgery. Half-life data from medication prescribing information.

terial infections have not been observed in rituximab-treated RA patients. With little supporting data, it has been suggested that elective surgery be held until B-cell numbers normalize.[56] We are not convinced this is necessary.

Abatacept, an anti-T-cell agent, has been approved for use in RA. As with rituximab, there are little data regarding perioperative dosing. Infections have not been a major issue. The authors suggest waiting to the end of the dosing interval (1 month, which equals 2 half-lives) for elective surgery and then 10–14 days following to restart.

There are two small studies evaluating tocilizumab, a new anti-IL-6 receptor antagonist, in the perioperative period.[57,58] Both are reassuring with regard to wound healing and infection, but both noted that the normal postoperative rise in temperature and CRP were both suppressed, potentially masking signs and symptoms of infection. Tocilizumab has an 11- to 13-day half-life depending on dose and requires planning elective surgery for at least 3 weeks after the last dose and waiting 10–14 days to restart. It does not need to be held for minor procedures.

Anakinra, an IL-1 inhibitor, has been mentioned in the context of treating postoperative gout. It may impact wound healing, and it should be used with caution in the early phases of wound healing.[56]

REFERENCES

1. Helmick CG, Felson DT, Lawrence RC, et al. Estimates of the prevalence of arthritis and other rheumatic conditions in the United States. Part I. *Arthritis Rheum.* Jan 2008;58(1):15–25.
2. Drossaers-Bakker KW, Kroon HM, Zwinderman AH, Breedveld FC, Hazes JM. Radiographic damage of large joints in long-term rheumatoid arthritis and its relation to function. *Rheumatology (Oxford).* Sep 2000;39(9):998–1003.
3. da Silva E, Doran MF, Crowson CS, O'Fallon WM, Matteson EL. Declining use of orthopedic surgery in patients with rheumatoid arthritis? Results of a long-term, population-based assessment. *Arthritis Rheum.* Apr 15 2003;49(2):216–220.
4. Weiss RJ, Stark A, Wick MC, Ehlin A, Palmblad K, Wretenberg P. Orthopaedic surgery of the lower limbs in 49,802 rheumatoid arthritis patients: results from the Swedish National Inpatient Registry during 1987 to 2001. *Ann Rheum Dis.* Mar 2006;65(3):335–341.
5. Ward MM. Decreases in rates of hospitalizations for manifestations of severe rheumatoid arthritis, 1983–2001. *Arthritis Rheum.* Apr 2004;50(4):1122–1131.
6. Poldermans D, Hoeks SE, Feringa HH. Pre-operative risk assessment and risk reduction before surgery. *J Am Coll Cardiol.* May 20 2008;51(20):1913–1924.
7. Peters MJ, Symmons DP, McCarey D, et al. EULAR evidence-based recommendations for cardiovascular risk management in patients with rheumatoid arthritis and other forms of inflammatory arthritis. *Ann Rheum Dis.* Feb 2010;69(2):325–331.
8. Metafratzi ZM, Georgiadis AN, Ioannidou CV, et al. Pulmonary involvement in patients with early rheumatoid arthritis. *Scand J Rheumatol.* Sep–Oct 2007;36(5):338–344.
9. Lynch DA. Lung disease related to collagen vascular disease. *J Thorac Imaging.* Nov 2009;24(4):299–309.
10. Neva MH, Hakkinen A, Makinen H, Hannonen P, Kauppi M, Sokka T. High prevalence of asymptomatic cervical spine subluxation in patients with rheumatoid arthritis waiting for orthopaedic surgery. *Ann Rheum Dis.* Jul 2006;65(7):884–888.
11. Segebarth PB, Limbird TJ. Perioperative acute upper airway obstruction secondary to severe rheumatoid arthritis. *J Arthroplasty.* Sep 2007;22(6):916–919.
12. Brazeau-Lamontagne L, Charlin B, Levesque RY, Lussier A. Cricoarytenoiditis: CT assessment in rheumatoid arthritis. *Radiology.* Feb 1986;158(2):463–466.

13. Bandi V, Munnur U, Braman SS. Airway problems in patients with rheumatologic disorders. *Crit Care Clin*. Oct 2002;18(4):749–765.

14. Neva MH, Kauppi MJ, Kautiainen H, et al. Combination drug therapy retards the development of rheumatoid atlantoaxial subluxations. *Arthritis Rheum*. Nov 2000;43(11):2397–2401.

15. Kauppi MJ, Neva MH, Laiho K, et al. Rheumatoid atlantoaxial subluxation can be prevented by intensive use of traditional disease modifying antirheumatic drugs. *J Rheumatol*. Feb 2009;36(2):273–278.

16. Nguyen HV, Ludwig SC, Silber J, et al. Rheumatoid arthritis of the cervical spine. *Spine J*. May–Jun 2004;4(3):329–334.

17. Kubiak EN, Moskovich R, Errico TJ, Di Cesare PE. Orthopaedic management of ankylosing spondylitis. *J Am Acad Orthop Surg*. Jul–Aug 2005;13(4):267–278.

18. Lofin I, Levine B, Badlani N, Klein GR, Jaffe WL. Psoriatic arthritis and arthroplasty: a review of the literature. *Bull NYU Hosp Jt Dis*. 2008;66(1):41–48.

19. Strauss EJ, Alfonso D, Baidwan G, Di Cesare PE. Orthopedic manifestations and management of psoriatic arthritis. *Am J Orthop*. Mar 2008;37(3):138–147.

20. McCarey D, Sturrock RD. Comparison of cardiovascular risk in ankylosing spondylitis and rheumatoid arthritis. *Clin Exp Rheumatol*. Jul–Aug 2009;27(4 Suppl 55):S124–S126.

21. Dik VK, Peters MJ, Dijkmans PA, et al. The relationship between disease-related characteristics and conduction disturbances in ankylosing spondylitis. *Scand J Rheumatol*. 2010;39(1):38–41.

22. Eder L, Sadek M, McDonald-Blumer H, Gladman DD. Aortitis and spondyloarthritis—an unusual presentation: case report and review of the literature. *Semin Arthritis Rheum*. 2010;39(6):510–514.

23. Rosenow E, Strimlan CV, Muhm JR, Ferguson RH. Pleuropulmonary manifestations of ankylosing spondylitis. *Mayo Clin Proc*. Oct 1977;52(10):641–649.

24. Iorio R, Healy WL. Heterotopic ossification after hip and knee arthroplasty: risk factors, prevention, and treatment. *J Am Acad Orthop Surg*. Nov–Dec 2002;10(6):409–416.

25. Tani Y, Nishioka J, Inoue K, Hukuda S, Tsujimoto M. Relation between ectopic ossification after total hip arthroplasty and activity of general inflammation in patients with ankylosing spondylitis. *Ann Rheum Dis*. Oct 1998;57(10):634.

26. Romano CL, Duci D, Romano D, Mazza M, Meani E. Celecoxib versus indomethacin in the prevention of heterotopic ossification after total hip arthroplasty. *J Arthroplasty*. Jan 2004;19(1):14–18.

27. Gladman DD, Ang M, Su L, Tom BD, Schentag CT, Farewell VT. Cardiovascular morbidity in psoriatic arthritis. *Ann Rheum Dis*. Jul 2009;68(7):1131–1135.

28. Sciubba DM, Nelson C, Hsieh P, Gokaslan ZL, Ondra S, Bydon A. Perioperative challenges in the surgical management of ankylosing spondylitis. *Neurosurg Focus*. 2008;24(1):E10.

29. Domsic RT, Lingala B, Krishnan E. Systemic lupus erythematosus, rheumatoid arthritis, and postarthroplasty mortality: a cross-sectional analysis from the nationwide inpatient sample. *J Rheumatol*. Jun 1 2010;37(7):1467–1472.

30. Esdaile JM, Abrahamowicz M, Grodzicky T, et al. Traditional Framingham risk factors fail to fully account for accelerated atherosclerosis in systemic lupus erythematosus. *Arthritis Rheum*. Oct 2001;44(10):2331–2337.

31. Wu H, Birmingham DJ, Rovin B, et al. D-dimer level and the risk for thrombosis in systemic lupus erythematosus. *Clin J Am Soc Nephrol*. Nov 2008;3(6):1628–1636.

32. Ruffatti A, Del Ross T, Ciprian M, et al. Risk factors for a first thrombotic event in antiphospholipid antibody carriers. A multicentre, retrospective follow-up study. *Ann Rheum Dis*. Mar 2009;68(3):397–399.

33. Massoudy P, Cetin SM, Thielmann M, et al. Antiphospholipid syndrome in cardiac surgery—an underestimated coagulation disorder? *Eur J Cardiothorac Surg*. Jul 2005;28(1):133–137.

34. Erkan D, Lockshin MD. New approaches for managing antiphospholipid syndrome. *Nat Clin Pract Rheumatol*. Mar 2009;5(3):160–170.

35. Sheth NP, Lieberman JR, Della Valle CJ. DVT prophylaxis in total joint reconstruction. *Orthop Clin North Am*. Apr 2010;41(2):273–280.

36. Thygesen K, Alpert JS, White HD. Universal definition of myocardial infarction. *Eur Heart J*. Oct 2007;28(20):2525–2538.

37. Park JH, Sung YK, Bae SC, Song SY, Seo HS, Jun JB. Ulnar artery vasculopathy in systemic sclerosis. *Rheumatol Int.* Jul 2009;29(9):1081–1086.
38. Craig MH, Poole GV, Hauser CJ. Postsurgical gout. *Am Surg.* Jan 1995;61(1):56–59.
39. Yu KH, Luo SF, Liou LB, et al. Concomitant septic and gouty arthritis—an analysis of 30 cases. *Rheumatology (Oxford).* Sep 2003;42(9):1062–1066.
40. Terkeltaub RA, Furst DE, Bennett K, Kook KA, Crockett RS, Davis MW. High versus low dosing of oral colchicine for early acute gout flare: twenty-four-hour outcome of the first multicenter, randomized, double-blind, placebo-controlled, parallel-group, dose-comparison colchicine study. *Arthritis Rheum.* Apr 2010;62(4):1060–1068.
41. So A, De Smedt T, Revaz S, Tschopp J. A pilot study of IL-1 inhibition by anakinra in acute gout. *Arthritis Res Ther.* 2007;9(2):R28.
42. Slappendel R, Weber EW, Benraad B, Dirksen R, Bugter ML. Does ibuprofen increase perioperative blood loss during hip arthroplasty? *Eur J Anaesthesiol.* Nov 2002;19(11):829–831.
43. Robinson CM, Christie J, Malcolm-Smith N. Nonsteroidal antiinflammatory drugs, perioperative blood loss, and transfusion requirements in elective hip arthroplasty. *J Arthroplasty.* Dec 1993;8(6):607–610.
44. Meunier A, Lisander B, Good L. Effects of celecoxib on blood loss, pain, and recovery of function after total knee replacement: a randomized placebo-controlled trial. *Acta Orthop.* Oct 2007;78(5):661–667.
45. Meunier A, Aspenberg P, Good L. Celecoxib does not appear to affect prosthesis fixation in total knee replacement: a randomized study using radiostereometry in 50 patients. *Acta Orthop.* Feb 2009;80(1):46–50.
46. Salem M, Tainsh RE, Jr., Bromberg J, Loriaux DL, Chernow B. Perioperative glucocorticoid coverage. A reassessment 42 years after emergence of a problem. *Ann Surg.* Apr 1994;219(4): 416–425.
47. Axelrod L. Perioperative management of patients treated with glucocorticoids. *Endocrinol Metab Clin North Am.* Jun 2003;32(2):367–383.
48. Howe CR, Gardner GC, Kadel NJ. Perioperative medication management for the patient with rheumatoid arthritis. *J Am Acad Orthop Surg.* Sep 2006;14(9):544–551.
49. Pieringer H, Stuby U, Biesenbach G. The place of methotrexate perioperatively in elective orthopedic surgeries in patients with rheumatoid arthritis. *Clin Rheumatol.* 2008;27(10):1217–1220.
50. Grennan DM, Gray J, Loudon J, Fear S. Methotrexate and early postoperative complications in patients with rheumatoid arthritis undergoing elective orthopaedic surgery. *Ann Rheum Dis.* Mar 2001;60(3):214–217.
51. Sathi N, Ackah J, Dawson J. Methotrexate induced neutropenia associated with coprescription of penicillins: serious and under-reported? *Rheumatology (Oxford).* Mar 2006;45(3):361–362; author reply 363–364.
52. Fuerst M, Mohl H, Baumgartel K, Ruther W. Leflunomide increases the risk of early healing complications in patients with rheumatoid arthritis undergoing elective orthopedic surgery. *Rheumatol Int.* Oct 2006;26(12):1138–1142.
53. Tanaka N, Sakahashi H, Sato E, Hirose K, Ishima T, Ishii S. Examination of the risk of continuous leflunomide treatment on the incidence of infectious complications after joint arthroplasty in patients with rheumatoid arthritis. *J Clin Rheumatol.* Apr 2003;9(2):115–118.
54. Loudon JR. Hydroxychloroquine and postoperative thromboembolism after total hip replacement. *Am J Med.* Oct 14 1988;85(4A):57–61.
55. Pappas DA, Giles JT. Do antitumor necrosis factor agents increase the risk of postoperative orthopedic infections? *Curr Opin Rheumatol.* Jul 2008;20(4):450–456.
56. Mushtaq S, Goodman SM, Scanzello CR. Perioperative management of biologic agents used in treatment of rheumatoid arthritis. *Am J Ther.* 2011;18(5):426–434.
57. Hirao M, Hashimoto J, Tsuboi H, et al. Laboratory and febrile features after joint surgery in patients with rheumatoid arthritis treated with tocilizumab. *Ann Rheum Dis.* May 2009;68(5):654–657.
58. Hiroshima R, Kawakami K, Iwamoto T, et al. Analysis of C-reactive protein levels and febrile tendency after joint surgery in rheumatoid arthritis patients treated with a perioperative 4-week interruption of tocilizumab. *Mod Rheumatol.* 2011;21(1):109–111.

CHAPTER *17*

ASSESSING AND MANAGING PSYCHIATRIC DISEASE

Elias A. Khawam, Anjala V. Tess, and Leo Pozuelo

INTRODUCTION

Patients with psychiatric illnesses can pose challenges in the perioperative period that require upfront management strategies to assure the best outcomes.[1,2] This chapter will review practical considerations for the patient with anxiety, mood, and psychotic disorders as well as the patient with chemical dependency. Finally, practical considerations will be outlined in the perioperative period of the patient undergoing electroconvulsive therapy (ECT). The detection and management of delirium is covered separately in Chapter 30.

THE PATIENT WITH AN ANXIETY DISORDER

General Considerations

In the general population, anxiety diseases such as panic disorder, generalized anxiety disorder, and social phobia are the most common psychiatric disorders. When an anxious patient is about to undergo a medical procedure, there is risk that the underlying anxiety may be heightened perioperatively. As a general rule, these patients should continue their anxiolytic regimen of antidepressants and/or benzodiazepines (BZDs) throughout the perioperative course.

Particular attention should be given to the patient's past hospital experiences to determine if any triggers of anxiety were present. The medical team should then inquire into how the current hospital visit can be made less anxiety provoking. In burn patients, for example, the prevalence of posttraumatic stress disorder (PTSD) is reported to be as high as 20%,[3] warranting consultation with behavioral specialists to minimize symptoms in current and future procedures. The PTSD spectrum of intrusive memories, nightmares, flashbacks, and psychological distress can be seen

---

Perioperative Medicine: Medical Consultation and Co-Management, First Edition.
Edited by Amir K. Jaffer and Paul J. Grant.
© 2012 Wiley-Blackwell. Published 2012 by John Wiley & Sons, Inc.

in patients who have suffered serious medical events such as motor vehicle accidents, cardiovascular surgery,[4] cancer,[5] and severe neurological insults. Finally, patients with firings of implantable cardioverter-defibrillator (ICD) devices[6] can experience heightened anxiety preoperatively, which may warrant medical and behavioral management.

Medication Management

Patients are commonly prescribed BZDs for acute and/or chronic management of their anxiety disorder. These medications are of various half-life duration and can all provoke a BZD withdrawal syndrome (anxiety, dizziness, tremors) when ceased abruptly, and escalate to autonomic instability and delirium as seen in alcohol withdrawal syndromes (AWSs). Ideally, the patient should be continued on his or her home dose of BZD during the perioperative hospital course. When the patient will be "nil per os" (NPO) for a significant period of time (more than 4–6 h), the patient should have his or her home BZD regimen administered in a parenteral route.

Using an equivalency chart of common BZDs (Table 17.1) allows for easy conversion of the various BZDs into the desired dosage and route of administration. A recommended approach is to convert the patient's home BZD regimen into a total daily dose of "per os" (PO or by mouth) oral lorazepam and then administering half of the daily dose intravenously during the NPO period. (i.e., a patient on alprazolam 0.25 mg PO every 6 h at home is taking the equivalent of lorazepam 1 mg PO every 6 h or a total oral dose of lorazepam 4 mg. This is equivalent to 2 mg of intravenous [IV] lorazepam, which can be administered to this patient over a 24-h period as 0.5 mg intravenously every 6 h). As far as potency equivalents, lorazepam PO is equal to lorazepam given intramuscularly. However, lorazepam IV is double the potency of PO and intramuscular (IM) preparations.

Clinicians may encounter perioperative scenarios where BZD use is limited such as in respiratory insufficiency. A non-BZD alternative that offers cross coverage for BZD is the anticonvulsant agent gabapentin.[7] Gabapentin can be titrated as

TABLE 17.1. Benzodiazepine Equivalency

Generic name	Trade name	Oral dose (mg)
Chlordiazepoxide	Librium	10
Diazepam	Valium	5
Lorazepam	Ativan	1
Clonazeapm	Klonopin	0.5
Alprazolam	Xanax	0.25

Adapted from:
- Goldberg RJ. Alcohol and substance abuse. In: *Practical Guide to the Care of the Psychiatric Patient*, 3rd edition, Goldberg RJ (ed.), p. 247. St. Louis, MO: Mosby; 2008.
- Renner JA, Gastfriend DR. Drug-addicted patients. In: *Massachusetts General Hospital Handbook of General Hospital Psychiatry*, 5th edition, Stern TA, Fricchione GL, Cassem NH, et al. (eds.), pp. 128–129, 224–228. Philadelphia: Mosby; 2004.

needed with caution in patients with renal insufficiency as this drug is cleared by the kidneys. For additional anxiolytic control, small dosages of atypical antipsychotics may be used (i.e., quetiapine 25–50 mg or olanzapine 2.5–5 mg); however, these agents do not offer cross coverage for BZDs and therefore will not prevent BZD withdrawal. Neither gabapentin nor atypical antipsychotics are formally approved by the U.S. Food and Drug Administration (FDA) for anxiety disorders and larger randomized controlled studies are still needed.

When the BZD-dependent patient is sedated with IV drips such as fentanyl, dexmedetomidine, or propofol, they are still at risk for active BZD withdrawal as none of sedative agents confer benzodiazepine cross coverage.

Selective serotonin reuptake inhibitors (SSRIs) and serotonin–norepinephrine reuptake inhibitors (SNRIs) are commonly used frontline medications to treat chronic anxiety disorders. The onset of action is 2–3 weeks and thus will not be effective in treating acute anxiety in the perioperative patient. However, if the patient was previously taking one of these medications, prompt resumption is recommended during the hospital stay. A list of the various routes of administration for antidepressants and psychotropics is provided in Table 17.2.

Abrupt discontinuation of the SSRIs or SNRIs may lead to a non-life-threatening but uncomfortable "discontinuation" syndrome consisting of dizziness, lightheadedness, flu-like symptoms, and paresthesias. Prompt resumption of the antidepressant medication will resolve these symptoms. The long-acting antidepressant fluoxetine with an extended half-life is the only antidepressant that does not routinely cause a discontinuation syndrome.

Behavior Management

Patients with anxiety disorders have benefited from short-term, problem-focused psychotherapies such as cognitive behavioral therapy (CBT). CBT has shown to be effective in treating the underlying disorder as well as providing relapse prevention. Prior to elective surgery, a patient with anxiety may benefit from a CBT session to reduce catastrophic worry as well as to provide relaxation skills for the hospital course. Progressive relaxation techniques and guided imagery[8] as well as basic mindfulness mediation techniques can be of assistance in dealing with the patient's anxiety perioperatively. Some medical centers are offering on-site "healing services," which can encompass some of these therapies at the bedside to help patients cope with the hospitalization and medical illness, potentially reducing anxiety levels and promoting overall wellness.

THE PATIENT WITH A MOOD DISORDER

General Considerations

The hospitalist will frequently encounter patients being treated for a mood disorder. The majority are unipolar depression (monopolar depression or major depression), and less common will be bipolar affective disorder (bipolar depression or manic

TABLE 17.2.   Various Routes of Administration of Common Psychiatric Medications

Generic name	Trade name	Administration route	Initial dose range	Target dose range (mg)
Fluoxetine	Prozac	Liquid oral	10 mg	20–40
Setraline	Zoloft	Liquid oral	50 mg	50–200
Paroxetine	Paxil	Liquid oral	10 mg	20–40
Citalopram	Celexa	Liquid oral	10 mg	20–40
Escitalopram	Lexapro	Liquid oral	10 mg	20–40
Mirtazapine	Remeron Sol-Tab	Oral dissolvable tablets	15 mg	30–45
Olanzapine	Zyprexa Zydis	Oral dissolvable tablets	5–10 mg	
Olanzapine	Zyprexa	IM (for acute agitation)	10 mg IM × 1 (maximum dose 30 mg/24-h period)	
Risperidone	Risperdal M-tab	Oral dissolvable tablets	1 mg/day	
Ziprasidone	Geodon	IM (for acute agitation)	10 mg	
Aripiprazole	Abilify Discmelt	Oral dissolvable tablet	10 or 15 mg/day	
Aripiprazole	Abilify	IM (for acute agitation)	5.25–9.75 mg dose	

Information from:
– Beliles KE. Alternative routes of administration of psychotropic agents. In *Psychiatric Care of the Medical Patient*, 2nd edition, Stoudemire A, Fogel BS, Greenberg DB (eds.), pp. 393–403. New York: Oxford University Press; 2000.
– Robinson MJ, Owen JA. Psychopharmacology. In: *Textbook of Psychosomatic Medicine*, 1st edition, Levenson JL (ed.), pp. 894–898. Washington, DC: American Psychiatric Publishing; 2005.
– Pozuelo L, et al. Preoperative evaluation and perioperative management of the psychiatric patient. In: *Textbook of Comprehensive Hospital Medicine*, Williams MV, Hayward R (eds.), pp. 863–871. Elsevier; 2007.
    IM, intramuscular.

depressive illness). The prescription and use of antidepressants has increased dramatically. The reasons for this include improved diagnosis, more treatment options, increased indications for these medications including anxiety disorders and pain syndromes, and improved safety and side effect profiles.[9] Although beyond the scope of this chapter, there is growing evidence of the deleterious effect of comorbid depression in the medically ill patient, manifest by increased medical morbidity and mortality, as well as less adherence to treatment recommendations and lifestyle modification. Key issues in medication management will be addressed, as will the use of behavioral techniques to ensure patients with a mood disorder are optimally managed in the perioperative period.

Medication Management

Unipolar Depression   The patient with unipolar depression should have their antidepressant medication continued as much as possible in the perioperative period, independent if they are receiving acute treatment or a maintenance medication regimen (to prevent relapse or recurrence of depression). SSRIs, SNRIs, mirtazapine, and bupropion are generally well tolerated when readministered to the postoperative patient. Aside from the "discontinuation syndrome" previously mentioned, there are no major physiological consequences from temporarily being off an antidepressant for 1–2 days. For longer periods of time without antidepressant continuation (i.e., weeks), the patient is at risk of relapse or recurrence of the depression. Abrupt discontinuation of home BZDs over 2 or 3 days can provoke a clinical breakthrough of anxiety as well as a BZD withdrawal syndrome with physical and psychiatric symptoms.

Parenteral preparations of antidepressants are limited. As previously stated, all SSRIs are available in liquid form. There is a dissolvable tablet form for mirtazapine that can be useful when the patient has difficulty swallowing. The only transdermal antidepressant available is a selegiline patch, a selective monoamine oxidase inhibitor type B (MAOI-B). Selegiline has minimal drug–drug and dietary interactions at lower dosages, but loses its selectivity at higher dosages posing challenges in medication and diet management typical for the monoamine oxidase inhibitors (MAOIs) (see below).

The SSRIs are generally well tolerated in the medically ill. On the consultation liaison service, our preference for prescribing an antidepressant *de novo* is citalopram, escitalopram, or sertraline due to the least drug–drug interactions and effects on the cytochrome P450 enzyme system. However, if a patient was taking another SSRI prior to hospital admission, the patient should be continued on their home regimen.

SSRIs should be used in caution in the perioperative period among patients at high risk for gastrointestinal (GI) bleeding, especially when given concomitantly with aspirin or nonsteroidal anti-inflammatory agents.[10] At baseline, SSRIs can prolong the bleeding time. In large epidemiologic studies, SSRIs have been associated with increased risk of upper GI bleeding. Additionally, case reports have shown similar findings with SNRIs such as venlafaxine. Clinically, both of these antidepressant classes should be stopped in the setting of active GI bleeding. Likewise, the international normalized ratio (INR) should be monitored when an SSRI is coadministered with oral anticoagulants such as warfarin.

The SNRI venlafaxine has a low incidence but known risk of blood pressure elevation. Conversely, the SNRI duloxetine can have a more profound interaction with medications cleared by the P450 cytochrome system such as lipophilic beta-blockers (i.e., propranolol and metoprolol) increasing the risk for hypotension and bradycardia. With higher dosages of bupropion (over 300 mg/day), there is potential for lowering the seizure threshold and thus should be avoided in the perioperative period for patients at risk for seizures.

The older tricyclic antidepressants (TCAs) and MAOIs[11] used in the treatment of depression are particularly cumbersome in the perioperative period. TCAs have strong anticholinergic effects (which can predispose to delirium) and hypotensive effects, in addition to potential toxicity on the cardiac conduction system. In this regard, it is advisable that patients have the TCA tapered off 1–2 weeks prior to elective surgery. If it is determined that the patient's depression warrants resumption of a TCA, the medication can be restarted at half the dose to minimize hypotensive and tachycardic effects. It is also advisable to restart TCAs outside the risk period for delirium. TCAs should not be used in patients with any cardiac conduction abnormalities given the higher risk of morbidity and mortality.[12]

MAOIs have a pronounced overall side effect profile in addition to significant drug interactions with sympathomimetic pressor agents and analgesics that potentiate a serotonergic effect. As such, MAOIs should be stopped 2 weeks prior to any elective surgery. The MAOIs available in the United States are all irreversible, which dictates a 2-week period off the medication before introducing a substitute antidepressant.

Finally, the herbal antidepressant *hypericum perforatum* (St. John's wort) should also be discontinued at a minimum of 2 weeks before elective surgery given the many potential drug–drug interactions.[13] This is a recommendation by the American Society of Anesthesiologists (ASA).

Bipolar Affective Disorder   A major objective of treating a medical patient with a preexisting bipolar affective disorder is resuming the patient's psychiatric medication(s) as soon as possible in the perioperative period. It is not unusual for a patient with this diagnosis to be managed pharmacologically with more than one class of medications. Typically, the patient will be on a "mood stabilizer" such as one of the anticonvulsants (i.e., valproic acid, carbabamazepine, or oxacarbamazepine) or the non-anticonvulsant lithium carbonate. In addition, the patient may be taking an antipsychotic that can minimize the tendency for any mood elevation (mania) as well as periodic use of an antidepressant to treat a depression phase of the illness, should one occur. In contrast to unipolar depression, if a bipolar affective disorder patient were to be maintained only on an antidepressant without a mood stabilizer or antipsychotic, the patient runs the risk of going into mania.

Patients with bipolar disorder require vigilance as they are predisposed to mood changes with psychological distress, sleep deprivation, and major physical illnesses. Consequently, coordinated care with a mental health provider is advisable when managing a bipolar affective disorder patient in the perioperative period.

Some specific considerations for bipolar patients are as follows. Prior to elective admission for surgery, all bipolar medication should be continued with the exception of lithium. Given its narrow therapeutic window, dehydration, and hemodynamic considerations, as well as its propensity to cause confusion in the medically ill, it is advisable to discontinue lithium prior to elective surgery. In the immediate perioperative period, consultation with a mental health professional is recommended as to what medications can be used to confer mood stability. Options include another mood stabilizer or antipsychotic agent that can be continued until the patient is clinically stable and the lithium can be resumed. Lithium resumption should be at a lower dosage while monitoring fluid and renal function with measuring lithium levels during titration. The only parenteral mood stabilizer available is valproate sodium, which can be given intravenously.

Most disruptions in sleep, breakthrough of mania, or significant mood lability of a bipolar patient can be managed with an antipsychotic in the perioperative period. Parenteral antipsychotic agents are available and referenced in Table 17.2. Among the older medications (i.e., first-generation or typical antipsychotics), the higher-potency parenteral haloperidol (IV or IM) is preferred over the lower-potency parenteral antipsychotics (i.e., thioridazine or chlorpromazine) as the latter group have a pronounced hypotensive and anticholinergic side effect profile.

Among the newer antipsychotic preparations (i.e., second-generation or atypical antipsychotics), olanzapine, ziprasidone, or aripiprazole are all parenteral considerations that can be administered intramuscularly. In addition, oral dissolvable tablets are available for olanzapine, risperidone, and aripiprazole. Some caveats are that olanzapine is more sedating, and risperidone will need dose titration due to hypotensive potential. Aripiprazole does not appear to cause sedation. A newer antipsychotic, asenapine, is exclusively administered sublingually and has extensive hepatic metabolization.

The only IV antipsychotic available is haloperidol, which has less potential for extrapyramidal effects when compared with oral or IM routes of administration. Administration of all antipsychotics, whether first or second generation, should include routine electrocardiogram (ECG) monitoring to assess for prolongation of the QTc interval.

Behavioral Management

Key tenants for the treatment of unipolar depression and bipolar affective disorder are supportive emotional therapy in the context of the medical illness, identification and treatment of coexisting anxiety, and preservation of a normal sleep–wake cycle. Specifically, overt sleep deprivation in bipolar patients can precipitate drastic mood changes.

Increased vigilance of steroid administration in the bipolar patient is warranted given its potential to exacerbate mood and behavior changes, including breakthrough mania. Optimal sleep hygiene with judicious use of antipsychotics to minimize any mania tendencies will help mitigate major mood disruptions. Consultation with a psychiatric team in these perioperative cases is recommended.

THE PATIENT WITH A PSYCHOTIC DISORDER

General Considerations

Patients with an active psychotic disorder may endorse delusions, hallucinations, and distortional thinking and may also exhibit personality changes.[14] Depending on the degree of psychosis, these patients may present with bizarre behaviors and have difficulty with social interaction with impairment in daily life activities. Schizophrenia, the most common of the psychotic disorders, is a treatable illness with a prevalence of about 1% in the general population.

Patients with adequately treated psychotic illness can comply with preoperative consultations and preparations. Depending on their state of illness, they can provide informed consent for their planned procedure. In other circumstances, surrogate decision-making steps must be enacted. However, it is not unusual for the schizophrenic patient to experience an exacerbation or breakthrough of psychosis during periods of stress such as the perioperative period.

Certain challenges affect the perioperative management of patients with psychotic disorders. Active paranoid delusions might affect the patient's capacity to consent for the procedure and to comply with the perioperative process. Concrete reasoning and cognitive impairment seen in chronic schizophrenia may also impact obtaining consent. In addition to exhibiting potential communication difficulties with medical providers, patients with schizophrenia can also present with altered pain sensitivities.[15]

In the preoperative period, it is important to obtain a baseline psychiatric history, information on past hospitalization experiences, an up-to-date psychiatric medication list, and recognize comorbid psychiatric conditions such as substance abuse. Patients with psychosis may not always be considered reliable historians; thus, involvement of family members and the patient's support system is essential in order to obtain collateral information as well as emotional support throughout the perioperative period. Finally, postoperative delirium can exacerbate an underlying psychotic disorder mandating aggressive treatment of both clinical conditions.

Medication Management

Similar to patients with established mood and anxiety disorders, the general principle of continuing home medications in the perioperative period also applies to patients with schizophrenia. In addition, postoperative confusion can be more pronounced in patients who discontinue antipsychotic medications prior to surgery.[16] The patient's regularly scheduled home medications, as well as any scheduled long-acting IM antipsychotic injections, should be continued. Examples of long-acting IM agents are the typical antipsychotics haloperidol and fluphenazine (given every 4 weeks and 2 weeks, respectively) and the atypical antipsychotic risperidone (given every 2 weeks).

There are a few medications to consider discontinuing in the immediate postoperative period, particularly if the patient is exhibiting or is at high risk for delirium. These are medications with anticholinergic properties such as benztropine or trihexyphenidyl that are often used to prevent extrapyramidal effects. These medications should be held for their potential deliriogenic properties.

Antipsychotic medications are divided in two classes: typical or first-generation, and atypical or second-generation antipsychotics.[11] Typical antipsychotics block histamine, α1-adrenergic, and muscarinic receptors, which can cause sedation, hypotension, and anticholinergic side effects. High-potency antipsychotics (such as haloperidol and fluphenazine) have less antihistamine, α1-adrenergic, and anticholinergic blockade compared with low-potency antipsychotic medications (such as chlorpromazine and thioridazine). In addition, typical antipsychotics block dopamine-D2 receptors with the high-potency agents more at risk for causing acute extrapyramidal symptoms, such as dystonias, rigidity, and akathisia.

Atypical antipsychotics have less potency to dopamine-D2 receptors. Thus, they have fewer extrapyramidal symptoms and, in general, have a better side effect profile than older typical antipsychotics. However, metabolic abnormalities such as weight gain, diabetes, and hyperlipidemia can occur, and all patients on these medications should be monitored.

In a prolonged NPO status, parenteral options are available as well as oral dissolving tablets (Table 17.2). Haloperidol is available in IM and IV formulations with the IV form used widely in the hospital setting for treatment of agitation and psychosis. It should be noted that the IV form is not approved by the FDA. Other IM preparations of the typical antipsychotics, chlorpromazine and thioridazine, are not recommended in the perioperative period due to their strong anticholinergic and hypotensive effects.

Short-acting IM preparations of the atypical antipsychotics are generally well tolerated. These are available for olanzapine, ziprasidone, and aripiprazole. These agents can be effective for the treatment of both underlying psychosis and agitation. As a precaution with IM olanzapine, concomitant lorazepam use should be avoided due to excess side effects, and be given at least 1 h after the olanzapine dose. Self-dissolving tablets for olanzapine, risperidone, and aripiprazole are quickly absorbed and are useful when patients are of NPO status. There is limited experience in the medically ill patient with the newer antipsychotic asenapine, which is given sublingually.

All patients on antipsychotics should be monitored for QTc prolongation, which can lead to dangerous arrhythmias such as torsades de pointes.[17] Discontinuation of antipsychotics is warranted if the QTc is greater than 500 ms.

Behavior Management

Understanding the patient's baseline functional level is key in helping clinicians distinguish chronic versus new psychosis during the perioperative period. A brief telephone consultation with the patient's established mental health provider team can be invaluable in managing the patient. Enlisting the family, and any members of the patient's mental health team, can facilitate this management and enhance postsurgical outcomes. Prompt follow-up with mental health providers in the discharge process is recommended for further observation and management of the psychotic disorder.

During the perioperative stay, patients with psychotic disorders can benefit from occupational therapy, supportive therapy, and daily reassurance from the medical team. Redirection to the medical issues at hand, decreasing overstimulation, and good sleep hygiene are important management techniques.

If the patient were to experience a breakthrough of psychosis, prompt consultation with a psychiatric team is essential for co-management. Emergency administration of a short-acting antipsychotic, placement in a safe setting (single occupancy room if possible), and use of a sitter for 1:1 observation are key measures. The actively psychotic patients can pose a danger to themselves (i.e., pulling out IV lines or catheters and contamination of the surgical wound site) and may necessitate physical restraints. Hospitals are obliged to have restraint protocols in place, starting with the least restrictive measure. Physical restraints are designed to provide adequate safety for both the patient and hospital staff.

For patients in an active psychotic state, supportive verbal therapy and reassurance are recommended, with a general nonconfrontational stance about delusions or beliefs systems. Gentle reassurance by the treatment team, employing a conciliatory communication style, is also recommended when acute hallucinations are present. These measures can assist the patient's impaired reality testing and promote a safe environment for both the patient and healthcare team. While violence is uncommon in schizophrenics, providers should always take appropriate safety precautions when the potential for escalating violence or aggressive behavior is perceived. In these situations, an urgent consultation with the psychiatric team should be sought.

THE PATIENT WITH CHEMICAL DEPENDENCY

General Considerations

Substance abuse disorders are commonly encountered in the hospital setting. It is estimated that at least 25% of hospitalized patients use alcohol, while approximately 30% of Americans use tobacco and 8% use illicit drugs.[18] Substance abuse is associated with significant morbidity and mortality. Careful preoperative care is needed, especially in patients using alcohol and sedatives. Providers should obtain a careful chemical dependence history and inquire about past hospitalization experiences to determine if any alcohol or drug withdrawal occurred as well as its severity and associated complications. Simple screening instruments such as the CAGE questionnaire (Table 17.3) can be used effectively to identify alcohol use disorders.[19] Laboratory tests such as urine and blood toxicology, liver function testing, gamma-glutamyl transpeptidase (GGT), basic metabolic panel, prothrombin time (PT), complete blood count including mean corpuscular volume (MCV), and carbohydrate-deficient transferrin (CDT) are used to identify substance use problems and possible organ damage secondary to alcohol and substance abuse.[20]

AWS is encountered in up to 25% of intensive care patients[21] and can present with a variety of signs and symptoms (Table 17.4). Manifestations of AWS typically occur within 24–48 h after consumption of the last alcoholic drink. Abrupt cessation of alcohol may cause potentially life-threatening complications such as delirium tremens (DTs) and withdrawal seizures. Attention should be given to the prevention and management of other alcohol-related complications such as Wernicke–Korsakoff encephalopathy, alcohol hallucinosis, depression, and malnutrition.

TABLE 17.3.   CAGE Questionnaire

C: Have you ever felt you should Cut down on your drinking?

A: Have people Annoyed you by criticizing your drinking?

G: Have you ever felt bad or Guilty about your drinking?

E: Have you ever had a drink first thing in the morning to steady your nerves or to get rid of a hangover (Eye opener)?

Scoring: Item responses on the CAGE are scored 0 or 1, with a higher score indicative of alcohol problems. A score of 2 or more is considered clinically significant.

Adapted from Stern TA, Herman JB. Alcoholism and alcohol abuse. In: *Massachusetts General Hospital Psychiatry Update and Board Preparation*, 2nd edition, pp. 73–84. New York: McGraw-Hill; 2004.

TABLE 17.4.   Chemical Dependency Signs and Symptoms of Intoxication and Withdrawal

	Intoxication	Withdrawal
Alcohol	• Inappropriate or aggressive behavior • Mood lability • Impaired judgment • Slurred speech • Incoordination • Unsteady gait and ataxia • Nystagmus • Impairment in attention and memory • Stupor or coma	• Autonomic hyperactivity (sweating, elevated heart rate and blood pressure) • Hand tremors • Insomnia • Nausea and vomiting • Transient visual, tactile, and auditory hallucinations or illusions • Psychomotor retardation • Anxiety • Grand mal seizures
Opioid	• Euphoria followed by apathy • Dysphoria • Psychomotor agitation or retardation • Impaired judgment • Impairment in attention and concentration • Decrease gastrointestinal motility • Pupil constriction (pinpoint pupils) • Sedation, drowsiness, or coma • Slurred speech	• Anxiety • Dysphoric mood • Nausea and vomiting • Abdominal pain • Muscle aches • Diarrhea • Insomnia • Fever • Mild hypertension • Tachycardia • Hot and cold flashes • Pupillary dilation • Piloerection • Sweating • Lacrimination or rhinorrhea • Yawning

Adapted from:
– Franklin JE, Levenson JL, Williams CS. Substance related disorders. In: *Textbook of Psychosomatic Medicine*, 1st edition, pp. 387–420. Washington, DC: American Psychiatry Publishing; 2005.
– Diagnostic Criteria from DSM-IV-TR. Washington, DC. American Psychiatric Association; 2000.

BZD withdrawal signs and symptoms are very similar to that of alcohol. Severe withdrawal symptoms and seizure activity may result in a life-threatening scenario requiring emergent treatment. The onset of withdrawal symptoms mainly depends on the elimination half-life of the drug. Alprazolam withdrawal symptoms occur within 1–2 days of last use, but longer-acting agents, such as diazepam, may be seen much later.

Management of opioid-abusing patients can be challenging in the perioperative period. High pain tolerance, drug-seeking behavior, apparent exaggeration of pain complaints, and possible comorbid personality traits might interfere with perioperative care.[22] Opioid withdrawal signs and symptoms are generally uncomfortable but not life threatening (Table 17.4). The onset of withdrawal symptoms during the perioperative period varies and depends on the drug's elimination half-life.

Cocaine cessation is usually associated with an uncomplicated withdrawal; however, the physiological effects of cocaine on multiple organs can have an impact on anesthetic management.

Medication Management

Early identification of patients with a history of alcohol use disorders is essential to prevent significant perioperative complications. Alcohol users who meet the criteria for alcohol abuse or dependence should be encouraged to seek abstinence with possible referral to alcohol abuse counseling.[23] Patients who abuse or are dependent on alcohol are at significant risk for withdrawal. Before elective surgery, patients may be referred to an addiction program for detoxification and rehabilitation.

BZDs are used as first-line agents for prevention and treatment of alcohol withdrawal and seizures.[24] However, medications are not always needed during alcohol detoxification for the dependent patient. The Clinical Institute Withdrawal Assessment for Alcohol—revised (CIWA-Ar)[25] (see Appendix) is a helpful scale that is used to objectively assess and quantify withdrawal symptoms. BZDs are then administered depending on the symptomatic indices of the scale (Table 17.5). Nonetheless, the use of a fixed benzodiazepine regimen can be used in any patient with history of alcohol withdrawal seizure, DTs, history of complicated withdrawal, and for patients with significant comorbid medical conditions.

Long-acting BZDs, such as chlordiazepoxide, have been effective in treating alcohol withdrawal; however, caution is required in patients with liver impairment. The use of short-acting BZDs, such as lorazepam, is preferred in patients with liver disease and in the elderly due to its method of metabolization.[23] Anticonvulsants, such as carbamazepine and valproic acid, may be needed for patients with a history of seizure. Nutritional supplements including thiamine, folic acid, and multivitamins should be given to all alcohol-dependent patients. Many authors recommend the use

---

TABLE 17.5. **Pharmacological Management of Alcohol Withdrawal**

1 Symptom-triggered medication regimens:
    When CIWA-Ar score >10, administer one of the following medications every 2–4 h:
    – Chlordiazepoxide 50–100 mg orally
    – Oxazepam 30–60 mg orally
    – Lorazepam 1–2 mg orally
    Repeat CIWA-Ar every 2–4 h after every dose
2 Structured medication regimens:
    Chlordiazepoxide 50 mg orally every 6 h for 4 doses
    Then 50 mg orally every 12 h for 24 h
    Then 25 mg orally every 12 h for 24 h and then discontinue
    Lorazepam 2 mg every 6 h for 4 doses
    Then 1 mg every 6 h × 8 doses
    Then0.5 mg every 6 h for 4 doses, and then discontinue

of parenteral thiamine for patients who are at high risk for Wernicke's encephalopathy and for those with poor nutrition.[24,26]

The mainstay treatment for AWS is BZDs, which should be administered around the clock if full-blown DTs are present, and are given intramuscularly or intravenously if the patient is unable to cooperate with PO administration. In this regard, lorazepam is the best choice as it can be administered intramuscularly or intravenously (chlordiazepoxide can only be given orally). Sedatives and alcohol dependence have similar intoxication/withdrawal symptoms and identical treatment regimens when managing the acute withdrawal period.

When encountering opioid abuse in the perioperative period, detoxification is often needed for heroin and prescription drug abusers. Methadone is the opioid commonly used to prevent withdrawal symptoms. However, methadone dosages of 60 mg/day or higher have been noted to prolong the QTc interval and therefore monitoring is required. Buprenorphine, a high-affinity partial agonist of the μ-opioid receptor, is approved by the U.S. FDA for treatment of opioid dependence. However, only providers with special training and who receive a waiver from the Center for Substance Abuse Treatment (CSAT) can prescribe this medication. Clonidine is helpful in symptomatic relief of opioid withdrawal; however, it is not FDA approved for this indication. Chronic pain patients with opioid dependence should be advised to take their prescribed pain medications before surgery.[22] Increasing the intraoperative and postoperative opioid dose is needed to compensate for tolerance. Recovering opioid-dependent patients who are on methadone maintenance should continue taking their usual methadone dose perioperatively. It is important to remember that these patients have developed tolerance and may need higher doses of opioids in the immediate postoperative period.

Behavior Management

Prevention, diagnosis, and treatment of AWS should be started early during the perioperative process in order to reduce the incidence of agitation and delirium that can be seen in acute alcohol withdrawal. In addition to general discomfort and delayed convalescence from surgery, patients with alcohol withdrawal typically require increased use of hospital personnel (i.e., 1:1 supervision) and are at increased risk of self-harm if the AWS is severe.

DTs will require intense hemodynamic monitoring and IV fluid support, and usually necessitate transfer to an intensive care unit setting. Physical restraints, according to the hospital's protocol, may be needed until the degree of acute delirium and agitation is under adequate control.

Patients with opioid abuse will require higher dosages of analgesics and should not be deprived of appropriate perioperative pain medications. Reassurance that the patient's pain level will be adequately treated is paramount for a favorable hospital course, with careful attention given to signs of opioid intoxication as well as withdrawal. However, as the patient's hospital course progresses, emphasis should be given to adequate chronic pain management and referral to outpatient chemical dependency programs.

THE PATIENT UNDERGOING ECT

General Considerations

ECT is used to treat patients with psychiatric conditions (i.e., depression, mania, catatonia) when medical treatment fails or is not acceptable due to side effects or risk.[27] The procedure itself entails delivery of an electrical current across unilateral or bilateral temporal positions to induce a generalized seizure. The patient receives anesthesia, a muscle relaxant with airway control, and continuous electrocardiographic monitoring. Patients typically undergo treatment three times a week for 2–4 successive weeks.[28] Most inpatient and outpatient centers require a preprocedure assessment by a physician. ECT is generally a safe procedure with two reported deaths per 100,000 treatments.[29] The procedure does carry associated morbidity and evaluation should focus on identifying patients who need intervention and management of acute or chronic conditions.

ECT can have significant effects on cardiac hemodynamics. As the electrical stimulus is applied, vagal tone increases causing bradycardia or even asystole. After the patient seizes, serum catecholamines rise, and heart rate and blood pressure can increase by up to 25% and 53%, respectively.[30] This increase in cardiac stress can occasionally cause significant arrhythmias or ischemia, but more commonly causes transient arrhythmias including asystole, premature ventricular or atrial contractions, transient severe hypertension, transient depressed ejection fraction, or chest pain without enzyme elevation.[31] There are few reported cardiac deaths that are related to ECT and most patients complete their course of ECT once the cardiac issue is managed. Intracerebral pressure increases during ECT, and though early retrospective studies of patients with brain tumors suggested that ECT leads to poor outcome, more recent though small prospective series have been more reassuring. Patients may suffer from memory dysfunction and disorientation after ECT. In some studies, these deficits can last beyond 6 months.[32] Some of this morbidity may be related to the type of electrode and/or shock used.

Initial evaluation should include a history, physical examination, and tailored laboratory testing. An ECG should be obtained in patients over 50 years of age. The assessment should focus on identifying chronic medical conditions, cardiac or neurological symptoms, pulmonary disease that may affect airway management, and history of anesthetic use.[31]

Patient-Focused Management

ECT is equivalent to a low-risk procedure as described in the clinical guideline for the perioperative management of patients undergoing noncardiac surgery written by the American College of Cardiology and American Heart Association. This guideline suggests that barring acute cardiac conditions, most patients can proceed to a low-risk procedure without further testing (see Chapter 9).[33] However, given the increased cardiac stress from hypertension and tachycardia, patients with coronary artery disease, aortic stenosis, aortic or intracerebral aneurysms, and congestive heart failure should be managed carefully (see section on "Medication Management"). Patients with acute cardiac conditions, severe aortic stenosis, or with implantable cardiac defibrillators should be evaluated by a cardiologist before proceeding with ECT.

The American Psychiatric Association (APA) lists pregnancy as a potential indication for ECT, and most patients can undergo treatment safely with close monitoring of the patient and fetus.[27,34] Evaluation and consent of these patients should involve an obstetrician and anesthesiologist as there are rare reports of fetal and maternal complications.

Patients with a history of stroke or intracranial vascular abnormalities need careful periprocedural control of blood pressure and heart rate. Based on older data, most patients can proceed with ECT 1 month after a stroke.[35] Patients with intracranial tumors or vascular lesions should be evaluated by a neurosurgeon before proceeding because the literature on these groups of patients is limited.[27]

Elderly patients are at risk for falls post-ECT and need to be watched carefully to maintain their safety with ambulation. Increased age may also be a risk factor for cognitive deficits in the posttreatment period.[36]

Medication Management

The medicine consultant should defer decisions about periprocedural seizure medication to a neurologist. The psychiatry team should manage all psychiatric medications and treatment of interictal delirium should it develop. With respect to prophylactic medication, the use of beta-blockers is controversial. Some data suggest that this class of medication may shorten the seizure or increase the risk of asystole.[37] Other more recent studies do not confirm these side effects, suggesting that short-acting beta-blockers can be used in high-risk patients to minimize cardiac stress.[38] Calcium channel blockers, nitrates, and other antihypertensive medications can lower blood pressure as well as heart rate. Any recommendation for new periprocedure cardiac medications should be made in consultation with the anesthesiologist who will be managing the patient acutely.

For diabetic patients, oral hypoglycemic agents should be held on the morning of ECT treatment until they are cleared to eat safely. Patients on long-acting insulin should receive at least half of their morning dose. If possible, the consultant should advocate for morning ECT to allow these patients to resume their diabetes regimen promptly. Patients with cardiac disease including arrhythmias, ischemic heart disease, and hypertension should continue on their chronic medications, including beta-blockers. Patients on warfarin can continue as long as the INR is less than 3.5. Theophylline should be tapered in patients with asthma given the risk of status epilepticus. Other chronic medications for asthma including inhaled bronchodilators and steroids should be continued.

Patients may complain of headache post-ECT. Nonsteroidal anti-inflammatory drugs (NSAIDs) or intranasal sumatriptan have been found to be useful in this setting.[39,40]

REFERENCES

1. Desan PH, Powsner S. Assessment and management of patients with psychiatric disorders. *Crit Care Med.* 2004;32:S166–S173.
2. Ziring B. Issues in the perioperative care of the patient with psychiatric illness. *Med Clin North Am.* 1993;77:443–452.
3. Powers PS, Cruse CW, Daniels S, Stevens B. Posttraumatic stress disorder in patients with burns. *J Burn Care Rehabil.* 1994;15:147–153.
4. Doerfler LA, Pbert L, DeCosimo D. Symptoms of posttraumatic stress disorder following myocardial infarction and coronary artery bypass surgery. *Gen Hosp Psychiatry.* 1994;16:193–199.
5. Cordova MJ, Studts JL, Hann DM, Jacobsen PB, Andrykowski MA. Symptom structure of PTSD following breast cancer. *J Trauma Stress.* 2000;13:301–319.
6. Kapa S, Rotondi-Trevisan D, Mariano Z, et al. Psychopathology in patients with ICDs over time: results of a prospective study. *Pacing Clin Electrophysiol.* 2010;33:198–208.
7. Kong VKF, Irwin MG. Gabapentin: a multimodal perioperative drug? *Br J Anaesth.* 2007;99:775–786.
8. Kshettry VR, Carole LF, Henly SJ, Sendelbach S, Kummer B. Complementary alternative medical therapies for heart surgery patients: feasibility, safety, and impact. *Ann Thorac Surg.* 2006;81:201–205.
9. Olfson M, Marcus SC. National patterns in antidepressant medication treatment. *Arch Gen Psychiatry.* 2009;66:848–856.
10. Turner MS, May DB, Arthur RR, Xiong GL. Clinical impact of selective serotonin reuptake inhibitors therapy with bleeding risks. *J Intern Med.* 2007;261:205–213.
11. Huyse FJ, Touw DJ, van Schijndel RS, de Lange JJ, Slaets JPJ. Psychotropic drugs and the perioperative period: a proposal for a guideline in elective surgery. *Psychosomatics.* 2006;47:8–22.
12. Cohen HW, Gibson G, Alderman MH. Excess risk of myocardial infarction in patients treated with antidepressant medications: association with use of tricyclic agents. *Am J Med.* 2000;108:2–8.
13. Ang-Lee MK, Moss J, Yuan CS. Herbal medicines and perioperative care. *JAMA.* 2001;286:208–216.
14. Lehman AF, Lieberman JA, Dixon LB, et al. Practice guideline for the treatment of patients with schizophrenia, second edition. *Am J Psychiatry.* 2004;161:1–56.
15. Kudoh A. Perioperative management for chronic schizophrenic patients. *Anesth Analg.* 2005;101:1867–1872.
16. Kudoh A, Katagai H, Takase H, Takazawa T. Effect of preoperative discontinuation of antipsychotics in schizophrenic patients on outcome during and after anaesthesia. *Eur J Anaesthesiol.* 2004;21:414–416.
17. Haddad PM, Anderson IM. Antipsychotic-related QTc prolongation, torsade de pointes and sudden death. *Drugs.* 2002;62:1649–1671.
18. Colpe LJ, Barker PR, Karg RS, et al. The national survey on drug use and health mental health surveillance study: calibration study design and field procedures. *Int J Methods Psychiatr Res.* 2010;19(Suppl 1):36–48.
19. Ewing JA. Screening for alcoholism using CAGE. Cut down, annoyed, guilty, eye opener. *JAMA.* 1998;280:1904–1905.
20. Kleber HD, Weiss RD, Anton RF, Jr., et al. Treatment of patients with substance use disorders, second edition. American Psychiatric Association. *Am J Psychiatry.* 2007;164:5–123.
21. Spies CD, Rommelspacher H. Alcohol withdrawal in the surgical patient: prevention and treatment. *Anesth Analg.* 1999;88:946–954.
22. Mitra S, Sinatra RS. Perioperative management of acute pain in the opioid-dependent patient. *Anesthesiology.* 2004;101:212–227.
23. Gordon AJ, Olstein J, Conigliaro J. Identification and treatment of alcohol use disorders in the perioperative period. *Postgrad Med.* 2006;119:46–55.
24. McKeon A, Frye MA, Delanty N. The alcohol withdrawal syndrome. *J Neurol Neurosurg Psychiatry.* 2008;79:854–862.
25. Busto UE, Sykora K, Sellers EM. A clinical scale to assess benzodiazepine withdrawal. *J Clin Psychopharmacol.* 1989;9:412–416.

26. Kopelman MD, Thomson AD, Guerrini I, Marshall EJ. The Korsakoff syndrome: clinical aspects, psychology and treatment. *Alcohol Alcohol.* 2009;44:148–154.
27. *The Practice of Electroconvulsive Therapy: Recommendations for Treatment, Training, and Privileging.* A Task Force Report of the American Psychiatric Association. Weiner R, Chair. 2nd edition, Washington, DC: American Psychiatric Association; 2001.
28. Lisanby SH. Electroconvulsive therapy for depression. *N Engl J Med.* 2007;357:1939–1945.
29. Shiwach RS, Reid WH, Carmody TJ. An analysis of reported deaths following electroconvulsive therapy in Texas, 1993–1998. *Psychiatr Serv.* 2001;52:1095–1097.
30. Takada JY, Solimene MC, Da Luz PL, et al. Assessment of the cardiovascular effects of electroconvulsive therapy in individuals older than 50 years. *Braz J Med Biol Res.* 2005;38:1349–1357.
31. Tess AV, Smetana GW. Medical evaluation of patients undergoing electroconvulsive therapy. *N Engl J Med.* 2009;360:1437–1444.
32. Rose D, Fleischmann P, Wykes T, Leese M, Bindman J. Patients' perspectives on electroconvulsive therapy: systematic review. *BMJ.* 2003;326:1363.
33. Fleisher LA, Beckman JA, Brown KA, et al. ACC/AHA 2007 Guidelines on perioperative cardiovascular evaluation and care for noncardiac surgery: a report of the American College of Cardiology/American Heart Association Task Force on Practice Guidelines (Writing Committee to Revise the 2002 Guidelines on Perioperative Cardiovascular Evaluation for Noncardiac Surgery). *Circulation.* 2007;116:e418–e499.
34. Miller LJ. Use of electroconvulsive therapy during pregnancy. *Hosp Community Psychiatry.* 1994;45:444–450.
35. Martin M, Figiel G, Mattingly G, Zorumski CF, Jarvis MR. ECT-induced interictal delirium in patients with a history of a CVA. *J Geriatr Psychiatry Neurol.* 1992;5:149–155.
36. Cattan RA, Barry PP, Mead G, Reefe WE, Gay A, Silverman M. Electroconvulsive therapy in octogenarians. *J Am Geriatr Soc.* 1990;38:753–758.
37. van den Broek WW, Leentjens AF, Mulder PG, Kusuma A, Bruijn JA. Low-dose esmolol bolus reduces seizure duration during electroconvulsive therapy: a double-blind, placebo-controlled study. *Br J Anaesth.* 1999;83:271–274.
38. Howie MB, Hiestand DC, Zvara DA, Kim PY, McSweeney TD, Coffman JA. Defining the dose range for esmolol used in electroconvulsive therapy hemodynamic attenuation. *Anesth Analg.* 1992;75:805–810.
39. Leung M, Hollander Y, Brown GR. Pretreatment with ibuprofen to prevent electroconvulsive therapy-induced headache. *J Clin Psychiatry.* 2003;64:551–553.
40. Markowitz JS, Kellner CH, DeVane CL, et al. Intranasal sumatriptan in post-ECT headache: results of an open-label trial. *J ECT.* 2001;17:280–283.

APPENDIX

Clinical Institute Withdrawal Assessment of Alcohol Scale, Revised (CIWA-Ar)

Patient: _____

Date: _____ Time: _____

Pulse or heart rate, taken for one minute: _____

Blood pressure: _____

Nausea and Vomiting

Ask "Do you feel sick to your stomach? Have you vomited?"

0 no nausea and no vomiting

1 mild nausea with no vomiting

2

3

4 intermittent nausea with dry heaves

5

6

7 constant nausea, frequent dry heaves and vomiting

Tactile Disturbances

Ask "Have you any itching, pins and needles sensations, any burning, any numbness, or do you feel bugs crawling on or under your skin?"

0 none
1 very mild itching, pins and needles, burning or numbness
2 mild itching, pins and needles, burning or numbness
3 moderate itching, pins and needles, burning or numbness
4 moderately severe hallucinations
5 severe hallucinations
6 extremely severe hallucinations
7 continuous hallucinations

Tremor

Ask the patient to extend arms with fingers spread apart.

0 no tremor
1 not visible, but can be felt fingertip to fingertip
2
3
4 moderate, with patient's arms extended
5
6
7 severe, even with arms not extended

Auditory Disturbances

Ask "Are you more aware of sounds around you? Are they harsh? Do they frighten you? Are you hearing anything that is disturbing to you? Are you hearing things you know are not there?"

0 not present
1 very mild harshness or ability to frighten
2 mild harshness or ability to frighten
3 moderate harshness or ability to frighten
4 moderately severe hallucinations
5 severe hallucinations
6 extremely severe hallucinations
7 continuous hallucinations

Paroxysmal Sweats

0 no sweat visible
1 barely perceptible sweating, palms moist
2
3
4 beads of sweat obvious on forehead

5
6
7 drenching sweats

Visual Disturbances

Ask "Does the light appear to be too bright? Is its color different? Does it hurt your eyes? Are you seeing anything that is disturbing to you? Are you seeing things you know are not there?"

0 not present
1 very mild sensitivity
2 mild sensitivity
3 moderate sensitivity
4 moderately severe hallucinations
5 severe hallucinations
6 extremely severe hallucinations
7 continuous hallucinations

Anxiety

Ask "Do you feel nervous?"

0 no anxiety, at ease
1 mild anxious
2
3
4 moderately anxious, or guarded, so anxiety is inferred
5
6
7 equivalent to acute panic states as seen in severe delirium or acute schizophrenic reactions

Headache, Fullness in Head

Ask "Does your head feel different? Does it feel like there is a band around your head?" Do not rate for dizziness or lightheadedness. Otherwise, rate severity.

0 not present
1 very mild
2 mild
3 moderate
4 moderately severe
5 severe
6 very severe
7 extremely severe

Agitation

0 normal activity
1 somewhat more than normal activity
2
3

4 moderately fidgety and restless
5
6
7 paces back and forth during most of the interview, or constantly thrashes about

Orientation and Clouding of Sensorium

Ask "What day is this? Where are you? Who am I?"

0 oriented and can do serial additions
1 cannot do serial additions or is uncertain about date
2 disoriented for date by no more than 2 calendar days
3 disoriented for date by more than 2 calendar days
4 disoriented for place/or person

Total CIWA-Ar Score _____
Rater's Initials _____
Maximum Possible Score 67
CIWA-Ar: Clinical institute withdrawal assessment for alcohol—revised

Adapted from Franklin JE, Leveson JL, Williams CS. Substance related disorders. In: *Textbook of Psychosomatic Medicine*, 1st edition, pp. 387–420. Washington, DC: American Psychiatry Publishing; 2005.

CHAPTER 18

THE PREGNANT SURGICAL PATIENT

Michael P. Carson

EPIDEMIOLOGY

Frequency and Types of Nonobstetric Surgery

Nonobstetric surgery is necessary in approximately 1/500 pregnancies, and healthy pregnant women generally have surgical outcomes similar to nonpregnant women. While surgery has the potential to increase the risk of fetal complications including miscarriage and preterm labor, one should not discount the obvious benefits to the patient and her fetus, or the lack of any data showing an increased risk of congenital anomalies in women who had surgery during early pregnancy.[1-4] A case-control study matched 2565 women who underwent incidental surgery during pregnancy to a pregnant female cohort who did not have surgery. No difference existed in the rate of congenital anomalies.[4]

Appendectomy and cholecystectomy are common surgical procedures that will be necessary during pregnancy. Appendectomy is the most common nonobstetric surgical procedure with rates varying from 1 to 2 per 2000 pregnancies, followed by cholecystectomy (1–6 per 10,000 pregnancies).[5,6] Appendicitis is a surgical emergency, and surgery cannot be delayed due to pregnancy. Similarly, delaying cholecystectomy can increase the risk of an open procedure.

A series of 9793 appendectomies performed between 1974 and 2000 identified 94 done in pregnant women (rate of 0.2% of all pregnancies). In this series, there were no maternal deaths, infant mortality was 3.2% ($n = 3$), and the reported postoperative spontaneous abortion rate was 13%. Although the spontaneous abortion rate seems unusually high, it may be related to the fact that 15% were complicated by perforation.[7]

HISTORY

During the first two trimesters, the position of the appendix is generally the same as in the nonpregnant population, so presentation of this disease can be

Perioperative Medicine: Medical Consultation and Co-Management, First Edition.
Edited by Amir K. Jaffer and Paul J. Grant.
© 2012 Wiley-Blackwell. Published 2012 by John Wiley & Sons, Inc.

straightforward. However, the appendix can be displaced into the right upper quadrant during the third trimester, tenderness may be difficult to localize, and the pain may be in the right upper quadrant. The presentation of gallstones and/or gallstone pancreatitis is not altered by pregnancy. The hormonal changes and increased bile stasis in the gallbladder due to pregnancy-induced decrease in smooth muscle tone are the factors that increase the risk for gallstones during pregnancy.

The preoperative evaluation should inquire about a personal or family history of bleeding and anesthesia-related complications such as malignant hyperthermia. Additionally, appropriate blood testing of organ function should be obtained if there are known or suspected abnormalities.

PHYSICAL EXAM AND NORMAL PHYSIOLOGICAL CHANGES OF PREGNANCY

It is helpful to recognize that most of the normal physiological changes in pregnancy are in the 50% range when compared with the nonpregnant patient (i.e., cardiac output, glomerular filtration rate [GFR]), and most decreases are due to something else being increased. For example, the increase in tidal volume causes a drop in the pCO_2, and the increase in blood volume causes the dilutional drop in hemoglobin and serum albumin level. However, hepatic blood flow and metabolism of medications are not significantly altered.[8] As a reference, normal laboratory values are listed in Table 18.1.

Cardiovascular Physiology

Cardiac output and stroke volume increase by 50% and peak at about 16 weeks' gestation. Probably the most important change of which one should be aware is that plasma volume increases to 50% above the nonpregnant state with the peak occurring at 28–32 weeks. It is at this gestational age when undiagnosed cardiac disorders such as mitral stenosis may present with heart failure or atrial fibrillation.[9] Therefore, any murmur not consistent with the normal pulmonary arterial flow murmur of pregnancy (see below) should be evaluated with an echocardiogram to exclude severe mitral or aortic stenosis. Regurgitant valve lesions do not pose as severe a risk for the pregnant patient.

Due to the fact that plasma volume increases to an extent greater than the normal increase in red blood cell mass, there is a physiologic (dilutional) anemia of pregnancy. The lowest hemoglobins (10–11 g/dL) are seen between 30 and 34 weeks of gestation. Systolic blood pressure will decrease by 10–20 mm Hg and diastolic blood pressure by 10 mm Hg, reaching a nadir about 20 weeks of gestation. The blood pressure then rises to prepregnancy levels by late pregnancy. The heart rate (HR) increases by 10% and plateaus at about 32 weeks of gestation. The HR may be higher when measured in the left lateral decubitus position.[10]

Cardiovascular Physical Exam

During pregnancy, the jugular venous pressure (JVP) remains normal, while the point of maximal impulse (PMI) will shift leftward and cephalad. Preexisting cardiac

TABLE 18.1. Laboratory Changes in Pregnancy

Parameter	Effect
Albumin and total protein	Decrease by 1 mg/dL: dilutional effect (albumin ~3.0, total protein ~6.0)
Alkaline phosphatase	Increases due to output by the placenta
Bicarbonate (serum)	Decreases to about 20 mEq; decreased ability to buffer acid loads; other electrolyte levels should be normal
Blood urea nitrogen	Should be <14 mg/dL
C-reactive protein	Normally elevated; not useful during pregnancy
Creatinine	Should be <0.8 mg/dL, mean is 0.5 mg/dL
Creatinine clearance	Increases by 50% to about 150 cc/min
Creatinine kinase-myocardial	May be elevated after cesarean section. The MB fraction makes up 6% of the total enzyme from the uterus and placenta
D-dimer	Increased false-positive rate during pregnancy; however, a negative value may be useful (similar to the nonpregnant population)
Erythrocyte sedimentation rate	Normally elevated; not useful during pregnancy
Fibrinogen	Should be high-normal range to elevated
Glomerular filtration rate	50% increase
Hemoglobin	Decreases to 10–12 g/dL, dilutional effect
Leukocyte count	Slight increase; mean 8–10 k/mm^3 and up to 14 k/mm^3 after delivery
Partial pressure of carbon dioxide (pCO$_2$)	Decreases to 28–32 mm Hg as a result of normal hyperventilation
pH	Mildly alkalotic, approximately 7.44
Platelets	No change
Partial pressure of oxygen (pO$_2$)	Increases slightly due to hyperventilation
Thyroid labs (thyroid-stimulating hormone [TSH], free T4, free T3)	No change; normal TSH values during pregnancy are lower than prepregnancy, but still in the normal range; free T4 may be elevated during the first trimester in 40% of women with hyperemesis gravidarum
Liver transaminases (AST/ALT) and bilirubin	No change
Urine protein—24-h collection	Up to 300 mg is normal

AST, aspartate aminotransferase; ALT, alanine aminotransferase.

murmurs may increase in intensity throughout pregnancy due to the increase in blood volume, and diastolic murmurs always warrant further evaluation. The most significant finding is that 96% of women will develop a grade I–II early systolic murmur over the pulmonary and tricuspid areas generated by rapid blood flow through the pulmonary artery. This pulmonary arterial flow murmur will become softer with inspiration (ask her to take a deep breath and hold it as you listen) as the chest wall and stethoscope move away from the source of the murmur. A nonsustained S3 gallop is reported to be a normal finding, but we have not found it to be common.

A sustained third or fourth heart sound, however, warrants further evaluation. About one-third of women will develop lower extremity edema during pregnancy as a normal variant. If the onset of the edema is sudden and/or increasing, evaluation for preeclampsia and/or venous thromboembolism should be considered.

Pulmonary Physiology

There is a progesterone-mediated increase in tidal volume (about 40–50%), without an increase in respiratory rate, that causes a respiratory alkalosis during normal pregnancy (normal pCO_2 is 28–32 mm H_2O). Spirometry, particularly the forced expiratory volume in 1 s (FEV_1), does not change, but there might be a slight drop in functional residual capacity (FRC) caused by diaphragmatic limitation by the gravid uterus. The FRC may decrease up to 70% when a pregnant woman is supine resulting in a lower oxygen reserve prior to the induction of anesthesia, so supplemental oxygen should be administered at that time. As in nonpregnant patients, preoperative pulmonary function testing is unlikely to alter management for a patient with an urgent surgical issue.

Renal Physiology

GFR increases by 50% over the nonpregnant level and contributes to more rapid clearance of some medications. Normal 24-h urine protein excretion is up to 300 mg, where only 150 mg is acceptable for nonpregnant women.[11] The kidneys compensate for the respiratory alkalosis and the normal serum bicarbonate is about 20 mEq/L.

TESTING

Diagnosis of Surgical Issues during Pregnancy

A retrospective case series reported that magnetic resonance imaging (MRI) was positive in 14/14 patients with confirmed appendicitis, while preoperative ultrasound was positive in 5/14.[12] This suggests that MRI can aid clinicians in making the sometimes challenging diagnosis of appendicitis during pregnancy. One study found that an MRI was positive in 4/4 patients with appendicitis, negative in 41/41 without it, and inconclusive in 3, yielding an overall sensitivity, specificity, negative predictive value, and accuracy for MRI of 100%, 93.6%, 100%, and 94.0%, respectively.[13] A case series of 13 women found that an abdominal computed tomography (CT) scan after inconclusive ultrasound imaging was associated with an 8% rate of negative appendectomies compared with 54% in women with no imaging ($n = 13$), and 36% among women who only had an ultrasound ($n = 55$).[14] Therefore, if additional imaging is desired, and an ultrasound is not diagnostic, we recommend an abdominal MRI as the next best study. If that is not conclusive, then an abdominal CT has been shown (in a small series) to add useful clinical information.

When the diagnosis of a cystic duct stone remains unclear after imaging with ultrasound, a hepatobiliary iminodiacetic acid (HIDA) scan is a reasonable next step. As listed in Table 18.2, one could theoretically obtain 33 HIDA scans before

TABLE 18.2.   Estimated Fetal Radiation Exposure Related to Maternal Radiological Studies

Study	Fetal exposure (rads)	Permissible in pregnancy
Radiation exposure during transcontinental flight	0.015[48]	333
Chest radiograph (CXR) single (with abdomen shielding)	0.00007[49,50]	Up to 71,429
V/Q scan	0.02–0.05[43]	100
HIDA	0.15[50]	33
ERCP	0.310[51]	16
CT head	<0.013	385
CT chest first trimester	0.002[52]	2500
CT chest helical third trimester	0.013[52]	385
CT abdomen	~2.0	2
Arteriogram (pulmonary/coronary) via femoral vessels	0.2–0.4[53]	12
Arteriogram (pulmonary/coronary) via brachial vessels	0.05[53]	100
MRI	Appears to have no adverse effect on the fetus[54,55]	

The upper limit of recommended fetal exposure is 5.0 rads (5000 mrad). Physicians and patients find this information useful to put the benefits of the test into proper perspective.
ECRP, endoscopic retrograde cholangiopancreatography.

reaching the upper limit of fetal radiation exposure felt to be within safe limits. These data give perspective to patients and physicians and allow them to make an appropriate benefit/risk assessment.

Preoperative Evaluation and Testing to Stratify Risk

Cardiac Testing   An echocardiogram should be considered if a patient has a sustained gallop, or an undiagnosed murmur suggesting a stenotic lesion, significant regurgitation, or hypertrophic cardiomyopathy. Preoperative cardiac stress testing is not likely to be indicated or useful. The approach is the same as for nonpregnant patients utilizing the American College of Cardiology/American Heart Association (ACC/AHA) guidelines, which generally do not recommend preoperative stress testing in low- or moderate-risk patients.[15] The randomized Coronary Artery Revascularization Prophylaxis (CARP) trial found that revascularization in high-risk patients before high-risk vascular procedures did not decrease mortality.[16] While listed as "elective," surgery during pregnancy is generally performed for urgent conditions, so it is unlikely that it can be delayed. Similarly, it is unlikely that cardiac stress testing results will alter the care plan. If it is determined that a preoperative stress test is indicated, perhaps in a patient who recently had a myocardial infarction, stress echocardiography is the preferred study as there is no radiation exposure.

Nuclear cardiac stress testing may be obtained if stress echocardiography is unavailable. Cardiac catheterization should only be performed if the stress test results are worrisome (Table 18.2).

Pulmonary Testing This may be indicated for patients with undiagnosed lung disease, but is not likely to offer useful information regarding the perioperative management of women whose disease is appropriately treated.

Use of Low-Dose Aspirin Women with a history of multiple pregnancy losses may be taking low-dose aspirin. The Collaborative Low-dose Aspirin Study in Pregnancy (CLASP) trial randomized 9364 pregnant women to 81 mg aspirin or placebo. Aspirin was not associated with an increase in bleeding during preparation for epidural anesthesia, but there was a slight increase in blood transfusions after delivery.[17]

Diagnostic Imaging Clinical diagnosis without appropriate radiological confirmation may lead to inappropriate treatment. Therefore, it is important to educate patients about the safety of radiographic studies and the importance of obtaining adequate clinical information in making treatment decisions. Fetal radiation exposure and data on the number of studies permissible during pregnancy are listed in Table 18.2. The number of "permissible" studies is valuable information that can put the patient, and the treating physician, at ease regarding these evaluations. Obtain chest radiographs, ventilation/perfusion (V/Q) lung scans, CT angiography, MRI studies, fluoroscopic procedures, and other tests as you would in a nonpregnant patient if the test result will clearly affect the treatment plan and benefit the patient. Most common radiographic investigations confer much less than the acceptable limit of 5.0 rads (5000 mrad) of fetal radiation exposure, cumulative over the course of the pregnancy. For reference, the typical fetal radiation exposure during a 2-h flight is 0.015 mrad versus 0.0007 with a maternal chest X-ray. According to the Centers for Disease Control (CDC), exposures less than 5.0 rads do not carry any risk of fetal demise, nor do they increase the risk that the child exposed in utero will develop cancer later in life.[18]

The intravenous iodinated contrast agents iobitridol and iohexol did not cross the placenta of pregnant rabbits in doses similar to those used for human angiography, and should be used when indicated during pregnancy or in breast-feeding mothers.[19,20] It is important to remember that the avoidance of indicated testing can lead to improper clinical decision making based on inadequate data.

PREDICTING RISK

Congenital Anomalies

The data are conflicting, but the overriding factor is realizing that a healthy fetus depends on a healthy mother. A study of 5405 operations in a Swedish population of 720,000 pregnant women (operation rate, 0.75%) found that the incidence of congenital malformations and stillbirths was not increased in the offspring of women who underwent surgery.[21] Additionally, a case-control study identified 694 mothers of infants with neural tube defects and 2984 controls. The odds ratio (OR) of a neural tube defect after the first trimester exposure to anesthesia was not significantly different (OR 1.7, confidence interval [CI]: 0.8–3.3). While this study found that a strong association existed between the first trimester anesthesia exposure and the combination of hydrocephalus *and* an eye defect (OR 39.6, CI: 7.5–209.2), this event is very rare, and still must be balanced against the consequences of delaying or not performing the surgery.[22] Barbiturates, ketamine, and benzodiazepines have not been associated with teratogenesis in humans.[23,24] No evidence supports a teratogenic risk when any local anesthetics, such as procaine, lidocaine, or bupivacaine, are used in humans.[24] One study reported an association between use of nitrous oxide during the first trimester and an increased incidence of spontaneous abortion; however, a larger study did not confirm this.[3,21]

Obstetric Complications (Preterm Labor/Loss)

The data regarding the perioperative risk of preterm labor/loss are not clear due to conflicting findings of case series. One study found that surgery early in pregnancy significantly increased the rate of spontaneous abortion compared with a control group that did not have surgery, another study did not find any spontaneous abortions among a cohort of 22 women with cholelithiasis, and a third reported no difference in the mean Apgar scores among neonates born subsequent to cholecystectomy compared with neonates born to patients in whom cholecystectomy was deferred.[3,25] While another series found surgery to be associated with an increased risk of preterm labor, there was no benefit to the prophylactic use of tocolytic agents.[26]

Some concern was raised by a reported increased risk of spontaneous fetal loss in those undergoing surgery with general anesthesia in the first or second trimester. This increased risk was most notable after gynecologic procedures (estimated relative risk [RR] 2.0), but also following procedures anatomically remote from the pelvis (estimated RR 1.54). It is unclear which factors account for the observed increase in fetal risk, but again, the consequences of *not* performing the procedure must be considered.[4] Among 5405 operations in a Swedish population of 720,000 pregnant women, the incidence of low- and very low-birth-weight infants was increased due to prematurity and intrauterine growth restriction. The incidence of infants that were born alive but died within 7 days was also increased. No specific types of anesthesia or operations were associated with increased risk of adverse reproductive outcomes.[21]

Terbutaline is often used as a tocolytic agent when a woman has preterm contractions. It has been associated with noncardiogenic pulmonary edema and atrial fibrillation[27]; therefore, using it to treat contractions without actual cervical change should be discouraged.

Maternal Complications

The primary cause for perioperative maternal mortality has shifted from complications of regional anesthesia to airway complications such as failed intubation.[14,28,29] While rare, loss of the maternal airway is the most common anesthesia-related cause of maternal death and the fifth or sixth most common cause of overall maternal mortality, depending on the study. During a 14-year study, there were 135 maternal deaths in 822,591 hospital admissions for delivery, and anesthesia-related complications were the sixth most common cause accounting for 5.2% of the deaths.[28,30] Factors that complicate airway management in normal pregnancy include edema of the hypopharynx and vocal cords, hypervascularity of the airway leading to bleeding with relatively minor trauma, and cephalad migration of the endotracheal tube caused by mechanical pressure from the gravid uterus.[31] Perioperative supplemental oxygen should be administered because while lung mechanics and airway flow are not altered during pregnancy, the FRC can be reduced by 70% when a woman is supine, resulting in less oxygen reserve during periods of apnea, as compared with the nonpregnant state. For these reasons, it is best to enlist the services of an anesthesiologist with training in obstetric anesthesia whenever possible.

Other risks for maternal complications include venous thromboembolism due to reduced venous flow and increased clotting factors, aspiration due to decreased gastric motility (during labor) and reduced competence of the gastroesophageal sphincter, and urinary tract infection (UTI)—especially with catheterization due to dilatation of the urinary collecting system.

Approach to Prescribing

Several principles should guide the selection of medications during pregnancy. When a drug is indicated, consider the consequences if you do *not* administer the medication. This perspective can be invaluable in providing the clinician and the patient with the proper perception. Fetal well-being is dependent on maternal well-being. Overly cautious restriction of medications in pregnancy could lead to a decline in maternal health, and thereby put the fetus at risk. Medications that have been used for long periods of time and proven to be safe to the fetus should be used over newer medications. Avoid underdosing in an effort to "minimize fetal exposure" because the increased maternal renal clearance and/or volume of distribution may necessitate higher doses or more frequent administration. With few exceptions, the *absolute* risk to the fetus of prescribing medications to pregnant women is mostly unknown, but the maternal benefits of most medications are obvious. The U.S. Food and Drug Administration (FDA) categorization system is oversimplified. A reference text such as *Drugs in Pregnancy and Lactation* by Briggs et al.[32] may prove to be more helpful for information on medication teratogenicity.

MINIMIZING RISK

Surgical Technique: Laparoscopy versus Laparotomy

Surgical experience should be the guiding force in the decision as to which surgical approach is best for an individual patient. Preterm delivery has been reported as a complication of pancreatitis in 26% of cases, which seems to justify performing a cholecystectomy to prevent another case of gallstone pancreatitis.[33] The Society of American Gastrointestinal Endoscopic Surgeons (SAGES) have published guidelines for laparoscopic surgery during pregnancy and indicate that a laparoscopic approach is preferred to decrease both maternal risk (decreased blood loss, less analgesic use) and fetal risk (preterm labor) when compared with open laparotomy.[1,34]

Laparotomy in the pregnant patient leads to a higher risk of preterm labor than laparoscopy.[5] Both laparoscopy and laparotomy are associated with an increased risk of delivering a fetus <2500 g, preterm delivery (<37 weeks), and growth restriction when compared with the general population. The explanation for these morbidities remains unclear.[1] During pregnancy, laparoscopy results in lower estimated blood loss, less analgesic use, and less need for tocolytics compared with open laparotomy.[20,35] A case series of 16 women who underwent laparoscopic cholecystectomy during pregnancy found that 9 of 11 whose surgery was performed more than 5 weeks after the onset of symptoms had recurrent attacks requiring 15 hospital admissions and 4 visits to the emergency department. Three of four women whose surgery was delayed until the third trimester developed premature contractions that were treated with tocolytics.[36] Delay of surgical therapy is associated with longer operative times, higher conversion rates to open cholecystectomy, and prolonged hospitalization.[37] A prospective, randomized trial compared early cholecystectomy with delayed cholecystectomy in pregnant patients with acute cholecystitis. In the delayed group, 13% of patients required emergent surgery within 90 days due to cholangitis, empyema, or peritonitis. Another 15% of patients developed acute recurrent symptoms within the 90-day period.[38]

Before considering the complications of an intervention, we must consider the consequences of *withholding* an indicated treatment such as surgery for cholecystitis. Limited data obtained from the case series of open cholecystectomy during pregnancy includes 0.1% maternal mortality, 5% fetal death, and 7% preterm labor and preterm delivery. Older case series of cholecystitis and cholecystectomy reported higher fetal mortality, but more recent studies found rates of 5–10%. Overall, the risk of morbidity and mortality is likely related to the severity of pancreatitis rather than the procedure to prevent another episode.[5,39]

Timing of Surgery

It is important not to unnecessarily delay surgery. As stated before, a healthy fetus depends on a healthy mother; thus, it is reasonable to proceed if clinical judgment points toward the benefits of intervention outweighing the potential risks to the fetus. Consider the clear benefits of a procedure (exclusion of appendicitis, avoidance of rupture/sepsis, decreasing the risk of recurrent pancreatitis, decreasing the risk of a more complicated procedure) before considering the *potential*, theoretical, and less likely issues such as an obstetric complication or future lawsuit. Overall, the risk of perioperative complications is dictated by the clinical circumstances and patient demographics, and there are no data to suggest that pregnancy alters those risks.

The ideal time for semi-elective surgery is the second trimester when possible. While a study found an association among the first trimester anesthesia, neural tube defects, and hydrocephalus, the risks to the mother and fetus of *not* doing a procedure must be considered.[26,40] Third trimester intra-abdominal surgical procedures are more technically difficult due to the enlarged uterus and are associated with preterm labor.

Intraoperative Issues

Abdominal CO_2 Insufflation   Consider limiting the intra-abdominal insufflation pressure to 12–15 mm Hg during the laparoscopic procedure to minimize a further decrease of the pulmonary FRC and cardiac preload.[41] There are no studies available to determine if exposure to CO_2 insufflation has any effects on the fetus, but intra-operative maternal monitoring with capnography could theoretically address some short-term exposure issues. Gasless laparoscopy involves placing a 1.2-mm wire in the subcutaneous tissue between the umbilicus and the pubis. This wire is attached to a lifting bar to pull the abdominal wall away from the pelvic organs. However, few operating rooms have the necessary equipment to perform gasless laparoscopy, and it could limit the field of exposure, thus increasing the risk of complications or prolonged operating room time.

Cesarean Section Carries Higher Maternal Risks   Occasionally, a compli-cated maternal issue will prompt the consultants to consider delivery in order to more "safely" initiate maternal care. However, outside of severe preeclampsia, the need for preterm delivery is generally made for obstetric indications rather than maternal ones. The recovery is faster and complication rates lower after a vaginal delivery. In one study, 60% of pregnancy-associated pulmonary emboli occurred postpartum, and 80% of those emboli were associated with cesarean section.[42] After vaginal delivery, the reported incidence of postpartum endometritis ranges from 0.9% to 3.9%, and the incidence after cesarean section ranges from 10% or less in most private services to 50% or more in large teaching services caring for indigent patients.[19,43]

Type of Anesthesia   Consider regional anesthesia when possible to avoid the morbidity associated with intubation and airway management of the pregnant surgi-cal patient. As discussed above, loss of the maternal airway is the most common anesthesia-related cause of maternal death, and the fifth or sixth most common cause overall, depending on the study. No increase in fetal morbidity or spontaneous abor-tion exists among patients who undergo surgery with general anesthesia during pregnancy.

Obstetric anesthesiologists are aware that pregnancy-induced changes in response to anesthesia exist, including decreases of 25–40% in minimal alveolar concentration of inhalational anesthetics. This is thought to be caused by progester-one and increased sensitivity to local anesthetics.[14,44]

Perioperative Collaboration   In centers with less exposure to obstetric care, it is always prudent to take a multidisciplinary approach and obtain input from the patient's obstetrician, perinatologists (maternal fetal medicine specialists) or obstet-ric internists, medical subspecialists, and the appropriate surgeon. A group meeting to document the group's rationale and plan of care can be placed in the chart. When available, obstetric anesthesiologists will be familiar with the physiological changes, alterations in sensitivity to anesthetic agents, and high risk of airway complications. Perinatologists or the patient's general obstetrician will decide on the most appropriate way to monitor the fetus intra- and postoperatively. Consider delaying surgery if possible for medical diseases that are not optimized.

Patient Positioning All pregnant patients undergoing surgery should be placed in the left lateral decubitus position using a "pelvic wedge" or pillow under the right hip. This position will prevent a decrease in cardiac output and venous return secondary to aortic/vena caval compression by the gravid uterus.[45] Similar compression of the vessels can occur if the mother is placed in a "fetal" position prior to a lumbar puncture or placement of an epidural catheter.

Fetal Monitoring When the fetus is less than 24 weeks' gestation, fetal heart rate (FHR) monitoring is less reliable at assessing fetal well-being. FHR monitoring was designed for use during labor and can only detect severe alterations in fetal perfusion. FHR changes suggestive of fetal stress can give the clinician an additional assessment of uterine perfusion, but these changes are not likely to occur without other obvious signs of maternal distress such as prolonged hypotension or hypoxia.

Avoid Overresponding to Contractions Tocolytic medications such as beta-adrenergic agonists are associated with maternal complications such as pulmonary edema, tachycardia, atrial fibrillation, chest pain, and electrocardiogram (ECG) changes.[8,27] A review of 49,567 births over a 10-year period revealed 78 cases of surgery during pregnancy. While surgery was associated with an increased risk of preterm labor, there was no demonstrable benefit from the prophylactic use of tocolytic agents.[26] Magnesium, a medication used in the past to treat uterine irritability, was found to prolong the *in vitro* bleeding time, inhibit ADP- and collagen-induced platelet aggregation , and inhibit the binding of fibrinogen to the platelet glycoprotein IIb/IIIa receptor.[9]

Determine the Plan of Care as if She Was Not Pregnant In critically ill patients, do not risk maternal well-being by withholding a medication that poses a theoretical risk to the fetus. If needed, ephedrine causes less uterine artery spasm than other pressor agents and is the vasopressor of choice with phenylephrine as the second-line agent.[10] One should not equate a potential for uterine artery vasoconstriction with complete loss of blood flow to the uterus.

POSTOPERATIVE CARE

Minimizing atelectasis by encouraging deep breathing, incentive spirometry, and early ambulation are important risk-reduction strategies. Until the patient becomes ambulatory, keeping the patient in the left lateral decubitus position can prevent the gravid uterus from compressing the vena cava.

Because 80% of pulmonary emboli that occur after delivery are associated with cesarean section, deep venous thrombosis (DVT) prophylaxis should be ordered. Unfractionated heparin (UFH) and low-molecular-weight heparin (LMWH) do not cross the placenta. In spite of a lack of prospective trials, pregnancy is a hypercoagulable state, and it is reasonable to generalize data from the nonpregnant population. The dose of UFH shown to decrease the risk of perioperative DVT in nonpregnant patients is 5000 units subcutaneously three times a day (not twice daily). There are no prospective data in pregnancy to support one dose over another, but due to the increased rate of heparin clearance, some practitioners will use 7500 units BID in the second trimester, and 10,000 units BID in the third trimester. Alternatively, enoxaparin 40 mg daily or BID may be used. Nonpharmacological methods can be used such as compression stockings, pneumatic compression boots, early ambulation, and maintaining an optimal volume status, but these are typically given in addition to pharmacologic therapy.

Hypertension

A medical consultant may be called to evaluate postoperative hypertension in a patient who recently underwent a cesarean section. As in the nonpregnant population, pain should be the first item on the differential, but be aware that preeclampsia complicates approximately 10% of all deliveries and may have been the indication for the surgery.

Classically, preeclampsia involves new systolic blood pressure >140 mm Hg or diastolic blood pressure >90 mm Hg, combined with proteinuria (>300 mg per 24 h collection or new proteinuria > "+1" on a urine dip). In the history, ask about a new headache, visual changes, right upper quadrant pain, or new-onset edema of the hands or face. Physical exam findings include retinal vasospasm, a sustained S3 or S4 gallop, pulmonary edema, tender liver, severe edema, and clonus. Laboratory abnormalities may include elevated transaminases, thrombocytopenia, proteinuria, hemolysis, or elevated hemoglobin and serum creatinine (>0.8 mg%) from hemoconcentration. These patients may have intravascular volume depletion from the capillary leak.

Common medications used to treat hypertension in preeclampsia patients include labetalol (orally 200 mg BID/TID, the dose can be doubled if the response is inadequate, to a maximum of 2400 mg/day; or 20 mg IV bolus with subsequent increases to 40 mg then 80 mg at 10- to 20-min intervals if the pressure remains elevated; or it may be infused at 1 mg/kg/h). Methyldopa is widely considered the first-line agent for treatment of hypertension during pregnancy with no adverse effects on cognitive development among children with in utero exposure, but it is limited to oral dosing (250 mg PO BID/TID, increasing every 2 days as needed, not to exceed 3 g/day). A good resource is the report of the National High Blood Pressure Education Program Working Group on High Blood Pressure in Pregnancy.[46]

If tocolytics were administered or if hypoxia were detected, it is imperative to monitor for noncardiogenic pulmonary edema. The chest X-ray may show bilateral pulmonary infiltrates because pulmonary edema in this setting is due to low oncotic pressure of normal pregnancy and increased capillary permeability from the medication, and not increased hydrostatic pressure from left heart failure. Therefore, the X-ray finding of pulmonary vein "cephalization" may be absent.

Peripartum Fever

Medical consultants may also be called to evaluate a fever after surgery. In a pregnant woman, especially one who had a cesarean section, there is a differential diagnosis with some unique issues. UTI and pyelonephritis are more frequent during pregnancy and are a common source of fever. Chorioamnionitis and meningitis can be caused by *Listeria* (associated with certain foods such as soft cheese) and can rapidly lead to transplacental fetal infection and death. When treating meningitis, ampicillin must be included to the antibiotic regimen. Noninfectious etiologies of fever such as postpartum thyroiditis, pulmonary embolism (PE), DVT, endometritis (more common after prolonged rupture of membranes, assisted delivery, and cesarean section), ovarian vein thrombosis (macroscopic clot visible on pelvic CT or MR venogram), and septic pelvic thrombophlebitis (SPT) (more common after cesarean section) should be considered in the right clinical setting or when a patient fails to defervesce after antibiotic treatment.

The approach to these patients is unchanged and starts with an appropriate history. Historical questions should include family history/sick contacts, unusual food ingestions, recent travel (malaria exposure), and symptoms of DVT/PE. In addition to the standard physical exam (IV sites, signs of meningitis, thyroid, costovertebral angle tenderness, lungs), palpate the uterus during the normal abdominal exam. It should be firm and palpable below the level of the umbilicus. A tender uterus on the general abdominal exam suggests endometritis, pelvic hematoma, ovarian vein thrombosis, or SPT. Unexplained tachycardia or tachypnea warrants a workup for PE.

Diagnostic testing should be obtained as one would for the nonpregnant person. CT angiography and/or abdominal/pelvic CT scan with oral and IV contrast are important tests to consider. This can exclude PE, ovarian vein thrombosis, abscess, and hematoma. SPT is a diagnosis of exclusion made after ruling out PE and other pelvic pathology. Consider laboratory testing such as a complete blood count, comprehensive metabolic panel, and a thyroid-stimulating hormone level when indicated. A maternal chest radiograph can also be helpful when considering a pulmonary source. Lower extremity Doppler ultrasound is the test of choice to exclude DVT, but not PE. If the leg ultrasound is positive, you may consider avoiding the pulmonary CT angiogram or V/Q scan, but realize that a negative lower extremity ultrasound does not rule out lung pathology, only leg pathology. If you obtain a CT pulmonary angiogram or abdominal CT scan, realize that iodinated CT contrast may be given antepartum and during lactation, and breast-feeding does not have to be interrupted. After a maternal V/Q scan, postpartum mothers should "pump and dump" breast milk for 24 h.

Recognize that the reported incidence of postpartum endometritis after vaginal delivery ranges from 0.9% to 3.9%, and the incidence after cesarean section ranges from 10% or less in most private services to 50% or more in large teaching services caring for indigent patients.[47] Always treat endometritis as a polymicrobial infection and provide coverage for anaerobes and enteric gram-negative organisms. In the absence of other pathology, treat until the patient is afebrile for 48 h, then stop all antibiotics. For treatment of SPT, older approaches suggested adding heparin to antibiotics and if defervescence occurred within 2 days, this was suggestive of SPT. However, any venous thromboembolism (VTE) (ovarian, pelvic, pulmonary) could respond to heparin, so one must exclude those first. If imaging is negative, full-dose heparin (LMWH or UFH) should be added to the antibiotics. Consider CT angiography immediately followed by CT abdomen/pelvis with prior administration of oral contrast. If negative, drug fever or pelvic thrombophlebitis should be considered. If a macroscopic thrombosis is visualized in an ovarian or other pelvic vein, treat with full-dose anticoagulation for 3 months.

CONCLUSION

By understanding the anatomic and physiologic changes that occur during pregnancy, and the approach to testing and treatment in this population, surgery in the pregnant patient can be performed safely with the morbidity and mortality approaching that in a nonpregnant woman.

It is important to educate the patient that the best measure to insure a healthy fetus is to keep the mother as healthy as possible. The patient and sometimes the other members of the healthcare team often worry about the potential, theoretical, and usually miniscule negative consequences of any medical intervention. However, using the evidence presented here, it is much easier to quantify the risk of an adverse outcome if the test or surgery is not considered. In this way, the medical consultant is ideally positioned to serve as a "quarterback" for the care team and advocate for the patient in a highly effective manner.

REFERENCES

1. Reedy MB, Kallen B, Kuehl TJ. Laparoscopy during pregnancy: a study of five fetal outcome parameters with use of the Swedish Health Registry. *Am J Obstet Gynecol.* Sep 1997;177(3): 673–679.
2. Mazze RI, Kallen B. Appendectomy during pregnancy: a Swedish registry study of 778 cases. *Obstet Gynecol.* Jun 1991;77(6):835–840.
3. Brodsky JB, Cohen EN, Brown BW, Jr., Wu ML, Whitcher C. Surgery during pregnancy and fetal outcome. *Am J Obstet Gynecol.* Dec 15 1980;138(8):1165–1167.
4. Duncan PG, Pope WD, Cohen MM, Greer N. Fetal risk of anesthesia and surgery during pregnancy. *Anesthesiology.* Jun 1986;64(6):790–794.
5. Curet MJ. Special problems in laparoscopic surgery. Previous abdominal surgery, obesity, and pregnancy. *Surg Clin North Am.* Aug 2000;80(4):1093–1110.
6. Kazim SF, Pal I. Appendicitis in pregnancy: experience of thirty eight patients diagnosed and managed at a tertiary care hospital in karachi. *Int J Surg.* Aug 2009;7(4):365–367.
7. Ueberrueck T, Koch A, Meyer L, Hinkel M, Gastinger I. Ninety-four appendectomies for suspected acute appendicitis during pregnancy. *World J Surg.* May 2004;28(5):508–511.
8. Pisani RJ, Rosenow EC, 3rd. Pulmonary edema associated with tocolytic therapy. *Ann Intern Med.* May 1 1989;110(9):714–718.

9. Gries A, Bode C, Gross S, Peter K, Bohrer H, Martin E. The effect of intravenously administered magnesium on platelet function in patients after cardiac surgery. *Anesth Analg.* 1999;88(6): 1213–1219.

10. Carson MP, Powrie RO, Rosene-Montella K. The effect of obesity and position on heart rate in pregnancy. *J Matern Fetal Neonatal Med.* 2002;11(1):40–45.

11. Williams KP, Galerneau F. Fetal heart rate parameters predictive of neonatal outcome in the presence of a prolonged deceleration. *Obstet Gynecol* Nov 2002;100(5 Pt 1):951–954.

12. Pedrosa I, Lafornara M, Pandharipande PV, Goldsmith JD, Rofsky NM. Pregnant patients suspected of having acute appendicitis: effect of MR imaging on negative laparotomy rate and appendiceal perforation rate. *Radiology.* Mar 2009;250(3):749–757.

13. Pedrosa I, Levine D, Eyvazzadeh AD, Siewert B, Ngo L, Rofsky NM. MR imaging evaluation of acute appendicitis in pregnancy. *Radiology.* Mar 2006;238(3):891–899.

14. Wallace CA, Petrov MS, Soybel DI, Ferzoco SJ, Ashley SW, Tavakkolizadeh A. Influence of imaging on the negative appendectomy rate in pregnancy. *J Gastrointest Surg.* Jan 2008;12(1):46–50.

15. Fleisher LA, Beckman JA, Brown KA, et al. ACC/AHA 2007 guidelines on perioperative cardiovascular evaluation and care for noncardiac surgery: a report of the American College of Cardiology/ American Heart Association Task Force on Practice Guidelines (Writing Committee to Revise the 2002 Guidelines on Perioperative Cardiovascular Evaluation for Noncardiac Surgery). *J Am Coll Cardiol.* Oct 23 2007;50(17):e159–e241.

16. McFalls EO, Ward HB, Moritz TE, et al. Coronary-artery revascularization before elective major vascular surgery. *N Engl J Med.* Dec 30 2004;351(27):2795–2804.

17. CLASP: a randomised trial of low-dose aspirin for the prevention and treatment of pre-eclampsia among 9364 pregnant women. CLASP (Collaborative Low-dose Aspirin Study in Pregnancy) Collaborative Group. *Lancet.* Mar 12 1994;343(8898):619–629.

18. CDC. Prenatal Radiation Exposure: A Fact Sheet for Physicians. 2010; Prenatal Radiation Exposure: A Fact Sheet for Physicians. Available at: http://www.bt.cdc.gov/radiation/prenatalphysician.asp. Accessed September 27, 2010.

19. Chan WS, Ray JG, Murray S, Coady GE, Coates G, Ginsberg JS. Suspected pulmonary embolism in pregnancy: clinical presentation, results of lung scanning, and subsequent maternal and pediatric outcomes. *Arch Intern Med.* May 27 2002;162(10):1170–1175.

20. Shay DC, Bhavani-Shankar K, Datta S. Laparoscopic surgery during pregnancy. *Anesthesiol Clin N Am.* Mar 2001;19(1):57–67.

21. Mazze RI, Kallen B. Reproductive outcome after anesthesia and operation during pregnancy: a registry study of 5405 cases. *Am J Obstet Gynecol.* Nov 1989;161(5):1178–1185.

22. Sylvester GC, Khoury MJ, Lu X, Erickson JD. First-trimester anesthesia exposure and the risk of central nervous system defects: a population-based case-control study. *Am J Public Health.* Nov 1994;84(11):1757–1760.

23. Friedman JM. Teratogen update: anesthetic agents. *Teratology.* Jan 1988;37(1):69–77.

24. Shepard LN (ed.). *Catalog of Teratogenic Agents,* 7th edition, Baltimore, MD: John Hopkins University Press; 1992.

25. McKellar DP, Anderson CT, Boynton CJ, Peoples JB. Cholecystectomy during pregnancy without fetal loss. *Surg Gynecol Obstet.* Jun 1992;174(6):465–468.

26. Kort B, Katz VL, Watson WJ. The effect of nonobstetric operation during pregnancy. *Surg Gynecol Obstet.* Oct 1993;177(4):371–376.

27. Carson MP, Fisher AJ, Scorza WE. Atrial fibrillation in pregnancy associated with oral terbutaline. *Obstet Gynecol.* 2002;100(5 Pt 2):1096–1097.

28. Hawkins JL, Koonin LM, Palmer SK, Gibbs CP. Anesthesia-related deaths during obstetric delivery in the United States, 1979–1990. *Anesthesiology.* Feb 1997;86(2):277–284.

29. Walsh CA, Tang T, Walsh SR. Laparoscopic versus open appendicectomy in pregnancy: a systematic review. *Int J Surg.* Aug 2008;6(4):339–344.

30. Panchal S, Arria AM, Labhsetwar SA. Maternal mortality during hospital admission for delivery: a retrospective analysis using a state-maintained database. *Anesth Analg.* Jul 2001;93(1):134–141.

31. Sadot E, Telem DA, Arora M, Butala P, Nguyen SQ, Divino CM. Laparoscopy: a safe approach to appendicitis during pregnancy. *Surg Endosc.* Feb 2010;24(2):383–389.

32. Briggs GG, Freeman RK, Yaffe SJ. *Drugs in Pregnancy and Lactation.* Baltimore, MD: Lippincott Williams & Wilkins; 2005.
33. Baldwin RM, Pritchard JA, Dickey JC. Blood volume changes in pregnancy and the puerperium. *Am J Obstet Gynecol.* 1962;84:1271–1281.
34. Guidelines for laparoscopic surgery during pregnancy. *Surg Endosc.* Feb 1998;12(2):189–190.
35. Akira S, Yamanaka A, Ishihara T, Takeshita T, Araki T. Gasless laparoscopic ovarian cystectomy during pregnancy: comparison with laparotomy. *Am J Obstet Gynecol.* Mar 1999;180(3 Pt 1):554–557.
36. Muench J, Albrink M, Serafini F, Rosemurgy A, Carey L, Murr MM. Delay in treatment of biliary disease during pregnancy increases morbidity and can be avoided with safe laparoscopic cholecystectomy. *Am Surg.* Jun 2001;67(6):539–542; discussion 542–533.
37. Rutledge D, Jones D, Rege R. Consequences of delay in surgical treatment of biliary disease. *Am J Surg.* Dec 2000;180(6):466–469.
38. Date RS, Kaushal M, Ramesh A. A review of the management of gallstone disease and its complications in pregnancy. *Am J Surg.* Oct 2008;196(4):599–608.
39. Ramin KD, Ramin SM, Richey SD, Cunningham FG. Acute pancreatitis in pregnancy. *Am J Obstet Gynecol.* Jul 1995;173(1):187–191.
40. Kallen B, Mazze RI. Neural tube defects and first trimester operations. *Teratology.* Jun 1990;41(6):717–720.
41. Bhavani-Shankar K, Steinbrook RA, Mushlin PS, Freiberger D. Transcutaneous PCO_2 monitoring during laparoscopic cholecystectomy in pregnancy. *Can J Anaesth.* Feb 1998;45(2):164–169.
42. Powrie RO, Larson L, Rosene-Montella K, Abarca M, Barbour L, Trujillo N. Alveolar-arterial oxygen gradient in acute pulmonary embolism in pregnancy. *Am J Obstet Gynecol.* Feb 1998;178(2):394–396.
43. Marcus CS, Mason GR, Kuperus JH, Mena I. Pulmonary imaging in pregnancy. Maternal risk and fetal dosimetry. *Clin Nucl Med.* Jan 1985;10(1):1–4.
44. Ueland K, Novy MJ, Peterson EN, Metcalfe J. Maternal cardiovascular dynamics. IV. The influence of gestational age on the maternal cardiovascular response to posture and exercise. *Am J Obstet Gynecol.* Jul 15 1969;104(6):856–864.
45. Endler GC, Mariona FG, Sokol RJ, Stevenson LB. Anesthesia-related maternal mortality in Michigan, 1972 to 1984. *Am J Obstet Gynecol.* Jul 1988;159(1):187–193.
46. Report of the National High Blood Pressure Education Program Working Group on High Blood Pressure in Pregnancy. *Am J Obstet Gynecol.* 2000;183(1):S1–S22.
47. Seaward PG, Hannah ME, Myhr TL, et al. International Multicentre Term Prelabor Rupture of Membranes Study: evaluation of predictors of clinical chorioamnionitis and postpartum fever in patients with prelabor rupture of membranes at term. *Am J Obstet Gynecol.* Nov 1997;177(5):1024–1029.
48. Barish RJ. Radiation risk from airline travel. *J Am Coll Radiol.* Oct 2004;1(10):784–785.
49. Jankowski CB. Radiation and pregnancy. Putting the risks in proportion. *Am J Nurs.* Mar 1986;86(3):260–265.
50. Toppenberg KS, Hill DA, Miller DP. Safety of radiographic imaging during pregnancy. *Am Fam Physician.* 1999;59(7):1813–1818, 1820.
51. Tham TC, Vandervoort J, Wong RC, et al. Safety of ERCP during pregnancy. *Am J Gastroenterol.* Feb 2003;98(2):308–311.
52. Winer-Muram HT, Boone JM, Brown HL, Jennings SG, Mabie WC, Lombardo GT. Pulmonary embolism in pregnant patients: fetal radiation dose with helical CT. *Radiology.* 2002;224(2):487–492.
53. Rosene-Montella K, Larson L. Diagnostic imaging. In: *Medical Care of the Pregnant Patient,* Lee RV (ed.), pp. 103–115. Philadelphia: American College of Physicians; 2000.
54. Kanal E, Gillen J, Evans JA, Savitz DA, Shellock FG. Survey of reproductive health among female MR workers. *Radiology.* May 1993;187(2):395–399.
55. Kanal E. Pregnancy and the safety of magnetic resonance imaging. *Magn Reson Imaging Clin N Am.* May 1994;2(2):309–317.

CHAPTER 19

THE PATIENT WITH CANCER

Sunil K. Sahai and Marc A. Rozner

EPIDEMIOLOGY

For 2012, the American Cancer Society estimates that more than 1.6 million Americans will be diagnosed with cancer, and more than 577,000 deaths will be attributable to cancer. Three-quarters of all cancers are diagnosed in persons 55 years old and older, so as the population in the United States ages, the numbers of cancer diagnoses and deaths are expected to increase.[1] Furthermore, with successful treatment becoming more common, more cancer survivors live to present with either new primary cancers or with medical conditions that require surgery.

For nonhematologic cancers, surgery plays a vital role from diagnosis to cure (Table 19.1).[2] The evaluation and preoperative preparation of the cancer patient must always balance the urgency of operative intervention and the need to treat any concurrent medical problem that could affect the patient's perioperative course.[3] For example, a patient with pancreatic cancer who has a mean life expectancy of 12 months as well as unstable coronary artery disease might not benefit from a Whipple procedure (pancreatectomy) if he or she experiences a myocardial infarction and dies shortly after the surgery. The issues that should be considered during a preoperative assessment are similar between cancer patients and patients without cancer, but for cancer patients, this assessment frequently includes extensive discussions with other physicians who will care for the patient, as multidisciplinary care has become the norm for treating cancer.

Several important points should be considered when preoperative cancer patients are being evaluated. First, many consultant physicians and medical care providers believe, albeit without data, that multiple preoperative consultations and interventions will reduce or eliminate the possibility of perioperative complications. Yet rarely does a preoperative consultation identify *new* disease that affects perioperative outcome.[4] In some centers, preoperative consultation might result in reduced postoperative length of stay but not in perioperative mortality.[5] Second, many practitioners continue in their previously learned ways, ignoring new or expert consensus

Perioperative Medicine: Medical Consultation and Co-Management, First Edition.
Edited by Amir K. Jaffer and Paul J. Grant.
© 2012 Wiley-Blackwell. Published 2012 by John Wiley & Sons, Inc.

TABLE 19.1. Reasons for Surgery for Patients with Cancer[2]

Surgery type	Purpose
Preventive	Removal of organs in genetically acquired conditions
Diagnostic	Biopsy, endoscopy, and so on
Staging	Exploratory surgery
Curative	Performed with the intent to cure
Debulking	Removal of part of the tumor (cytoreduction)
Palliative	Performed to relieve discomfort, pain, or organ dysfunction
Supportive	Placement of vascular access devices or feeding tubes; reconstruction or restoration
Unrelated	Surgery for an unrelated medical condition during cancer treatment or for a cancer survivor

Adapted from *Surgery*, American Cancer Society. Published: August 25, 2011. Available at: http://www.cancer.org/Treatment/TreatmentsandSideEffects/TreatmentTypes/Surgery/surgery-and-cancer. Accessed: April 27, 2012.

guidelines and believing that "some study" does not apply to their patients. One needs to look no further than the consultant's recommendation to place pulmonary artery catheters, which have never been shown to benefit patients and might actually harm them.[6-8] Third, the role of the consultant is not always clearly delineated. Unclear expectations from poor communication can lead to controversy over who will inform a patient of his or her perioperative risk or whether the consultant should follow the patient postoperatively on a daily basis.[9] And fourth, reviews in this area show that perioperative internal medicine consultation continues to produce inconsistent effects on efficiency and quality of care in surgical patients.[10,11]

For postoperative care, the role of the medical consultant, or hospitalist, is not well defined in the general surgical population and has not as yet been explored with cancer patients. For orthopedic (but not cancer) patients, a recent review supported co-management by hospitalists, which appears to reduce time to surgery, time to consultation, and length of stay.[12] Whether co-management provides better outcomes in all hospital settings remains to be determined,[13] and no studies have been published that describe the co-management of postoperative cancer patients.

HISTORY

During the preoperative evaluation of a cancer patient, two distinct elements of the patient's history are important: the cancer history and the medical comorbidities. Usually (and especially in a cancer center), the cancer history and related cancer surgical history will be well documented and the chemotherapeutic history less well documented. On the other hand, the presence of medical comorbidities, the extent to which they interfere with the patient's physiology, prior treatments, and optimization attempts, and the possible extent to which they could affect the perioperative course are frequently missing from the patient's chart.

In addition, the assessment of each organ system needs to be documented, and the extent of control and compliance with treatment determined. Any prior diagnostic studies and invasive treatments should be documented as well.

CANCER HISTORY

A cancer patient may undergo chemotherapy, radiotherapy, or surgery in any combination and order. For the presurgical patient, all prior treatment history must be taken into account. For a patient currently undergoing evaluation for a new cancer or a recurrence, the history of prior therapy may guide surgical decision making. For example, a patient with a history of abdominal radiotherapy for colon cancer who now presents with ovarian cancer may have developed adhesions, precluding a laparoscopic approach.

For patients who had prior chemotherapy, the agents that were used and any medical side effects that were experienced should be noted, as they may affect perioperative care. For example, the patient with a history of anthracycline administration may be at risk for cardiomyopathy. While a thorough discussion of adverse effects from chemotherapy is beyond the scope of this chapter, it is important to note that the effects tend to be similar within broad classes of chemotherapeutic agents.

MEDICAL CONDITIONS

Cardiovascular Conditions

Radiotherapy and many chemotherapeutic agents can trigger or influence cardiovascular system disease. Several agents can cause direct myocardial injury leading to decreased left ventricular performance, and some agents can exacerbate hypertensive disease. Radiotherapy that falls on myocardial vessels can create or exacerbate atherosclerotic disease. With the identification of prior chemotherapy or radiotherapy, an appropriate workup can be initiated for the patient symptomatic for cardiovascular disease. Similarly, the presence or absence of cardiac symptoms before the cancer is diagnosed can assist in the decision for further testing for cardiovascular disease. For example, a patient who is undergoing cancer treatment and develops fatigue with exertion, but had previously been vigorous, may be experiencing a side effect of chemotherapy rather than preexisting cardiac symptoms (Figure 19.1).

Some chemotherapeutic agents cause the development of dilated cardiomyopathy with typical signs and symptoms of ventricular dysfunction (dyspnea, peripheral edema, jugular venous distention, and pulmonary edema) (Table 19.2). The risk of developing cardiomyopathy can vary for each agent and is often dose dependent. The risk of developing cardiomyopathy also depends on several other factors, including preexisting cardiac disease or cardiomyopathy, the use of additional chemotherapeutic agents, and radiotherapy to the chest.

A cancer patient with a treatment-related cardiomyopathy should be considered for evaluation by a cardiologist who knows that the patient is a surgical

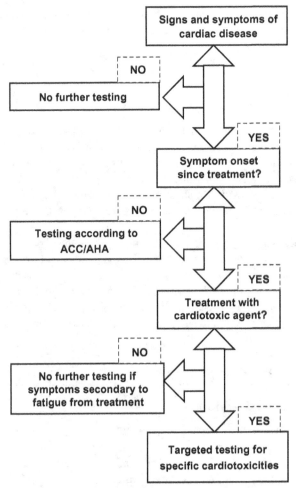

Figure 19.1.   Approach to the cancer patient with cardiovascular symptoms prior to surgery. ACC/AHA, American College of Cardiology/American Heart Association.

TABLE 19.2.   Chemotherapeutic Agents Associated with Cardiotoxicity

Anthracyclines	Taxanes	Monoclonal Antibodies	Tyrosine Kinase Inhibitors
Daunorubicin	Paclitaxel	Trastuzumab	Imatinib
Doxorubicin	Docetaxel	Rituximab	Gefitinib
Epirubicen		Bevacizumab	Sunitinib
Idarubicin			Dasatinib
Mitoxantrone			Erlotinib
Valrubicin			Sorafenib

TABLE 19.3. Chemotherapeutic Agents that may Cause Ischemia[52-54]

Capecitabine

5-Fluorouracil (5-FU)

Gemcitabine

Vincristine

Vinblastine

Vinorelbine

Paclitaxel

Docetaxel

Bevacizumab

Erlotinib

Sorafenib

TABLE 19.4. Cardiovascular Side Effects of Radiotherapy[55]

Cardiac condition	Symptom	Evaluation
Acute pericarditis	Chest pain	Electrocardiography, echocardiography
Constrictive pericarditis	Dyspnea, edema	Echocardiography, computed tomography of chest
Coronary atherosclerosis	Chest pain, dyspnea	Electrocardiography, stress testing, cardiac catheterization
Valvular stenosis and regurgitation	Chest pain, dyspnea	Echocardiography
Restrictive cardiomyopathy	Dyspnea, edema	Echocardiography
Conduction system defects	Dizziness, syncope	Electrocardiography

Reprinted with permission from Sahai SK. Perioperative Management of the Cancer Patient. Available at: http://www.perioperativecancermedicine.org/uploads/Perioperative_Management_of_the_Cancer_Patient_2010.pdf. Published: March 1, 2010. Accessed: April 27, 2012.

candidate. Any patient who develops chest pain during chemotherapy administration needs to be evaluated for possible underlying coronary artery disease, as there are several agents that can cause coronary vasospasm and ischemia (Table 19.3).

Radiotherapy to the chest wall or neck area may also initiate or accelerate cardiovascular disease (Table 19.4). The potential adverse effects of mediastinal or mantle irradiation include coronary artery disease, pericarditis, cardiomyopathy, valvular disease, and conduction abnormalities.[14] A significantly higher risk of death due to ischemic heart disease has been reported for patients who had been treated with radiotherapy to the chest for Hodgkin's disease or breast cancer,[15] although not all investigators are convinced that breast irradiation leads to increased heart disease.[16] Coronary artery endothelial cell damage from chest irradiation has been proposed as one mechanism for heart disease; the factors that may affect the development of coronary artery disease include the percentage of the left ventricle irradiated, concurrent hormonal treatment, and a history of hypercholesterolemia.[17] As previously noted, the risk of cardiomyopathy increases when radiotherapy is combined with doxorubicin (or any of the anthracyclines). This combination appears to have a synergistic toxic effect on the myocardium.[15]

Pulmonary Conditions

The cancer patient with underlying pulmonary disease should be evaluated based on the current symptoms and the stability of the disease. Patients with new pulmonary symptoms should undergo chest radiography, as it may reveal metastatic disease or the presence of pleural effusions. Pulmonary function testing can be considered in symptomatic patients with a history of chest irradiation or exposure to chemotherapy that had resulted in pulmonary toxicity. Preoperative thoracentesis may optimize lung function for patients with malignant pleural effusions. Patients with chronic obstructive pulmonary disease who are undergoing neoadjuvant chemotherapy may benefit from pulmonary rehabilitation before surgery.[18] The administration of pulmotoxic chemotherapeutic agents, the best known of which is bleomycin, may result in symptoms years after the fact (Table 19.5). Those with a history of radiation therapy to the chest wall are also at risk for developing pulmonary fibrosis.

Because of the increased risk of venous thromboembolism (VTE) in the patient with cancer, the presence of unexplained shortness of breath or dyspnea should prompt an investigation for pulmonary embolism. The decision to evaluate a patient for VTE needs to be made in light of the patient's clinical presentation. A patient who presents with new-onset shortness of breath and edema may undergo echocardiography in a search for heart failure. An incidental finding of enlarged right ventricle size or elevated systolic pressure may be consistent with an undiagnosed pulmonary embolus.[19]

Diabetes

For the cancer patient who has diabetes, the severity of this condition appears to affect the outcome of surgery. A recent meta-analysis found that among cancer

TABLE 19.5. Pulmotoxic Chemotherapeutic Drugs[56–60]

Bronchospasm		Pneumonitis or pulmonary fibrosis	Pleural or pericardial effusion
Busulfan	Gemcitabine	Bleomycin	Dasatinib
Cyclophosphamide	Methotrexate	Chlorambucil	Imatinib
Cytosine arabinoside (ARA-C)	Mitomycin	Carmustine	Nilotinib
Doxorubicin	Procarazine		
Etoposide	Taxanes (paclitaxel, docetaxel)		
Fludarabine	Vinca alkaloids		

patients, those with diabetes were 50% more likely than those who do not have diabetes to die in the postoperative period.[20]

Hyperglycemia is a common response to metabolic stress and critical illness, and it is associated with increased inflammation, susceptibility to infection, and multiorgan dysfunction.[21–23] For this reason, many cancer patients will experience *de novo* glucose intolerance, whereas others will develop hyperglycemia due to the corticosteroid therapy given concomitantly with the chemotherapeutic regimen or to the reduce intracranial pressure associated with neurologic cancers (primary or metastatic).[24] The glycosylated hemoglobin A1c (HbA1c) determined at the time of the preoperative consultation can assist in determining a patient's compliance with diabetic medication regimens. For patients at risk for metabolic syndrome, the HbA1c assay might also be used to identify patients with impaired glucose tolerance.[25]

Renal Conditions

A focus on renal issues in the cancer patient is warranted, as chemotherapy may have adverse affects on renal function (Table 19.6). In addition, a patient with renal insufficiency who undergoes partial or complete nephrectomy may need urgent consultation in the postoperative period for temporary or permanent dialysis.

Perioperative acute kidney injury occurs in approximately 1% of patients with a prior history of normal kidney function who undergo noncardiac general surgery.[26] Acute kidney injury is also associated with significant postoperative and long-term morbidity and mortality.[27] Risk factors for postoperative acute kidney injury include preexisting renal insufficiency, diabetes mellitus, patient age over 65 years, major vascular surgery, cardiopulmonary bypass time longer than 3 h, and recent exposure to nephrotoxic agents (such as contrast dyes, bile pigments, aminoglycoside antibiotics, and nonsteroidal anti-inflammatory drugs).[28] The literature offers little guidance for pre- or intraoperative management for these patients. In a meta-analysis of 20 studies that had been conducted over 20 years (1988–2008), Brienza et al. stated that "preoperative hemodynamic optimization" resulted in reduced perioperative renal dysfunction.[29] However, no consistent optimization regimen could be identified because the various therapies included administration of fluids and the use of inotropes, vasodilators, and vasopressors.

The literature also offers little guidance on perioperative renal management. Experts have suggested maintenance of euvolemia, control of blood pressure, limited

TABLE 19.6. Renal Side Effects of Chemotherapy[61–63]

Agent	Side effect
Cisplatin, carboplatin	Nephrotoxicity is dose limiting; hypomagnesemia can persist
Methotrexate	Nephrotoxicity due to precipitation in lumen is reversible
Ifosfamide	Proximal tubular dysfunction
Cyclophosamide	Hemorrhagic cystitis

use of diuretics, and avoidance of nephrotoxic agents. Although preoperative statin use has been associated with reduced postoperative acute kidney injury in cardiac surgery patients,[30] their effect on renal function in noncardiac surgery (e.g., cancer surgery) has not been studied.

Patient Age

As the general population ages, the need to assess life expectancy against the possibility of perioperative mortality becomes more important. Many people believe, mistakenly, that age represents a direct risk factor for perioperative complications. However, age alone might not be an independent risk factor. Pisanu et al. followed 94 patients undergoing gastrectomy with curative intent and reported that compared with the younger patients, those aged 75 years and older had more comorbidities and poorer nutritional status.[31] Although the elderly patients experienced greater medical mortality, the only independent factor was the presence of medical comorbidities. The 5-year survival rate was 56% in the older group and 62% in the younger group with tumor stage being the only prognostic factor influencing survival. Holmes reminded us that a balance must be sought between overzealous application of advanced surgical treatment and long-term quality of life and functional outcomes, even as current surgical techniques are replaced by newer and less invasive procedures.[32]

Several tools exist that may assist the clinician in assessing elderly cancer patients prior to surgery.[33-35] However, in every case, the presence and severity of medical comorbidities should be given greater weight than the patient's age.

Nutrition Status

A common issue affecting cancer patients is suboptimal nutritional status. This status may be due to the malignancy itself, nausea from chemotherapy, or poor dietary choices. For the patient with gastrointestinal cancer, poor nutritional status, coupled with delayed and inadequate postoperative nutrition practices, appears to worsen clinical outcomes.[36] Poor nutritional status also puts the elderly patient at risk for postoperative delirium, which can extend the length of stay and increase postoperative morbidity.[37] For these reasons, the medical history needs to include the patient's nutritional status and nutrition should be optimized preoperatively. This may or may not include supplementation via an enteral or parental route prior to surgery.[38,39] Evaluation by a nutritionist in the perioperative period may be useful.[40]

Type of Surgery

A cancer patient typically undergoes several procedures during the course of treatment, from biopsies to radical surgeries that require multiple surgical teams. When a patient is assessed for a particular procedure, the future care should be anticipated as well. For example, a patient with suspected bladder cancer may need no additional care following a diagnostic low-risk cystoscopy, whereas more consideration would be needed before a patient with prostate cancer undergoes a radical cystoprostatectomy. In addition, certain types of surgery may require co-management with considerable communication between the consultant and various teams caring for the patient over the entire course of treatment.

PHYSICAL EXAMINATION

The physical examination of a cancer patient who is expected to undergo surgery does not differ from that of any patient undergoing surgery, with the exception that the site of the cancer needs to be addressed in some detail.

Head and Neck

Examination of the head and neck is particularly important for patients with head and neck cancers. For example, a patient with a cancer in the neck or oropharynx who has previously undergone radiotherapy likely has post-irradiation changes in the neck area, which can affect swallowing (i.e., risk of perioperative aspiration) as well as access for airway control, an issue of particular importance for the anesthesiologist. In addition, radiotherapy may have accelerated previously undiagnosed carotid artery disease, resulting in a bruit. Patients with thyroid masses may have deviation and compression of the trachea, which results in upper airway sounds that mimic wheezing.

Thorax

In patients who have received radiotherapy to the chest wall, auscultation might reveal crackles, which may point to the presence of pulmonary fibrosis. Pleural effusions from the cancer or the chemotherapy may be discernable secondary to decreased breath sounds and dullness to percussion.

Cardiovascular System

In rare cases, chest or mantle field irradiation may accelerate valvular disease, leading to the presence of murmurs. Pericarditis may be present secondary to effusions from cancer or irradiation. Examination of the chest wall may reveal excoriation or scarring from irradiation.

Gastrointestinal System

Ascites may interfere with the physical examination of patients with hepatocellular cancer, and constipated patients may have impaction and thus palpable masses on examination. Bowel obstruction is a common complication in patients with gastrointestinal malignancies, especially if they have had prior radiotherapy or surgery. Bowel sounds may be variable, especially for patients who use opioids for pain control. Moreover, many cancer patients have feeding tubes, and examination of the tube site may detect infection or other pathology that will need evaluation.

Neurologic System

Neurologic examination of a patient with a brain tumor may provide additional information about the cancer and will provide a baseline should any neurologic deficits develop in the postoperative period. Any seizure history should be documented (e.g., first seizure, most recent seizure, seizure activity, and any precipitating factors). Signs or symptoms of increased intracranial pressure (e.g., headache, nausea or vomiting, gait disturbance, or papilledema) should be sought with the intention of instituting treatment if they are discovered. Additionally, a new focal neurologic finding such as facial droop, cranial nerve palsy, incontinence, or foot drop needs evaluation for undiagnosed metastatic disease affecting the central nervous system.

Extremities

The presence of edema may be the only sign of cardiomyopathy secondary to chemotherapy. Unilateral swelling of the extremities should prompt evaluation for venous thrombosis. Lower extremity weakness should prompt evaluation for possible spinal cord compression.

Skin

Skin injury secondary to prior radiotherapy is common among patients with new cancer. Acute findings include erythema, pruritis, and desquamation. Many patients with cancer have paraneoplastic changes secondary to the disease process or from the treatment received.

Psychological System

For an elderly patient, postoperative delirium can be a source of significant morbidity. One common cause of cognitive dysfunction is the syndrome known as "chemobrain."[41,42] Although its exact mechanism is unknown, chemobrain is thought to be secondary to adverse effects from chemotherapy. It may mimic early onset dementia, and as such may be difficult to distinguish them apart. Cognitive dysfunction that occurs in close proximity to the chemotherapy administration should not be confused with dementia. The extent to which chemobrain affects immediate postoperative cognitive function is unknown. Presurgical use of a cognitive assessment tool may help to identify patients at risk for postoperative delirium.

PERIOPERATIVE TESTING

In general, testing before surgery should be limited and targeted. In contrast to persons undergoing elective procedures, most patients with cancer already have a wealth of presurgical laboratory and radiological data available. The challenge for the physician who is evaluating the patient in the preoperative setting is obtaining the relevant data from the various sources to avoid unnecessarily exposing patients to duplicate tests. For example, a staging chest radiograph is routinely obtained for most cancer patients. If it has already been performed and there is no history of intervening treatments or pulmonary symptoms, there is no need to repeat chest radiography. The decision to obtain a staging chest X-ray image should be left to the oncologist. In addition, unless a lung resection is planned, the need for pulmonary function testing is limited. As another example, the cancer patient tends to undergo laboratory testing on a routine basis during chemotherapy. These tests do not need to be repeated unless a suspicion of derangement is present (e.g., hypomagnesemia in the face of platin chemotherapy).

According to the American College of Cardiology/American Heart Association (ACC/AHA) guidelines, little information can be gained from the routine use of preoperative echocardiography to determine ejection fraction and thus should be avoided.[43] Echocardiography does appear to be warranted for patients with new or worsening symptoms of cardiac decompensation, but in the absence of a valid indication, this procedure can delay surgery. Such testing should also be discouraged for patients with adequate functional status, normal cardiac examination results, and no history of cardiomyopathy. Similarly, a routine electrocardiogram might be indicated for cancer patients at risk for cardiovascular disease but offers little benefit for patients without cardiovascular risk factors despite exposure to cardiotoxic chemotherapy.

POSTOPERATIVE MANAGEMENT

Postoperative management of the cancer patient should follow the established norms at the hospital where the surgery is taking place. Close attention to wound healing is prudent, especially for patients with a history of radiotherapy or diabetes. Patients with preoperative renal dysfunction due to use of a chemotherapeutic drug (e.g., cisplatin) might need to have electrolyte and magnesium levels monitored after surgery.

A key concept with any surgical patient is optimal nutrition, as stated previously. Patients with cachexia and a decreased nutritional reserve may experience delayed and complicated recovery. Early initiation of postsurgical nutrition should be employed, including total parental nutrition if enteral feeding is not possible.

Guidelines from the American Society of Clinical Oncology (ASCO) and the National Comprehensive Cancer Network (NCCN) specifically address the cancer patient in the postoperative setting.[44,45] Of particular concern is the daily assessment of the need for VTE prophylaxis. For some patients, VTE prophylaxis within 24 h of surgery is withheld secondary to concerns about bleeding. However, initiation of VTE prophylaxis on postoperative day 2 or 3 sometimes fails to be addressed.

Another concern is the need to address postdischarge or extended VTE prophylaxis for patients at high risk for developing this condition (Figure 19.2). The ASCO and NCCN guidelines each address the need for extended deep venous thrombosis prophylaxis beyond the date of discharge in the cancer patient. The recommendations are mirrored in the most recent American College of Chest

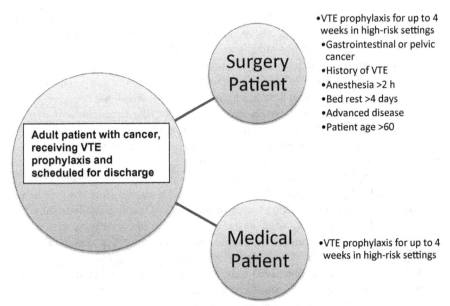

Figure 19.2.   National Comprehensive Cancer Network (NCCN) practice guidelines risk factors indicating a need for extended VTE prophylaxis. Adapted with permission from NCCN 2.2011 venous thromboembolic disease: clinical practice guidelines in oncology. National Comprehensive Cancer Network, 2011. Available at: http://www.nccn.org. Accessed: April 27, 2012. To view the most recent and complete version of the guideline, go online to: http://www.nccn.org/professionals/physician_gls/f_guidelines.asp.

Physicians (ACCP) guidelines for abdominal cancer surgery.[46] We recommend adherence to the Surgical Care Improvement Project (SCIP) recommendations with respect to VTE prophylaxis as well as perioperative antibiotic coverage.[47]

QUALITY INDICATORS

Established quality measures of the care provided for patients undergoing cancer surgery are the same for any patient undergoing noncancer surgery, namely, adherence to the SCIP protocols, of which VTE prophylaxis is arguably the most important. Current regulations mandate reporting of these core measures to the federal government for subsequent publication on the http://hospitalcompare.hhs.gov website. What is not captured at this site, however, is the extent to which the ASCO, ACCP, and NCCN guidelines for extended VTE prophylaxis after surgery are implemented.

PATIENT EDUCATION

Educating a patient after a thorough presurgical evaluation remains the most important aspect of perioperative care. The perioperative consultant provides a risk assessment to not only the surgeon but also the patient and family. As a result of this information, a patient at particularly high risk for a poor outcome may choose to forego surgical resection of the cancer and opt for another treatment modality. All treatment decisions made by the physician must respect the expectations and wishes of the patient and family.

Multidisciplinary cancer programs routinely take into account a patient's medical comorbidities when formulating a course of treatment. Patients diagnosed with cancer, however, tend to focus on the malignancy with the exclusion of their other comorbidities. It may be necessary to educate the patient about the importance of optimizing their chronic diseases (e.g., adequate control of diabetes improves surgical outcomes) and of physical fitness and activity during neoadjuvant treatment (e.g., maintaining good functional status will likely improve the surgical outcome).[48] In addition, patients who use tobacco products can be referred to a tobacco treatment program to assist in cessation efforts.

CONCLUSION

In summary, evaluation of the cancer patient undergoing surgery requires a thoughtful understanding of the cancer diagnosis in addition to the patient's perioperative risks. Frequently, chemotherapeutic complications can masquerade as cardiovascular symptoms and vice versa. Familiarity with a patient's prior treatment history will enable the physician to provide a comprehensive and accurate risk assessment and evaluation. Furthermore, the unique risks of cancer patients, especially in regards to malnutrition and thrombosis risk, need to be considered and optimally managed. In addition to medical optimization by pharmacologic means, lifestyle interventions such as smoking cessation and maintaining the best possible functional status should be part of the perioperative evaluation of the cancer patient.

REFERENCES

1. American Cancer Society. *Cancer Facts and Figures 2012*. Atlanta, GA: American Cancer Society; 2012. Available at http://www.cancer.org/Research/CancerFactsFigures/CancerFactsFigures/cancer-facts-and-figures-2012. Accessed April 27, 2012.
2. American Cancer Society. *Surgery*. Available at http://www.cancer.org/Treatment/TreatmentsandSide Effects/TreatmentTypes/Surgery/index. Accessed April 27, 2012.
3. Ewer MS. Specialists must communicate in complex cases. *Int Med World Rep*. 2001;16(5):17.
4. Katz RI, Cimino L, Vitkun SA. Preoperative medical consultations: impact on perioperative management and surgical outcome. *Can J Anaesth*. 2005;52(7):697–702.
5. Wijeysundera DN, Austin PC, Beattie WS, Hux JE, Laupacis A. A population-based study of anesthesia consultation before major noncardiac surgery. *Arch Intern Med*. 2009;169(6):595–602.
6. Sandham JD, Hull RD, Brant RF, et al. A randomized, controlled trial of the use of pulmonary-artery catheters in high-risk surgical patients. *N Engl J Med*. 2003;348(1):5–14.
7. Barone JE, Tucker JB, Rassias D, Corvo PR. Routine perioperative pulmonary artery catheterization has no effect on rate of complications in vascular surgery: a meta-analysis. *Am Surg*. 2001;67(7): 674–679.

8. Bonazzi M, Gentile F, Biasi GM, et al. Impact of perioperative haemodynamic monitoring on cardiac morbidity after major vascular surgery in low risk patients. A randomised pilot trial. *Eur J Vasc Endovasc Surg.* 2002;23(5):445–451.

9. PausJenssen L, Ward H, Card S. An internist's role in perioperative medicine: a survey of surgeons' opinions. *BMC Fam Pract.* 2008;9(4):1–6.

10. Auerbach AD, Rasic MA, Sehgal N, Ide B, Stone B, Maselli J. Opportunity missed—medical consultation, resource use, and quality of care of patients undergoing major surgery. *Arch Intern Med.* 2007;167(21):2338–2344.

11. Macpherson DS, Lofgren RP. Outpatient internal medicine preoperative evaluation: a randomized clinical trial. *Med Care.* 1994;32(5):498–507.

12. Peterson MC. A systematic review of outcomes and quality measures in adult patients cared for by hospitalists vs nonhospitalists. [Review]. *Mayo Clin Proc.* 2009;84(3):248–254.

13. Centor RM. A hospitalist inpatient system does not improve patient care outcomes. *Arch Intern Med.* 2008;168(12):1257–1258.

14. Adams MJ, Hardenbergh PH, Constine LS, Lipshultz SE. Radiation-associated cardiovascular disease. *Crit Rev Oncol Hematol.* 2003;45(1):55–75.

15. Basavaraju SR, Easterly CE. Pathophysiological effects of radiation on atherosclerosis development and progression, and the incidence of cardiovascular complications. *Med Phys.* 2002;29(10):2391–2403.

16. Vallis KA, Pintilie M, Chong N, et al. Assessment of coronary heart disease morbidity and mortality after radiation therapy for early breast cancer. *J Clin Oncol.* 2002;20(4):1036–1042.

17. Lind PA, Pagnanelli R, Marks LB, et al. Myocardial perfusion changes in patients irradiated for left-sided breast cancer and correlation with coronary artery distribution. *Int J Radiat Oncol Biol Phys.* 2003;55(4):914–920.

18. Sekine Y, Chiyo M, Iwata T, et al. Perioperative rehabilitation and physiotherapy for lung cancer patients with chronic obstructive pulmonary disease. *Jpn J Thorac Cardiovasc Surg.* 2005;53(5):237–243.

19. Mookadam F, Jiamsripong P, Goel R, Warsame TA, Emani UR, Khandheria BK. Critical appraisal on the utility of echocardiography in the management of acute pulmonary embolism. [Review]. *Cardiol Rev.* 2010;18(1):29–37.

20. Barone BB, Yeh HC, Snyder CF, et al. Postoperative mortality in cancer patients with preexisting diabetes: systematic review and meta-analysis. *Diabetes Care.* 2010;33(4):931–939.

21. Lipshutz AK, Gropper MA. Perioperative glycemic control: an evidence-based review. *Anesthesiology.* 2009;110(2):408–421.

22. Ouattara A, Lecomte P, Le Manach Y, et al. Poor intraoperative blood glucose control is associated with a worsened hospital outcome after cardiac surgery in diabetic patients. *Anesthesiology.* Oct 2005;103(4):687–694.

23. Umpierrez GE, Isaacs SD, Bazargan N, You X, Thaler LM, Kitabchi AE. Hyperglycemia: an independent marker of in-hospital mortality in patients with undiagnosed diabetes. *J Clin Endocrinol Metab.* 2002;87(3):978–982.

24. Sahai SK, Zalpour A, Rozner MA. Preoperative evaluation of the oncology patient. *Anesthesiol Clin.* 2009;27(4):805–822.

25. Osei K, Rhinesmith S, Gaillard T, Schuster D. Is glycosylated hemoglobin A1c a surrogate for metabolic syndrome in nondiabetic, first-degree relatives of African-American patients with type 2 diabetes? *J Clin Endocrinol Metab.* 2003;88(10):4596–4601.

26. Kheterpal S, Tremper KK, Englesbe MJ, et al. Predictors of postoperative acute renal failure after noncardiac surgery in patients with previously normal renal function. *Anesthesiology.* 2007;107(6):892–902.

27. Bihorac AMD, Yavas SMD, Subbiah SBA, et al. Long-term risk of mortality and acute kidney injury during hospitalization after major surgery. *Ann Surg.* 2009;249(5):851–858.

28. Sear JW. Kidney dysfunction in the postoperative period. *Br J Anaesth.* 2005;95(1):20–32.

29. Brienza N, Giglio MT, Marucci M, Fiore T. Does perioperative hemodynamic optimization protect renal function in surgical patients? A meta-analytic study. *Crit Care Med.* 2009;37(6):2079–2090.

30. Virani SS, Nambi V, Polsani VR, et al. Preoperative statin therapy decreases risk of postoperative renal insufficiency. *Cardiovasc Ther.* 2010;28(2):80–86.

31. Pisanu A, Montisci A, Piu S, Uccheddu A. Curative surgery for gastric cancer in the elderly: treatment decisions, surgical morbidity, mortality, prognosis and quality of life. *Tumori*. 2007;93(5): 478–484.

32. Holmes HM. Quality of life and ethical concerns in the elderly thoracic surgery patient. *Thorac Surg Clin*. 2009;19(3):401–407.

33. Audisio RA, Pope D, Ramesh HS, et al. Shall we operate? Preoperative assessment in elderly cancer patients (PACE) can help. A SIOG surgical task force prospective study. *Crit Rev Oncol Hematol*. 2008;65(2):156–163.

34. Audisio RA, Ramesh H, Longo WE, Zbar AP, Pope D. Preoperative assessment of surgical risk in oncogeriatric patients. *Oncologist*. 2005;10(4):262–268.

35. Pope D, Ramesh H, Gennari R, et al. Pre-operative assessment of cancer in the elderly (PACE): a comprehensive assessment of underlying characteristics of elderly cancer patients prior to elective surgery. *Surg Oncol*. 2006;15(4):189–197.

36. Garth AK, Newsome CM, Simmance N, Crowe TC. Nutritional status, nutrition practices and post-operative complications in patients with gastrointestinal cancer. *J Hum Nutr Diet*. 2010;23(4): 393–401.

37. Tei M, Ikeda M, Haraguchi N, et al. Risk factors for postoperative delirium in elderly patients with colorectal cancer. *Surg Endosc*. 2010;24(9):2135–2139.

38. Wu GH, Liu ZH, Wu ZH, Wu ZG. Perioperative artificial nutrition in malnourished gastrointestinal cancer patients. *World J Gastroenterol*. 2006;12(15):2441–2444.

39. Wu MH, Lin MT, Chen WJ. Effect of perioperative parenteral nutritional support for gastric cancer patients undergoing gastrectomy. *Hepatogastroenterology*. 2008;55(82–83):799–802.

40. Antoun S, Baracos V. Malnutrition in cancer patient: when to have a specialized consultation?. *Bull Cancer*. 2009;96(5):615–623.

41. Boykoff N, Moieni M, Subramanian SK. Confronting chemobrain: an in-depth look at survivors' reports of impact on work, social networks, and health care response. *J Cancer Surviv*. 2009;3(4): 223–232.

42. Wefel JS, Lenzi R, Theriault R, Buzdar AU, Cruickshank S, Meyers CA. "Chemobrain" in breast carcinoma?: a prologue. *Cancer*. 2004;101(3):466–475.

43. Fleisher LA, Beckman JA, Brown KA, et al. ACC/AHA 2007 guidelines on perioperative cardiovascular evaluation and care for noncardiac surgery: a report of the American College of Cardiology/American Heart Association Task Force on practice guidelines (writing committee to revise the 2002 guidelines on perioperative cardiovascular evaluation for noncardiac surgery). *J Am Coll Cardiol*. 2007;50:e159–e241.

44. Lyman GH, Khorana AA, Falanga A, et al. American Society of Clinical Oncology guideline: recommendations for venous thromboembolism prophylaxis and treatment in patients with cancer. *J Clin Oncol*. 2007;25(34):5490–5505.

45. Wagman LD, Baird MF, Bennett CL, et al. Venous thromboembolic disease. NCCN. Clinical practice guidelines in oncology. *J Natl Compr Canc Netw*. 2008;6(8):716–753.

46. Geerts WH, Bergqvist D, Pineo GF, et al. Prevention of venous thromboembolism: American College of Chest Physicians Evidence-Based Clinical Practice Guidelines (8th Edition). *Chest*. 2008;133(6 Suppl):381S–453S.

47. Gold JA. The Surgical Care Improvement Project. *Wis Med J*. 2005;104(1):73–74.

48. Adamsen L, Quist M, Andersen C, et al. Effect of a multimodal high intensity exercise intervention in cancer patients undergoing chemotherapy: randomised controlled trial. *BMJ*. 2009;339:b3410.

49. Chu TF, Rupnick MA, Kerkela R, et al. Cardiotoxicity associated with tyrosine kinase inhibitor sunitinib. *Lancet*. 2007;370(9604):2011–2019.

50. Gharib MI, Burnett AK. Chemotherapy-induced cardiotoxicity: current practice and prospects of prophylaxis. *Eur J Heart Fail*. 2002;4(3):235–242.

51. Khakoo AY, Yeh ET. Therapy insight: management of cardiovascular disease in patients with cancer and cardiac complications of cancer therapy. *Nat Clin Pract Oncol*. 2008;5(11):655–667.

52. Yeh ETH, Bickford CL. Cardiovascular complications of cancer therapy: incidence, pathogenesis, diagnosis, and management. *J Am Coll Cardiol*. 2009;53(24):2231–2247.

53. Webster DR. Microtubules in cardiac toxicity and disease. *Cardiovasc Toxicol*. 2002;2(2):75–89.

54. Lapeyre-Mestre M, Gregoire N, et al. Vinorelbine-related cardiac events: a meta-analysis of randomized clinical trials. *Fundam Clin Pharmacol.* 2004;18(1):97–105.
55. Sahai SK. Perioperative Management of the Cancer Patient [Lecture], 2010. Available at http://www.perioperativecancermedicine.org/uploads/Perioperative_Management_of_the_Cancer_Patient_2010.pdf. Accessed April 27, 2012.
56. Copper JA, Jr. Drug-induced lung disease. *Adv Intern Med.* 1997;42:231–268.
57. Einhorn L, Krause M, Hornback N, Furnas B. Enhanced pulmonary toxicity with bleomycin and radiotherapy in oat cell lung cancer. *Cancer.* 1976;37(5):2414–2416.
58. Kelly K, Swords R, Mahalingam D, Padmanabhan S, Giles FJ. Serosal inflammation (pleural and pericardial effusions) related to tyrosine kinase inhibitors. *Target Oncol.* 2009;4(2):99–105.
59. Klein DS, Wilds PR. Pulmonary toxicity of antineoplastic agents: anaesthetic and postoperative implications. *Can Anaesth Soc J.* 1983;30(4):399–405.
60. Tashiro M, Izumikawa K, Yoshioka D, et al. Lung fibrosis 10 years after cessation of bleomycin therapy. *Tohoku J Exp Med.* 2008;216(1):77–80.
61. Stohr W, Paulides M, Bielack S, et al. Nephrotoxicity of cisplatin and carboplatin in sarcoma patients: a report from the late effects surveillance system. *Pediatr Blood Cancer.* 2007;48(2):140–147.
62. Stohr W, Paulides M, Bielack S, et al. Ifosfamide-induced nephrotoxicity in 593 sarcoma patients: a report from the Late Effects Surveillance System. *Pediatr Blood Cancer.* 2007;48(4):447–452.
63. Widemann BC, Balis FM, Kempf-Bielack B, et al. High-dose methotrexate-induced nephrotoxicity in patients with osteosarcoma. *Cancer.* 2004;100(10):2222–2232.

POSTOPERATIVE CARE AND CO-MANAGEMENT BY SURGERY TYPE

CHAPTER 20

CARDIAC SURGERY

Uzma Abbas and Andres F. Soto

BACKGROUND

Cardiac surgery, including coronary artery bypass grafting (CABG), represents one of the most common procedures performed worldwide. The Society of Thoracic Surgeons (STS) National Cardiac Database (NCD) is one the largest specialty-specific clinical data registries in the world. It currently has more than 926 participants enrolled, representing just under 90% of the cardiac surgery providers in the United States, with data on more than 3.6 million procedures.[1] Most cardiac surgeries are considered high-risk procedures and require careful preoperative and postoperative care to ensure optimal outcomes. Although a cardiologist is inevitably involved in the care of cardiac surgery patients, generalists such as hospitalists are commonly engaged given the multiple medical comorbidities typically present in this patient population.

SURGERY SPECIFIC RISK

According to the STS National Database for Cardiac Surgery, isolated CABG is one of the most common procedures in the United States with approximately 160,000 surgeries performed each year.[1] Aortic valve replacement (AVR) is the second most common cardiac surgery performed.[1-3] The STS National Database for the year 2009 indicated an unadjusted operative mortality for isolated CABG at just above 2%. It is approximately 3.8% for AVR and 6% for mitral valve replacement (MVR). The mortality substantially increases for combined procedures and is approximately 7% and 12% for AVR + CABG and MVR + CABG, respectively.[1,4]

The primary determinants of success of cardiac surgery go beyond what occurs in the operating room and includes long-term postoperative outcomes. Hence, efforts should be aimed at understanding the contributing factors of patient mortality and morbidity following cardiac surgery.[5] Advances in cardiac surgical techniques have led to improved outcomes, but older and more morbid patients are undergoing

Perioperative Medicine: Medical Consultation and Co-Management, First Edition.
Edited by Amir K. Jaffer and Paul J. Grant.
© 2012 Wiley-Blackwell. Published 2012 by John Wiley & Sons, Inc.

cardiac surgery.[6] Forty percent of the annual hospital cost for CABG is consumed by 10–15% of the patients who suffer serious nonfatal complications after cardiac surgery. Therefore, optimizing perioperative practice patterns is critical in order to achieve optimal outcomes.

PREOPERATIVE ASSESSMENT

The preoperative history and physical examination is an important aspect of patient evaluation.[7,8] It provides an opportunity to assess and modify perioperative risk, as well as identify any potential contraindications. Examination of the head, neck, and oral cavity for signs of infection is important to assess the risk for endocarditis, especially for patients undergoing valvular surgery. Particular attention should be paid to assessment of the cardiac and vascular systems. Peripheral vascular insufficiency, abdominal aortic aneurysm, and aortic insufficiency can be potential contraindications for using an intra-aortic balloon pump. Additionally, aortic regurgitation can worsen during cardiopulmonary bypass for patients undergoing CABG. Examination of the lower extremities may provide useful information regarding patency of the venous system, which is important when assessing their use as a conduit. The presence of a carotid bruit may require further evaluation by carotid ultrasound to assess the need for revascularization. A preoperative neurologic assessment provides a baseline for comparison in the event of a postoperative cerebrovascular event with neurologic deficit.[9]

LABORATORY EVALUATION

Basic preoperative laboratory testing should include a complete blood count, chemistry profile, coagulation screen, and stool hemoccult test. Patients with anemia and/or occult gastrointestinal (GI) bleeding should be identified prior to surgery as postoperative antiplatelet and anticoagulation use is common. A patient's bleeding risk may also influence decisions regarding the type of prosthetic valve used.[7,8] Patients with coagulopathies can be challenging and may necessitate further testing and preoperative hematology consultation.[10] A chemistry profile can identify patients with electrolyte abnormalities and provide baseline assessment of renal and liver function, which are important predictors of mortality and morbidity. Nutrition status should be assessed with serum albumin and prealbumin levels as malnutrition increase risk of postoperative sepsis and respiratory failure.

Ventricular and valvular cardiac function is routinely evaluated with preoperative echocardiography. A carotid artery ultrasound should be performed in high-risk patients as combined CABG/endarterectomy procedures are considered in patients with severe carotid disease or prior history of stroke.[9,11] Additional preoperative testing should be individualized with consideration of the type of cardiac surgery planned.[7]

PREOPERATIVE ESTIMATION OF MORBIDITY AND MORTALITY RISK

Assessing surgical risk and predicting patient outcomes are important aspects of perioperative medicine. In an era of widespread concerns about variations in the quality of care and use of healthcare resources, methods to assess the risks of cardiac surgery are of increasing importance. Cardiac surgery is resource intensive and has a moderately high in-hospital mortality rate. As a result, considerable effort has gone into the development of perioperative risk models to predict outcomes from cardiac surgery interventions.[12] Risk stratification has several potential benefits. In addition to informing the patient, primary care physician, surgeon, and anesthesiologist of the patient's perioperative risks, it also allows for a tailored approach for patient optimization prior to surgery.

Several risk models and risk scoring systems are available to predict the risk for morbidity and mortality of patients undergoing cardiac surgery.[13,14] Selection of any risk model should be based on the study population, accuracy, validity, and physician's choice.[5,15] The STS cardiac risk stratification scoring system is the most commonly used scoring system in the United States.[1,4]

Although the STS risk models are based on excellent clinical data and large sample sizes, there are shortfalls. Certain risk factors that may be less common, such as liver disease and functional status, were not considered in STS risk models despite being important predictors of surgical outcomes. As data for any risk model are derived from large patient populations, application to a single patient should be supplemented by professional judgment. Another caveat to using risk models is that the prevalence of risk factors may change over time, which may influence their predictive accuracy. Additionally, their utility may be limited when applied to a different procedure.

POSTOPERATIVE ASSESSMENT AND MANAGEMENT

Many systems have the potential for derangement postoperatively; therefore, a systems-based approach may be necessary when caring for the postcardiac surgery patient. Major postoperative complications usually fall into two categories: worsening of a preexisting comorbidity, and new complications that occur as a consequence of the operation and/or cardiopulmonary bypass. Many perioperative complications can be anticipated allowing for early and aggressive management in an attempt to reduce morbidity and shorten convalescence.

CARDIAC

Although cardiac surgery such as CABG is performed to improve cardiac function and myocardial flow, multiple complications can occur that impair perfusion and cause postoperative myocardial ischemia, low cardiac output, and even sudden death. Postoperative ischemia and infarction should be suspected in the presence of unexplained heart failure, or electrocardiogram (ECG) findings such as new ST-wave changes, arrhythmias, and new bundle branch or complete heart block. Any of these findings should lead to prompt evaluation including serial cardiac enzymes, serial ECGs, echocardiogram, and cardiac catheterization if indicated. Assessment and optimization of hemodynamics should be a principal focus of immediate postoperative care.

The predominant goal should be maintenance of adequate oxygen delivery to vital tissues. Initial assessment should carefully review current medications, heart rate and rhythm, mean arterial pressure, central venous pressure, pulmonary capillary wedge pressure, and mixed venous oxygen saturation. Trends in hemodynamic parameters are usually more important than any single reading.

HEART RATE AND RHYTHM

Cardiac arrhythmias can cause significant clinical deterioration; thus, optimization of heart rate and rhythm requires prompt assessment and intervention. Cardiac pacing is one option to control heart rate with atrial pacing preferred over atrioventricular pacing, which is preferred over ventricular pacing. Internal permanent pacemakers can often be reprogrammed to improve output.

Nonsustained ventricular tachycardia is a common arrhythmia following cardiac surgery. It is generally a reflection of underlying reperfusion injury, electrolyte imbalance, or excessive sympathetic stimulation. Therefore, a focused approach is needed to correct the underlying problem. Sustained ventricular tachycardia is a more serious and potentially life-threatening issue that requires emergent assessment and aggressive treatment. Atrial fibrillation is one of the most common arrhythmias following cardiac surgery and will be discussed in more detail below.

ATRIAL FIBRILLATION

Incidence

The incidence of atrial fibrillation after cardiac surgery varies widely with estimates ranging from 5% to 50%, depending on patient characteristics, type of surgery, duration of postoperative monitoring, and criteria used to define atrial fibrillation.[15–19] A meta-analysis of 24 trials estimated the incidence at 26.7%.[17] Patients undergoing CABG alone have a lower incidence of atrial fibrillation than patients undergoing valve surgery. The highest incidence is found in combined CABG and valve surgery.

Atrial fibrillation most commonly develops on postoperative day 2 or 3, but can occur at any point in the recovery period. Many patients (25–80%) spontaneously convert to sinus rhythm within 24 h. Most patients convert to normal sinus rhythm by 6 weeks.[15,20]

Morbidity and Mortality

Atrial fibrillation is associated with prolonged hospitalization, hemodynamic instability, and increased risk for cardiac thromboembolism. The risk of stroke increases threefold in patients with postoperative atrial fibrillation. It has been estimated that hospital charges are increased by $10,000 to $11,000 per patient with atrial fibrillation.[21] Even after adjustment for severity of illness, patients with atrial fibrillation have longer intensive care unit and total hospital lengths of stay.[21] Moreover, patients who develop postoperative atrial fibrillation have significantly higher 30-day and 6-month mortality rates compared with patients who do not develop this arrhythmia.

Risk Stratification

Several preoperative, intraoperative, and postoperative factors are associated with the development of atrial fibrillation with cardiac surgery. Increasing age is the most consistent predictor of postoperative atrial fibrillation with patients 65 years of age and older being 2.7 times more likely to develop postoperative atrial fibrillation than younger patients. Multiple studies have shown that patients with a history of chronic obstructive pulmonary disease, hypertension, hyperlipidemia, valve surgery, preoperative withdrawal of beta-blockers, and atrial fibrillation are at increased risk for developing postoperative atrial fibrillation.[15-19] A multicenter prospective observational study of 4757 patients undergoing CABG surgery allowed for the development of a risk index to identify patients at risk of developing postoperative atrial fibrillation.[19] This risk index may help identify patients for whom prophylactic therapy can be considered.

Prophylaxis and Treatment

Current guidelines from the American Heart Association/American College of Cardiology (ACC/AHA) and the European Society of Cardiology (ESC) recommend prophylactic beta-blocker therapy for all patients without contraindications undergoing CABG as it decreases the incidence of postoperative atrial fibrillation by as much as 70–80%. Prophylaxis with amiodarone or sotalol is reserved for patients at high-risk for developing postoperative atrial fibrillation (i.e., those with a history of atrial fibrillation, left atrial enlargement, or valvular heart disease).[15-23] Management strategies for persistent and recurrent atrial fibrillation are usually targeted at rate control, electrolyte repletion, and rhythm control for patients at high risk for bleeding with anticoagulation therapy.[20-23] Although spontaneous conversion within 24 h is common after cardiac surgery, patients with atrial fibrillation for more than 48 h should be considered for anticoagulation.

RENAL DISEASE

Incidence

Acute renal failure (ARF) after cardiac surgery is a well-recognized complication. It develops in approximately 5–30% of patients undergoing cardiac surgery, depending on the type of surgery, definition used for ARF, and duration of postoperative period studied. ARF requiring dialysis occurs in approximately 1% of patients. The mortality rate in this group is 63.7% versus 4.3% without ARF.[24–26] CABG has the lowest incidence of ARF followed by valvular surgery with the highest incidence noted in combined CABG/valvular procedures.

Approximately 2–5% of patients undergoing CABG have prior renal dysfunction. This comorbidity has been steadily increasing over the last decade due to an aging population and an increasing incidence of diabetes and hypertension.[6]

Patients who develop ARF have higher rates of mortality, complicated hospital course, risk of infections, and resource utilization, with the worst outcomes seen in patients requiring hemodialysis.[25,26] Emerging evidence suggests that even mild renal dysfunction (serum creatinine 1.47–2.25 mg/dL) is associated with increased rates of perioperative and long-term mortality, need for postoperative dialysis, and postoperative stroke.[27]

Risk Stratification

Prediction of ARF can provide an opportunity to develop a strategy for early diagnosis, risk modification, and prevention. Chertow et al. were among the first to develop a risk algorithm to predict postoperative ARF.[24] More recently, the Cleveland Clinic Foundation has developed a clinical risk scoring system to better identify these patients.[28] This risk index is discussed in more detail in Chapter 34. Increasing age, preexisting renal dysfunction, severity of heart failure, and cardiopulmonary bypass time are some of the significant risk factors noted in several studies.[24–28] Criteria to predict ARF has been studied in patients after cardiothoracic surgery by Lassnigg et al.[29] and found to be effective in finding patients at risk of adverse postoperative outcomes.

Management

Efforts to minimize renal injury include decreasing contrast load and optimizing patient volume status. There are not enough data to conclusively demonstrate the benefits of pharmacological therapy in the prevention of ARF. The basic tests for renal function evaluation include a urinalysis, serum creatinine (Cr), blood urea nitrogen (BUN)/Cr ratio, urine and plasma osmolality, fractional excretion of sodium (FENa), and free water clearance. Free water clearance is a simple and accurate method of identifying early subclinical renal dysfunction.

Ensuring the patient is not obstructed is an appropriate initial step in evaluating and managing ARF. Differentiating between prerenal and intrinsic renal causes of renal failure can be challenging. However, given that prerenal etiologies of ARF are more common, it is prudent to optimize hemodynamics by ensuring adequate cardiac output, avoiding hypotension, and confirming appropriate blood volume. It is also important to avoid nephrotoxins and renally dose medications. Once renal failure is established, early and aggressive hemofiltration/hemodialysis decreases mortality in cardiac surgery patients. This intervention may also decrease time on mechanical ventilation, shorten intensive care unit stay, and possibly improve the rate of renal recovery.

PULMONARY DISEASE

Incidence

Pulmonary complications after cardiac surgery are common and range from 8% to 79%. Atelectasis, pleural effusion, and pneumonia are the most frequent pulmonary complications post CABG.[30,31] Other complications include hemothorax, pulmonary edema, and diaphragmatic dysfunction.

The high incidence of pulmonary complications is in part due to the disruption of normal ventilatory function, performance of pleurotomy, trauma to the chest wall, and use of an internal mammary artery graft. Furthermore, patients undergoing cardiac surgery often have underlying lung disease and/or pulmonary dysfunction secondary to cardiac disease that increases their susceptibility for postoperative respiratory complications. Bando et al. found that a major determinant of poor pulmonary outcomes after cardiac surgery is poor cardiac function.[32]

Developments in minimally invasive surgery, non-bypass techniques, and advances in anesthesia have reduced the physiologic stress of surgery and subsequent risk of postoperative pulmonary complications. However, pulmonary complications remain an important cause of postcardiac surgical morbidity, prolonged hospital stays, and increased healthcare cost.

Risk Factors

Risk factors for postoperative atelectasis include age >65 years, diabetes, and an American Society of Anesthesiologists (ASA) classification >3. The development of postoperative pneumonia has been associated with previous myocardial infarction, mechanical ventilation >10 h, and a hospital stay >5 days. Cohen and colleagues found that patients with significant chronic obstructive pulmonary disease (COPD) undergoing CABG have higher rates of arrhythmias, reintubation, and longer lengths of stay in the ICU.[33] Fuster and colleagues noted that a forced expiratory volume in 1 s (FEV_1) of <60% of predicted is associated with higher mortality during CABG.[34] COPD is the most common cause of perioperative pulmonary dysfunction. Hence, clinical assessment of lung function and severity of COPD is a critical component of the preoperative assessment. The most common cause of postoperative pulmonary edema is preexisting left ventricular dysfunction, coupled with the negative inotropic effects of anesthesia.[30–32,35,36] No significant risk factors have been related to the development of pleural effusion.

Prolonged mechanical ventilation is a common complication after cardiac surgery. Prolonged mechanical ventilation not only increases the duration of ICU length of stay, but also increases total hospital stay and resource utilization. Among few other risk scoring systems, the Spivack Scoring System (SSS) helps to predict the risk of prolonged mechanical ventilation for patients undergoing CABG.[37] It has been validated by Yende and Wunderink[38] and can be used as a preoperative screening tool. Risk factors for prolonged mechanical ventilation include advanced age, postoperative renal dysfunction, severe left ventricular dysfunction, and pulmonary hypertension.[37-39] Preoperative screening of arterial oxygen concentration on room air can provide guidance in respiratory management postoperatively. The roles of preoperative spirometry and perioperative bronchodilators remain unclear in stable patients, and thus cannot be recommended on a routine basis.

Prevention and Treatment

Preoperative effort should be directed toward smoking cessation, optimizing the management of COPD, and aggressively treating any respiratory infections. Preoperative inspiratory muscle training is associated with reduction in postoperative pulmonary complications and can be considered in high-risk patients undergoing cardiac surgery.[40] Intraoperative improvement of respiratory function can be aided by maintaining an intact pleura, especially during harvesting of the internal mammary graft.

Postoperatively, interventions focusing on airway management, endotracheal suctioning, and physical therapy that includes deep breathing and coughing exercises are highly recommended. Incentive spirometry is one of the most effective methods to reduce the risk of pulmonary complications after surgery.[40]

NEUROLOGIC COMPLICATIONS AND CAROTID ARTERY DISEASE

Incidence

Neurological complications after cardiac surgery include encephalopathy, intellectual and memory functional decline, and focal neurological dysfunction. Perioperative stroke carries significant morbidity and mortality with an incidence ranging from 1% to 6% after cardiac surgery.[41] Carotid artery disease is responsible for as many as 30% of postoperative strokes. It is believed that neurologic complications are often related to the effects of cardiopulmonary bypass. Cerebral microembolization from the arterial tree during CABG is likely the most common culprit.

Risk Factors

Risk factors for stroke likely depend more on a patient's preoperative condition rather than intraoperative factors. An analysis from Boeken and colleagues showed that among 783 patients undergoing cardiac surgery, the predictors of central nervous system complications included symptomatic cerebrovascular disease, advanced age, diabetes, advanced renal failure, urgent surgery, and aortic atheroma.[42] He developed a risk prediction tool, which can be used preoperatively to asses the risk of neurological complications following cardiac surgery.

The independent risk factors predictive of stroke as determined by Aboyans et al. included history of stroke or transient ischemic attack (TIA), neck bruit, clinically apparent peripheral arterial disease (PAD) or subclinical PAD (ankle brachial index [ABI] <0.85 or >1.5), and age >70 years.[11] Charlesworth and colleagues also developed a prediction model to estimate the perioperative risk of stroke.[43]

Prevention and Treatment

Efforts should be focused on the identification and management of significant carotid artery disease, perioperative hemodynamics, and arrhythmias such as atrial fibrillation. The ACC/AHA guidelines state that selective carotid artery screening should be considered in high-risk patient populations. According to these guidelines, carotid endarterectomy (CEA) should be considered either prior to, or as a combined procedure with CABG.

DIABETES

Diabetes is an important risk factor for atherosclerotic heart disease and a significant predictor of in-hospital mortality after CABG. Although the Bypass Angioplasty Revascularization Investigation (BARI) did not evaluate patients with coronary artery stents, it demonstrated that diabetic patients with multivessel disease have greater survival with CABG compared with those who receive percutaneous coronary intervention (PCI).

Postoperative mortality is higher in diabetic patients with vascular and/or renal disease compared with those without these complications.[44] Furthermore, diabetic patients who undergo CABG have more renal and neurologic complications, longer ICU stays, require more blood transfusions, and have higher reopening rates. Diabetic patients who undergo valve operations have a fivefold increased risk of a major pulmonary complication.[45]

Patients with undiagnosed diabetes are also at higher risk perioperatively. Undergoing CABG with undiagnosed diabetes leads higher rates of resuscitation and reintubation, longer periods of ventilatory support, and a higher 30-day mortality rate compared with known diabetic patients. These findings underscore the importance of screening patients for diabetes in the preoperative setting.[46]

HEMATOLOGICAL COMPLICATIONS

There are several hematological complications related to cardiothoracic surgery procedures with anemia and thrombocytopenia being the most common. Approaches to identify these conditions as well as methods to minimize the untoward complications have been described in the literature.

Anemia

Anemia is an independent risk factor for perioperative complications and mortality in cardiothoracic surgery patients.[47] Patients with mean hematocrit values below

25% during CABG had higher morbidity than those with mean values above 28%.[48] The use of blood conservation techniques is recommended to avoid complications related to blood transfusions. The management of anemia varies according to the etiology.

Preoperative Period Hemoglobin values of 13 mg/dL for men and 12 mg/dL for women should be the goal before sending the patient to the operation room,[47] and a variety of techniques can be used to achieve this goal. Increasing the red blood cell mass with erythropoietin-stimulating agents can reduce the number of blood transfusions.[49] However, the safety and cost-effectiveness of using these agents has been a source of debate. Using these agents in cardiothoracic surgery patients would be considered an "off-label" use.

Autologous donation in the weeks preceding surgery is the safest form of transfusion by decreasing the risk for infection and autoimmune reaction. Although the risk of mismatch during storage exists, the overall risk of transfusion reaction is definitively less when compared with allogeneic donation.[50] The downside of autologous donation is the uncertainty of the number of units needed to donate in addition to the high percentage of wasted blood product. Autologous donation is contraindicated in patients with bacteremia, unstable angina, uncontrolled heart failure, severe aortic stenosis, anemia, and carotid artery disease with recent TIA.[50]

Intraoperative Period During the procedure, a patient may become anemic from either acute blood loss or hemolysis. Some of the agents that have been used to control intraoperative blood loss include antifibrinolytics such as aminocaproic acid, tranexamic acid, desmopressin, and aprotinin. Additionally, cell saver technique can be used when the expected blood loss is equal to 20% of the total body blood volume. Another technique is acute normovolemic hemodilution in which a volume of blood is replaced with colloid or crystalloid at the beginning of the surgical procedure and then transfused back to the patient when hemostasis has been achieved or when the hematocrit drops below 18%.

Postoperative Period Blood transfusion thresholds should be individualized and match the patients' clinical condition. Patients with a hemoglobin level less than 6 g/dL usually require transfusion. In patients with a hemoglobin more than 10 g/dL, transfusion should be avoided. Between 6 and 10 g/dL, blood transfusions should only be administered after careful evaluation of the clinical scenario to determine if the benefits will outweigh the potential risks (i.e., mismatched units, allergic reactions, infection transmission).

Recent publications have shown an increased use of blood products (packed red blood cells and fresh frozen plasma) in patients taking antiplatelet medications such as clopidogrel and aspirin in the days prior to surgery. These results continue to support the idea of holding antiplatelet treatment for 7 days before elective cardiothoracic surgery.[51]

Hemolysis

The use of minimized extracorporeal circulation (MECC) continues to show less hematological effects (such as hemolysis) when compared with conventional cardiopulmonary bypass. Additionally, recent studies suggest MECC poses less of an effect on platelet aggregation when compared with conventional cardiopulmonary bypass circuits (CCEC).

Thrombocytopenia

Thrombocytopenia is frequent in the cardiothoracic surgery population and the potential etiologies are diverse. It is well known that 25–50% of patients exposed to cardiopulmonary bypass during heart surgery are positive for heparin-dependent antibodies and 1–3% develop heparin-induced thrombocytopenia (HIT).[52] A decrease of 50% or more in the platelet count or an unexpected arterial or venous thrombotic event should trigger a high suspicion of HIT. Cessation of all heparin products (including low-molecular-weight heparins) should occur while confirmatory studies are obtained. Anticoagulation with a direct thrombin inhibitor agent such as bivalirudin or argatroban should be initiated as treatment for HIT and avoidance of thrombotic complications.

Patients with confirmed HIT after cardiothoracic surgery have increased morbidity and mortality. The incidence of sepsis in cardiothoracic surgery patients with HIT is significantly higher than those without HIT. The incidence of renal failure and limb ischemia are also reported to be higher in patients with HIT.

Thrombocytopenia can also occur after AVR. The literature suggests that bioprosthetic valves decrease the incidence of thrombocytopenia when compared with mechanical valves.[53]

GI COMPLICATIONS AFTER CARDIOTHORACIC SURGERY PROCEDURES

GI complications are present in 1.2–1.5 % of cardiothoracic procedures.[54] In addition to increasing hospital length of stay and costs, GI complications are also associated with increased mortality. Although the specific etiology of GI complications is not completely understood, the pathophysiology likely involves some level of gut ischemic due to pump failure, vascular disease, and release of vasoactive mediators.

Upper GI Bleeding

Although the overall incidence of upper GI bleeding as a complication from cardiothoracic surgery has shown to be approximately 1% in published series, the mortality can be up to 15–20%. This highlights the importance of early diagnostic studies (such as endoscopy) and aggressive resuscitation with transfusion when indicated.[55]

Lower GI Bleeding

In contrast to upper GI bleeding, bleeding from the lower GI tract has a much higher incidence of up to 10%. The mortality associated with lower GI bleeding in the cardiothoracic surgery patient is similar at approximately 17%.[55] In the stable patient, identifying the bleeding source with a tagged red blood cell scan is a reasonable first step, followed by embolization if the source is identified. Urgent surgery is indicated in the presence of massive bleeding, often defined by the use of 5 or more units of packed red blood cells in the first 24 h.

Ischemic Bowel

Ischemic bowel is a rare but potentially catastrophic complication. Although ischemic bowel is an infrequent finding at less than 0.2% of all cardiothoracic surgery cases, its mortality is roughly 50% in conservative case series. While the more common nonocclusive type due to hypoperfusion can present more insidiously, occlusive mesenteric ischemia from thrombus formation is acute and leads to rapid clinical deterioration.[55]

In the presence of nonocclusive ischemic bowel, the goal is to improve perfusion with efforts directed toward adequate resuscitation. Occlusive ischemia requires an early diagnosis and a prompt multidisciplinary treatment approach with vascular surgery and interventional radiology.

CONCLUSION

Cardiac surgeries are high-risk procedures that require careful preoperative and postoperative management. Given the multiple medical comorbidities often present in this patient population, general internists such as hospitalists are commonly involved in their perioperative care. By understanding a patient's preoperative risk, in addition to preparing for common postoperative complications, the hospitalist's partnership with the cardiothoracic surgeon will be poised to optimize medical care and surgical outcomes.

REFERENCES

1. The Society of Thoracic Surgeons National database. Executive Summaries, Adult Cardiac Surgery Database, 2011. Available at http://www.sts.org/national-database/database-managers/executive-summaries. Accessed June 2, 2011.
2. Edwards FH. The STS database at 20 years: a tribute to Dr Richard E Clark. *Ann Thorac Surg.* 2010;89(1):9.
3. Edwards FH. Evolution of the Society of Thoracic Surgeons National Cardiac Surgery Database. *J Invasive Cardiol.* 1998;10:485–488.
4. Welke KF, Peterson ED, Vaughan-Sarrazin MS, et al. Comparison of cardiac surgery volumes and mortality rates between the Society of Thoracic Surgeons and Medicare databases from 1993 through 2001. *Ann Thorac Surg.* 2007;84:1538–1546.
5. Granton J, Cheng D. Risk stratification models for cardiac surgery. *Semin Cardiothorac Vasc Anesth.* 2008;12:167–174.
6. Bacchetta MD, Ko W, Girardi LN, et al. Outcomes of cardiac surgery in nonagenarians: a 10-year experience. *Ann Thorac Surg.* 2003;75:1215–1220.
7. Cohn LH, Edmunds LH, Jr. (eds.). *Cardiac Surgery in the Adult.* New York: McGraw-Hill; 2003, pp. 235–248.

8. Eagle KA, Guyton RA, Davidoff R, et al. ACC/AHA 2004 guideline update for coronary artery bypass graft surgery: summary article. A report of the American College of Cardiology/American Heart Association task force on practice guidelines (committee to update the 1999 guidelines for coronary artery bypass graft surgery). *Circulation*. 2004;110:1168–1176.

9. Schwartz LB, Bridgman AH, Kieffer RW, et al. Asymptomatic carotid artery stenosis and stroke in patients undergoing cardiopulmonary bypass. *J Vasc Surg*. 1995;21:146–153.

10. Hogan WJ, McBane RD, Santrach PJ, et al. Antiphospholipid syndrome and perioperative hemostatic management of cardiac valvular surgery. *Mayo Clin Proc*. 2000;75:971–976.

11. Aboyans V, Lacroix P, Guilloux L, et al. A predictive model for screening cerebrovascular disease in patient undergoing coronary artery bypass grafting. *Interact Cardiovasc Thorac Surg*. 2005;4:90–95.

12. Hammermeister KE, Burchfiel C. Identification of patients at greatest risk for developing major complications at cardiac surgery. *Circulation*. 1990;82(5):380–389.

13. Dewey TM, Brown D, Ryan WH, Herbert MA, Prince SL, Mack MJ. Reliability of risk algorithms in predicting early and late operative outcomes in high-risk patients undergoing aortic valve replacement. *J Thorac Cardiovasc Surg*. 2008;135:180–187.

14. Kurki TS, Jarvinen O, Kataja MJ, Laurikka J, Tarkka M. Performance of three preoperative risk indices; CABDEAL, EuroSCORE and Cleveland models in a prospective coronary bypass database. *Eur J Cardiothorac Surg*. 2002;21:406–410.

15. Maisel WH, Rawn JD, Stevenson WG. Atrial fibrillation after cardiac surgery. *Ann Intern Med*. 2001;135:1061–1073.

16. Funk M, Richards SB, Desjardins J, Bebon C, Wilcox H. Incidence, timing, symptoms, and risk factors for atrial fibrillation after cardiac surgery. *Am J Crit Care*. 2003;12:424–433.

17. Andrews TC, Reimold SC, Berlin JA, Antman EM. Prevention of supraventricular arrhythmias after coronary artery bypass surgery. A meta-analysis of randomized control trials. *Circulation*. 1991;84(5 Suppl):III236–III244.

18. Kailasam R, Palin CA, Hogue CW, Jr. Atrial fibrillation after cardiac surgery: an evidence-based approach to prevention. *Semin Cardiothorac Vasc Anesth*. 2005;9:77–85.

19. Mathew JP, Fontes ML, Tudor IC, et al. A multicenter risk index for atrial fibrillation after cardiac surgery. *JAMA*. 2004;291:1720–1729.

20. Aranki SF, Shaw DP, Adams DH, et al. Predictors of atrial fibrillation after isolated coronary artery surgery. Current trends and impact on hospital resources. *Circulation*. 1996;94:390–397.

21. Hravnak M, Hoffman LA, Saul MI, Zullo TG, Whitman GR, Griffith BP. Predictors and impact of atrial fibrillation after isolated coronary artery bypass grafting. *Crit Care Med*. 2002;30:330–337.

22. Echahidi N, Pibarot P, O'Hara G, Mathieu P. Mechanisms, prevention, and treatment of atrial fibrillation after cardiac surgery. *J Am Coll Cardiol*. 2008;51:793–801.

23. Durham SJ, Gold JP. Late complications of cardiac surgery. In: *Cardiac Surgery in the Adult*, Cohn LH (ed.), pp. 535–548. New York: McGraw-Hill; 2008.

24. Chertow GM, Lazarus JM, Christiansen CL, et al. Preoperative renal risk stratification. *Circulation*. 1997;95:878–884.

25. Mangano CM, Diamondstone LS, Ramsay JG, et al. Renal dysfunction after myocardial revascularization: risk factors, adverse outcomes, and hospital resource utilization. *Ann Intern Med*. 1998;128:194–203.

26. Rosner MH, Okusa MD. Acute kidney injury associated with cardiac surgery. *Clin J Am Soc Nephrol*. 2006;1:19–32.

27. Devbhandari MP, Duncan AJ, Grayson AD, et al. Effect of risk-adjusted, non-dialysis-dependent renal dysfunction on mortality and morbidity following coronary artery bypass surgery: a multicentre study. *Eur J Cardiothorac Surg*. 2006;29:964–970.

28. Thakar CV, Arrigain S, Worley S, Yared JP, Paganini EP. A clinical score to predict acute renal failure after cardiac surgery. *J Am Soc Nephrol*. 2005;16:162–168.

29. Lassnigg A, Schmid ER, Hiesmayr M, et al. Impact of minimal increases in serum creatinine on outcome in patients after cardiothoracic surgery: do we have to revise current definitions of acute renal failure? *Crit Care Med*. 2008;36:1129–1137.

30. Wynne R, Botti M. Postoperative pulmonary dysfunction in adults after cardiac surgery with cardio-pulmonary bypass: clinical significance and implications for practice. *Am J Crit Care.* 2004;13: 384–393.
31. Ng CSH, Wan S, Yim APC, Arifi AA. Pulmonary dysfunction after cardiac surgery. *Chest.* 2002;121:1269–1277.
32. Bando K, Sun K, Binford RS, Sharp TG. Determinants of longer duration of endotracheal intubation after adult cardiac operations. *Ann Thorac Surg.* 1997;63:1026–1033.
33. Cohen A, Katz M, Katz R, Hauptman E, Schachner A. Chronic obstructive pulmonary disease in patients undergoing coronary artery bypass grafting. *J Thorac Cardiovasc Surg.* 1995;109: 574–581.
34. Fuster RG, Argudo JAM, Albarova OG, et al. Prognostic value of chronic obstructive pulmonary disease in coronary artery bypass grafting. *Eur J Cardiothorac Surg.* 2006;29:202–209.
35. Rady MY, Ryan T, Starr NJ. Early onset of acute pulmonary dysfunction after cardiovascular surgery: risk factors and clinical outcome. *Crit Care Med.* 1997;25:1831–1839.
36. Higgins TL, Yared JP, Paranandi L, Baldyga A, Starr NJ. Risk factors for respiratory complications after cardiac surgery. *Anesthesiology.* 1991;75:A258.
37. Spivack SD, Shinozaki T, Albertini JJ, Deane R. Preoperative prediction of postoperative respiratory outcome: coronary artery bypass grafting. *Chest.* 1996;109:1222–1230.
38. Yende S, Wunderink R. Validity of scoring systems to predict risk of prolonged mechanical ventilation after coronary artery bypass graft surgery. *Chest.* 2002;122:239–244.
39. Doering LV, Imperial-Perez F, Monsein S, Esmailian F. Preoperative and postoperative predictors of early and delayed extubation after coronary artery bypass surgery. *Am J Crit Care.* 1998;7:37–44.
40. Hulzebos EH, Helders PJ, Favie NJ, et al. Preoperative intensive inspiratory muscle training to prevent postoperative pulmonary complications in high-risk patients undergoing CABG surgery: a randomized clinical trial. *JAMA.* 2006;296:1851–1857.
41. Roach GW, Kanchugar M, Mangano CM, et al. Adverse cerebral outcomes after coronary bypass surgery. Multicenter study of Perioperative Ischemia Research Group and the Ischemia Research and Education Foundation Investigators. *N Engl J Med.* 1996;335:1857–1863.
42. Boeken U, Litmathe J, Feindt P, Gams E. Neurological complications after cardiac surgery: risk factors and correlation to the surgical procedure. *Thorac Cardiovasc Surg.* 2005;53(1):33–36.
43. Charlesworth DC, Likosky DS, Marrin CA, et al. Development and validation of a prediction model for strokes following coronary artery bypass grafting. *Ann Thorac Surg.* 2003;76:436–443.
44. Leavitt BJ, Sheppard L, Maloney C, et al. Effects of diabetes and associated conditions on long-term survival after coronary artery bypass graft surgery. *Circulation.* 2004;110(11 Suppl 1):II41–II44.
45. Albacker T, Carvalho G, Schricker T, Lachapelle K. High-dose insulin therapy attenuates systemic inflammatory response in coronary artery bypass grafting patients. *Ann Thorac Surg.* 2008;86: 20–27.
46. Lauruschkat AH, Arnrich B, Albert AA, et al. Prevalence and risks of undiagnosed diabetes mellitus in patients undergoing coronary artery bypass grafting. *Circulation.* 2005;112:2397–2402.
47. van Straten AHM, Hamad MAS, van Zundert AJ, Martens EJ, Schonberger JPAM, de Wolf AM. Preoperative hemoglobin level as a predictor of survival after coronary artery bypass grafting: a comparison with the matched general population. *Circulation.* 2009;120:118–125.
48. Ranucci M, Conti D, Castelvecchio S, et al. Hematocrit on cardiopulmonary bypass and outcome after coronary surgery in nontransfused patients. *Ann Thorac Surg.* 2010;89(1):11–17.
49. Podesta A, Parodi E, Dottori V, Crivellari R, Passerone GC. Epoetin alpha in elective coronary and valve surgery in Jehovah's Witnesses patients. Experience in 45 patients. *Minerva Cardioangiol.* 2002;50(2):125–131.
50. Owings DV, Kruskal MS, Thurer RL, et al. Autologous blood donations prior to elective cardiac surgery: safety and effect on subsequent blood use. *JAMA.* 1989;262:1963–1968.
51. Badreldin A, Koerner A, Kamiya H, Lichtenberg A, Hekmat K. Effect of clopidogrel on perioperative blood loss and transfusion in coronary artery bypass graft surgery. *Interact Cardiovasc Thorac Surg.* 2010;10:48–52.
52. Pouplard C, Regina S, May MA, Gruel Y. Heparin-induced thrombocytopenia: a frequent complication after cardiac surgery. *Arch Mal Coeur Vaiss.* 2007;100:563–568.

53. van Straten AH, Hamad MA, Berreklouw E, Ter Woorst JF, Martens EJ, Tan ME. Thrombocytopenia after aortic valve replacement: comparison between mechanical and biological valves. *J Heart Valve Dis*. 2010;19(3):394–399.

54. Diaz-Gomez JL, Nutter B, Xu M, et al. The effect of postoperative gastrointestinal complications in patients undergoing coronary artery bypass surgery. *Ann Thorac Surg*. 2010;90:109–115.

55. Rodriguez R, Robich MP, Plate JF, Trooskin SZ, Sellke FW. Gastrointestinal complications following cardiac surgery: a comprehensive review. *J Card Surg*. 2010;25:188–197.

CHAPTER 21

INTRA-ABDOMINAL AND PELVIC SURGERY

M. Chadi Alraies and Franklin Michota

BACKGROUND

Every year, 20 million Americans undergo surgery; almost half are abdominal and pelvic surgeries. Lately, and because of the increased incidence of obesity and early cancer screening, the number of abdominal and pelvic surgeries increased. Respiratory complications (i.e., pneumonia, atelectasis, and respiratory failure with prolonged ventilation) are common complications of upper abdomen surgeries especially for obese patients or patients with chronic lung disease (i.e., chronic obstructive pulmonary disease [COPD] and asthma). Furthermore, 20–30% of these surgeries are cancer related, which by itself increases the risk for other complications including delayed wound healing and venous thromboembolism (VTE). The frequency of these complications can be reduced with proper preoperative evaluation and postoperative preventive measures.

SURGERY-SPECIFIC RISK

Overall, intra-abdominal and pelvic surgery is considered an intermediate risk surgery with respect to cardiovascular risk and is associated with a <5% risk for cardiovascular complications. However, there are unique aspects of intra-abdominal and pelvic surgery that may increase the risk for postoperative pulmonary complication (PPC) compared with other types of surgery. For intra-abdominal cases, surgery-specific risk factors for PPCs include surgical sites close to the diaphragm, duration of surgery over 3 h, and the use of general anesthesia. In addition, many intra-abdominal surgery patients have comorbidities that can further increase PPC rates and should be factored into the overall risk equation. For example, an albumin of <4 g/dL is an independent risk factor for PPC and may be found in intra-abdominal surgery patients with cancer or inflammatory bowel disease (IBD). Chronic lung

Perioperative Medicine: Medical Consultation and Co-Management, First Edition.
Edited by Amir K. Jaffer and Paul J. Grant.
© 2012 Wiley-Blackwell. Published 2012 by John Wiley & Sons, Inc.

disease also increases the risk for PPC and may present in bariatric surgery patients with concomitant obstructive sleep apnea (OSA).

PREOPERATIVE ASSESSMENT

The preoperative assessment for intra-abdominal and pelvic surgery is no different than that performed for other surgical procedures. Cardiovascular risk should be determined using the American Heart Association/American College of Cardiology (AHA/ACC) guidelines for preoperative assessment of cardiac risk for patients undergoing noncardiac surgery.[1] Emphasis should be placed on the history and physical with targeted laboratory testing. Unique aspects to the preoperative assessment include increased risk for PPCs and two special patient groups—those with IBD and morbid obesity (bariatric surgery patients).

As stated in the previous section, PPCs are common in patients undergoing intra-abdominal procedures, particularly upper abdomen surgeries. These complications include pneumonia, respiratory failure with prolonged mechanical ventilation, bronchospasm, symptomatic atelectasis, and exacerbation of underlying chronic lung disease. Patients that smoke should be strongly encouraged to stop. Smoking increases PPCs even in the absence of underlying pulmonary disease, and this risk declines only if smoking is stopped 8 weeks prior to surgery. Patients with underlying pulmonary disease should be at their baseline lung function prior to proceeding with elective surgery. Patients with COPD should be treated with daily ipratropium or tiotropium with an as needed beta-agonist agent. These medications should be continued the morning of surgery and throughout the perioperative period. COPD patients with active lung disease may benefit from corticosteroids and/or antibiotics perioperatively.[2] Lung expansion maneuvers, such as deep breathing exercises or the use of incentive spirometry, should be taught to all patients at risk for PPC in the preoperative visit. Preoperative education of lung expansion maneuvers has been shown to reduce the risk for PPC compared with postoperative education.[3]

One-half of patients with IBD need at least one abdominal surgery during the course of their disease.[4] Patients with IBD are typically young and have no underlying medical problems that need to be addressed prior to surgery. However, IBD surgery may have a significant psychological effect, particularly in patients who will receive an ostomy. Counseling and education prior to ostomy surgery are important components to a successful postoperative outcome. Individuals with severe cases of IBD who require surgical intervention are frequently sick, anemic from persistent gastrointestinal (GI) bleeding and/or coagulopathy, immunosuppressed from medication, and/or have ongoing infection. If possible, all comorbidities should be optimized prior to surgery. Anemia and coagulopathy should be treated appropriately including the potential use of supplemental iron, erythropoietin, and vitamin K. Malnutrition prior to surgery is associated with a number of complications perioperatively including poor surgical wound healing, prolonged ventilation and ICU stay. Parenteral nutrition may be beneficial prior to surgery, especially in patients who need variable degrees of bowel rest. Perioperative infection associated with immunosuppressive therapy (prednisone, azathioprine and 6-mercaptopurine, mesalamine,

TABLE 21.1.   STOP-BANG Questionnaire for Obstructive
Sleep Apnea Screening

S	Snoring
T	Tiredness during the daytime
O	Observed apnea
P	Hypertension (pressure)
B	Body mass index (BMI) >35 kg/m^2
A	Age >50 years
N	Neck circumference >17" for males or >16" for females
G	Male gender or postmenopausal female

cyclosporine, and tumor necrosis factor-alpha [TNF-α] inhibitors) remains a concern as the available literature is conflicting. The majority of IBD patients is on extended systemic steroids prior to surgery and will need stress dose steroids perioperatively to avoid adrenal insufficiency and hypotension. High-dose steroids (hydrocortisone 125 g IV once on the day of surgery) are required for any patient prescribed prednisone ≥20 mg/day for 30 days in the last 12 months. Steroids can be tapered after surgery if the disease is not active. In addition, IBD patients are at even greater risk for arterial and venous thrombosis compared with other intra-abdominal surgery patients and need appropriate VTE prophylaxis with pharmacologic agents.

Bariatric surgery patients also have some unique preoperative features. There is an increased prevalence of undiagnosed OSA in bariatric surgery patients.

OSA has been associated with an increased rate of postoperative atrial fibrillation, lung infection, encephalopathy, and longer intensive care unit stay. Compliance with noninvasive positive pressure ventilation (CPAP, BiPAP) has been shown to reduce morbidity, particularly if treatment is begun 6 weeks prior to surgery. Screening by history with the use of a validated instrument, such as the STOP-BANG questionnaire (Table 21.1),[5] followed by confirmatory testing (polysomnogram) and subsequent preoperative treatment (nightly continuous positive airway pressure) should be included in the preoperative assessment of morbidly obese surgery patients. Much like IBD patients, bariatric surgery patients have an increased risk for VTE above that associated with surgery and anesthesia alone. In addition, appropriate pharmacologic prophylaxis may include drug doses that are greater than that used in other normal weight surgical patients. Finally, the preoperative assessment should include consideration for the resources and equipment of the surgical center. Morbidly obese patients often require special equipment (magnetic resonance imaging, computed tomography (CT), stretchers, operating table, beds and toilets, etc.) that can accommodate their size.

POST-OP ASSESSMENT

The postoperative assessment is no different than that performed for other surgical procedures. Evaluation of any preoperative comorbidities along with a general examination of mental status, the cardiopulmonary system, abdomen, surgical site, and signs and symptoms of VTE should be performed daily until hospital discharge.

MEDICAL MANAGEMENT

Postoperative pain control is important to prevent respiratory complications, along with aggressive use of lung expansion maneuvers (deep breathing exercises, incentive spirometry, intermittent positive pressure breathing, CPAP).[3] CPAP is considered a secondary intervention in patients with refractory atelectasis, yet should be a primary prevention strategy in patients who are less cooperative and unable to perform regular deep breathing exercises or incentive spirometry.[6]

Postoperative ileus (POI) is a common and costly complication of intra-abdominal surgery. POI is a nonmechanical bowel obstruction that disrupts the normal coordinated motor activity of the GI tract.[7] POI can happen with any surgical intervention; however, it happens in 15% in patients undergoing abdominal hysterectomy and 3% of bowel resection surgeries.[8] Duration of ileus varies with the part of the GI involved. Small bowel ileus lasts 0–24 h, while colonic ileus may last up to 72 h. Prolonged ileus increases postoperative morbidity by delaying oral intake and predisposing the patient to poor wound healing, infection, and the need for parental nutrition. Also, an ileus will further decrease patient mobility translating into an increased risk for VTE and prolonged hospital stay.[9,10] POI presents with abdominal distention, diffuse abdominal pain, nausea and vomiting, inability to pass flatus, and inability to tolerate oral intake. Prolonged POI is defined when any of the above symptoms last longer than 3 days. Reversible causes for ileus (i.e., hypokalemia, hypomagnesemia) should be treated, and mechanical bowel obstruction and ischemia should be ruled out with appropriate imaging studies. A CT scan of the abdomen with oral contrast should be considered when the ileus is not responding to conventional treatment or when the clinical picture is suggestive of small bowel obstruction (SBO) or bowel perforation. It is important to rule out SBO in patients with POI. Compared with POI, SBO is associated with more severe sequelae (bowel perforation, ischemia, necrosis with peritonitis, and sepsis) and will often need early surgical intervention. Risk factors for POI include long-standing diabetes (especially when associated with gastroparesis), previous abdominal and pelvic surgery, and certain patient medications (i.e., opioids, antacids, warfarin, amitriptyline, and chlorpromazine). POI may be reduced with good surgical technique, gentle handling and minimal manipulation of the intestine. In addition, the use of local anesthetics, minimally invasive surgery, limiting the length of abdominal incision, and minimizing opioid use may reduce the risk for POI. There is a misconception that general anesthesia is associated with higher rate of POI; this is not well proven.[11] However, epidural thoracic anesthesia using local anesthetic has been associated with lower rate of POI and reduced mean time for return of GI function.[12] Laparoscopic and minimally invasive surgeries performed through small skin incisions are associated with a lower rate of POI and quicker recovery of the GI function defined by return of flatus or first bowel movement.[13,14] Alvimopan, a peripheral acting μ-opioid receptor antagonist, has been shown to reduce the incidence of POI in patients undergoing bowel surgery and abdominal hysterectomy.[15] Alvimopan studies also demonstrate an earlier return to bowel function as measured by time to first stool, tolerance to an oral regular diet, and hospital length of stay.[16] However, alvimopan has been linked to adverse cardiovascular outcomes and increased neoplastic risk. As a result, strict indication criteria have been initiated by the U.S. Food and Drug Administration to restrict its use for small and large bowel resection with primary anastomosis.

Routine use of a postoperative nasogastric tube (NGT) has been associated with slower return of the bowel function[17] and increased pulmonary complications including pneumonia and atelectasis.[17,18] We recommend avoiding routine NGT placement after abdominal surgery unless clinically indicated. NGT should be considered in the patient with severe abdominal distention or continuous nausea and vomiting. NGT should be placed in the stomach and position confirmed with a plain abdominal X-ray. When using an NGT, the patient should be started on intravenous fluids (half normal saline with 20 mEq/L potassium) along with daily recording patient input and output. Concomitant oral feeding with an NGT is associated with an increased risk of aspiration and therefore not advised. The NGT should be removed when the abdomen is decompressed and bowel sounds are present or when the patient passes flatus.

As mentioned previously, abdominal surgery patients are at increased risk for VTE and should be on pharmacologic VTE prophylaxis postoperatively unless there is a contraindication such as poor hemostasis, severe thrombocytopenia, or coagulopathy. The duration of prophylaxis is usually 7–10 days or until hospital discharge. Cancer patients are a special patient population in regards to VTE risk, and the duration of VTE prophylaxis may need to be extended. Randomized trials have confirmed that VTE prophylaxis with daily subcutaneous low-molecular-weight heparin (LMWH) for up to 4 weeks reduces postoperative VTE.[19,20] Recent VTE prophylaxis guidelines by the American Society of Clinical Oncology recommends 4 weeks of LMWH following major abdominal and pelvic surgery with residual malignant disease, morbid obesity, or previous history of VTE.[21]

DISCHARGE RECOMMENDATIONS

Discharge considerations are similar for intra-abdominal procedures as they would be for other types of surgery. The patient should be able to tolerate an oral diet (liquid to solid food), maintain hydration with oral intake, and demonstrate that they can pass gas and stool. Pain control should be achieved using oral medications. All comorbidities should be optimized prior to discharge. Those patients that require ongoing VTE prophylaxis should be instructed on how to self-inject subcutaneous medications. Some patients will have restrictions on lifting and other physical activities. Patient education regarding activity restrictions as well as the discharge medications should be provided.

SUMMARY

The number of intra-abdominal and pelvic surgeries is increasing yearly. These surgeries are associated with higher rate of VTE and respiratory complications, which increase morbidity, mortality, and hospital length of stay. For patients who are obese, going for upper abdomen or cancer surgeries needs special attention perioperatively, which includes adequate control of underlying lung disease, postoperative pain control, incentive spirometry, and deep vein thrombosis (DVT) prophylaxis.

REFERENCES

1. Fleisher LA, Beckman JA, Brown KA, et al. ACC/AHA 2007 guidelines on perioperative cardiovascular evaluation and care for noncardiac surgery: a report of the American College of Cardiology/American Heart Association Task Force on Practice Guidelines (Writing Committee to Revise the 2002 Guidelines on Perioperative Cardiovascular Evaluation for Noncardiac Surgery) developed in collaboration with the American Society of Echocardiography, American Society of Nuclear Cardiology, Heart Rhythm Society, Society of Cardiovascular Anesthesiologists, Society for Cardiovascular Angiography and Interventions, Society for Vascular Medicine and Biology, and Society for Vascular Surgery. *J Am Coll Cardiol.* Oct 2007;50(17):e159–e241.
2. Celli BR. Perioperative respiratory care of the patient undergoing upper abdominal surgery. *Clin Chest Med.* Jun 1993;14(2):253–261.
3. Celli BR, Rodriguez KS, Snider GL. A controlled trial of intermittent positive pressure breathing, incentive spirometry, and deep breathing exercises in preventing pulmonary complications after abdominal surgery. *Am Rev Respir Dis.* Jul 1984;130(1):12–15.
4. Cima RR, Pemberton JH. Medical and surgical management of chronic ulcerative colitis. *Arch Surg.* Mar 2005;140(3):300–310.
5. Abrishami A, Khajehdehi A, Chung F. A systematic review of screening questionnaires for obstructive sleep apnea. *Can J Anaesth.* May 2010;57(5):423–438.
6. Gold MI, Helrich M. A study of complications related to anesthesia in asthmatic patients. *Anesth Analg.* Mar–Apr 1963;42:238–293.
7. Miedema BW, Johnson JO. Methods for decreasing postoperative gut dysmotility. *Lancet Oncol.* Jun 2003;4(6):365–372.
8. Wolff BG, Viscusi ER, Delaney CP, Du W, Techner L. Patterns of gastrointestinal recovery after bowel resection and total abdominal hysterectomy: pooled results from the placebo arms of alvimopan phase III North American clinical trials. *J Am Coll Surg.* Jul 2007;205(1):43–51.
9. Prasad M, Matthews JB. Deflating postoperative ileus. *Gastroenterology.* Aug 1999;117(2):489–492.
10. Kehlet H, Holte K. Review of postoperative ileus. *Am J Surg.* Nov 2001;182(5A Suppl):3S–10S.
11. Condon RE, Cowles V, Ekbom GA, Schulte WJ, Hess G. Effects of halothane, enflurane, and nitrous oxide on colon motility. *Surgery.* Jan 1987;101(1):81–85.
12. Jorgensen H, Wetterslev J, Moiniche S, Dahl JB. Epidural local anaesthetics versus opioid-based analgesic regimens on postoperative gastrointestinal paralysis, PONV and pain after abdominal surgery. *Cochrane Database Syst Rev.* 2000;(4):CD001893.
13. Bohm B, Milsom JW, Fazio VW. Postoperative intestinal motility following conventional and laparoscopic intestinal surgery. *Arch Surg.* Apr 1995;130(4):415–419.
14. Schwenk W, Bohm B, Haase O, Junghans T, Muller JM. Laparoscopic versus conventional colorectal resection: a prospective randomised study of postoperative ileus and early postoperative feeding. *Langenbecks Arch Surg.* Mar 1998;383(1):49–55.
15. Camilleri M. Alvimopan, a selective peripherally acting mu-opioid antagonist. *Neurogastroenterol Motil.* Apr 2005;17(2):157–165.

16. Traut U, Brugger L, Kunz R, et al. Systemic prokinetic pharmacologic treatment for postoperative adynamic ileus following abdominal surgery in adults. *Cochrane Database Syst Rev.* 2008;(1): CD004930.
17. Nelson R, Edwards S, Tse B. Prophylactic nasogastric decompression after abdominal surgery. *Cochrane Database Syst Rev.* 2005;(1):CD004929.
18. Cheatham ML, Chapman WC, Key SP, Sawyers JL. A meta-analysis of selective versus routine nasogastric decompression after elective laparotomy. *Ann Surg.* May 1995;221(5):469–476; discussion 476–468.
19. Bergqvist D, Agnelli G, Cohen AT, et al. Duration of prophylaxis against venous thromboembolism with enoxaparin after surgery for cancer. *N Engl J Med.* Mar 2002;346(13):975–980.
20. Rasmussen MS, Jorgensen LN, Wille-Jorgensen P, et al. Prolonged prophylaxis with dalteparin to prevent late thromboembolic complications in patients undergoing major abdominal surgery: a multicenter randomized open-label study. *J Thromb Haemost.* Nov 2006;4(11):2384–2390.
21. Lyman GH, Khorana AA, Falanga A, et al. American Society of Clinical Oncology guideline: recommendations for venous thromboembolism prophylaxis and treatment in patients with cancer. *J Clin Oncol.* Dec 2007;25(34):5490–5505.

CHAPTER 22

MAJOR ORTHOPEDIC SURGERY

Barbara Slawski

BACKGROUND

Medical consultants are commonly involved in the care of orthopedic patients, with medical/surgical co-management models becoming common. Orthopedic surgeries are performed in high volumes and account for 11% of all inpatient hospital costs in the United States. The most common orthopedic procedures in the United States are total knee arthroplasty (TKA), total hip arthroplasty (THA), spinal fusion, and hip fracture surgeries (HFSs).[1]

HFS/Orthopedic Trauma

Hip fractures are primarily a disease of the elderly, with 86% of these fractures occurring in patients over age 64.[2] Incidence of hip fractures has declined steadily since 1995,[1] with lifetime risk of hip fracture 17.5% for women and 6.0% for men.[3] Hip fractures and hospitalizations for repair carry significant morbidity and mortality, with 1-year mortality rates reported over 30%. Mortality is higher in males than in females.[1]

Arthroplasty

Over 700,000 joint arthroplasties are performed in the United States annually. Patients with advanced arthritis warranting arthroplasty are usually elderly and have medical comorbidities that may increase surgical risk.

Orthopedic Oncology

Primary bone and soft tissue tumors are rare, representing less than 1% of malignancies,[4,5] and there is limited literature regarding medical management of these patients. Metastatic bone tumors are much more common and represent patients

Perioperative Medicine: Medical Consultation and Co-Management, First Edition.
Edited by Amir K. Jaffer and Paul J. Grant.
© 2012 Wiley-Blackwell. Published 2012 by John Wiley & Sons, Inc.

with significant comorbidities. These patients are diagnostic challenges when they present with unidentified primary tumors.

Other Orthopedic Surgeries

Procedures such as spine surgery are discussed in Chapter 24. Additionally, arthroscopy is primarily an outpatient surgery and will not be addressed in this chapter.

SURGERY-SPECIFIC RISK

Overall Risk

In general, inpatient orthopedic operations carry a mortality rate of 0.9% with half of these deaths in HFS patients. The majority of deaths occur in patients over age 70, with a mortality of almost 5% in patients over age 90 after any orthopedic surgery.[6]

Predictors of mortality after orthopedic surgery are listed in Table 22.1. A linear increase in mortality is seen with increasing numbers of risk factors. Without

TABLE 22.1. Risks for Postoperative Complications of Orthopedic Surgery

Risk factor	Odds ratio for mortality
Preoperative risk factors	(95% CI)
Chronic renal failure	6.0 (3.3–11.0)
Bone metastases	5.8 (3.7–9.1)
Age over 70	4.5 (3.5–5.8)
Congestive heart failure	3.0 (2.8–3.9)
Osteomyelitis	2.2 (1.2–3.8)
Chronic obstructive pulmonary disease	1.9 (1.1–3.2)
Atrial fibrillation	1.4 (1.0–1.9)
Hypertension	0.32 (0.2–0.5)
Postoperative risk factors	
Pulmonary embolus	26.2 (15.4–44.6)
Acute renal failure	20.2 (12.8–32.0)
Myocardial infarction	7.3 (4.5–11.8)
Cerebrovascular event	6.3 (3.7–10.5)
Pneumonia	5.0 (3.5–7.2)

Risks have a $P < 0.05$.
CI, confidence interval.
Adapted from Bhattacharyya et al.[6]

any of these critical risk factors, mortality is 0.25%. Among orthopedic surgical categories, surgeries for cancer, trauma, and infection carry the highest risks for mortality.

Patients undergoing orthopedic surgery are at particularly high risk for venous thromboembolism (VTE). Postoperative pulmonary embolus (PE) in orthopedic surgery patients carries a significantly increased risk of mortality, with an odds ratio of 26.[6] Fatal PE is not common when routine thromboprophylaxis is employed.[7]

HFS/Trauma

HFS is associated with substantial morbidity, mortality, and costs. In addition to noted predictors of morbidity and mortality for orthopedic surgery in general, surgical delay, poor prefracture walking ability, albumin <3.5 mg/dL, and male gender also predict poor outcomes in HFS patients.[8–10]

The term "hip fracture" is a misnomer, as these injuries are fractures of the proximal femur or acetabulum, which require different management. These are primarily low-velocity fractures that occur in the geriatric population due to low bone mass. In this text, "hip fracture" refers to proximal femur fractures.

Proximal femur fractures are further divided into femoral neck fractures, intertrochanteric fractures, and subtrochanteric fractures. The femoral neck and head have limited blood supply that is disrupted when a fracture is displaced. The intertrochanteric region has good blood supply, so fractures in this area are less prone to avascular necrosis than femoral neck fractures, but associated with more blood loss.[11]

Surgical management of hip fractures is based on characteristics such as prefracture mobility, age, preexisting degenerative changes, type of fracture, and whether displacement of fracture is present. Surgical management options include intramedullary nailing, open reduction/internal fixation, hemi-arthroplasty, and THA[12] (see Figures 22.1 and 22.2).

Patients likely have high rates of morbidity and mortality after HFS because frailty and medical illness led to their fall, rather than resulted from surgery. Acute inpatient mortality for HFS patients has declined over time and is now reported at 5.2% in women and 9.3% in men. One-year mortality rates are 21.9% and 32.5%, respectively.[1]

Open fractures are considered surgical emergencies and have higher infection rates than closed fractures. Current practice is to provide antibiotics and proceed to surgery within 6 h.[13]

Pelvic ring injuries tend to have a bimodal distribution of young patients with high-velocity trauma and elderly patients with low-velocity traumas. These fractures are associated with a high rate of hemorrhage.[14]

Fat emboli are not specific to orthopedic surgery but are most common in this population. Fat emboli occur from dislodged fat deposits, usually triggered by trauma of long bones. These may embolize and result in hypoxemia, coagulopathy, mental status changes, hypovolemic shock, and petechial hemorrhages. Early fixation decreases the risk of fat embolization syndrome.[15]

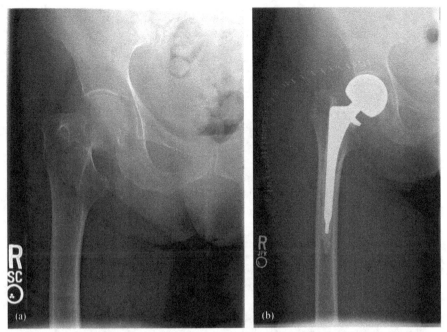

Figure 22.1.   Pre- (a) and postoperative (b) views of a right femoral neck fracture with subsequent hemiarthroplasty.

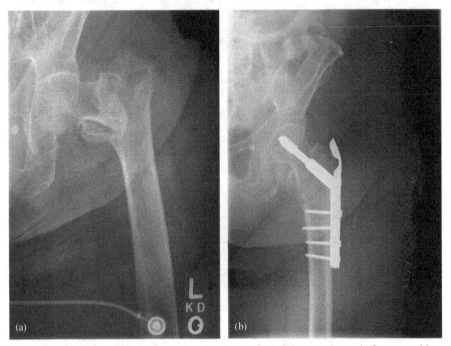

Figure 22.2.   Pre- (a) and postoperative (b) views of a left intertrochanteric fracture with subsequent dynamic hip screw.

Arthroplasty

Arthroplasties of the hip and knee are often elective procedures performed in geriatric patients with advanced osteoarthritis and patients with inflammatory arthropathies. Rheumatoid arthritis and other autoimmune diseases are associated with many medical complications. The medications commonly used to treat these conditions (immunosuppressants and/or immunomodulators) may also directly affect perioperative outcomes. Thirty-day mortality after arthroplasty is less than 1%.[16]

Orthopedic Oncology

Patients with malignancy undergoing surgery are at substantial risk for postoperative complications. Orthopedic oncology includes patients with primary bone and soft tissue malignancies, as well as metastatic bone disease. Prostate, breast, lung, kidney, and thyroid cancers account for the majority of metastatic bone disease.[17] The overall inpatient mortality rate is 5.2% for acute orthopedic oncology surgeries.[6]

PREOPERATIVE ASSESSMENT

The preoperative assessment includes assessment of all organ systems performed in standard preoperative evaluations. Issues specific to orthopedic inpatients also include determining the urgency of surgery, recognizing potential cardiac and pulmonary risk factors, and employing a VTE prophylaxis strategy preoperatively.

Urgent/emergent orthopedic surgeries are common and patients are evaluated and optimized differently than elective surgery patients. The geriatric population undergoing orthopedic surgery is at risk for perioperative cardiac complications. The American College of Cardiology/American Heart Association (ACC/AHA) guidelines for perioperative cardiac assessment[18] provides valuable risk assessment and risk-reduction strategies. However, it should be recognized that stress testing is generally avoided in urgent surgeries. Pulmonary risk factors in this population including advanced age, functional dependence, chronic obstructive pulmonary disease (COPD), congestive heart failure (CHF), impaired sensorium, and exposure to general anesthesia[19] also place patients at higher risk for postoperative complications.

Determining the plan for VTE prophylaxis preoperatively is important and requires recognizing risks specific to the patient and the planned procedure. For HFS, preoperative VTE prophylaxis should be administered as the risk for VTE starts at the time of fracture, rather than the time of surgery. VTE prophylaxis is discussed in detail in the "Postoperative Assessment" section.

HFS/Trauma

Falls can be classified as either mechanical or medical. Patients with new or uncontrolled medical illness causing a fall require further evaluation preoperatively (i.e., syncope or stroke). Patients should also be evaluated for additional trauma that may have been sustained during a fall. It is important to determine the patient's prefracture ambulatory status because nonambulatory patients may not require surgery, unless required for pain control or stabilization of the fracture for transfers. A randomized trial comparing nonoperative and surgical treatment of hip fractures is unlikely. It appears that there are higher mortality rates with nonoperative treatment of hip fractures,[9] with probable selection bias.

Multiple studies have examined the preoperative evaluation of hip fracture patients, how extensive this should be, and the relationship of surgical delay to postoperative morbidity and mortality. Mortality is probably increased when surgery is delayed beyond 24–48 h.[20] Delays to surgery postpone weight bearing; decrease full functional recovery; cause prolonged pain; and increase risk for VTE, pneumonia, urinary tract infections, and skin breakdown.[21,22] Based on available data, it is reasonable to treat significant comorbid medical illness, avoid testing that will not change decision making, and proceed to surgery within 24–48 h.

In regard to preoperative cardiac testing, HFS patients who undergo preoperative cardiac stress testing have no difference in mortality than patients who do not have testing.[23] Additionally, patients who have preoperative stress testing wait over 24 h longer for surgery than patients who do not undergo testing.

Creatinine clearance needs to be calculated in every hip fracture patient, even those with normal serum creatinine levels. Some of the risks for osteoporotic fractures are also factors that cause poor renal function (gender, low body weight, age). Patients who live alone may not procure medical care for hours or days after injury and potentially have volume depletion, electrolyte abnormalities, and acute kidney injury.

HFS patients require analgesia preoperatively. Preoperative skeletal traction does not improve pain or quality of fracture reduction.[24] Perioperative regional anesthesia may be related to lower mortality in HFS patients and lower risks of VTE,[25] and improves postoperative pain control. Nonsteroidal anti-inflammatory drugs (NSAIDs) should generally be avoided because of potential renal toxicity.

Arthroplasty

Joint replacement surgery patients report substantial improvement in symptoms and quality of life, but these surgeries do not prolong life.[26] These are elective procedures and preoperative evaluation should focus on appropriate patient selection, along with maximal medical optimization. The average age of an arthroplasty patient is 69 years.[27] Cardiac, pulmonary, and renal diseases are common in this age group, so careful assessment of these risks with preoperative counseling regarding potential adverse outcomes is advised.

Bilateral knee arthroplasties may sound appealing to patients; however, they are associated with higher rates of PE, cardiac complications, and mortality. Complication rates with staged knee arthroplasties at least 3 months apart are not different from unilateral arthroplasties.[28]

Prosthetic joint infection is a morbid complication of arthroplasty, and the preoperative evaluation should identify risks for infection including active infections, elevated body mass index, open skin near the surgical site, bilateral surgery, anemia, and rheumatoid arthritis.[29]

Orthopedic Oncology

Preoperative evaluation and decision making in the cancer patient is challenging. Expected survival, comorbidities, ability to participate in rehabilitation, and quality of life all contribute to complicated decision making. The preoperative evaluation can risk-stratify patients, as well as identify opportunities for optimization. Furthermore, the preoperative evaluation can sometimes influence whether the decision to proceed to surgery is appropriate.

In patients with metastatic bone disease, surgery is often palliative, and the goal is to restore function in a short period of time with minimal morbidity.[17] Patients with impending or pathologic fractures are best surgically managed because non-surgical treatments are generally not effective. In some patients, postoperative radiation therapy increases return to functional status and decreases need for further orthopedic procedures.[17] The evaluation of undiagnosed skeletal metastases is beyond the scope of this chapter.

Metastatic disease, chemotherapy, and radiation treatment are associated with cardiomyopathy, cardiac ischemia, pulmonary and renal toxicity, and electrolyte and hematologic derangements. Patients should be evaluated based on the type of therapy received and symptomatology.

Osteosarcomas tend to occur in younger patients and are commonly treated with surgery and chemotherapy. Adult patients are more likely to have soft tissue sarcomas, treated with surgery and radiation. The role of chemotherapy in soft tissue sarcoma is less well established.[4,5] See Table 22.2 for common chemotherapeutic agents used in this patient population.

TABLE 22.2. Chemotherapies Commonly Used for Soft Tissue Sarcomas and Osteosarcomas

Warnings/precautions	Ifosfamide	Doxorubicin	Methotrexate	Cisplatin
Cardiotoxic		X		
Myelosuppression	X	X	X	X
Pulmonary toxicity			X	
Neurotoxic	X		X	X
Nephrotoxic	X		X	X
Acidosis or electrolytes	X			X
GI/hepatotoxic	X	X	X	X
Tumor lysis		X	X	
Dermatologic	X	X	X	
Anaphylaxis				X
Infections			X	
Ototoxic				X
Hemorrhagic cystitis	X			
Inhibited wound healing	X			

Drug information derived from Micromedex 1.0 (Healthcare Series).

POSTOPERATIVE ASSESSMENT

Initial Postoperative Assessment

The patient's intraoperative course, immediate postoperative stability, and plan for postoperative management should be the initial focus of the postprocedure assessment. This evaluation should include reviewing the patients' hemodynamic monitoring records during surgery and in recovery, as well as their cardiopulmonary status, particularly in patients with underlying disease. Also, consider wound status/hemostasis/drains, anesthetic delivered, and remaining regional anesthesia catheters. It is common for orthopedic patients to receive regional anesthesia. In addition, review all perioperative medications ordered and provided, including VTE and antibiotic prophylaxis.

VTE Prophylaxis

VTE is a serious complication in orthopedic surgery patients. Recommendations noted in this chapter are consistent with those from the American College of Chest Physicians (ACCP).[7] The American Academy of Orthopedic Surgeons (AAOS) has guidelines for arthroplasty patients.[30] These guidelines, in contrast to the ACCP guidelines, recommend pharmacologic and/or mechanical prophylaxis for prevention of VTE. Specific recommendations for the type of pharmacologic prophylaxis are not provided in the AAOS guidelines.

Recent guideline updates by the ACCP do not differentiate among HFS, THA, and TKA. These surgeries are categorized as "major orthopedic surgery." In patients undergoing major orthopedic surgery, recommendations suggest the use of prophylaxis as opposed to no antithrombotic prophylaxis. Recommended pharmacologic agents include low-molecular-weight heparin (LMWH), fondaparinux, dabigatran, apixaban, rivaroxaban (THA or TKA but not HFS), low-dose unfractionated heparin, adjusted-dose vitamin K antagonist, or aspirin (all Grade 1B). LMWH is recommended in preference to other agents. In patients who decline injections, apixaban or dabigatran are suggested (Grade 1B). In patients receiving pharmacologic prophylaxis, intermittent pneumatic compression devices (IPCDs) are suggested during the hospital stay (Grade 2C). IPCDs are also noted as acceptable prophylaxis (Grade 1C). Prophylaxis is recommended for a minimum of 10–14 days, with a suggestion to extend thromboprophylaxis for up to 35 days (Grade 2B). In patients at increased bleeding risk, IPCDs or no prophylaxis is suggested (Grade 2C).

Oncology There are no ACCP VTE prophylaxis guidelines for patients with orthopedic malignancies. Patients often have VTE risk factors in addition to malignancy and surgery that include recent chemotherapy, central venous catheters, hormonal therapy, and use of erythropoiesis-stimulating agents. Small studies show that VTE rates are highest when tumor resections are performed in the pelvis, thigh, and lower extremity.[31,32] Proximal VTE rates after hip replacement for oncologic indications are significantly lower when LMWH is used in addition to mechanical devices.[31] Based on minimal data, it is reasonable to consider pharmacologic prophylaxis with postdischarge prophylaxis. Carefully consider bleeding risk in these patients as tumor resections and limb salvage surgeries have substantial bleeding risk.

Special VTE Prophylaxis Considerations   Consider the presence of neuraxial anesthesia catheters when providing pharmacologic VTE prophylaxis, due to the potential for epidural/spinal hematoma. It is also important to consider body weight and renal function when providing LMWHs or fondaparinux.

MEDICAL MANAGEMENT

Co-Management Models

Examples of medical/surgical co-management are common in orthopedic surgery. This model is based on the several principles including effective communication between physicians provides expedited care and decreases overall and iatrogenic complications, shorter times to surgery result in better outcomes, and use of protocols and order sets provides standardized care.

Although the literature is inconsistent, some orthopedic co-management models have shown to improve mortality, length of stay, complication rates, readmission rates, cost, and patient and provider satisfaction. Outcomes are better with provision of direct care rather than writing recommendations.[33]

Incidence of major postoperative complication after HFS is 12–62%.[33,34] The most common postoperative complications are[33,35,36] delirium, pressure ulcers, CHF, VTE, pneumonia, infection, arrhythmia, and urinary tract infection. Given the frequency and variety of several potential postoperative complications, co-management models employing the expertise of a hospitalist have gained significant popularity in recent years.

Postoperative Medical Care

Delirium   Delirium is an acute confusional state with alteration of consciousness and is a frequent complication of orthopedic surgery, particularly HFS. More than 65% of patients develop delirium postoperatively. Elderly patients with underlying brain disease, most notably dementia, are at highest risk for postoperative delirium. Delirium is associated with poor functional recovery, even after adjusting for pre-fracture mobility.[37] These patients are more likely to be placed in nursing homes, have higher mortality rates, and longer lengths of stay. It is important to note that although delirium typically lasts for several days, it may persist for months.[38]

The confusion assessment method (CAM) is a validated clinical assessment tool designed for the identification of delirious patients.[39] The basic evaluation of delirium in postoperative patients is described in Figure 22.3.

Postoperative delirium can be reduced in hip fracture patients using a structured protocol and with co-management.[37,40] Measures for reduction of delirium incidence include supplemental oxygen if indicated, maintenance of fluid and

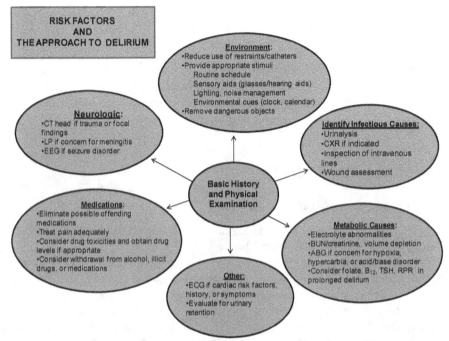

Figure 22.3. The approach to postoperative delirium. CT, computed tomography; LP, lumbar puncture; EEG, electroencephalography; ECG, electrocardiography; CXR, chest X-ray; BUN, blood urea nitrogen; ABG, arterial blood gas; TSH, thyroid-stimulating hormone; RPR, rapid plasma reagin.

electrolyte balance, pain control, and reduction of polypharmacy. The protocol also includes management of bowel and bladder function, nutritional supplements, early mobilization, early identification and treatment postoperative complications, and environmental stimulation.

There are minimal data regarding the efficacy of pharmacologic prophylaxis of delirium. One randomized trial of low-dose haloperidol did not reduce the incidence of delirium in hip fracture patients. Low-dose neuroleptics such as haloperidol, risperidone, and olanzapine may provide symptom control in delirious patients.[37]

Surgical Site Infection (SSI) SSIs are serious complications of orthopedic surgery that often require additional surgical procedures and prolonged antibiotics, and result in periods of disability. Staphylococcal organisms are the most common causes of orthopedic SSI. First- or second-generation cephalosporins are the antibiotics of choice for SSI prophylaxis. Vancomycin and clindamycin are alternatives for patients with penicillin or cephalosporin allergies.[41] The first dose of antibiotics is given within 1 h of surgical incision and then discontinued within 24 h postoperatively.

TABLE 22.3.   Common Causes of Osteoporosis

Lifestyle	Poor calcium intake
	Caffeine and alcohol consumption
	Smoking
	Low body weight
Endocrine disorders	Vitamin D deficiency
	Hyperprolactinemia
	Thyrotoxicosis
	Androgen/estrogen deficiency and insensitivity
	Hyperparathyroidism
	Cushing's syndrome
	Corticosteroid use
Gastrointestinal disorders	Celiac disease, malabsorption
	Inflammatory bowel disease
	Primary biliary cirrhosis
Hematologic disorders	Multiple myeloma
	Sickle-cell disease
	Leukemia, lymphomas
Metabolic	Chronic acidosis
	Chronic renal disease

Derived from the 2008 National Osteoporosis Foundation Guidelines.[44]

Osteoporosis Only about 10–25% of recent HFS patients receive adequate osteoporosis treatment.[42] A clinical diagnosis of osteoporosis can be made in at-risk individuals with a low-trauma fracture. Bone mineral density testing in these cases is obtained as a baseline to guide future therapy.

Elderly patients with fractures should be evaluated for secondary causes of osteoporosis (Table 22.3). Vitamin D deficiency is extremely common in adults and is a risk factor not only for hip fractures, but also for muscle weakness and falls that may precipitate fractures.[43]

Current pharmacologic options for osteoporosis treatment according to the 2008 Guidelines from the National Osteoporosis Foundation include providing adequate amounts of calcium (at least 1200 mg/day) and vitamin D (800–1000 IU/day).[44] Other therapies such as bisphosphonates, calcitonin, estrogens and/or hormone therapy, and parathyroid hormone are more likely to be initiated as an outpatient.

Renal Function Renal function should be taken into account, as noted in the "Preoperative Assessment" section, with medications properly dosed for renal function and avoidance of intravenous contrast studies as appropriate. Low urine output in the postoperative period is almost always a volume issue and should not be treated with diuretics unless a patient demonstrates obvious signs of volume overload. Diuretic use is commonly associated with postoperative renal insufficiency. Urinary catheters should be promptly removed after surgery (typically on the first postoperative day) to decrease the risk of urinary tract infection.

Pain Management   Pain control is challenging as it has been demonstrated that both excessive pain and excessive opiate use contribute to delirium. Meperidine, in particular, causes increased delirium risk compared with other opiates and should be avoided.[38] Measures to prevent constipation should be initiated when using opioid pain medications.

Anemia   Perioperative anemia is associated with poor outcomes; however, transfusion in many cases does not ameliorate this risk and is associated with increased risk of morbidity and mortality. Studies in HFS patients have not found benefit or harm of packed red cell transfusion, even in patients with preexisting cardiovascular disease.[45] Preoperative autologous donation wastes blood in many cases, is costly, and induces anemia, causing excess subsequent transfusion in up to 21% of cases.

Preoperative therapy with erythropoeitin and iron reduces perioperative transfusion in arthroplasty patients.[45] Supplemental oral iron therapy does not significantly increase postoperative hemoglobin or improve mortality in hip fracture patients,[46] but does increase the risk of constipation. If erythropoietin is used in the postoperative period, this should be done cautiously due to VTE risk.[47]

Nutrition   The use of postoperative nutritional supplements should be considered. There is some evidence that demonstrates that high-protein feeds may improve outcomes in hip fracture patients.[48]

Rehabilitation   For almost all orthopedic surgeries, early mobilization is encouraged and improves functional and medical outcomes. Physical therapy should be initiated within 24 h postoperatively with session occurring twice daily. Almost all TKA, THA, and HFS patients are weight bearing postoperatively. This should be confirmed with the orthopedic surgeon and patients should be mobilized appropriately.

DISCHARGE RECOMMENDATIONS

Placement

A safe discharge plan is required for all hospitalized patients. For patients who require physical assistance, discharge to a skilled nursing facility that can offer physical therapy is a common practice. Almost 95% of HFS patients are discharged to facilities other than home.[1]

Rehabilitation

Supervised physical therapy exercise programs after discharge have shown to improve functional recovery. There is no specific program that has demonstrated to be superior to others.[49] Physical therapy can be offered in the inpatient setting (i.e., at a skilled nursing facility), at an outpatient center, or in the patient's home.

Treat Osteoporosis

Discharging patients on calcium and vitamin D supplementation is a recommended practice in the appropriate patient. Additional pharmacologic therapies may be needed, but are best initiated as an outpatient by the patient's primary care provider.

VTE Prophylaxis

Given that many orthopedic surgery patients require extended pharmacologic VTE prophylaxis, it is important to ensure that a supervised follow-up plan is in place upon hospital discharge. This typically involves clear communication with the orthopedic surgery team and the patient's primary care provider.

REFERENCES

1. Brauer CA, Coca-Perraillon M, Cutler DM, Rosen AB. Incidence and mortality of hip fractures in the United States. *JAMA*. 2009;302(14):1573–1579.
2. Braithwaite RS, Col NF, Wong JB. Estimating hip fracture morbidity, mortality and costs. *J Am Geriatr Soc*. 2003;51:364–370.
3. Huddleston JM, Whitford KJ. Medical care of elderly patients with hip fractures. *Mayo Clin Proc*. 2001;76:295–298.
4. Mendenhall WM, Indelicato DJ, Scarborough MT, et al. The management of adult soft tissue sarcomas. *Am J Clin Oncol*. 2009;32(4):436–442.
5. Messerschmitt PJ, Garcia RJ, Abdul-Karim FW, Greenfield EM, Petty PJ. Osteosarcoma. *J Am Acad Orthop Surg*. 2009;17(8):515–527.
6. Bhattacharyya T, Iorio R, Healy WL. Rate of and risk factors for acute inpatient mortality after orthopaedic surgery. *J Bone Joint Surg Am*. 2002;84:562–572.
7. Falck-Ytter Y, Francis CW, Johanson NA, et al. Prevention of VTE in orthopedic surgery patients antithrombotic therapy and prevention of thrombosis, 9th ed: American College of Chest Physicians Evidence-Based Clinical Practice Guidelines. *Chest*. 2012;141(2 Suppl):e278S–e325S.
8. Radcliffe TA, Henderson WG, Stoner TJ, Khuri SF, Dohm M, Hutt E. Patient risk factors, operative care, and outcomes among older community-dwelling male veterans with hip fracture. *J Bone Joint Surg Am*. 2008;90:34–42.
9. Bottle A, Aylin P. Mortality associate with delay in operation after hip fracture. *BMJ*. 2006;332(7547):947–951.
10. Grimes JP, Grefory PM, Noveck H, Butler MS, Carson JL. The effects of time-to-surgery on mortality and morbidity in patients following hip fracture. *Am J Med*. 2002;112:702–709.
11. Kaplan K, Miyamoto R, Levine BR, Egol KA, Zuckerman JD. Surgical management of hip fractures: an evidence-based review of the literature. *J Am Acad Orthop Surg*. 2008;16(11):665–673.
12. Flierl M, Gerhardt DC, Hak DJ, Morgan SJ, Stahel PF. Key issues in the acute management of hip fractures. *Orthopedics*. 2010;33:102.
13. Kanu Okike BA, Bhattacharyya T. Trends in the management of open fracture. *J Bone Joint Surg Am*. 2006;88:2739–2748.
14. Failinger MS, McGanity PL. Unstable fractures of the pelvic ring. *J Bone Joint Surg Am*. 1992;74:781–791.
15. Bone LB, Johnson KD, Weigelt J, Scheinberg R. Early versus delayed stabilization of femoral fractures: a prospective randomized study. *Clin Orthop Relat Res*. 2004;422:11–16.

16. Huddleston JL, Maloney WJ, Wang Y, Verzier N, Hunt DR, Herndon JH. Adverse events after total knee arthroplasty: a national Medicare study. *J Arthroplasty.* 2009;24(6 Suppl):95–100.
17. Bickels J, Dadia S, Lidar Z. Surgical management of metastatic bone disease. *J Bone Joint Surg Am.* 2009;91:1503–1516.
18. Fleischer LA, Beckman JA, Brown KA, et al. Perioperative cardiovascular evaluation and care for noncardiac surgery. *J Am Coll Cardiol.* 2009;54(22):e13.
19. Smetana GW. Postoperative pulmonary complications: an update on risk assessment and reduction. *Cleve Clin J Med.* 2009;76(Suppl 4):S60–S65.
20. Khan SK, Kalra S, Khanna A, Thiruvengada MM, Parker MJ. Timing of surgery for hip fractures: a systematic review of 52 published studies involving 291,413 patients. *Injury.* 2009;40(7):692–697.
21. Orosz GM, Magaziner J, Hannan EL, et al. Association of timing of surgery for hip fracture and patient outcomes. *JAMA.* 2004;291(14):1738–1743.
22. Lefaivre KA, Macadam SA, Davidson DJ, Gandhi R, Chan H, Broekhuse HM. Length of stay, mortality, morbidity, and delay to surgery in hip fractures. *J Bone Joint Surg Br.* 2009;91:922–928.
23. Ricci WM, Della Rocca GJ, Combs C, Borrelli J. The medical and economic impact of preoperative cardiac testing in elderly patients with hip fractures. *Injury.* 2007;38(Suppl 3):S49–S52.
24. Parker MJ, Handoll HHG. Pre-operative traction for fractures of the proximal femur in adults. *Cochrane Database Syst Rev.* 2009;(3):CD000168.
25. Parker MJ, Handol HHG, Griffiths R. Anaesthesia for hip fracture surgery in adults. *Cochrane Database Syst Rev.* 2004;(4):CD000521.
26. Hamel MB, Toth M, Legedza A, Rosen MP. Joint replacement surgery in elderly patients with severe osteoarthritis of the hip or knee. *Arch Intern Med.* 2008;168(13):1430–1438.
27. Roder C, Staub LP, Eggli S, Dietrich D, Busato A, Muller U. Influence of preoperative functional status on outcome after total hip arthroplasty. *J Bone Joint Surg Am.* 2007;89:11–17.
28. Restrepo C, Parvizi J, Dietrich T, Einhorn TA. Safety of simultaneous bilateral total knee arthroplasty: a meta-analysis. *J Bone Joint Surg Am.* 2007;89:1220–1226.
29. Pulido L, Ghanem E, Joshi A, Purtill JJ, Parvizi J. Periprosthetic joint infection. *Clin Orthop Relat Res.* 2008;466:1710–1715.
30. American Academy of Orthopaedic Surgeons. *Guideline on Preventing Venous Thromboembolic Disease in Patients Undergoing Elective Hip and Knee Arthroplasty. Evidence-Based Guideline and Evidence Report.* Available at http://www.aaos.org/Research/guidelines/VTE/VTE_full_guideline.pdf. Accessed May 2012.
31. Nathan SS, Simmons KA, Lin PP, et al. Proximal deep vein thrombosis after hip replacement for oncologic indications. *J Bone Joint Surg Am.* 2006;88(5):1066–1069.
32. Mitchell SY, Lingard EA, Kesteven P, McCaskie AW, Gerrand CH. Venous thromboembolism in patients with primary bone or soft tissue sarcomas. *J Bone Joint Surg Am.* 2007;89:2433–2439.
33. Friedman SM, Mendelson DA, Kates SL, McCann RM. Geriatric co-management of proximal femur fractures: total quality management and protocol-driven care result in better outcomes for a frail patient population. *J Am Geriatr Soc.* 2008;56(7):1349–1356.
34. Vidan M, Serra JA, Concepcion M, Riquelme G, Ortiz J. Efficacy of a comprehensive geriatric intervention in older patients hospitalized for hip fracture: a randomized, controlled trial. *J Am Geriatr Soc.* 2005;53:1476–1482.
35. McLaughlin MA, Orosz GM, Magaziner J, et al. Preoperative status and risk of complications in patients with hip fracture. *J Gen Intern Med.* 2006;21:219–225.
36. Moran CG, Wenn RT, Sikand M, Taylor AM. Early mortality after hip fracture: is delay before surgery important? *J Bone Joint Surg Am.* 2005;87:483–489.
37. Marcantonio ER, Flacker JM, Wright RJ, Resnick NM. Reducing delirium after hip fracture: a randomized trial. *J Am Geriatr Soc.* 2001;49:516–522.
38. Robertson BD, Robertson TJ. Postoperative delirium after hip fracture. *J Bone Joint Surg.* 2006;88:2060–2068.
39. Inouye SK, van Dyck CH, Alessi CA, Balkin S, Siegal AP, Horwitz RI. Clarifying confusion: the confusion assessment method. *Ann Intern Med.* 1990;113:941–948.
40. Siddiqi N, Holt R, Britton AM, Holmes J. Interventions for preventing delirium in hospitalised patients. *Cochrane Database Syst Rev.* 2007;(2):CD005563.

41. The Medicare Quality Improvement Community (MedQIC). Specifications Manual Version 3.2b, Section 2.4. The Surgical Care Improvement Project, update April 2010. Available at http://www.qualitynet.org. Accessed April 2010.

42. Siris ES. Patients with hip fracture: what can be improved? *Bone.* 2006;38(2):8–12.

43. Holick MF. Vitamin D deficiency. *N Engl J Med.* 2007;357:266–281.

44. *National Osteoporosis Foundation Clinician's Guide to Prevention and Treatment of Osteoporosis. 2010.* Available at http://www.nof.org/professionals/clinical-guidelines. Accessed May 2012.

45. Carson JL, Terrin ML, Magaziner J, et al. Transfusion trigger trail for functional outcomes in cardiovascular patients undergoing surgical hip fracture repair. *Transfusion.* 2006;46:2192–2205.

46. Parker MJ. Iron supplementation for anemia after hip fracture surgery: a randomized trial of 300 patients. *J Bone Joint Surg Am.* 2010;92:265–269.

47. Kumar A. Perioperative management of anemia: limits of blood transfusion and alternatives to it. *Cleve Clin J Med.* 2009;76(Suppl 4):S112–S118.

48. Avenell A, Handoll HHG. Nutritional supplementation for hip fracture aftercare in older people. *Cochrane Database Syst Rev.* 2010;(1):CD001880.

49. Handoll HHG, Sherrington C. Mobilisation strategies after hip fracture surgery in adults. *Cochrane Database Syst Rev.* 2007;(1):CD001704.

CHAPTER 23

TRAUMA SURGERY

Fahim A. Habib, Nikolay Buagev, and Mark G. McKenney

BACKGROUND

In the United States, injury is the leading cause of death in the first four decades of life.[1] It is also the leading cause of premature death resulting in the greatest amount of years of potential life lost, more than heart disease, stroke, and cancer combined.[2]

Injury is gaining increasing significance as a major healthcare problem among older Americans. This is for several reasons: older persons are becoming an increasing proportion of the population, are retiring later, and are living more physically active lives. As a consequence, the injured population is now more likely to have significant comorbidities that must be taken into account.

To further compound the issue, other unique characteristics of the trauma patient makes the delivery of perioperative care challenging. Imaging performed for trauma may identify incidental lesions that require further workup.[3] Also, a number of systemic diseases may be discovered as a consequence of injury. Hypertension, diabetes, cardiac arrhythmias, coronary artery disease, and cerebral vascular disease are some examples. In such instances, adequate communication must be established to ensure appropriate continuity of care for their medical conditions.[4]

MEDICAL DISEASE PRESENTING WITH TRAUMA

Medical diseases may cause acute alteration of consciousness that result in traumatic injury. Common examples include seizures,[5] syncope,[6] cerebrovascular accidents, cardiac arrhythmias, acute coronary syndromes, undiagnosed diabetic ketoacidosis, undiagnosed renal failure with uremia, and obstructive sleep apnea.[7] A prior diagnosis may not always be present. Obtaining a history of the events preceding the injury may allow for the diagnosis of a medical condition to be made.

A seizure disorder, as the basis for a traumatic event, should be considered in those with an underlying history of seizures, when a history of abnormal movements prior to the event is present, or in those with a characteristic postictal appearance. The initial approach follows the tenets of the American College of Surgeon's

Perioperative Medicine: Medical Consultation and Co-Management, First Edition.
Edited by Amir K. Jaffer and Paul J. Grant.
© 2012 Wiley-Blackwell. Published 2012 by John Wiley & Sons, Inc.

Advanced Trauma Life Support guidelines.[8] In addition, computed tomography (CT) of the brain to evaluate for possible intracranial injuries as the cause of the seizures must be rapidly performed. If the patient is still actively seizing, lorazepam or diazepam is administered for seizure control.[9] Prevention of additional seizure activity is achieved by administration of and anticonvulsant medication such as phenytoin.[10] Rapid administration of phenytoin, however, can result in significant hypotension. Hence, in the acute setting, fosphenytoin is the preferred drug for the loading dose.[11] Drug levels must be obtained to ensure adequate serum levels and because approximately 50% of phenytoin is protein bound, an albumin level must be obtained so the drug level can be corrected appropriately. In patients with seizure disorder who remain unresponsive, the possibility of status epilepticus must be considered. An electroencephalogram remains the only means of establishing the diagnosis, and early consultation with the neurologist is recommended.[12]

With advancing age, syncope due to a multitude of causes is common. The patient is often "found-down" unresponsive, or falls from a standing position with evidence of modest trauma to the head. The initial approach again involves a rapid, accurate, and priority-based assessment of the traumatic injury. A thorough workup for syncope must then follow.

Patients who are suspected to have suffered a cerebrovascular accident pose a greater challenge. In a proportion of these patients, the underlying event is an ischemic stroke. Here, the presence of significant trauma must be rapidly ascertained as the patient may be a candidate for thrombolytic therapy.

An underlying cardiac condition must also be considered in patients presenting with trauma. A history of coronary artery disease, clinical symptomology of ischemic heart disease, the presence of a median sternotomy scar, and electrocardiogram abnormalities are all ways to help determine if a cardiac etiology may be contributory. When considering the administration of antiplatelet agents, injuries at high-risk bleeding sites (i.e., brain, solid viscera) must be carefully evaluated as this may prohibit the administration of aspirin and/or clopidogrel.

SPECIFIC ISSUES IN THE PERIOPERATIVE MANAGEMENT OF THE INJURED PATIENT

Trauma poses unique challenges to management in the perioperative period. Each injury pattern has its own particular characteristics, which must be understood in order to assure an optimal outcome. Issues specific to different types of injuries are outlined in the subsequent sections.

Traumatic Brain Injury (TBI)

TBI is not only a major cause of mortality and morbidity, but also imposes a significant economic cost to society. There are two distinct phases of TBI: primary and secondary. Primary TBI occurs at the time of injury and can only be reduced by promotion of preventative measures. Secondary TBI occurs in the time period following the primary insult and results from physiologic events that compromise brain tissue metabolism, potentially worsening outcome.

It is hence the prevention, early recognition, and prompt and aggressive management of these secondary insults that has had the greatest impact on improving outcomes following TBI. The main goals of management include maintaining adequate brain tissue perfusion by preventing hypotension, maintaining oxygenation by preventing hypoxia, providing adequate calories, and aggressively managing conditions that increase metabolism of the already damaged brain tissue such as fever and seizures.

Imaging with CT is fundamental. It allows the determination of the presence of intracranial injury and characterization of the nature and severity of injury, as well as the presence of midline shift. A midline shift of greater than 5 mm is an indication for surgical intervention.

The key management principles for TBI are outlined in the guidelines of the Brain Trauma Foundation.[13] Maintenance of adequate brain tissue oxygenation remains a key principle. Data from the Traumatic Coma Data Bank reveal that hypoxemia occurs in over 22% of patients with severe TBI and is associated with a significant increase in morbidity and mortality.[14,15] Hence, close monitoring of oxygenation using pulse oximetry and frequent arterial blood gas analysis is critical, with a minimal target PaO_2 of >60 mm Hg or SaO_2 of >90%. This is achieved by administrating supplemental oxygen to those not requiring mechanical ventilation. In the presence of coma (Glasgow coma scale [GCS] <8), or the presence of associated injuries that potentially impair oxygenation, the airway is secured and mechanical ventilation is provided. Excessive positive end-expiratory pressure (PEEP) must be avoided as this impairs venous drainage from the brain and has the propensity to increase brain edema. Sedation and analgesic medications must be provided to alleviate agitation, treat pain, and improve patient–ventilator synchrony. Adequate sedation also reduces the metabolic requirements of the brain tissue, potentially improving outcome. Short-acting intravenous agents are preferred for sedation as they can be temporarily discontinued to perform frequent neurologic assessments.

Under normal circumstances, the brain autoregulates its blood flow; that is, brain flow is maintained proportional to its metabolic requirements over a range of mean arterial pressures, typically between 50 and 150 mm Hg. In the injured brain, this ability to autoregulate is lost, and blood flow becomes directly proportional to the cerebral perfusion pressure (CPP). The CPP is described by the formula CPP = MAP − ICP, where MAP is the mean arterial pressure and ICP is the intracranial pressure. The latter is measured directly by a catheter placed in the ventricles or the brain parenchyma. A CPP between 50 and 70 mm Hg is targeted. Improvements in CPP can be achieved by either increasing the MAP, decreasing the ICP, or both. In order to maintain an adequate MAP, the systolic blood pressure (SBP) must be maintained greater than 90 mm Hg. In fact, even a single episode of hypotension, defined as SBP <90 mm Hg, doubles the mortality from TBI.[15] The target ICP is <20 mm Hg. As stated earlier, this can be measured using a catheter placed either into the ventricle or into the brain parenchyma. The key advantage of the former approach is that it allows the removal of cerebrospinal fluid (CSF) as a means of lowering the ICP. ICP monitoring is indicated in all patients with a GCS of <9 who have findings on CT of intracranial hematomas, contusion, swelling, compressed basal cisterns, or evidence of impending herniation. It is also indicated in patients with a GCS <9 with a normal CT in those over 40 years of age, SBP <90 mm Hg, and unilateral posturing.

Mannitol is useful in the management of elevated ICP. It exerts its effects by expanding plasma volume, decreasing blood viscosity, and thereby improving brain perfusion. In addition, mannitol has osmotic properties, drawing fluid out from the brain tissue. Its use is recommended in patients with clinical signs or measured evidence of elevated ICP. It is administered in an initial loading dose of 1 g/kg, then at 0.25–0.5 g/kg every 6 h. Serum osmolality is measured prior to each dose, and the drug is discontinued if it reaches 320 mOsm. It should be avoided or used with caution in patients with sepsis, preexisting renal failure, and with concomitant use of nephrotoxic agents.

Seizures may occur in the immediate postinjury period (defined as within 1 week following the TBI), or thereafter. The development of seizures can negatively impact recovery by increasing metabolic requirements, altering oxygen delivery and consumption, increasing neurotransmitter release, and increasing the ICP. The incidence of early posttraumatic seizures in untreated patients varies from 4% to 25% depending on the severity of the injury, and reduces to 3% when prophylactic antiseizure medication is administered.[16] While antiseizure prophylaxis is effective in reducing the incidence of seizures in the early period following TBI, it has no beneficial effect on late-onset seizures, death, or neurologic disability.[17] Their use is hence recommended for the first 7 days following injury. Phenytoin is the most commonly employed agent. Rapid administration of the loading dose is associated with a risk of adverse effects including hypotension, local tissue injury, and cardiac toxicity. Fosphenytoin, a water-soluble prodrug of phenytoin is hence often used for provision of the initial loading dose following TBI. This formulation, however, is 10-fold more expensive. Hence, once the loading dose has been provided, phenytoin can be used for maintenance, as there is no longer the need for rapid administration. Due to the narrow therapeutic index of phenytoin, drug monitoring is essential.

Nutritional support should be initiated once the patient has been adequately resuscitated. Enteral feeds are preferred and caloric goals should be attained by day 7.

Sedation and Analgesia

Goals of therapy include keeping the patient comfortable and free of pain, relieving anxiety, and minimizing the psychological effects of a hostile and invasive environment on the patient.

The ideal agent to achieve this is one, which provides both sedation and analgesia, has a rapid onset of action, a short half-life, no bioaccumulation, no drug interactions, and is easy to titrate.[18] No such drug exists. Each drug possesses one or more of these features, and one chooses an agent based on the particular clinical circumstance and side effect profile.

Analgesia is best achieved by the administration of small doses of the drug intravenously. Morphine is the most commonly used agent; however, fentanyl may be employed. Morphine is best avoided in patients with renal and hepatic insufficiency where there is accumulation of its metabolites. In such cases, hydromorphone is preferred. Nonsteroidal agents are best avoided due to the potential for increased bleeding. Pain management depends on the severity of the injuries and the patient's pain threshold. For intubated patients, either intermittent doses of morphine or hydromorphone can be used. Alternatively, a continuous infusion of fentalyl can be administered. Unresponsive patients may not be able to express experiencing pain. Subtle clues such as tachycardia, hypertension, and agitation may be the only indication of pain. Transdermal or intramuscular administration of narcotics is not recommended in the acute setting as absorption is unpredictable.

Sedation in conjunction with analgesia is often required in most trauma patients. Factors that must be considered in selecting the appropriate sedative are the duration of sedation required, whether the airway is secure, age, and comorbidities. Small doses of midazolam may be provided for short procedures such a reduction of a closed fracture or debridement of a burn wound. While it can be administered to the nonintubated patient, care must be taken to monitor oxygenation with continuous pulse oximetry. Midazolam may cause hypotension and has an active metabolite, which can accumulate causing prolonged effects, especially in the elderly. This drug may also exhibit unpredictable kinetics in the hemodynamically quasistable trauma patient.[19]

Propofol is a short-acting intravenous hypnotic agent that can be utilized for short procedures as well as for continuous sedation. It causes respiratory depression and should not be administered unless the airway has been secured. Additionally, propofol may cause hypertriglyceridemia, increase risk for infection due to immune modulation, and, although rare, produce the characteristic propofol infusion syndrome. This syndrome was initially described in children receiving high doses of propofol for prolonged periods, but is also now recognized in adults. It is characterized by cardiac failure, rhabdomyolysis, severe metabolic acidosis, and renal failure.[20–22] Hence, use for over 48 h in doses greater than 5 µg/kg/min is strongly discouraged. Should longer duration of sedation be required, lorazepam is the preferred agent. The occurrence of toxicity due to accumulation of the dilutent of lorazepam, propylene glycol, must be recognized.[23] It presents with an increase in anion gap (≥15), decrease in bicarbonate, elevated osmolar gap (≥10 mOsm/L), acidemia, and eventually lead to shock and organ failure. Dexmedetomidine, a centrally acting alpha-2 agonist is another agent that may be used. It has the advantage of not requiring the patient to be intubated as it does not suppress respiratory drive.

Sedation must be titrated to effect using a sedation scale, such as the Ramsey Sedation Scale[24] or the Richmond Agitation Sedation Scale (RASS).[25] Failure to titrate sedation to effect using a predefined scale often leads to over sedation, which prolongs the duration of mechanical ventilation and overall length of hospital stay.[26–28] A daily sedation vacation must be provided to all mechanically ventilated patients whose lung injury is stable or resolving, and who are hemodynamically stable (heart rate [HR] < 100, MAP > 65), have reasonable FiO2 requirements (<0.5), are on modest

PEEP (<8), and are able to initiate spontaneous breaths. When the patients are awake and able to follow instructions, a spontaneous breathing trial can be attempted. This "wake up and breathe" approach has led to a significant decrease in duration of mechanical ventilation, ICU stay, and mortality.[29] If the patient fails the sedation vacation, the infusion of sedative is restarted at half the original dose.

Thoracic Trauma

Pulmonary contusion is a common sequela of blunt trauma to the chest. Associated skeletal injury is almost uniformly present except in children who have pliable ribs and in blast injuries. The blunt force results in hemorrhage into the alveolar spaces as well as interstitial edema secondary to increased vascular permeability resulting in reduced lung compliance, ventilation–perfusion mismatch, and increased vascular resistance. The extent of the contusion worsens over the first 24–72 h and resolves over a period of 7 days if no complications ensue.[30] This anticipated worsening of respiratory function must be taken into account when assessing the respiratory status and the need for mechanical ventilation, and in deciding on patient disposition.

Rib fractures are often associated with some degree of underlying pulmonary contusion. In addition to the aforementioned, the pain of rib fractures leads to splinting, atelectasis, and retention of secretions with worsening of pulmonary function. Adequate analgesia to prevent splinting and pulmonary toilet to prevent collapse and help mobilize secretions are key principles.

Flail chest describes a severe complex pattern of rib fractures associated with significant pulmonary contusion, where three or more ribs are fractured in two more places. The disrupted mobile segment of the thoracic cage transmits a blunt force to the underlying lung causing significant pulmonary contusion.

Diagnosis of these conditions can be made by a careful clinical examination looking for localized chest wall tenderness, crepitus, and reduced breath sounds over the affected lung fields. The initial chest X-ray obtained in the trauma bay may demonstrate the associated skeletal injury, pneumothorax, hemothorax, and opacification of the lung fields. However, the contusion may not have had adequate time to evolve and may be underappreciated on the initial X-ray. CT of the chest has superiority in assessing the presence and severity of the injury.[31]

Management principles for this group of injuries are generally supportive and include pain management of associated skeletal injuries, supplemental oxygen, mechanical ventilatory support, pulmonary toilet, and judicious fluid management.[32]

Blunt Cardiac Injury

Due to the absence of a clear, widely accepted clinical definition, the exact incidence of blunt cardiac injury remains unknown.[33] It should be considered in patients with blunt trauma to the chest, physical evidence of thoracic trauma, chest wall crepitus, jugular venous distention, electrocardiographic (EKG) changes, and elevation of cardiac enzymes.[34] While any cardiac rhythm abnormality is possible, sinus tachycardia, premature atrial contractions, and premature ventricular contractions remain the most common.[35]

Patient evaluation involves obtaining an electrocardiogram and cardiac enzymes. In patients with a normal electrocardiogram and without elevation of serum troponin I, further evaluation is unnecessary and the patient can be safely discharged.[36] Hemodynamically stable patients with EKG changes or elevation of troponin I should be admitted to a monitored setting and observed for 24–48 h. Transthoracic echocardiography should be performed to assess cardiac function as well as to evaluate for possible structural damage. Unstable patients should be emergently evaluated with transthoracic or transesophageal echocardiography.

Cardiac arrhythmias should be managed as is appropriate. Medical therapy is employed in hemodynamically stable patients while unstable patients should be cardioverted. Coronary angiography with percutaneous coronary intervention (PCI) may be required in patients with posttraumatic acute coronary syndromes. The inability to routinely use dual antiplatelet therapy makes PCI challenging in this group of patients. The decision to use aspirin, clopidrogel, and/or glycoprotein IIb/ IIIa inhibitors must be highly individualized based on the patients' associated injuries and the attendant risk of bleeding, especially in the face of TBI. Emergent cardiac surgical intervention is needed in cases with structural damage including blunt cardiac rupture and septal defects.

POSTOPERATIVE ISSUES

Delirium Tremens

A significant proportion of critically injured patients have a history of alcohol misuse and abuse.[37] The development of delirium tremens significantly increases the morbidity and mortality following trauma. Consequences include increased risk of infection, delayed wound healing, increased risk of hemorrhage requiring blood transfusions, pancreatitis, longer durations of mechanical ventilation, and longer ICU stays.[38–41] Delirium tremens is characterized by the development of tremors, diaphoresis, autonomic instability, and hallucinations. These symptoms typically manifest 2–4 days after the last ingestion of alcohol. Prediction involves patient history and short interview tools such as the AUDIT and CAGE questionnaires.[42]

Management includes correction of fluid and electrolyte abnormalities, and the use of benzodiazepines,[43] particularity lorazepam. Adjunctive propofol and neuroleptic agents may also be used. Anticonvulsive agents have not been shown to be effective. The use of alcohol is not widely recommended as it is difficult to titrate, has a narrow therapeutic index, and a poorly predictable pharmacokinetic profile.[44–46]

Venous Thromboembolism following Trauma

Trauma patients are particularly prone to develop venous thromboembolism. This results as a consequence of stasis, endothelial damage, and hypercoagulability, an etiologic constellation termed "Virchow's triad."

Sequential compression devices are often employed to overcome venous stasis; however, these provide inadequate protection when used alone (but should still be applied in all patients without lower extremity injury). Hypercoagulability is addressed by using prophylactic doses of anticoagulants. Unfractionated heparin (UFH) was the first agent available; however, this has unpredictable pharmacokinetics and exposes the patient to the risk of heparin-induced thrombocytopenia (HIT). Low-molecular-weight heparins (LMWHs) have largely replaced UFH, and have predictable pharmacokinetics and a lower incidence of HIT. LMWHs are inadequately cleared in patients with renal disease leading to unpredictable prolongation of effect. This precludes their use in this patient population. In addition, due to the large volume of distribution from the typical fluid resuscitation needs, the once daily dosing employed in medical and surgical patients is inappropriate and twice daily dosing is advised. Fondaparinux, a heparin pentasaccharide, consists of five saccharide molecules that bind to antithrombin III leading to its activation. Its use is associated with virtually no risk of HIT. However, its prolonged half-life, accumulation in patients with renal disease, and absence of an antagonist make its utility in the trauma patient limited.

In patients who have a contraindication to anticoagulation, such as injury involving the central nervous system, or when nonoperative management of solid organs such as the liver or spleen is being attempted, an inferior vena cava filter may be employed. Even in patients in whom a filter has been placed, pharmacologic anticoagulation should begin as soon as appropriate. This is in an effort to prevent the development of lower extremity deep vein thrombosis (DVT) with possible subsequent postphlebitic syndrome as well as showering of the pulmonary circulation with small nonfatal emboli that may result in pulmonary hypertension.

Thromboprophylaxis should be continued until discharge from the hospital, including any period of inpatient rehabilitation.[47]

Glycemic Control

Tight glycemic control, with maintenance of blood sugars between 80 and 110 mg/dL, has been shown to lower mortality and reduce the incidence of infectious complications.[48] Subsequent studies, however, have shown that the detrimental effects of hypoglycemia that occurs in an effort to maintain such tight control results in increased mortality that effectively precludes any benefit.[49] Intensive insulin control also requires significant resources and is challenging to implement at the majority of institutions. As a consequence, attempts at tight glycemic control have largely been abandoned. A more reasonable goal is to maintain the blood sugar levels at 140 ± 20 mg/dL. Hypoglycemia most commonly results when there is a disconnection between the delivery of insulin and the delivery of calories. This most commonly occurs when feeds are held because of intolerance, loss of access, or planned procedures. Frequent blood glucose monitoring and ensuring the insulin administration is stopped whenever calorie supply is suspended will help prevent this potentially fatal complication.

Renal

Most injured patients undergo imaging studies including CT where intravenous contrast media is almost universally administered to reliably exclude active hemorrhage. As the patient's premorbid clinical history is often not available, and laboratory test results may not become available in a timely manner, patients are at risk for developing contrast-induced acute kidney injury. The resulting kidney injury is a combination of cell death as a direct consequence of exposure to contrast media, and accentuated by the effect of the contrast media causing vasoconstriction resulting in a reduction of medullary blood flow. A creatinine increase of 0.5 mg/dL (or a 25% increase in patients with an elevated baseline creatinine) that occurs within 48–72 h following exposure to contrast defines contrast-induced acute kidney injury. The elderly, diabetics, and patients who are volume depleted are at highest risk. Key preventative strategies include intravenous volume expansion.[50] Antioxidant therapy using acetylcysteine is also an option. The infusion of sodium bicarbonate is another therapeutic modality that may ameliorate the development of contrast-induced acute kidney injury. This results in alkalinization of the urine and neutralization of reactive oxygen species. In extremely high-risk patients or those with advanced chronic kidney disease, hemodialysis may be provided in an effort to remove contrast agent.

Anemia

Anemia is a common clinical problem in critically injured patients. The cause of anemia in these patients is often multifactorial in etiology. Initially, anemia is the result of blood loss secondary to hemorrhage caused by the injury. Additional causes include phlebotomy for diagnostic laboratory testing, gastrointestinal bleeding, surgical blood loss, and as a result of underlying chronic diseases such as renal failure.

Transfusion of packed red blood cells has remained the standard approach to the management of anemia in critically injured patients. Most of these transfusions are administered in response to a particular hemoglobin level, the "transfusion trigger." Earlier recommendations were based on tradition and suggest that a transfusion may be indicated if the hemoglobin concentration is less than 10 g/dL. However, recently generated scientific evidence refutes this position and clearly suggests that most critically ill patients can safely tolerate low hemoglobin levels.[51] Also, packed red blood cell transfusions are associated with numerous potential complications. Finally, blood is a scarce and costly resource that may not always be available; hence, its use must be limited to those most likely to benefit. Transfusion of packed red blood cells must therefore be used for a physiologic indication and not in response to a "transfusion trigger." The only absolute indication for packed red blood cell transfusion is in the treatment of hemorrhagic shock.[52] Here, the number of units transfused is based not on a particular hemoglobin level but on the physiologic state of the patient. Transfusion is also indicated in the presence of acute hemorrhage with either hemodynamic instability or evidence of inadequate oxygen delivery as demonstrated by elevated blood lactate levels or base deficit. In hemodynamically stable trauma patients, there is no strict transfusion strategy, but packed red blood cells are typically transfused when the hemoglobin falls below 7 g/dL. In patients with active cardiac disease, reduction in mortality can be achieved by transfusion to a hematocrit of 30–33% while no benefit is seen when higher levels are obtained. Transfusion to wean patients off mechanical ventilation has been proven to be of no benefit and hence is not indicated.

Nutrition

Injury results in the release of a host of mediators that activates a profound proin-flammatory state. In turn, this produces a highly catabolic state. In the absence of adequate nutritional support, the body rapidly consumes its glycogen stores, and begins to breakdown tissues to generate nutrients. Early provision of nutrition is therefore essential. However, in inadequately resuscitated patients or those receiving significant doses of vasopressor agents, blood flow to the gastrointestinal tract is often impaired. Enteral nutrition in this circumstance has the potential to cause gut ischemia or bowel necrosis. Enteral feeds are therefore instituted after the patient has been adequately resuscitated and the vasopressor agents have been weaned off. In the interim, a dextrose containing maintenance fluid is provided to meet the needs of tissues that are obligate glucose users. In most patients, except for those with severe malnutrition prior to the injury, a few days of dextrose supplementation is adequate. Enteral feeds should be started early within 24–48 h following injury, once the patient has been adequately resuscitated, and is hemodynamically stable. The feeds should then be rapidly advanced over the next 48–72 h. The presence of bowel sounds or passage of flatus or stool is not required to initiate feedings. Unless con-traindicated, the head of the bed should be elevated to 30° to reduce the risk of aspiration. In patients with high gastric residual volumes, a distal feeding tube can be placed and feeds delivered into the small bowel. When adequate nutrition using the enteral route cannot be administered for 7 days, parental nutrition should be provided.

Despite the availability of complex devices such as indirect calorimeters, provision of 25–35 kcal/kg is adequate for virtually all patients. Protein require-ments are proportional to the severity of the injury, and 1–2 g/kg/day is recom-mended. In patients unable to be given adequate enteral feeds, a minimum of 10 mL/h is given as this is trophic for intestinal epithelium and is believed to reduce the translocation of bacteria across the intestinal lumen. Parenteral nutrition is tra-ditionally indicated only when there is no functional gut. Immune-modulating for-mulations supplemented with agents such as arginine glutamine nucleic acid, omega-3 fatty acids, and antioxidants should be used in patients who develop sepsis subsequent to the injury. Soluble fiber containing small peptide formulations is indicated in patients with diarrhea. In patients with respiratory failure, high-lipid and low-carbohydrate formulations reduce carbon dioxide production and should be considered. In patients with acute respiratory failure, as well as those with significant cardiac disease, fluid-restricted calorie-dense formulations should be used. Electro-lytes including calcium, magnesium, and phosphate levels should be monitored closely and replaced as necessary. Patients requiring hemodialysis have an increased protein requirement, up to a maximum of 2.5 g/kg/day is administered.

Abdominal Compartment Syndrome

Fluid resuscitation is often required in an effort to maintain homeostasis following traumatic injury. However, due to the release of a multitude of inflammatory media-tors, there is an increased vascular permeability. As a consequence, the administered fluid often leaks out of the vascular system and accumulates in the interstitial spaces. In tissue spaces that are bound by inelastic, unyielding fascia, the accumulation of fluid results in a rise in compartment pressure. The clinical consequence of such elevated pressures is dependent on the nature of the fascia. In compartments where the fascia is exceedingly unyielding, the increased pressure ultimately exceeds perfusion pressure and results in ischemia of the compartment contents (i.e., fascial compartments of the lower extremity). In contrast, when the fascia is less unyielding, the increase in pressure is initially compensated for by distention of the compartment. However, as the volume of the compartment continues to increase, it compresses surrounding structures. The compression of adjacent viscera results in organ dysfunction producing the clinical constellation that characterizes the syndrome.[53] In the case of the abdomen, initial increases in pressure are compensated by abdominal distention. However, as the pressure continues to rise the distended abdomen results in an upward deflection of the diaphragm. This increases pressures within the chest cavity, increasing the peak airway pressures, and results in difficulties with ventilation. Compression of the inferior vena cava within the abdominal cavity results in a decrease in venous return; if this is compounded by increased intrathoracic pressures, return of blood to the heart is impaired. When filling is impaired, cardiac output falls and hypotension results. Compression of the renal parenchyma as well as that of the renal vessels results in oliguria. Hence, the combination of ventilatory difficulties due to elevated airway pressures, hypotension, and oliguria in the face of increased abdominal pressures characterizes the abdominal compartment syndrome.

Key to the management of these patients is early detection. Physical examination is notoriously unreliable, compounded by injuries or alterations in mental status. A high index of suspicion is essential, and intra-abdominal pressures must be measured liberally in patients at risk for the development of the abdominal compartment syndrome. For patients with intra-abdominal hypertension, efforts to decrease further increases in intra-abdominal pressure can be made by evacuating intra-abdominal contents (nasogastric tube, rectal tube, prokinetic agents, discontinuation of enteral feeds, etc.), evacuating intra-abdominal space-occupying lesions (ultrasound or CT-guided catheter drainage, surgical evacuation), improving abdominal wall compliance (sedation, paralysis, removal of constrictive dressings), optimizing fluid administration, and optimizing tissue perfusion. Once a compartment syndrome has developed, decompressive laparotomy remains the only definitive management. The procedure is potentially lifesaving and can be done at the bedside in the intensive care unit. Immediate improvement in organ physiology is often observed once decompression is performed. In pediatric burn patients, the use of percutaneous peritoneal dialysis catheters has been reported. In adults, this approach is currently under investigation and cannot currently be recommended.

Coagulopathy

Coagulation abnormalities are common and often multifactorial in etiology. Hemorrhage results in consumption of clotting factors and platelets. Furthermore, initial resuscitation with crystalloid results in a dilution of clotting factors. This can be exacerbated by transfusion of packed red blood cells in the absence of appropriate replacement of fresh frozen plasma and/or platelets. Additional factors that contribute to coagulopathy include activation of the fibrinolytic system, hypothermia, acidosis, and other metabolic changes.

The management of trauma-induced coagulopathy involves many components. The first step is to achieve normovolemia by fluid resuscitation. This may, however, result in dilution of clotting factors. Gelatin-containing products also impact fibrin polymerization and decrease clot elasticity. Hydroxyethyl starch-containing solutions result in hypocalcemia, blockade of the fibrinogen receptor, and disturbance in fibrin polymerization, all of which contribute to increased bleeding. Due to increased fibrinolysis, which results from tissue damage and subsequent release of tissue plasminogen activator, there is tendency for clot breakdown. This can be ameliorated by the administration of tranexamic acid.[54]

The development of acidosis also impairs clotting by altering enzyme activity, depleting fibrinogen levels, reducing platelet counts, prolonging the clotting time, and increasing bleeding time. Correction of acidosis and its effect on clotting is best achieved by reestablishing adequate tissue perfusion. At a pH of 7.1, there is a profound effect on enzyme activity; hence, at levels below this pH, administration of bicarbonate is indicated. Hypothermia also impairs coagulation by prolonging the prothrombin time, increasing the activated partial thromboplastin time, and reducing fibrinogen synthesis. In patients who become hypothermic as a consequence of trauma, management of the associated coagulopathy is limited until the hypothermia is corrected.

Thrombocytopenia, defined as platelet counts of less than 50,000, impairs clot formation. In such patients, platelet transfusions are required to prevent bleeding. Patients taking antiplatelet agents may have significant abnormalities of the clotting system despite normal platelet counts. This is especially critical in TBI associated with intracerebral hemorrhage, pelvic fractures, and significant bleeding into the soft tissues. In patients with a pre-injury history of aspirin or clopidogrel use, platelets are transfused irrespective of the platelet count. In patients on warfarin therapy, fresh frozen plasma must be administered to correct the international normalized ratio to a normal range.

SUMMARY

Injury is an important healthcare problem. Clinicians caring for trauma patients require a thorough understanding of the disturbances in homeostasis that accompany the injury. Furthermore, patients are now older, have more comorbidities, and have specific medical needs that must be recognized and addressed in order to restore health and optimize functional outcome.

REFERENCES

1. WISQARS Leading Causes of Death Reports, 1999–2007, Available at http://www.webappa.cdc.gov/sasweb.ncipc/leadcaus10.html. Accessed October 15, 2010.

2. WISQARS Years of Potential Life Lost (YPPL) before Age 65, ••. Available at http://www.webappa.cdc.gov/sasweb/ncipc/ypll10.html. Accessed October 15, 2010.

3. Ekeh AP, Walusimbi M, Brigham E, et al. The prevalence of incidental findings on abdominal computed tomography scans of trauma patients. *J Emerg Med.* 2010;38(4):484–489.

4. Munk MD, Peitzman AB, Hostier DP, Wolfson AB. Frequency and follow-up of incidental findings on trauma computed tomography scans: experience at a level one trauma center. *J Emerg Med.* 2010;38(3):346–350.

5. Kirby S, Sadler MR. Injury and death as a result of seizures. *Epilepsia.* 1995;36(1):25–28.

6. Bartoletti A, Fabiani P, Bagnoli L, et al. Physical injuries caused by transient loss of consciousness: main clinical characteristics of patients and diagnostic contribution of carotid sinus massage. *Eur Heart J.* 2008;29(5):618–624.

7. Fuchs BD, McMaster J, Smull G, et al. Underappreciation of sleep disorders as a cause of motor vehicle crashes. *Am J Emerg Med.* 2001;19(7):575–578.

8. Kortbeek JB, Turki SA, Ali J, et al. Advanced trauma life support, 8th edition, the evidence for change. *J Trauma.* 2008;64(1):1638–1650.

9. Riss J, Cloyd J, Gates J, Collins S. Benzodiazepines in epilepsy: pharmacology and pharmacokinetics. *Acta Neurol Scand.* 2008;118(2):69–86.

10. Frend V, Chetty M. Dosing and therapeutic monitoring of phenytoin in young adults after neurotrauma: are current practices relevant? *Clin Neuropharmacol.* 2007;30(6):362–369.

11. Eriksson K, Keranen T, Kalviainen R. Fosphenytoin. *Expert Opin Drug Metab Toxicol.* 2009;5(6):695–701.

12. Vespa PM, Nuwer MR, Nenov V, et al. Increased incidence and impact of nonconvulsive and convulsive seizures after traumatic brain injury as detected by continuous electroencephalographic monitoring. *J Neurosurg.* 1999;91(5):750–760.

13. Bullock MR, Povlishock JT. Guidelines for the management of severe traumatic brain injury. *J Neurotrauma.* 2007;24(Suppl 1):S1–S95.

14. Chesnut RM, Marshall LF, Klauber MR, et al. The role of secondary brain injury in determining outcome from severe head injury. *J Trauma.* 1993;34:216–222.

15. Marmarou A, Anderson RL, Ward JD, et al. Impact of ICP instability and hypotension in patients with severe head trauma. *J Neurosurg.* 1991;75:159–166.

16. Temkin NR, Dikmen SS, Wilensky AJ, et al. A randomized, double-blind study of phenytoin for the prevention of post-traumatic seizures. *N Engl J Med.* 1990;323:497–502.

17. Schierhout G, Roberts I. Antiepileptic drugs for preventing seizures following acute traumatic brain injury. *Cochrane Database Syst Rev.* 2001;(4):CD000173.

18. Mehta S, McCullagh I. Current sedation practices: lessons learned from international surveys. *Crit Care Clin.* 2009;25:471–488.

19. Spina SP, Ensom MHH. Clinical pharmacokinetic monitoring of midazolam in critically ill patients. *Pharmacotherapy.* 2007;27(3):389–398.

20. Kam PC, Cardone D. Propofol infusion syndrome. *Anesthesiology.* 2007;62:690–701.

21. Fong JJ, Sylvia L, Ruthazer R, et al. Predictors of mortality in patients with suspected propofol infusion syndrome. *Crit Care Med.* 2008;36(8):2281–2287.

22. Marik PE. Propofol: an immunomodulating agent. *Pharmacotherapy.* 2005;25:28S–33S.

23. Arroliga AC, Shehab N, McCarthy K, et al. Relationship of continuous infusion lorazepam to serum propylene glycol concentration in critically ill adults. *Crit Care Med.* 2004;32(8):1709–1714.

24. Ramsay MA, Savege TM, Simpson BR, et al. Controlled sedation with alphaxalone-alphadolone. *Br Med J.* 1974;2(920):656–659.

25. Sessler CN, Gosnell MS, Grap MJ, et al. The Richmond agitation-sedation scale: validity and reliability in adult intensive care unit patients. *Am J Respir Crit Care Med.* 2002;166(10):1338–1344.

26. Payen JF, Chanques G, Mantz J, et al. Current practices in sedation and analgesia for mechanically ventilated critically ill patients: a prospective multicenter patient-based study. *Anesthesiology.* 2007;106(4):687–695.

27. Weinert CR, Calvin AD. Epidemiology of sedation and sedation adequacy for mechanically ventilated patients in a medical and surgical intensive care unit. *Crit Care Med.* 2007;35(2):393–401.

28. Sessler CN, Varney K. Patient-focused sedation and analgesia in the ICU. *Chest.* 2008;133(2):552–565.

29. Girard TD, Kress JP, Fuchs BD, et al. Efficacy and safety of a paired sedation and ventilation weaning protocol for mechanically ventilated patients in intensive care (awakening and breathing controlled trial): a randomized controlled trial. *Lancet.* 2008;371:126–134.

30. Cohn SM, DuBose JJ. Pulmonary contusion: an update on recent advances in clinical management. *World J Surg.* 2010;34:1959–1970.

31. Pape HC, Remmers D, Rice J, et al. Appraisal of early evaluation of blunt chest trauma: development of a standardized scoring system for initial clinical decision making. *J Trauma.* 2000;49:496–504.

32. Truitt MS, Mooty RC, Amos J, Lorenzo M, Mangram A, Dunn E. Out with the old, in with the new: a novel approach to treating pain associated with rib fractures. *World J Surg.* 2010;34:2359–2362.

33. Pasquale MD, Nagy K, Clarke J. Practice management guidelines for screening of blunt cardiac injury. *J Trauma.* 1998;44(6):941–956.

34. Weyant MJ, Fullerton DA. Blunt thoracic trauma. *Semin Thorac Cardiovasc Surg.* 2008;20:26–30.

35. Elie MC. Blunt cardiac injury. *Mt Sinai J Med.* 2006;73:542–552.

36. Salim A, Velmahos GC, Jindal A, et al. Clinically significant blunt cardiac trauma: role of serum troponin levels combined with electrocardiographic findings. *J Trauma.* 2001;50(2):237–243.

37. Halpern NA, Bettes L, Greenstein R. Federal and nationwide intensive care units and healthcare costs: 1986–1992. *Crit Care Med.* 1994;22:2001–2007.

38. Jurkovich. GJ, Rivara FP, Gurney JG, et al. The effect of acute alcohol intoxication and chronic alcohol abuse on outcome from trauma. *JAMA.* 1993; 270:51–56.

39. Molina PE, Zambell KL, Norenberg K, et al. Consequences of alcohol-induced early dysregulation of responses to trauma/hemorrhage. *Alcohol.* 2004;33:217–227.

40. Spies CD, Kissner M, Neumann T, et al. Elevated carbohydrate- deficient transferrin predicts prolonged intensive care unit stay in traumatized men. *Alcohol Alcohol.* 1998;33:661–669.

41. Spies CD, Neuner B, Neumann T, et al. Intercurrent complications in chronic alcoholic men admitted to the intensive care unit following trauma. *Intensive Care Med.* 1996;22:286–293.

42. Reinert DF, Allen JP. The alcohol use disorders identification test (AUDIT): a review of recent research. *Alcohol Clin Exp Res.* 2002;26:272–279.

43. Amato L, Minozzi S, Vecchi S, Davoli M. Benzodiazepines for alcohol withdrawal. *Cochrane Database Syst Rev.* 2010;(3):CD005063.

44. Blondell RD, Dodds HN, Blondell MN, et al. Ethanol in formularies of US teaching hospitals. *JAMA.* 2003;289:552.

45. Hodges B, Mazur JE. Intravenous ethanol for the treatment of alcohol withdrawal syndrome in critically ill patients. *Pharmacotherapy.* 2004;24:1578–1585.

46. Mayo-Smith MF, Beecher LH, Fischer TL, et al. Management of alcohol withdrawal delirium. An evidence-based practice guideline. *Arch Intern Med.* 2004;164:1405–1412.

47. Geerts WH, Bergqvist D, Pineo GF, et al. Prevention of venous thromboembolism: American College of Chest Physicians evidence-based practice guidelines (8th edition). *Chest.* 2008;133(6 Suppl): 381S–453S.

48. Van Den Berghe G, Wilmer A, Hermans G, et al. Intensive insulin therapy in critically ill patients. *N Engl J Med.* 2001;345(19):1359–1367.

49. NICE-SUGAR Study Investigators, Finfer S, Chittock DR, Su SY, et al. Intensive versus conventional glucose control in critically ill patients. *N Engl J Med.* 2009;360(13):1283–1297.

50. Lepanto L, Tang A, Murphy-Lavallee J, Billiard JS. The Canadian Association of Radiologists guidelines for the prevention of contrast-induced nephropathy: a critical appraisal. *Can Assoc Radiol J.* 2010;62(4):238–242.

51. Hebert PC, Wells G, Blajchman MA, et al. A multicenter, randomized, controlled clinical trial of transfusion requirements in critical care. Canadian Critical Care Trials Group. *N Engl J Med.* 1999;340(6):409–417.

52. Napolitano LM, Kurek S, Luchette FA, et al. Clinical Practice Guideline: red cell transfusion in adult trauma and critical care. *J Trauma.* 2009;67(6):1439–1442.

53. Balogh ZJ, Butcher NE. Compartment syndromes from head to toe. *Crit Care Med.* 2010;38(9 Suppl):S445–S451.

54. CRASH-2 Trial Collaborators, Shakur H, Roberts I, Bautista R, et al. Effects of tranexamic acid on death, vascular occlusive events, and blood transfusion in trauma patients with significant haemorrhage (CRASH-2): a randomised, placebo-controlled trial. *Lancet.* 2010;376(9734):23–32.

CHAPTER 24

NEUROSURGERY

Christina Gilmore Ryan, Kamal S. Ajam,
and Rachel E. Thompson

BACKGROUND

Hospitalists are becoming increasingly involved in the neurosciences for many of the same reasons that led the hospitalist movement.[1] Neurosurgeons are constrained by the demands of outpatient clinics, operating rooms, and the care of medically complex inpatients. As the complexity of inpatient neurological care increases, many hospitals are looking to hospitalists to manage these patients. Hospitalists are well suited to assist in the care of neurosurgical patients given the wide variety of and frequent medical comorbidity and complications. There are few published evaluations of service lines employing hospitalists that work with neurosurgeons, although one study suggests that collaboration between surgical subspecialties and hospitalists can decrease time to surgery and length of stay.[2] Josephson et al. described their co-management model in which a hospitalist manages nonvascular neurosurgical patients and a neurologist manages vascular neurosurgical patients.[1] They suggested that this arrangement may allow for improved patient care and better availability of inpatient neurology consultation.

The perioperative care of a neurosurgery patient is challenging. Many of these patients are unable to communicate, and history is limited to collateral information or objective findings. The physical examination may be restricted due to the patient's inability to participate, the presence of devices or braces, or difficulty repositioning the patient. Moreover, neurosurgery patients are at risk for complications such as central fever or autonomic dysregulation and their medical comorbidities may be exacerbated and difficult to control in the setting of brain injury.

Hospitalists who co-manage neurosurgery patients must be aware that their own view and approach to certain medical problems may differ from their neurosurgical colleagues. Clear communication and collaboration are paramount. This chapter will describe the challenges and pitfalls inherent in the care of medically complex neurosurgery patients.

Perioperative Medicine: Medical Consultation and Co-Management, First Edition.
Edited by Amir K. Jaffer and Paul J. Grant.
© 2012 Wiley-Blackwell. Published 2012 by John Wiley & Sons, Inc.

SURGERY-SPECIFIC RISK

The spectrum of neurosurgical procedures may be as diverse and varied as those performed by general surgeons, especially when one considers the intricacy of spine surgery, intracranial surgery, and endovascular surgery. Clearly defining the risks for these procedures is difficult. The best way to estimate procedure-specific risks is through discussion with the operating neurosurgeon. Low-, intermediate-, and high-risk procedures that neurosurgeons perform can be generally categorized as follows:

- Lower-risk procedures include lumbar drain placement and lumbar punctures. Patients being evaluated for hydrocephalus or shunt dysfunction are also in this risk category. All of these procedures require little or no exposure to general anesthesia, though they are sometimes performed in the operating room. Duration is brief and blood loss is minimal.

- Intermediate-risk procedures include most elective craniotomies or craniectomies for tumor resection, and electroencephalogram lead placement. These procedures rarely require unusual positioning or prolonged exposure to anesthesia. Endoscopic neurosurgical procedures, including transsphenoidal pituitary tumor resection, are also intermediate-risk procedures. Placement of ventriculoperitoneal shunt is of intermediate risk, as access to multiple surgical sites and the use of general anesthesia are necessary.

- By the American College of Cardiology/American Heart Association (ACC/AHA) guidelines, spine surgery is considered intermediate risk for perioperative cardiac complications. We find this to be true of one- or two-level spinal fusions. Our impression is that multilevel spine fusions, especially staged procedures, are high risk for perioperative complications. For many spine surgeries, such as multilevel decompression and fusion, the patient must be prone for several hours. If an anterior approach is used, the patient may need a chest tube for postoperative pneumothorax. Often, there is sufficient blood loss to require perioperative transfusions. This example shows that communication with the surgeon preoperatively is essential to determining surgery-specific risk.

- Higher-risk intracranial procedures include craniotomy or craniectomy for trauma, cerebrovascular bypass grafting, and clipping of arteriovenous malformation or aneurysms. Given the difficult positioning, resection of skull base tumors is also a high-risk procedure. Craniotomy for traumatic brain injury is considered high risk by the American Surgical Association guidelines as managing intracranial hypertension can make anesthesia administration challenging.

PREOPERATIVE ASSESSMENT

Many neurosurgical procedures are urgent or emergent and patients must be taken directly to the operating room with minimal preoperative evaluation. For nonemergent surgeries, the general approach to the preoperative risk assessment for neurosurgical patients is similar to other surgical populations with the addition that it is essential for a member of the team to document a thorough neurologic exam. Preoperatively, after documenting the patient's neurologic function and defining the surgery-specific risk, hospitalists should consider challenges associated with the patient's intraoperative positioning. Are there any limitations to positioning and is the neck flexible and stable? The operative time and plan should also be considered: how long is the procedure, and how many stages are anticipated? What is an allowable and safe time for recovery between stages? Can the patient's surgery-specific risk be reduced if different methods of anesthesia are used? Hospitalists should raise and discuss these issues with their anesthesia colleagues to allow them to select appropriate intraoperative management. Assessing and reducing cardiovascular risk are crucial in caring for patients undergoing any procedure. Neurosurgery patients can be particularly difficult to evaluate because their limited mobility may prevent the ability to assess functional capacity. In the high-risk surgical patient (i.e., patients with multiple cardiovascular risk factors and/or a high Revised Cardiac Risk Index score), it may be prudent to pursue stress imaging to determine the extent of at-risk myocardium.

Postoperative pulmonary complications should also be considered and are particularly common after cervical spine surgeries and posttraumatic decompressive craniectomies. Risk factors for postoperative pulmonary complications include, but are not limited to, smoking, chronic lung disease, and congestive heart failure.[3] These patients can benefit from simple early interventions such as elevation of the head of the bed to greater than 30 degrees, aggressive pulmonary toilet, incentive spirometry, and selective nasogastric tube decompression.

Obesity has been associated with increased need for blood transfusions and discharge to assisted living or skilled nursing in postoperative spine patients.[4] A prospective analysis demonstrated that age greater than 70 years is associated with an increased complication rate (29.8% vs. 13.1%, $P < 0.0001$), length of stay (15.2 days vs. 10.9 days, $P < 0.0001$), and 30-day mortality (12% vs. 4.6%, $P < 0.0001$) in patients undergoing craniotomy for meningioma resection.[5] In this study, functionally dependent patients were 2.8 times more likely to die than functionally independent patients. These findings were independent of other medical comorbidities such as diabetes requiring insulin, chronic obstructive pulmonary disease (COPD), and renal failure.

POST-OP ASSESSMENT

Postoperative assessment of the neurosurgical patient should be guided by the neurologic exam. A thorough exam should be done and compared with the preoperative assessment—documenting expected and unexpected changes. Ideally, in the immediate postoperative setting, the patient should be monitored in the intensive care unit (ICU) where the patient can be assessed for recovery frequently. Unexpected changes should be communicated to the attending hospitalist, intensivist, or neurosurgeon and prompt an urgent examination. Patients at risk for vasospasm, or other acute neurologic deterioration, will require a prolonged ICU stay until they are clinically stable.

Comprehensive postoperative management of the neurosurgery patient also includes blood pressure control. Avoiding excessive hypertension and hypotension helps protect vulnerable brain tissue. Though permissive hypertension may be used to modulate postoperative vasospasm (particularly in patients with a subarachnoid hemorrhage [SAH]), excessive hypertension can lead to increased intracranial pressure, cerebral edema, and poor neurologic outcomes. Hypotension from overzealous blood pressure control, volume depletion, or other reasons can precipitate decreased cerebral perfusion pressure and cause peri-injury infarction.

After neurologic surgery, the hospitalist should assess the extubated patient's ability to protect his or her airway. Cervical spine procedures, particularly with an anterior approach, are associated with edema of the neck tissue, compromising both ventilation and swallowing. Altered mental status makes aspiration even more likely. Keeping the patient nil per os (NPO), raising the head of the bed, encouraging incentive spirometry, and considering early use of nasogastric tube decompression are ways to prevent postoperative pulmonary complications. Continuing ICU level of care for frequent assessment and monitoring from nursing and respiratory therapy is important.

The comprehensive and routine postoperative assessment should also include the following: (1) postoperative pain control and cautious use of pain medicines so as not to compromise the neurologic exam; (2) a safe plan for venous thromboembolism (VTE) prevention as discussed with the neurosurgeon; (3) monitoring for postoperative bleeding by routine examination of the surgical site, frequent neurological assessment, and monitoring postoperative hematocrit (checking platelet count and coagulation tests may be indicated following extensive spine surgeries, as these patients are at risk for consumptive coagulopathy); and (4) a thorough assessment of the patient's preexisting medical comorbidities, and outline of a safe plan for restarting outpatient medications.

MEDICAL MANAGEMENT

Medical complications in the neurosurgical patient are common and challenging. One must be watchful for the uncommon presentation of common problems and for perioperative issues unique to neurosurgery patients. We will review the problems commonly encountered in a postoperative neurosurgery patient.

Hyponatremia and Sodium Management

Sodium management is fundamental to comprehensive perioperative neurosurgical care. Sodium balance maintains adequate cerebral perfusion pressure and prevents cerebral edema, but this homeostasis is commonly altered in brain-injured patients. Hyponatremia is defined as a serum sodium less than 130 mEq/L. Among inpatients, it has a prevalence of 1–7% with two-thirds of cases developing after admission.[6,7] Hyponatremia has been associated with increased length of stay both in the general inpatient setting[8,9] and in neurosurgical inpatients.[10–12] It has also been associated with increased cerebral irritation that manifests as seizure activity and decreased level of consciousness.[10] To date, no significant association between mortality and hyponatremia has been demonstrated among neurosurgical patients. However, increased mortality of a general inpatient population was demonstrated in a large study.[8] Of note, mortality was greatest among patients who developed hyponatremia after admission.

Internists and neurosurgeons have different views on hyponatremia. To an internist, a sodium level of 130 mEq/L is not particularly alarming in the absence of symptoms. But the same sodium level may prompt a neurosurgeon to treat the patient for cerebral salt wasting (CSW) with salt tablets or, in the acute setting, transfer the patient to the ICU for hypertonic saline. Although the brain can adapt to sodium disturbances, this ability is limited by the rigid skull. If cerebral edema occurs (Figure 24.1) and intracranial pressure rises, brain damage and death may ensue.[13]

The brain responds to changes in osmolality by employing hypothalamic osmoreceptors. These cells signal magnocellular neurons to release arginine vasopressin (AVP; also known as antidiuretic hormone [ADH]). The magnocellular neurons also receive input from baroreceptors and will release AVP in response to moderate to severe volume loss. The net effect is for the kidney to retain water.[13]

Hyponatremia is common postoperatively. Two notable mechanisms include an increase in AVP induced by surgery and the administration of hypotonic saline.[6] Other common causes include the syndrome of inappropriate antidiuretic hormone (SIADH), polydipsia, and drug effects.[14] However, in hyponatremic neurosurgical

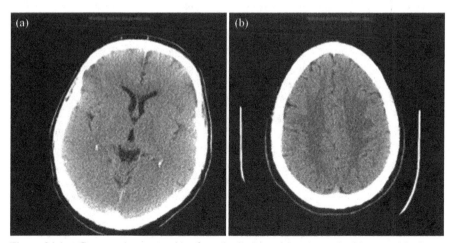

Figure 24.1.   Computed tomography of cerebral edema (a) compared with normal brain (b). Note loss of gray-white boarder in the presence of edema (a). *Images provided by Dr. Sung E. Logerfo, Assistant Professor of Radiology, University of Washington.* See color insert.

patients, scrupulous attention must be given to the possibility of CSW. This entity can look similar to SIADH but is treated differently. A failure to diagnose CSW may lead to increased morbidity and mortality.

One study from the Irish National Neurosciences Centre describes the course, pathophysiology, and associated outcomes of hyponatremia in neurosurgery patients.[10] Among the 1698 admitted patients, 187 developed hyponatremia after admission (serum sodium less than 130 mEq/L). On average, hyponatremia occurred 6.7 days after injury or 5.8 days after a procedure. The average time to resolution of hyponatremia was 3 days. The sodium level was between 126 and 130 mEq/L in 73% of patients and 121–125 mEq/L in 22% of patients. Only 5% had a serum sodium less than or equal to 120 mEq/L. Hyponatremia was more common among patients with SAH (19.6%) and tumor (15.8%) and less common in traumatic brain injury (9.6%) and pituitary surgery (6.2%). Only 0.8% of spine surgery patients developed documented hyponatremia. SIADH was the most common pathophysiology of hyponatremia <130 mEq/L in this study, identified in 62% of cases. Approximately 25% of patients with SIADH were noted to be on a medicine known to cause SIADH. Hypovolemic hyponatremia was the second most common cause. CSW was the etiology in 4.8% of cases, but the authors suggested this may be an underestimate of the true prevalence given the challenges in accurate volume assessment in the study's retrospective design.

Another study of SAH patients found similar rates of SIADH and CSW.[11] More recently, investigators from Stanford retrospectively studied a subset of patients with aneurysms and SAH with a sodium <135 mEq/L and found that CSW caused hyponatremia in 22.9% of patients and SIADH was the cause in 35.4% of patients.[12]

Both SIADH and CSW cause high urine sodium. Distinguishing the disorders can be difficult and treatment differs dramatically. Missing the diagnosis of CSW can lead to worsened cerebral vasospasm, ischemia, and infarction[15] because CSW causes negative sodium balance and volume contraction. The pathophysiology is unclear, but it is hypothesized that disrupted neural input or increased circulating natriuretic factors that act on the nephron may decrease sodium resorption.[13] In contrast, SIADH occurs when there is inappropriate antidiuresis that may occur in the presence of excessive ADH though this excess is not always seen.[7] In patients with SIADH, renal sodium handling is normal and water resorption is increased leading to an expansion of extracellular fluid.

A thorough evaluation of hyponatremia in the neurosurgical patient includes a review of fluid intake and output, medications, evaluation of volume status, and measurement of serum and urine osmolality and urine sodium. Hypovolemia distinguishes CSW from SIADH and is represented by decreased weight, negative fluid balance, low central venous pressures, increased hematocrit, rising blood urea nitrogen and bicarbonate, and possibly, increased creatinine and low fractional excretion of sodium (Table 24.1).[15,16]

If CSW is suspected, adequate volume repletion is the mainstay of therapy. Additionally, oral salt tablets or hypertonic saline may be necessary to replete total body sodium, although the evidence supporting this practice is limited. For refractory cases, one can consider adding fludrocortisone or hydrocortisone.[15] If SIADH is suspected, euvolemia should be confirmed before fluid restriction is ordered.

TABLE 24.1. Differentiating Cerebral Salt Wasting (CSW) and Syndrome of Inappropriate Antidiuresis Hormone (SIADH)[15,16]

Feature	CSW	SIAD
Hematocrit	Increased	Normal
Albumin	Increased	Normal
Blood urea nitrogen (BUN)/Cr	Increased	Decreased
Potassium	Normal/increased	Normal
Uric acid	Normal/decreased	Decreased
Central venous pressure	<6	>6
Treatment	Saline, salt tablets	Free water restriction[a]

[a] Caution must be taken when fluid restricting neurosurgical patients. One must first be certain that the patient is euvolemic and subsequently maintains euvolemia.

Symptomatic hyponatremia in a neurosurgical patient, regardless of etiology, necessitates intensive care and therapy with hypertonic saline. In acute hyponatremia (developed within 48 h), rate of correction is less of a concern. However, patients with subacute or chronic hyponatremia are at increased risk for osmotic demyelination if the sodium level increases too rapidly. The rate of correction should be no more than 10–12 mEq/L in a 24-h period. Frequent serum sodium monitoring (i.e., every 4–6 h) is imperative.

Fever: Infection, Central Fever, and Dysautonomia

Fever is common in the neurosurgical patient with a reported incidence of 50–70% in patients with acute ischemic stroke and more than 75% of ICU patients with intracranial hemorrhage. Fever usually occurs in the first 72 h of hospitalization and can be associated with the usual postoperative causes or be specific to the neurologic injury as in central fever. In the SAH population, fever in the ICU is more often related to nosocomial infection than noninfectious causes (odds ratio [OR] 2.96 vs. 2.78, $P = 0.05$).[17,18]

Fever is a normal physiologic response to a stimulus. The stimulus (usually bacteria or trauma) causes macrophage activation and release of cytokines that signal host cells to produce cyclooxygenase-2 (COX-2) and prostaglandin E2 (PGE2). COX-2 and PGE2 cross the blood–brain barrier and trigger warm sensitive neurons in the hypothalamus to increase the core temperature through shivering and increased metabolism. Fever can be beneficial to the body by releasing nitric oxide and heat shock proteins that support normal body functioning and response to insults. Some of this benefit is outweighed by the effect of fever on the brain: free radical production, increased intracranial hypertension, and increased permeability of the blood–brain barrier—all of which lead to increased tissue damage.[19]

Studies have shown that fever in neurosurgical patients correlates to poor clinical outcomes and longer ICU stays. One retrospective cohort study of 110 adults with traumatic brain injury found that ICU patients with fever had a length of stay increased by 7 days. Furthermore, fever was associated with increased intracranial pressure despite equivalent cerebral perfusion pressure. This study also showed that patients with fever were more likely to have a Glasgow coma scale less than 8, suggesting that fever is associated with poor neurologic outcome. It is unclear, however, whether fever is a cause or result of these findings.[18,20]

Fever in the neurosurgical patient can have many etiologies including infectious, thromboembolic, and iatrogenic processes. Physical examination, chest radiography, and urinalysis are an important part of the diagnostic workup. Other sources of infection include sinusitis from feeding tube placement, nosocomial meningitis, wound infection, and drain or line infection. If drain infection, ventriculitis, meningitis, or wound infection is suspected, prompt communication with the neurosurgery team is crucial.

Medications can also cause fever in neurosurgery patients. For posttrauma seizure prophylaxis, phenytoin, a common cause of drug-induced fever, is routinely prescribed. Phenytoin-associated fever usually starts within 5 days of the first dose, but can present up to 30 days after the first administration.[21] It can be associated with a rash, lymphadenopathy (54%), and alterations in liver function (71%), the latter is often referred to as anticonvulsant hypersensitivity syndrome. Once the medication is discontinued, it can take up to 2 weeks for the fevers to subside. Anticonvulsants such as carbamezepine and phenobarbital can also cause fever. Other less common drug-related fevers include heparin, thyroid hormone, anticholinergics, antihistamines, and hydralazine.

Two diagnoses specific to neurosurgical patients include central fever and dysautonomia. Central fever is generated by the hypothalamus in response to the presence of blood in the cerebrospinal fluid (CSF) or proximate tissue damage. It is a diagnosis of exclusion. Central fever is more commonly seen in patients with severe central nervous system injury and tends to have a long duration. Central fever is part of the cluster of autonomic dysregulation syndromes. These include dysautonomia (or autonomic storm), autonomic dysreflexia, and neuroleptic malignant syndrome. Dysautonomia occurs in up to 33% of traumatic brain injury patients, but it can also occur in patients with tumor, hydrocephalus, and anoxic brain injury.[22] The etiology is only theoretical and includes direct injury to the hypothalamus, disruption of connections between hypothalamus and cortex, or disruption of connection between the hypothalamus and brain stem controls. Central fever likely develops by a combination of all three mechanisms.

There are multiple definitions of dysautonomia in the literature, and making the diagnosis is challenging (Table 24.2). It variably presents with paroxysms of agitation, hyperthermia, hypertension, tachycardia, drenching sweats, and tachypnea. The patient may also have either extensor or flexor hypertonia and posturing.[23] Dysautonomia usually presents during the first week after brain injury, and it may last weeks or months. Longer periods of dysautonomia, when they occur, are characteristic of patients with anoxic brain injury, but these rarely last more than a year.

It is important to manage fever safely in the brain-injured patient. Reducing fever decreases the metabolic demands of the brain and helps prevent further brain injury. Acetaminophen should be scheduled, but sometimes, it is ineffective as monotherapy for fever in brain-injured patients. Ibuprofen and other nonsteroidal

TABLE 24.2. Dysautonomia (Storming) and Agitation Related to Brain Injury

	Dysautonomia	Agitation[a]

Diagnosis	• Onset within a week of injury
	• May persist for weeks to months
	• Clinical signs:
	  Temperature >38°C
	  Tachycardia 140–170
	  Hypertension 120–180/80–120
	  Diaphoresis
	  Posturing
		• Increases with fatigue or overstimulation
		• Restlessness
		• Purposeful movements
		• Picks at tubes and clothes
		• May have associated tachycardia and hypertension
		• Less commonly associated with high fever

Treatment	Morphine
	Propranolol
	Bromocriptine
	Clonidine
	Thorazine
		Acutely:
		  Benzodiazapines
		  Haloperidol
		Chronic:
		  Propranolol
		  Carbamazepine
		  Haloperidol
		  Valproic acid

These can be difficult to differentiate in a brain-injured patient.[22,23]

[a] In diagnosing agitation that relates to brain injury, one must first consider and evaluate for other causes including pain, infection, drug or alcohol withdrawal, increased intracranial pressures, and other causes of medical delirium.

anti-inflammatory drugs (NSAIDs) have antiprostaglandin mechanisms of therapy and are useful adjuncts to acetaminophen therapy if acceptable to the comanaging neurosurgeon.

Managing dysautonomia often requires the use of multiple agents. Morphine, benzodiazepines, clonidine, beta-blockers, bromocriptine, and gabapentin have all been used with variable success. One systematic review found a trend toward benefit from bromocriptine and baclofen. Propranolol and benzodiazepines also had trends toward benefit, but there was no effect with opiates.[22]

Neurocardiology

Morphologic changes on electrocardiogram (EKG) in patients with intracranial pathology have been described in the literature since the 1950s, primarily in patients with ruptured aneurysms (Figure 24.2). In fact, up to 80% of SAH patients may have EKG changes. Any abnormality may be seen, but the most common findings are repolarization abnormalities and T-wave inversions. In one study in which EKG changes were evaluated, ST depression correlated with poor outcomes. This relationship was lost after accounting for APACHE II scores, vasospasm, and intracranial hypertension.[24]

There are multiple theories about the causes of these EKG changes: (1) the patients have preexisting coronary artery disease, (2) nervous system-mediated coronary artery vasospasm occurs, or (3) catecholamines released directly into the myocardium from the sympathetic nervous system cause contraction band necrosis.[25,26]

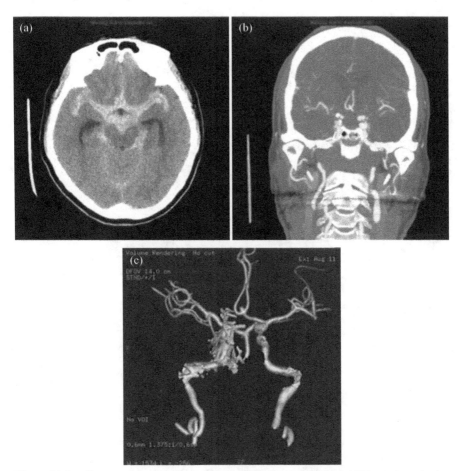

Figure 24.2.   Computed tomography angiogram (CTA) of subarachnoid hemorrhage in the setting of an aneurysm. (a) CTA sagittal view demonstrating blood in the subarachnoid space; (b) CTA coronal view showing aneurysm; (c) 3D reconstruction of vasculature demonstrating aneurysm. *Images provided by Dr. Sung E. Logerfo, Assistant Professor of Radiology, University of Washington.* See color insert.

Cardiac dysfunction may be noted on echocardiography, but the consequences of any findings in the setting of brain injury are poorly understood. In one prospective study of 39 patients with SAH, electrocardiogram and troponin I were ordered daily for 7 days. Echocardiograms were performed within 24 h of any documented abnormality. About 20% of patients had troponin elevation. Patients with a more severe Hunt–Hess score (a commonly used measure of neurologic injury ranging from 1 with at most mild symptoms or signs to 5 with coma or decerebrate posturing) were more likely to have abnormal troponins and myocardial dysfunction.[25]

Another study of 223 SAH patients confirmed troponin I elevation correlates with severity of SAH. Troponin release was most common in patients with Hunt–

Hess Grade 5. Troponin elevation correlated with left ventricular hypertrophy, hypotension, and tachycardia, and was more common in women and younger patients. There was no correlation between troponin elevation and serum catecholamine measurements.[26]

To differentiate neurocardiac injury from acute myocardial infarction, Bulsara et al. performed a retrospective analysis of 10 patients with SAH and severe cardiac dysfunction. These patients were compared with patients admitted with acute myocardial infarction and similar left ventricular ejection fractions. They found that EKG and echocardiographic findings did not correlate to a coronary vascular distribution in patients with SAH as they did in myocardial infarction patients. Furthermore, SAH patients had, on average, lower troponins—generally less than 2.8 ng/mL. They concluded that enzymes could not be trended to distinguish between the two etiologies. Those with neurocardiogenic left ventricular dysfunction recovered more quickly—in less than 5 days—compared with those with myocardial infarction.[27]

If neurocardiac injury is confirmed, routine supportive cardiac care is indicated. There is no specific additional care. However, the patient should be screened and treated for occult cardiovascular disease, and monitored closely in the outpatient setting for resolution of neurocardiac abnormalities.

Hypertension

In the neurosurgical patient, postoperative hypertension may be a necessity rather than a problem to be solved. The differential diagnosis includes untreated essential hypertension (new diagnosis vs. usual medications held), pain, anxiety, intravascular volume excess, endocrinopathy, and Cushing response. Knowing the etiologies and the effects of hypertension in the neurosurgical patient helps guide management.

Postoperative spine patients are frequently hypotensive in the immediate postoperative period. As they transition from intravenous to oral pain medications and become volume replete, blood pressure begins to rise. After ensuring their pain is well controlled, it is prudent to restart patients with essential hypertension on their outpatient medication regimens. If the hypertension is new and asymptomatic, starting a rapid onset medication for severe hypertension may help decrease the risk of surgical site bleeding. The primary care provider should be alerted to the fact that the patient is receiving a new medication, one that may not be effective, or even necessary, after discharge.

Patients with intracranial pathology and hypertension require a different overall approach. In the ICU, permissive hypertension is used to maintain cerebral perfusion pressure (cerebral perfusion pressure = MAP − intracranial pressure). The goal is to allow adequate cerebral perfusion pressure without increasing intracranial pressure which can cause secondary brain injury.[28] In SAH patients, hypertension may be used to treat vasospasm, and it represents one pillar of what is commonly known as "triple-H" therapy: hypervolemia, hemodilution, and hypertension. Each intervention improves cerebral perfusion. Triple-H protocols have never been studied in randomized clinical trials but are often favored based on evidence from observational studies.[29] The role of the hospitalist is to ensure the patient is hypervolemic and limit antihypertensive medications.

Subsequent to the acute phase of brain injury, many patients with intracranial hemorrhage (especially SAH patients) have severe hypertension requiring three or more drugs. The patient is often on a calcium channel blocker such as nimodipine for vasospasm management that is typically continued for a 21-day course. Beta-blockers, angiotensin-converting enzyme (ACE) inhibitors, diuretics, and alpha agents are all options that can be added as appropriate. The blood pressure should be reduced to less than 150–160/90 mm Hg with continued outpatient titration of medications until the target long-term blood pressure goal is achieved.

Glycemic Control

Diabetes is associated with a 4.2-fold increase in perioperative mortality.[30] Hyperglycemia among patients with diabetes as well as stress hyperglycemia in patients with no history of diabetes has been associated with increased neuronal damage following ischemia.[31] One study of patients with SAH found a sevenfold increase in poor neurologic outcome at 10 months in patients with persistent hyperglycemia, defined as having glucoses greater than 200 mg/dL for 2 or more days.[32] Increased morbidity has also been associated with diabetes and hyperglycemia among patients undergoing brain biopsy and spinal procedures.[33,34]

In the neurocritical care setting, intensive insulin therapy was associated with a decreased infection rate in one study,[35] but not in a subsequent study.[36] No long-term neurologic benefit was observed. Another intervention trial among patients with spontaneous intracranial hemorrhage and hyperglycemia found elevations in glucose correlated with increased mortality; however, early intensive insulin therapy did not improve prognosis.[37] Despite these findings, a meta-analysis of intensive insulin therapy found a mortality benefit among surgical ICUs (risk ratio 0.63 [95% confidence interval {CI} 0.44–0.91]); however, specific data for neurocritical care patients were not evaluated.[38] Among patients with traumatic brain injury, intensive insulin therapy is associated with increased hypoglycemia, intracranial pressure, and a trend toward worsened 21-day mortality.[39] Hypoglycemia has also been associated with increased mortality and morbidity in more generalized critical care settings.[40]

In the final analysis, both severe hyperglycemia *and* intensive insulin therapy with increased risk of hypoglycemia have been associated with poor outcomes in the neurosurgical patient population. What remains to be defined is an optimal range of glucose levels or another measure that better determines adequate control to prevent morbidity and maximize neurologic outcome. There is expert consensus that all blood sugars in the intensive care or the acute care setting should be less than 180 mg/dL and avoidance of low sugars is essential. It may be reasonable to aim for an upper limit of blood glucose closer to 150 mg/dL in neurocritical care settings, but there is insufficient evidence to support this practice.

To obtain these goals in the intraoperative and intensive care settings, we recommend intravenous insulin infusions for patients who are hyperglycemic to greater than 180 mg/dL. In less acute patients and in patients either eating or with enteral feedings, a combination of basal, prandial, and correction dose subcutaneous insulin is superior. Avoidance of sliding-scale insulin and oral hypoglycemics among inpatients is standard of care in our institution.

Anticoagulation

Approximately 10% of in-hospital deaths are due to pulmonary embolism (PE), making it the most common cause of inpatient mortality.[41] Fatal PE occurs most commonly in hip fracture patients (4–7%) and also significantly contributes to neurosurgical mortality (1%).[42] VTE prophylaxis can reduce this rate, but not without potentially serious consequences. The risk of worsening injury or death from bleeding is great enough that neurosurgeons are reluctant to anticoagulate patients perioperatively. Thus, there are little outcome data on the impact of heparin in these patients.

Compression devices and pharmacologic prophylaxis are effective in reducing risk of VTE. Elastic stockings and compression devices pose little or no risk of harm. One randomized controlled trial of stockings versus stockings and compression devices in 150 intracranial hemorrhage patients found that combination therapy significantly reduced the risk of asymptomatic lower extremity deep venous thrombosis.[43]

Low-dose unfractionated heparin decreases VTE incidence by at least 40% compared with compression devices alone in the neurosurgical population.[44] Despite these rather compelling data, heparin administration is frequently left to the surgeon's discretion due to the associated increased risk of intracranial bleeding.

Few randomized controlled studies have examined the consequences of pharmacologic prophylaxis for VTE in neurosurgery patients. One systematic review with a decision analysis evaluation showed an insignificant trend toward increased bleeding with pharmacologic prophylaxis.[44,45] This study suggested that unfractionated heparin may have less of a risk than LMWH. The authors noted that more studies are needed to determine safe use parameters. Additionally, a recent meta-analysis of neurosurgery patients demonstrated that prophylactic low-molecular-weight heparin (LMWH) was associated with a nonsignificant increase in bleeding risk compared with non-pharmacologic alternatives. Another study of 68 patients with brain tumors randomized to LMWH at the time of preanesthesia versus compression devices alone was stopped prior to completion due to five clinically significant postoperative hemorrhages (four intracerebral and one epidural) in the 44 patients assigned to the LMWH group. There was no significant difference in VTE incidence.[46] Patients with lobar hemorrhage, larger aneurysms, older age, and more severe Hunt–Hess grade may be at increased risk for rebleeding while on heparin prophylaxis.[28] Among polytrauma patients and patients with spinal cord injury with paralysis, LMWH is believed to be superior to unfractionated heparin. Our institutional guidelines reflect this and are available in Table 24.3.[47] Hospitalists should be knowledgeable of these risks and benefits of VTE prophylaxis modalities specific to the neurosurgical population and thus will be better equipped to engage in conversations about anticoagulation with our neurosurgical colleagues.

Delirium

Delirium in the inpatient is a known cause of inpatient mortality.[48,49] Hospitalists can anticipate which patients are at risk and help create environments that decrease the risk of delirium. One review of 224 patients identified independent risk factors for postoperative delirium lasting 14–60 days in patients over the age of 70 years. These

TABLE 24.3. University of Washington Guideline for Venous Thromboembolism Prophylaxis in Neurosurgical Patients[47]

Injury type	First line	Second line	SCD augmentation	Routine DVT screen with duplex
Spinal cord injury (when hemostasis is evident)	Enoxaparin 30 mg sq q12h	UF heparin 5000 sq q8h or q12h and SCDs	Yes	High risk for VTE (SCI, LE, or pelvic fracture, head injury) and suboptimal prophylaxis
Head injury/bleed (when hemorrhage is stable on CT)	UF heparin 5000 sq q8h or q12h	Enoxaparin 40 mg sq daily	Yes	No
Elective neurosurgery (generally considered safe to institute 48–72 h after surgery)	UF heparin 5000 sq q8h or q12h	Enoxaparin 40 mg sq daily	Yes	No

UF, unfractionated; SCD, sequential compression device; DVT, deep venous thrombosis; SCI, spinal cord injury; LE, lower extremity; CT, computed tomography.

were prior history of dementia and diabetes, surgery under local or regional anesthesia (the authors note this as a potential marker of higher risk patients), and severe postoperative pain requiring opioids. The incidence of delirium was 21.4%, 95% of whom had delirium by postoperative day 2.[50] Though the study had several limitations, it is the first that attempted to define a target population of neurosurgical patients at risk for delirium. Clearly, in all neurosurgical patients, deliriogenic medications and interventions should be avoided. A multidisciplinary team can help minimize nighttime interruptions, provide frequent reorientation, and maintain circadian patterns.

Once the diagnosis is made, the goal should be to determine the etiology of delirium. In the hospitalized medical patient, the differential includes drugs, infections, uncontrolled pain, metabolic derangements, low perfusion states, and recent surgery. The differential in the neurosurgical patient includes all of these in addition to a few others specific to the clinical situation: seizures, brain injury, new or worsening intracranial hemorrhage, vasospasm leading to cerebral ischemia, increased intracranial pressure, and dysautonomia.

Medical treatment of delirium has not been well studied in the neurosurgical patient population. Animal studies have shown that typical antipsychotics may delay motor function recovery when used in traumatic brain injury.[51] Case-based evidence suggests atypical antipsychotics cause less D2 receptor inhibition and more serotonergic receptor inhibition. In one randomized controlled trial of 28 inpatients, there was no difference in recovery between patients treated with haloperidol and those treated with risperidone. There were more extrapyramidal symptoms in the halo-peridol group.[52] Our neurosurgery colleagues prefer quetiapine scheduled in the evening.

Selective serotonin reuptake inhibitors (SSRIs) have been used to treat delirium in patients with traumatic brain injury because there is increased incidence of depression in these patients, which can contribute to delirium.[53] There is case-based and anecdotal evidence to support the use of SSRIs in treating agitated delirium in the traumatic brain injury patient.[54] If agitation or depression is not present, halo-peridol can also be used to treat delirium. Though haloperidol is widely accepted as a treatment option for delirium, it is not well studied in neurosurgery patients.

Hospitalists should maintain a high index of suspicion for other causes of delirium in the neurosurgery patient such as nonconvulsive epileptic seizures, recurrent intracranial hemorrhage, ventriculitis, meningitis, or shunt infection. In pursuit of an etiology and safe management plan for delirium in the neurosurgery patient, effective communication with neurosurgery colleagues is essential.

DISCHARGE RECOMMENDATIONS AND CONSIDERATIONS

Transitioning a neurosurgery patient from the inpatient to the outpatient setting requires precision. Clear communication between inpatient and outpatient providers of a documented care plan including medication changes and pending test results is paramount.[55] Hospitalists ensure a safe hand off to the patient's primary care provider by documenting the neurosurgical plan as well as summarize any medical developments that occurred in the hospital and updates on prehospitalization conditions.

Discharge documentation should include recommendations regarding nutrition, speech, physical and occupational therapies, and signs or symptoms that should prompt immediate attention. These might include fever, a change in mental status, a change in level of functioning, or signs of wound infection. For patients discharging to home, consider the need for visiting nurse services and evaluations. Additionally, the hospitalist should arrange for follow-up of sodium balance, blood pressure, and glycemic control as appropriate.

REFERENCES

1. Josephson SA, Engstrom JW, Wachter RM. Neurohospitalists: an emerging model for inpatient neurological care. *Ann Neurol.* Feb 2008;63(2):135–140.
2. Peterson MC. A systematic review of outcomes and quality measures in adult patients cared for by hospitalists vs nonhospitalists. *Mayo Clin Proc.* Mar 2009;84(3):248–254.
3. Qaseem A, Snow V, Fitterman N, Hornbake ER, Lawrence VA, Smetana GW, Weiss K, Owens DK, Aronson M, Barry P, Casey DE, Jr., Cross JT, Jr., Fitterman N, Sherif KD, Weiss KB, Clinical Efficacy Assessment Subcommittee of the American College of Physicians. Risk assessment for and strategies to reduce perioperative pulmonary complications for patients undergoing noncardiothoracic surgery: a guideline from the American College of Physicians. *Ann Intern Med.* Apr 2006; 144(8):575–580.

4. Shamji MF, Parker S, Cook C, Pietrobon R, Brown C, Isaacs RE. Impact of body habitus on perioperative morbidity associated with fusion of the thoracolumbar and lumbar spine. *Neurosurgery.* Sep 2009;65(3):490–498; discussion 498.

5. Patil CG, Veeravagu A, Lad S, Boakye M. Craniotomy for resection of meningioma in the elderly: a multicenter, prospective analysis from the National Surgical Quality Improvement Program. *J Neurol Neurosurg Psychiatry.* May 2010;81(5):502–505.

6. Anderson RJ, Chung HM, Kluge R, Schrier RW. Hyponatremia: a prospective analysis of its epidemiology and the pathogenetic role of vasopressin. *Ann Intern Med.* Feb 1985;102(2):164–168.

7. Ellison DH, Berl T. Clinical practice. the syndrome of inappropriate antidiuresis. *N Engl J Med.* May 2007;356(20):2064–2072.

8. Gill G, Huda B, Boyd A, Skagen K, Wile D, Watson I, van Heyningen C. Characteristics and mortality of severe hyponatraemia—a hospital-based study. *Clin Endocrinol (Oxf).* Aug 2006;65(2): 246–249.

9. Wald R, Jaber BL, Price LL, Upadhyay A, Madias NE. Impact of hospital-associated hyponatremia on selected outcomes. *Arch Intern Med.* Feb 2010;170(3):294–302.

10. Sherlock M, O'Sullivan E, Agha A, Behan LA, Owens D, Finucane F, Rawluk D, Tormey W, Thompson CJ. Incidence and pathophysiology of severe hyponatraemia in neurosurgical patients. *Postgrad Med J.* Apr 2009;85(1002):171–175.

11. Sherlock M, O'Sullivan E, Agha A, Behan LA, Rawluk D, Brennan P, Tormey W, Thompson CJ. The incidence and pathophysiology of hyponatraemia after subarachnoid haemorrhage. *Clin Endocrinol (Oxf).* Mar 2006;64(3):250–254.

12. Kao L, Al-Lawati Z, Vavao J, Steinberg GK, Katznelson L. Prevalence and clinical demographics of cerebral salt wasting in patients with aneurysmal subarachnoid hemorrhage. *Pituitary.* 2009; 12(4):347–351.

13. Diringer MN, Zazulia AR. Hyponatremia in neurologic patients: consequences and approaches to treatment. *Neurologist.* May 2006;12(3):117–126.

14. Adrogue HJ, Madias NE. Hyponatremia. *N Engl J Med.* May 2000;342(21):1581–1589.

15. Rahman M, Friedman WA. Hyponatremia in neurosurgical patients: clinical guidelines development. *Neurosurgery.* Nov 2009;65(5):925–935; discussion 935–936.

16. Palmer BF. Hyponatremia in patients with central nervous system disease: SIADH versus CSW. *Trends Endocrinol Metab.* May–Jun 2003;14(4):182–187.

17. Cormio M, Citerio G, Portella G, Patruno A, Pesenti A. Treatment of fever in neurosurgical patients. *Minerva Anestesiol.* Apr 2003;69(4):214–222.

18. Commichau C, Scarmeas N, Mayer SA. Risk factors for fever in the neurologic intensive care unit. *Neurology.* Mar 2003;60(5):837–841.

19. Thompson HJ, Tkacs NC, Saatman KE, Raghupathi R, McIntosh TK. Hyperthermia following traumatic brain injury: a critical evaluation. *Neurobiol Dis.* Apr 2003;12(3):163–173.

20. Stocchetti N, Rossi S, Zanier ER, Colombo A, Beretta L, Citerio G. Pyrexia in head-injured patients admitted to intensive care. *Intensive Care Med.* Nov 2002;28(11):1555–1562.

21. Mansur AT, Pekcan Yasar S, Goktay F. Anticonvulsant hypersensitivity syndrome: clinical and laboratory features. *Int J Dermatol.* Nov 2008;47(11):1184–1189.

22. Baguley IJ. Autonomic complications following central nervous system injury. *Semin Neurol.* Nov 2008;28(5):716–725.

23. Blackman JA, Patrick PD, Buck ML, Rust RS, Jr. Paroxysmal autonomic instability with dystonia after brain injury. *Arch Neurol.* Mar 2004;61(3):321–328.

24. Sakr YL, Lim N, Amaral AC, Ghosn I, Carvalho FB, Renard M, Vincent JL. Relation of ECG changes to neurological outcome in patients with aneurysmal subarachnoid hemorrhage. *Int J Cardiol.* Sep 2004;96(3):369–373.

25. Parekh N, Venkatesh B, Cross D, Leditschke A, Atherton J, Miles W, Winning A, Clague A, Rickard C. Cardiac troponin I predicts myocardial dysfunction in aneurysmal subarachnoid hemorrhage. *J Am Coll Cardiol.* Oct 2000;36(4):1328–1335.

26. Tung P, Kopelnik A, Banki N, Ong K, Ko N, Lawton MT, Gress D, Drew B, Foster E, Parmley W, Zaroff J. Predictors of neurocardiogenic injury after subarachnoid hemorrhage. *Stroke.* Feb 2004; 35(2):548–551.

27. Bulsara KR, McGirt MJ, Liao L, Villavicencio AT, Borel C, Alexander MJ, Friedman AH. Use of the peak troponin value to differentiate myocardial infarction from reversible neurogenic left ventricular dysfunction associated with aneurysmal subarachnoid hemorrhage. *J Neurosurg.* Mar 2003;98(3):524–528.

28. Greenberg MS. *Handbook of Neurosurgery*, 6th edition. London: Thieme; 2005.

29. Lazaridis C, Naval N. Risk factors and medical management of vasospasm after subarachnoid hemorrhage. *Neurosurg Clin N Am.* Apr 2010;21(2):353–364.

30. Acott AA, Theus SA, Kim LT. Long-term glucose control and risk of perioperative complications. *Am J Surg.* Nov 2009;198(5):596–599.

31. Clement S, Braithwaite SS, Magee MF, Ahmann A, Smith EP, Schafer RG, Hirsch IB, American Diabetes Association Diabetes in Hospitals Writing Committee. Management of diabetes and hyperglycemia in hospitals. *Diabetes Care.* Feb 2004;27(2):553–591.

32. McGirt MJ, Woodworth GF, Ali M, Than KD, Tamargo RJ, Clatterbuck RE. Persistent perioperative hyperglycemia as an independent predictor of poor outcome after aneurysmal subarachnoid hemorrhage. *J Neurosurg.* Dec 2007;107(6):1080–1085.

33. McGirt MJ, Woodworth GF, Coon AL, Frazier JM, Amundson E, Garonzik I, Olivi A, Weingart JD. Independent predictors of morbidity after image-guided stereotactic brain biopsy: a risk assessment of 270 cases. *J Neurosurg.* May 2005;102(5):897–901.

34. Olsen MA, Nepple JJ, Riew KD, Lenke LG, Bridwell KH, Mayfield J, Fraser VJ. Risk factors for surgical site infection following orthopaedic spinal operations. *J Bone Joint Surg Am.* Jan 2008;90(1):62–69.

35. Bilotta F, Spinelli A, Giovannini F, Doronzio A, Delfini R, Rosa G. The effect of intensive insulin therapy on infection rate, vasospasm, neurologic outcome, and mortality in neurointensive care unit after intracranial aneurysm clipping in patients with acute subarachnoid hemorrhage: a randomized prospective pilot trial. *J Neurosurg Anesthesiol.* Jul 2007;19(3):156–160.

36. Bilotta F, Caramia R, Cernak I, Paoloni FP, Doronzio A, Cuzzone V, Santoro A, Rosa G. Intensive insulin therapy after severe traumatic brain injury: a randomized clinical trial. *Neurocrit Care.* 2008;9(2):159–166.

37. Godoy DA, Pinero GR, Svampa S, Papa F, Di Napoli M. Hyperglycemia and short-term outcome in patients with spontaneous intracerebral hemorrhage. *Neurocrit Care.* 2008;9(2):217–229.

38. Griesdale DE, de Souza RJ, van Dam RM, Heyland DK, Cook DJ, Malhotra A, Dhaliwal R, Henderson WR, Chittock DR, Finfer S, Talmor D. Intensive insulin therapy and mortality among critically ill patients: a meta-analysis including NICE-SUGAR study data. *CMAJ.* Apr 2009;180(8):821–827.

39. Meier R, Bechir M, Ludwig S, Sommerfeld J, Keel M, Steiger P, Stocker R, Stover JF. Differential temporal profile of lowered blood glucose levels (3.5 to 6.5 mmol/l versus 5 to 8 mmol/l) in patients with severe traumatic brain injury. *Crit Care.* 2008;12(4):R98.

40. Egi M, Bellomo R, Stachowski E, French CJ, Hart GK, Taori G, Hegarty C, Bailey M. Hypoglycemia and outcome in critically ill patients. *Mayo Clin Proc.* Mar 2010;85(3):217–224.

41. Maynard G, Stein J. *Preventing Hospital-Acquired Venous Thromboembolism: A Guide for Effective Quality Improvement.* AHRQ Publication No. 08-0075. Rockville, MD: Agency for Healthcare Research and Quality; Aug 2008. Available at http://www.ahrq.gov/qual/vtguide/.

42. Geerts WH, Bergqvist D, Pineo GF, Heit JA, Samama CM, Lassen MR, Colwell CW, American College of Chest Physicians. Prevention of venous thromboembolism: American college of chest physicians evidence-based clinical practice guidelines (8th edition). *Chest.* Jun 2008;133(6 Suppl):381S–453S.

43. Lacut K, Bressollette L, Le Gal G, Etienne E, De Tinteniac A, Renault A, Rouhart F, Besson G, Garcia JF, Mottier D, Oger E. VICTORIAh (Venous Intermittent Compression and Thrombosis Occurrence Related to Intra-Cerebral Acute Hemorrhage) Investigators. Prevention of venous thrombosis in patients with acute intracerebral hemorrhage. *Neurology.* Sep 2005;65(6):865–869.

44. Collen JF, Jackson JL, Shorr AF, Moores LK. Prevention of venous thromboembolism in neurosurgery: a meta-analysis. *Chest.* 2008;134(2):237–249.

45. Danish SF, Burnett MG, Ong JG, Sonnad SS, Maloney-Wilensky E, Stein SC. Prophylaxis for deep venous thrombosis in craniotomy patients: a decision analysis. *Neurosurgery.* Jun 2005;56(6):1286–1292; discussion 1292–4.

46. Dickinson LD, Miller LD, Patel CP, Gupta SK. Enoxaparin increases the incidence of postoperative intracranial hemorrhage when initiated preoperatively for deep venous thrombosis prophylaxis in patients with brain tumors. *Neurosurgery.* Nov 1998;43(5):1074–1081.

47. UWMC. VTE Tool Kit [Internet], Available at http://www.uwmcacc.org. Accessed April 10, 2010.

48. Silva TJ, Jerussalmy CS, Farfel JM, Curiati JA, Jacob-Filho W. Predictors of in-hospital mortality among older patients. *Clinics (Sao Paulo).* 2009;64(7):613–618.

49. Gonzalez M, Martinez G, Calderon J, Villarroel L, Yuri F, Rojas C, Jeria A, Valdivia G, Marin PP, Carrasco M. Impact of delirium on short-term mortality in elderly inpatients: a prospective cohort study. *Psychosomatics.* May–Jun 2009;50(3):234–238.

50. Oh YS, Kim DW, Chun HJ, Yi HJ. Incidence and risk factors of acute postoperative delirium in geriatric neurosurgical patients. *J Korean Neurosurg Soc.* Mar 2008;43(3):143–148.

51. Goldstein LB, Bullman S. Differential effects of haloperidol and clozapine on motor recovery after sensorimotor cortex injury in rats. *Neurorehabil Neural Repair.* Dec 2002;16(4):321–325.

52. Han CS, Kim YK. A double-blind trial of risperidone and haloperidol for the treatment of delirium. *Psychosomatics.* Jul–Aug 2004;45(4):297–301.

53. Alderfer BS, Arciniegas DB, Silver JM. Treatment of depression following traumatic brain injury. *J Head Trauma Rehabil.* Nov–Dec 2005;20(6):544–562.

54. Jorge RE, Robinson RG, Moser D, Tateno A, Crespo-Facorro B, Arndt S. Major depression following traumatic brain injury. *Arch Gen Psychiatry.* Jan 2004;61(1):42–50.

55. Snow V, Beck D, Budnitz T, Miller DC, Potter J, Wears RL, Weiss KB, Williams MV. Transitions of Care Consensus policy statement: American College of Physicians, Society of General Internal Medicine, Society of Hospital Medicine, American Geriatrics Society, American College of Emergency Physicians, and Society for Academic Emergency Medicine. *J Hosp Med.* Jul 2009;4(6):364–370.

CHAPTER *25*

BARIATRIC SURGERY
Donna L. Mercado, Mihaela Stefan, and Xiao Liu

BACKGROUND

Due to the continued rise in the prevalence of obesity, bariatric surgical procedures have become commonplace. In 2008, it was estimated that 220,000 bariatric procedures were performed in the United States and Canada.[1] The major types of procedures currently performed are the laparoscopic gastric band (LAGB), which is restrictive in nature, and the Roux-en-Y gastric bypass (RYGB), which is both restrictive and malabsorptive. A newer restrictive surgery called the gastric sleeve is now becoming popular, and has some advantages over the other two procedures, especially in that it can be performed on larger patients who may not be good candidates for the other two procedures, and does not require the frequent adjustments necessary in the gastric band.[2] Decisions regarding which type of procedure is appropriate for a given patient are made by the surgeon. Patients eligible for surgery include all those with a body mass index (BMI) of >40 kg/m^2, and patients with a BMI of 35–39 kg/m^2 who have at least one obesity-associated comorbidity such as diabetes, hypertension (HTN), obstructive sleep apnea (OSA), obesity hypoventilation syndrome (OHS), severe arthritis of the lower extremities, hyperlipidemia, or cardiac disease.[3] In general, the procedures have a good safety record, with a reported 30-day mortality rate in most studies in the range of <1%. Mortality is generally caused by pulmonary embolism (PE), anastomotic leak (in the case of gastric bypass), and cardiac causes. A study of 4756 patients performed by the National Surgical Quality Improvement Program showed no difference in the 30-day mortality between LAGB and laparoscopic gastric bypass, although the LAGB is associated with a shorter postoperative stay and fewer major complications.[4]

SURGERY-SPECIFIC RISK

The LAGB has a 30-day mortality of 0.17% based on a 2-year study of the National Surgical Quality Improvement Program.[4] Early complications include acute stomal

Perioperative Medicine: Medical Consultation and Co-Management, First Edition.
Edited by Amir K. Jaffer and Paul J. Grant.
© 2012 Wiley-Blackwell. Published 2012 by John Wiley & Sons, Inc.

357

obstruction, band infection, gastric perforation, hemorrhage, and delayed gastric emptying. Acute stomal obstruction can occur in up to 6% of patients, and presents as persistent nausea and vomiting, and an inability to tolerate oral intake.[5] Late complications include band slippage or prolapse, band erosion (up to 7% occurrence rate), port or tubing malfunction including leakage, and pouch or esophageal dilatation. Slippage of the band requires urgent surgery.[6]

The RYGB (both open and laparoscopic) has a reported 30-day mortality of 0–1%. The main causes of death are the early complications of anastomotic leaks (50%) and pulmonary embolus (30%).[7] The general rates for occurrence of anastomotic leak are between 0.5% and 1%. Rates of occurrence for deep vein thrombosis (DVT) are between 0% and 5.4%, and between 0% and 0.4% for pulmonary embolus. Anastomotic leaks generally present within the first 48 h postoperatively. Common symptoms include tachypnea, tachycardia, hypotension, and abdominal pain. Other early complications include bleeding, wound infection, and rarely, gastric remnant distention. Late complications include stomal stenosis (6–20%), which generally presents as nausea, vomiting, dysphagia, gastroesophageal reflux, and eventually inability to tolerate oral intake.[8] Marginal ulcers (0.6–16%) present as pain, nausea, and sometimes bleeding.[9] Other late complications include cholelithiasis, ventral and internal hernias, nutrient deficiencies, postoperative hypoglycemia, and the dumping syndrome. The dumping syndrome occurs after malabsorptive procedures such as RYGB because there is rapid postprandial emptying of hyperosmolar gastric contents into the small intestine. This triggers a reflux of vascular fluid into the bowel lumen, causing a rapid decrease in circulating volume, with associated hypotension and tachycardia. In addition, patients can experience nausea, vomiting, diaphoresis, and an osmotic diarrhea.[10]

The gastric sleeve has a reported 30-day mortality of 0.39%. Early complications include leaks at the staple line, bleeding, abscess, stricture, and trocar site infection. Late complications include gastroesophageal reflux, stricture, and cholelithiasis.[2]

PREOPERATIVE ASSESSMENT

The preoperative evaluation should be comprehensive, with particular attention to cardiac function, pulmonary function, and risk for DVT and PE. The preoperative evaluation should also include a detailed review of systems with attention to symptoms suggestive of obesity-related comorbidities in an effort to identify undiagnosed conditions (Table 25.1).[11] Patients should also be screened for underlying causes of obesity such as thyroid disease and Cushing's syndrome. Some patients may have undiagnosed coronary artery disease, congestive heart failure (CHF), OSA, or OHS. Obese patients frequently report symptoms of dyspnea and palpitations with minimal exertion, as well as orthopnea, fatigue, lower extremity edema, and atypical chest pain. These symptoms are often multifactorial, and make it difficult to assess the presence and extent of cardiovascular and pulmonary disease during the preoperative evaluation. Physicians should specifically inquire about exercise patterns, duration,

TABLE 25.1.   Obesity-Related Review of System (Obesity-Associated Diseases)

Cardiovascular	Respiratory
Hypertension	Obstructive sleep apnea
Congestive heart failure	Hypoventilation syndrome
Coronary artery disease	Pickwickian syndrome
Pulmonary hypertension	Asthma
Venous stasis ulcers	

Venous thromboembolism	Endocrine
Deep venous thrombosis	Metabolic syndrome
Pulmonary embolism	Type 2 diabetes mellitus
	Gestational diabetes
	Nonalcoholic fatty liver disease
	Dyslipidemia
	Polycystic ovary syndrome
	Amenorrhea, infertility

Gastrointestinal	Genitourinary
Gastroesophageal reflux disease	Urinary stress incontinence
Cholelithiasis	Nephrolithiasis
Abdominal hernia	

Musculoskeletal	Neurologic
Degenerative joint disease	Pseudotumor cerebri
Low back pain	Stroke
Gout	Migraine
Skin	Psychiatric
Lymphedema	Depression
Cellulitis	Anxiety
Intertrigo	
Acanthosis nigricans	

and intensity to identify patients with poor functional capacity. Patients who are very inactive or who have a poor functional capacity are likely to benefit from preoperative cardiac testing. Patients may have occult cardiomyopathy of obesity, consisting of both systolic and diastolic dysfunction,[12] which can go undetected. Patients with unexplained dyspnea at rest or with minimum physical activities, fatigue, chest discomfort, or respiratory symptoms such as wheezing should be considered for a preoperative echocardiogram, a cardiac stress test, as well as resting pulmonary function testing (PFT) to rule out occult coronary artery disease, the cardiomyopathy of obesity, or occult pulmonary disease. Most bariatric surgery programs routinely evaluate patients for OSA since studies have shown that a higher incidence of postoperative complications is seen in patients with OSA. The polysomnogram is the preferred study since the Epworth sleepiness scale has been found in many studies to be an inadequate screening tool for OSA. In addition to routine screening labs, patients should be screened for iron deficiency and vitamin D deficiency; these conditions should be treated preoperatively since they frequently develop or worsen over time in the postoperative period. At the discretion of the surgeon, patients may be screened for gallbladder disease. Cholelithiasis may develop after surgery due to rapid weight loss; therefore, cholecystectomy may be done at the time of surgery if cholelithiasis is already present preoperatively. Patients should undergo a psychiatric evaluation both to identify possible contraindications to the surgery (substance abuse, eating disorders, major psychiatric diagnoses) and to identify potential postoperative challenges to the behavioral change necessary for long-term weight management. In addition to significant psychiatric illness, other absolute contraindications to surgery include central diabetes insipidus (because of the chronic need for large volumes of water taken orally), and any prohibitive pulmonary and cardiac conditions.

Physical Exam

All patients should undergo a careful preoperative physical exam, as for any surgery. In the morbidly obese patient, the cardiac exam can be particularly unreliable, and often underestimates the presence and extent of cardiac dysfunction. For example, heart sounds are often distant, and auscultation of an S3, S4, or a murmur can be difficult. The point of maximal intensity (PMI) is also less evident. Detection of jugular vein distention and hepatojugular reflux is also difficult due to lipid deposition around the neck. Auscultation of the lungs can be similarly difficult, with distant lung sounds. Examination of the abdomen is hampered by the presence of a large pannus, and palpation of masses or enlarged organs is generally difficult. While examining the abdomen, it is important to lift the pannus to look for skin breakdown or the presence of rashes. The lower extremities often have peripheral edema, lymphedema, and lipidema. Other aspects of the preoperative assessment for the obese patient include the following.

HTN   The patient's arm circumference should be measured to ensure accurate blood pressure measurement. The blood pressure cuff should be at least 80% of the arm circumference, and the width of the cuff should be at least 50% of the arm circumference at the midpoint of the upper arm. As with all patients, uncontrolled HTN may increase the risk for perioperative cardiovascular events, and a chronic blood pressure of 180/110 or greater is associated with a risk of intraoperative and postoperative hypertensive urgency. Angiotensin-converting enzyme inhibitors and angiotensin II antagonists are associated with intraoperative hypotension with induction of general anesthesia. On the morning of surgery, it may be advisable to discontinue these agents and diuretics, but patients should take all the other antihypertensive medications.

Cardiac Evaluation

Noninvasive Cardiac Testing   Morbid obesity induces structure changes such as atrial and ventricular enlargement, as well as ventricular hypertrophy as a result of chronic shear stress with increased cardiopulmonary workload. In addition, accumulation of adipose tissue around the chest wall, breast tissues, and epicardial fat also reduces imaging quality. Thus, the sensitivity and specificities of cardiac tests are reduced in morbidly obese individuals with BMI >50. Failure to recognize these limitations may result in unnecessary or inappropriate testing to confirm or compare findings from prior suboptimal procedures. These tests not only increase cost, but also delay the surgeries, and provoke anxiety in patients. Here, we provide a brief review to guide perioperative cardiovascular risk assessment in the morbidly obese population.

Electrocardiogram (ECG)   A routine preoperative ECG is recommended for men over 40 years of age, and women over 50, or individuals with cardiac risk factors. It is noted that women with morbid obesity have higher percentage of electrocardiographic (EKG) abnormalities. Common abnormalities associated with morbid obesity are summarized in Table 25.2.[13]

In addition to baseline EKG abnormalities, several factors limit the use of treadmill exercise stress testing: (1) inability to exercise due to osteoarthritis or deconditioning, (2) exceeding weight limit for treadmills (usually less than 400–450 lb), and (3) poor ECG quality in females or patients with a BMI of >50 due to breast movement with exercise. Some obese females may need a special elastic vest to secure ECG leads and reduce interference. Some stress labs use stationary bikes, which can be programmed to adapt morbidly obese patients with arthritis.

Although treadmill exercise can be used to access physical activity level and monitor symptoms during exercise, it is rarely used as a single modality in the

TABLE 25.2.   Common EKG Changes in Obese Individuals

$\uparrow$ Heart rate

$\uparrow$ PR interval

$\uparrow$ QRS interval

$\uparrow$ or $\downarrow$ QRS voltage

$\uparrow$ QT interval

$\uparrow$ QT dispersion

$\uparrow$ Signal-averaged electrocardiography (late potentials)

ST-T-wave abnormalities

ST depression

Left-axis deviation

Flattening of the T-wave (inferolateral leads)

Left atrial abnormalities

False-positive criteria for inferior myocardial infarction

Prior et al. *Circulation.* 2006;113:902.

preoperative setting with morbidly obese patients. However, it can be used in conjunction with other modalities such as echocardiography or myocardial perfusion to screen patients for coronary artery disease.

Echocardiography   Transthoracic echocardiography can be technically difficult in morbidly obese females with a BMI of >50 or patients with significant chronic obstructive lung disease. Contrast echocardiography has been shown to improve LV endocardial border resolution in patients with suboptimal imaging due to obesity or mechanical ventilation.[14] It is useful for the assessment of LV function, as well as LV global and regional wall motion after intravenous (IV) injection of microbubble contrast agents (i.e., Optison or Definity). Several studies have shown that this imaging modality is safe in the morbidly obese population. Therefore, this modality is useful in morbidly obese patients with intermediate probability for coronary artery disease or screening for CHF.

Transesophageal dobutamine stress echocardiography can also be used for the evaluation of myocardial ischemia in morbidly obese patients with the advantage of superior quality of echocardiogram windows. However, this is a semi-invasive procedure that typically requires sedation. In addition, a high incidence of hypotension during peak dobutamine infusion has been reported.[15] Thus, this modality must be used with caution.

Myocardial Perfusion Imaging   In general, myocardial perfusion imaging is the most commonly used method in obese patients for preoperative cardiac evaluation. However, diagnostic accuracy is reduced by attenuation from the diaphragm or breast tissue in patients with a BMI of >50. In such patients, higher false-positive rates have been observed. Weight limitation of nuclear imaging equipment may also limit its use in extremely obese patients.

Invasive Cardiac Testing

Cardiac Catheterization   Cardiac catheterization should be used in morbidly obese patients with high probability for clinically significant coronary artery disease. Cardiac catheterization can be safely performed in this population; however, the risk of vascular complications (such as large hematomas and arteriovenous fistulas) is higher.[16] The cardiac catheterization tables have a weight limit, so patients with super morbid obesity in whom a test is indicated must have the test performed in a catheterization lab that can accommodate their weight safely.

A comparison of the various cardiac tests available for bariatric patients is shown in Table 25.3.

Pulmonary Evaluation

Obese patients have a decreased expiratory reserve volume, decreased functional residual capacity (FRC), diaphragmatic dysfunction, and decreased compliance of the chest wall and lungs. After induction of anesthesia, and with the patient in the supine position, FRC is further decreased, which leads to atelectasis, increased

TABLE 25.3. Comparison of Different Cardiac Testing Modalities

	Indications	Advantages	Limitation
Treadmill exercise ECG	• Male patients who are able to exercise • Females with BMI <50 who are able to exercise • Normal ECG is required when it is used alone	• Low cost • Great tool to access functional capacity and symptoms induced by exercise • Can be used in conjunction with stress echo or myocardial perfusion imaging	• Weight limits • Poor quality of EKG tracing in females with BMI >50
Dobutamine stress echo with contrast agents	• Morbidly obese patients with intermediate suspicion for CAD or CHF or vavular diseases	• Cost-effective • Safe • Good tool to evaluate LVH, LV function, and valve function	• RV imaging quality may be poor • Poor echo windows with patients with significant COPD
Transesophageal dobutamine stress echo	• Morbidly obese patients with intermediate to high suspicion for CAD or valular diseases	• Superior imaging quality	• Semi-invasive, requires sedation • Caution in patients with significant OSA and other pulmonary conditions • Operator dependent
Myocardial perfusion imaging	• Morbidly obese patients with intermediate suspicion for CAD	• Most commonly used in preoperative setting	• Weight limit of table • Higher false-positive rate in females with BMI >50 • Less clinical data yield in comparison with contrast stress echo
Cardiac catheterization	• Morbidly obese patients with high suspicion for CAD • Confirm findings on noninvasive testing	• Gold standard for diagnosis of CAD	• Weight limit of table • High cost • Invasive
CT coronary angiography or PET	• Limited use in morbidly obese patients	• New modalities	• Weight limit of table • High cost • IV contrast exposure (for CT) • Limited data regarding sensitivity and specificity

ECG, electrocardiogram; EKG, electrocardiographic; BMI, body mass index; CAD, coronary artery disease; CHF, congestive heart failure; LVH, left ventricular hypertrophy; LV, left ventricle; RV, right ventricle; COPD, chronic obstructive pulmonary disease; OSA, obstructive sleep apnea; CT, computed tomography; PET, positron emission tomography.

shunting, and impaired oxygenation. During laparoscopic procedures, the intra-abdominal pressure increases due to the insufflation of air and further reduces lung volumes and ventilation–perfusion mismatch due to Trendelenburg positioning and insufflation of air.[17]

OSA is common in obese patients. One recent study showed that the prevalence of OSA in bariatric surgery patients was greater than 77%, irrespective of OSA symptoms, BMI, gender, age, or menopausal state.[18] Because the Epworth sleepiness scale, pulse oximetry, and BMI are not considered to be reliable indicators of OSA, many authors recommend preoperative polysomnography. Anesthetics and narcotics have an exaggerated respiratory depressant effect and thus worsen hypoventilatory episodes. They also decrease arousal responses. In addition, anesthetic agents alter REM sleep postoperatively, particularly on postoperative days 2 and 3. This increases the number of apneic episodes. Thus, OSA patients are likely to worsen postoperatively due to both changes in sleep architecture and medication effects.[19] There is no clear relationship between the severity of the OSA and perioperative outcome. The presence of OSA is a significant risk factor for postoperative anastomotic leak and PE[20] and is associated with both a longer length of stay and higher postoperative costs.[21]

OHS is an important disorder frequently associated with OSA in morbidly obese patients. OHS is defined as chronic daytime hypoxia ($PaO_2 < 65$) and hypercapnea ($PaCO_2 > 45$) without another explanation for hypoventilation and in the absence of chronic obstructive pulmonary disease. Patients with OHS can be screened by room air pulse oximetry. An arterial blood gas is indicated for O_2 saturation less than 96%. Patients with OHS are at higher risk for postoperative respiratory failure.

Preoperative Thrombotic Risk Assessment

Obesity is by itself a risk factor for venous thromboembolism (VTE) in general surgery patients, and some evidence suggests that morbid obesity is associated with a procoagulant state. During laparascopic procedures, the increase in intra-abdominal pressure affects venous return, further increasing the risk of DVT.

The incidence of PE after bariatric surgery is low (0.2–0.8%)[22] but is the leading cause of death in perioperative period (accounts for 30–50% of death). Autopsy studies have documented the high incidence of PE in patients who have died in the early postoperative period after gastric bypass. In a much-cited study, Melinek et al. reported a case series of 10 autopsies after Roux-en-Y anastomosis; three of the deaths were attributable to PE, and in eight patients, microscopic evidence of PE was present.[23] A prospective study on 3800 patients found that the incidence of PE was 0.85% at 60 days with a mortality of 27%. The average time from surgery to PE was 13 days, and one-third of the events occurred after hospital discharge.[24] Evidence from the literature identifies venous stasis, BMI ≥60, truncal obesity, OHS, and OSA as risk factors for VTE in bariatric surgery.

Recommendations to Reduce the Risk of DVT/PE The Eighth American College of Chest Physicians Conference on Antithrombotic and Thrombolytic Therapy endorse routine thromboprophylaxis with low-molecular-weight heparin (LMWH) or low-dose unfractionated heparin (LDUH three times daily), fondaparinux, or the combination of one of these pharmacologic methods with optimally used

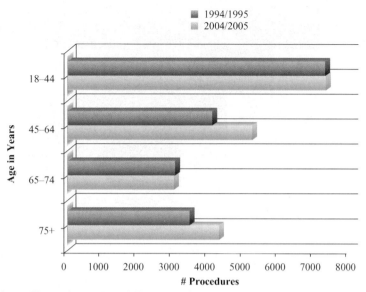

Figure 9.1. Change in number of discharges for surgical procedures by age group: 1994/1995 versus 2004/2005. Adapted from DeFrances et al.[6]

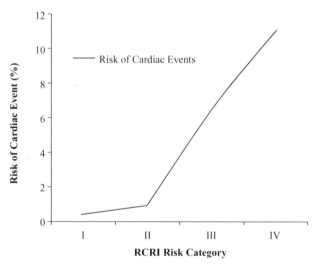

Figure 9.2. Risk of cardiac events by Revised Cardiac Risk Index class. Class I = zero points; Class II = 1 point; Class III = 2 points; Class IV = 3 or more points. Adapted from Lee et al.[24]

Perioperative Medicine: Medical Consultation and Co-Management, First Edition.
Edited by Amir K. Jaffer and Paul J. Grant.
© 2012 Wiley-Blackwell. Published 2012 by John Wiley & Sons, Inc.

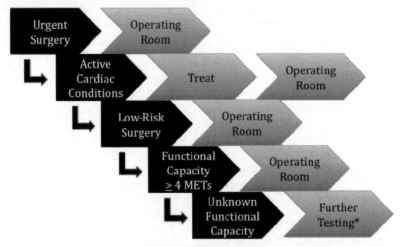

Figure 9.3. Simplified ACC/AHA algorithm for perioperative cardiac risk assessment and care. *Based on risk factors and risk of surgery. Adapted from Fleisher et al.[28]

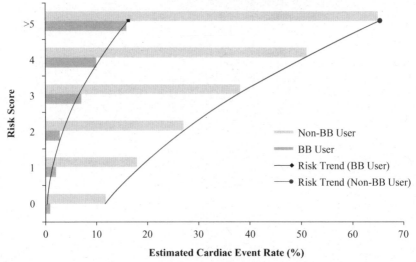

Figure 9.4. Association between beta-blocker (BB) use and cardiac events in patients undergoing vascular surgery (risk trend). Adapted from Boersma et al.[37]

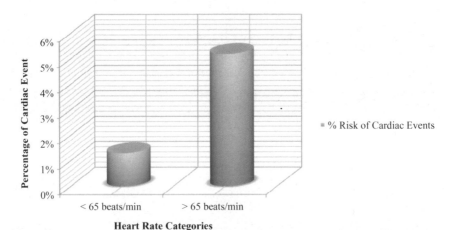

Figure 9.5. Relationship between heart-rate reduction and perioperative events. Adapted from Poldermans et al.[19]

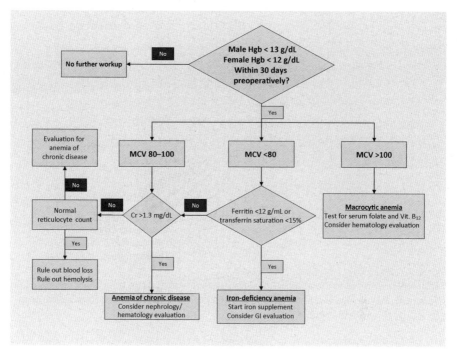

Figure 13.1. Evaluation of preoperative anemia.

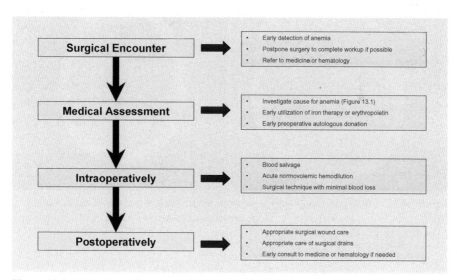

Figure 13.2. Multifaceted approach to perioperative blood conservation.

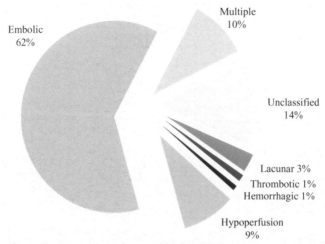

Figure 15.1. Proposed mechanisms for perioperative stroke. Data from Likosky DS, Caplan LR, Weintraub RM, et al. Heart Surg Forum 2004;7:E271–E276. Reproduced with permission from Selim,[12] figure 1.

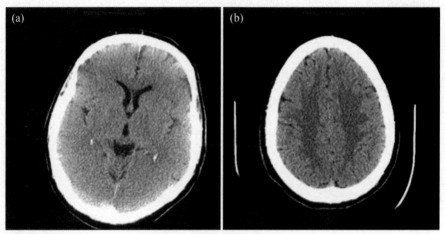

Figure 24.1. Computed tomography of cerebral edema (a) compared with normal brain (b). Note loss of gray-white boarder in the presence of edema (a). Images provided by Dr. Sung E. Logerfo, Assistant Professor of Radiology, University of Washington.

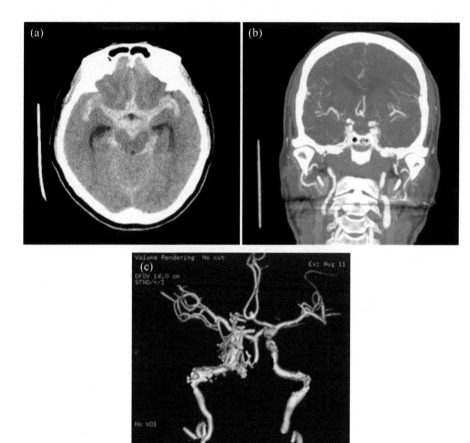

Figure 24.2. Computed tomography angiogram (CTA) of subarachnoid hemorrhage in the setting of an aneurysm. (a) CTA sagittal view demonstrating blood in the subarachnoid space; (b) CTA coronal view showing aneurysm; (c) 3D reconstruction of vasculature demonstrating aneurysm. *Images provided by Dr. Sung E. Logerfo, Assistant Professor of Radiology, University of Washington.*

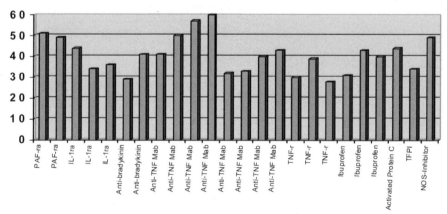

Figure 27.1. Variability in the mortality rate (percent) of control arms of clinical trials classified according to type of mediator-specific anti-inflammatory agent.

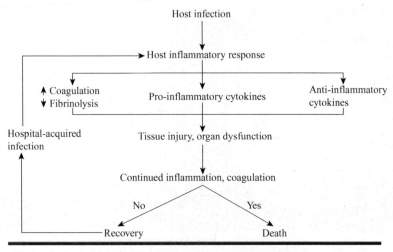

Figure 27.2.   Pathophysiology of severe sepsis.

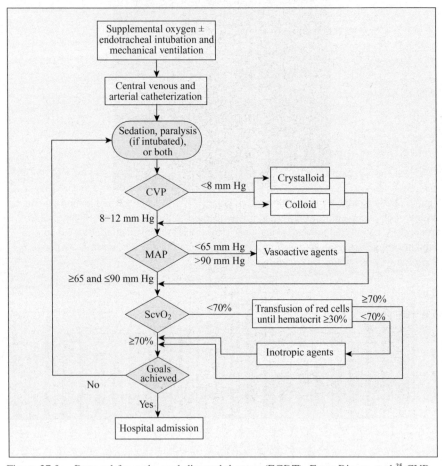

Figure 27.3.   Protocol for early goal-directed therapy (EGDT). From Rivers et al.[35] CVP, central venous pressure; MAP, mean arterial pressure; ScvO$_2$, central venous oxygen saturation.

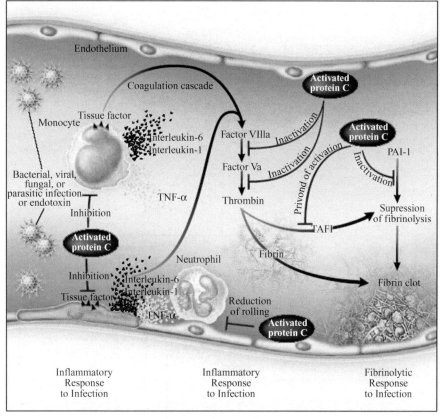

Figure 27.4. Proposed action of activated protein C in modulating the systemic inflammatory, procoagulant, and fibrinolytic host responses to infection. From Bernard et al.[51] TAFI, thrombin activatable fibrinolysis inhibitor.

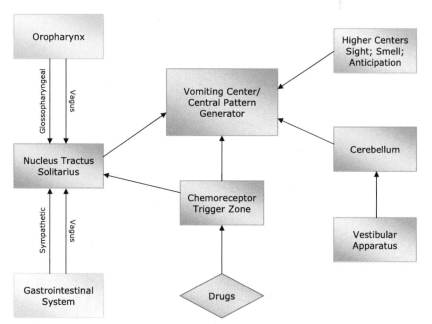

Figure 29.1. Mechanism of nausea and vomiting.

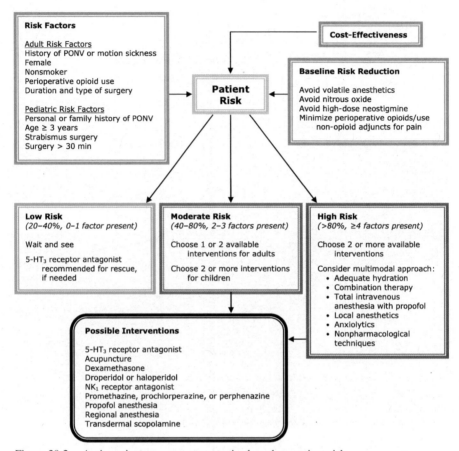

Figure 29.2. Antiemetic management strategies based on patient risk.

pneumatic compression devices (each Grade 1C).[25] The guidelines suggest that higher than usual doses of LMWH or LDUH be used, but no specific recommendations are given. There is not enough evidence to suggest optimal regimen, dosage, timing, and duration of thromboprophylaxis in bariatric surgery patients. Depending on the center, patients receive enoxaparin 30 mg preoperatively, 40 mg postoperatively every 12 or 24 h, or unfractionated heparin three times daily for up to 10 days upon discharge. Most centers combine the mechanical methods of prophylaxis with pharmacological therapy. Because evidence exists that majority of thromboembolic events take place after hospital discharge, consideration should be given to extend anticoagulation after hospitalization, but no consensus yet exists. Although controversial, prophylactic placement of a temporary inferior vena cava (IVC) filter is recommended by some authors for patients with respiratory failure (i.e., obesity–hypoventilation syndrome), pulmonary HTN (pulmonary artery pressure >40 mm Hg), super obesity with limited mobility, hypercoagulable states, previous history of VTE, or severe venous stasis.[26] Failure of IVC filters to prevent PE has been described with a frequency of as high as 6.0%.[27] Causes may be malposition or fracture of the filter, thrombi originating in the upper extremities or distal from the filter, or a hypercoagulable state.

Diabetes Mellitus (DM)

Obesity is a recognized cause for type 2 DM (T2DM), and DM management remains a challenge in clinical practice. Bariatric surgery has been shown to effectively reverse or ameliorate DM in most patients, with the RYGB being the most effective method.[28] Rapid resolution or marked improvement of DM is strongly associated with loss of insulin resistance through the mechanism shown in Figure 25.1.[29] These

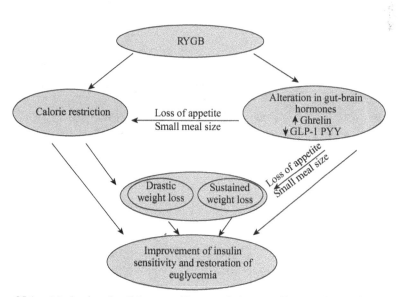

Figure 25.1.   Mechanism for diabetes mellitus resolution post Roux-en-Y gastric bypass (RYGB) surgery. GLP-1, glucagon-like peptide-1; PYY, peptide YY.

include (1) caloric restriction, (2) alterations of gastrointestinal (GI) anatomy and gut hormones, (3) robust and sustained fat loss, and (4) changes in adipokine signaling. Rapid resolution of T2DM occurs within days to weeks in patients with mild or well-controlled DM post-RYGB. Resolution of T2DM is defined as the following: (1) fasting glucose less than 126 mg/dL, (2) glycosylated hemoglobin levels less 7%, and (3) discontinuation of diabetic medications at some time after surgeries. However, there are currently no established guidelines or consensus available for managing insulin and oral hypoglycemic agents perioperatively.

In general, LAGB patients have a much slower course of weight loss and no need for major changes in DM management in the postoperative setting. For RYGB patients, however, the necessary changes to diabetic medications in the immediate postoperative period can be drastic. Before RYGB, patients are typically instructed to adhere to a low-calorie liquid diet (<1000 kcal) for approximately 2 weeks. It is well recognized that a low-calorie diet preoperatively reduces liver steatosis and overall liver size, thus allowing easier access to the stomach. Because the calorie intake during this period is significantly less, patients should be advised to stop premeal insulin and to decrease long-acting insulin by 40–60%. Dosages of oral hypoglycemics and incretin mimetics (i.e., exenatide) should also be decreased. High-dose metformin can cause lactic acidosis and worsened renal function in the setting of a catabolic state and should be decreased or discontinued. Sulfonylureas should also be decreased or discontinued to prevent hypoglycemia. Patients should be instructed to follow their blood glucoses frequently, and medication regimens should be titrated accordingly.

POSTOPERATIVE ASSESSMENT AND MANAGEMENT

HTN

As with other surgical patients, antihypertensives should be titrated according to the patient's postoperative blood pressures. Diuretics should be held unless the patient has known CHF or significant peripheral edema. Patients who are on perioperative beta-blockers should maintain their dosage as much as possible; therefore, they may need the doses of their other antihypertensives decreased. Patients may experience hypotension postoperatively, especially if they are experiencing vomiting or have poor oral intake. Weight loss after bariatric surgery is associated with long-term improvement of HTN, and two-thirds of patients decrease or discontinue their antihypertensives 2–3 years postsurgery.[30]

Cardiac

Patients should receive the standard postoperative monitoring for ischemia as for any surgical patient. Physicians should monitor any evidence of postoperative CHF, as obese patients can have occult diastolic dysfunction, or an occult obesity-related cardiomyopathy. CHF in the postoperative setting can also be provoked by injudicious use of IV fluids, ischemia, and HTN. All diuretics should be stopped to avoid electrolyte disturbances and dehydration unless active CHF or overwhelming symptoms of fluid retention are present.

Pulmonary

Patients should receive standard postoperative pulmonary toilet. In addition, for patients with OSA, they should be extubated only when fully awake, and preferably to their own CPAP or BiPAP equipment. This should also be used during regular sleep, as well as for naps, while in the hospital. For patients with suspected OSA but who have not had preoperative polysomograms, 24-h pulse oximetry is recommended. If periods of hypoxemia are observed, CPAP should be instituted. Patients with undiagnosed OSA are at risk for negative pressure pulmonary edema after extubation. This is caused by a markedly negative intrathoracic pressure due to forced inspiration against a closed glottis. The negative intrathoracic pressure causes transudation of fluid from pulmonary capillaries to the interstitium following relief of the upper airway obstruction. Predisposing factors for this syndrome include obesity, a short neck, and OSA. This syndrome presents as rapid onset of pulmonary edema, with hypoxemia, tachypnea, and tachycardia within 24 h of surgery. The chest X-ray generally reveals bilateral infiltrates in a pattern consistent with noncardiac pulmonary edema.[31] Treatment with diuretics can be tried but is of unclear benefit. General therapy for negative pressure pulmonary edema consists of supportive care.

Supplemental oxygen can mask hypoventilation in patients with OSA or OHS. Therefore, patients with unexplained confusion or somnolence postoperatively should have an arterial blood gas to detect hypercarbia.

Diabetes

In general, clinical improvement in DM control occurs in all patients following RYGB. However, some patients experience mild-to-moderate hyperglycemia during their postoperative hospital stay due to the stress response induced by surgery as well as the use of dextrose-containing IV fluids. Patients can be treated with a low-dose, long-acting insulin, or with a rapid-acting insulin correction scale. The average caloric intake after RYGB is between 300 and 500 kcal/day for the first month postoperatively, which results in a significantly decreased glycemic load and contributes to the decreased medication requirement.[32] A conservative insulin glargine regimen is the best choice for the majority of patients experiencing hyperglycemia postoperatively, with close observation and titration by their outpatient physician.

DM Regimens at the Time of Discharge   Diabetic management should be individualized and avoid "one size fits all." Therapy should be tailored to the changes in fasting glucose levels before or after RYGB and matched to the meal patterns/ caloric intake. With low calorie intakes, three to five small-size meals per day, postprandial hyperglycemia is no longer a concern. Checking glucose levels before meals and administering short-acting premeal insulin are not recommended in this population. For most patients, checking daily fasting glucose levels in the morning is sufficient for monitoring T2DM resolution:

- *Mild DM, Duration Less Than 5 Years, Well Controlled (Hemoglobin A1c [HbA1c] < 8), and Only Require One or Two Oral Agents.* About 30% of patients can discontinue all DM medications including insulin at the time of discharge. These patients typically have short duration of DM and are more likely to take oral DM medications or use only a small amount of insulin preoperatively. In general, these patients will have complete resolution of DM and do not require any medications following surgery, especially after recovery from perioperative stress-induced hyperglycemia. If patients develop transient postoperative hyperglycemia with glucose levels >200 mg/dL in the absence of dextrose infusion, short-term use of low-dose insulin glargine is a good choice. Patients should be advised to check daily fasting glucose levels and stop long-acting insulin therapy once they reach a euglycemic state. Although resuming oral diabetic agents is an alternative, it may not be as reliable or as effective in controlling hyperglycemia due to the potential of decreased bioavailability in patients immediately post-RYGB.

- *Moderate DM, Duration Less Than 10 Years, HbA1c 8–9, and Require More Than One Oral Agent with or without Insulin.* The majority of these patients will achieve resolution of DM over time. If patients developed persistent hyperglycemia with glucose >200 mg/dL, a conservative long-acting insulin glargine regimen can be offered at the time of discharge. Once patients become euglycemic, they should seek advice from their physicians regarding tapering their DM medications. A small percentage of patients will need long-term DM treatment. Once patients have established a stable insulin requirement (less than 20 U/day) approximately 6 months after RYGB, insulin therapy can be stopped and switch to oral diabetic medication.

- *Severe DM, Duration Greater Than 10 Years, Poor Controlled (HbA1c > 9–10), with a Large Insulin Requirement.* These patients are less likely to achieve complete resolution due to impaired beta cell function. Patients will often require small doses of basal insulin (approximately 20–30% of prior daily insulin requirement) and may require continuation of low-dose oral agents.

All patients should be followed closely postoperatively as they lose weight so that diabetic medications can be titrated.

Medication Management In addition to changes in diabetic medications outlined above, RYGB patients should also have alteration of their medications that are long acting. Because of the length of the small intestine that is bypassed, intestinal absorptive capacity is significantly decreased. Therefore, long-acting medications are not as effective and should be changed to short-acting formulation immediately postoperatively. In addition, with all bariatric surgeries, any pills that are large should be changed to chewable or liquid formulations, or changed to another medication to avoid obstruction of the pouch. For patients who have their gallbladders remaining postoperatively, some surgeons will treat prophylactically for 1 year with ursode-oxycholic acid to prevent the formation of new gallstones during the period of active weight loss.[33]

DISCHARGE RECOMMENDATIONS

Upon discharge, patients will have been given a very specific diet information by the surgical team depending on the type of surgery performed. Patients should have their antihypertensive medication doses titrated before discharge. As weight loss ensues, medications can be titrated downward by their primary care providers. Consideration should be given to stop diuretics unless patients have signs or symptoms of CHF. Due to significantly decreased fluid intake, continuing diuretics poses risks for dehydration, syncope, or acute renal failure. At the time of discharge, physicians should discuss the goal of diabetic care and outpatient regimens with the patients in detail. Therapy and monitoring should take the following into consideration: (1) diabetes severity and duration, (2) meal patterns/caloric intake, (3) the impact of caloric restriction and weight loss on fasting glucose levels after RYGB, and (4) simplicity of T2DM regimen and monitoring. It is important to recognize that patients have a very low calorie intake with profound loss of appetite, and almost complete elimination of high-sugar (trigger dumping syndrome) and high-fat food from their diet immediately post-RYGB. Thus, postprandial hyperglycemia is not a major concern for the patients shortly after RYGB. For long-term management, a small number of patients may "outeat" by frequent snacking of energy-dense food. Monitoring for weight regain, postprandial or fasting hyperglycemia, and recurrence of T2DM is required in these patients. In addition, although uncommon, a late complication of RYGB is a type of postprandial hypoglycemia due to pancreatic islet cell hyperplasia called nesidioblastosis. This condition is possibly induced by postoperative changes in GI hormones. The syndrome is generally treated by a low-carbohydrate diet and with the alpha-glucosidase inhibitor acarbose or the use of verapamil.[34] Patients with severe cases require subtotal pancreatectomy.

Pregnancy is strongly discouraged until 18–24 months postoperatively when weight loss has stabilized. At the time of discharge, female patients should be counseled about appropriate birth control. The complications of pregnancy after bariatric surgery include anemia, persistent vomiting, micronutrient deficiencies, intrauterine growth retardation, and neural tube defects.[35]

Patients who undergo bariatric surgery, especially RYGB, can develop several nutrient deficiencies. They are generally counseled by the surgical team to take vitamin D, vitamin A, calcium, iron, B complex vitamins, and folate, but the hospitalist can play a vital role in making sure the patient understands the vitamin requirements (Table 25.4).[36] In addition, although bariatric patients are expected to follow up with their surgeons every 3 months for the first year, and once a year thereafter, they often have poor attendance at appointments after the first year. It is thus important for the primary care physician to be aware of the vitamin regimen that these patients should be following.

TABLE 25.4. Recommended Nutritional Supplementation after Bariatric Surgery

Multivitamin with minerals	1 tablet daily
Calcium citrate or carbonate	1200–1500 mg daily
Vitamin D	1000 IU daily
Vitamin A	5000 IU daily
Vitamin B$_{12}$	500 µg daily
Ferrous sulfate or gluconate	325 mg twice a day

REFERENCES

1. Buchwald H, Oren D. Metabolic/bariatric surgery worldwide 2008. *Obes Surg.* 2009;19: 1605–1611.
2. Ab-Jaish W, Rosenthal RJ. Sleeve gastrectomy: a new surgical approach for morbid obesity. *Expert Rev Gastroenterol Hepatol.* 2010;4:101–119.
3. Consensus Development Conference Panel. NIH Conference: gastrointestinal surgery for severe obesity. Consensus Development Conference Panel. *Ann Int Med.* 1991;115:956–961.
4. Lancaster RT, Huttler MM. Bands and bypasses: 30 day morbidity and mortality of bariatric surgical procedures as assessed by prospective, multi-clear, risk adjusted ACS-NSQIP data. *Surg Endosc.* 2008;22:2554.
5. Gravante G, Araco A, Araco F, et al. Laparoscopic adjustable gastric bandings: a prospective randomized study of 400 operations performed with two different devices. *Arch Surg.* 2007;142:958.
6. DeMaria EJ, Sugerman HJ, Meador JG, et al. High failure rate after laparoscopic adjustable silicone gastric banding for treatment of morbid obesity. *Ann Surg.* 2001;223:809.
7. Wittgrove AC, Clark GW. Laparoscopic gastric bypass, Roux-en-Y patients: technique and results, with 3–60 month follow up. *Obes Surg.* 2000;10:233.
8. Schneider BE, Villegas L, Blackburn GL, et al. Laparoscopic gastric bypass surgery outcomes. *J Leparoendose Adv Surg Tech A.* 2003;13:247.
9. Sapala JA, Wood MH, Sapala MA, Flake TM, Jr. Marginal ulcer after gastric bypass: a prospective 3-year study of 173 patients. *Obes Surg.* 1998;8:505.
10. Presultti RJ, Gorman RS, Swain JM. Primary care perspective on bariatric surgery. *Mayo Clinic Proc.* 2004;79:1158.
11. Mechanick J, Kushner RF, Sugerman HJ, et al. American Association of Clinical Endocrinologists, The Obesity Society, and American Society for Metabolic and Bariatric Surgery Medical Guidelines for Clinical Practice for the perioperative nutritional, metabolic, and nonsurgical support of the bariatric surgery patient. *Surg Obes Relat Dis.* 2008;4(5 Suppl):S109–S184.
12. Alpert MA. Cardiac morphology and ventricular function. In: *Morbid Obesity Peri-Operative Management,* Alvarez A (ed.), p. 63. Cambridge, UK: Cambridge University Press; 2004.
13. Alpert MA, Terry BE, Cohen MV, et al. The electrocardiogram in morbid obesity. *Am J Cardiol.* 2000;85:908.
14. Saya S, Gupta R, Abu-Fadel M, Sivaram CA. Effect of body mass index on myocardial performance index, featured original research presentations at the 19th Annual Scientific Sessions of the American Society of Echocardiography. *J Am Soc Echocardiogr.* 2008;21:596.
15. Madu E. Transesophageal dobutamine stress echocardiography in the evaluation of myocardial ischemia in morbidly obese subjects. *Chest.* 2000;117:657–661.
16. McNulty PH, Ehinger SM, Field JM, et al. Cardiac catheterization in morbidly obese patients. *Catheter Cardiovasc Interv.* 2002;56:174–177.
17. Pelosi P, Croci M, Ravagnan I, et al. The effects of body mass on long volumes, respiratory mechanics and gas exchange during general anesthesia. *Anesth Analg.* 1998;87(3):654–660.
18. Sareli AE, Cantor CR, Williams NN, et al. Obstructive sleep apnea in patients undergoing bariatric surgery—a tertiary center experience. *Obes Surg.* 2011;21:316–327.

19. Tung A, Rock P. Perioperative concerns in sleep apnea. *Curr Opin Anaesthesiol.* 2001;14: 671–678.
20. Fernandez AZ, Jr., DeMaria EJ, Tichansky DS, et al. Experience with over 3000 open and laparoscopic bariatric procedures: multivariate analysis of factors related to leak and resultant mortality. *Surg Endosc.* 2004;18(2):193–197.
21. Ballantine GH, Svahn J, Capella RF, et al. Predictors of prolonged hospital stay following open and laparoscopic gastric bypass for morbid obesity: body mass index, length of surgery, sleep apnea, asthma, and the metabolic syndrome. *Obes Surg.* 2004;14(8):1042–1050.
22. Sapala JA, Wood MH, Schuhknecht MP, Sapala MA. Fatal pulmonary embolism after bariatric operations for morbid obesity: a 24-year retrospective analysis. *Obes Surg.* 2003;13(6):819–825.
23. Melinek J, Livingston E, Cortina G, Fishbein MC. Autopsy findings following gastric bypass surgery for morbid obesity. *Arch Pathol Lab Med.* 2002;126(9):1091–1095.
24. Carmody BJ, Surgeman HJ, Kellum JM, et al. Pulmonary embolism complicating bariatric surgery: detailed analysis of a single institution's 24-year experience. *J Am Coll Surg.* 2006;203(6): 831–837.
25. Geerts WH, Bergqvist D, Pineo GF, et al. Prevention of venous thromboembolism: American College of Chest Physicians evidence-Based Clinical Practice Guidelines (8th Edition). *Chest.* 2008;133(6 Suppl):381S–453S.
26. Sugerman HJ. Bariatric surgery for severe obesity. *J Assoc Acad Minor Phys.* 2001;12(3): 129–136.
27. John MS, Nemck AA, Benanati MD, et al. The safety and effectiveness of the retreivable option IVC filter: a United States prospective multicenter clinical study. *J Vasc Interv Radiol.* 2010;21: 1173–1184.
28. Greenway SE, Greenway FL, Klein S. Effects of obesity surgery on non-insulin dependent diabetes mellitus. *Arch Surg.* 2002;137:1109–1117.
29. Sjostrom L, Lindroos A-K, Peltonen M, et al. Lifestyle, diabetes, and cardiovascular risk factors 10 years after bariatric surgery. *NEJM.* 2004;351:2683–2693.
30. Sjostrom CD, Lissner L, Sjostrom L. Relationships between changes in body composition and changes in cardiovascular risk factors: the SOS Intervention Study, Swedish Obese Subjects. *Obes Res.* 1997;5(6):519–530.
31. Chuang Y-C, Wang C-H, Lin Y-S. Negative pressure pulmonary edema: report of three cases and review of literature. *Eur Arch Otorhinolaryngol.* 2007;264:1113–1116.
32. Flancbaum L, Choban FS, Bradley LR, Burge JC. Changes in measured resting energy expenditure after Roux-en-Y gastric bypass for clinically severe obesity. *Surgery.* 1997;122:943–949.
33. Bell BJ, Bour ES, Scott JD, et al. Management of complications after laparoscopic Roux-en-Y gastric bypass. *Minerva Chir.* 2009;64:265–276.
34. Goldfine AB, Mun E, Patti ME. Hyperinsulinemic hypoglycemia following gastric bypass surgery for obesity. *Curr Opin Endocrinol Diab Obes.* 2006;13:419.
35. AACE/TOS/ASMBS. Bariatric surgery guidelines. *Endocr Pract.* 2008;14(Suppl 1):1–79.
36. Malinowski SS. Nutritional and metabolic complications of bariatric surgery. *Am J Med Sci.* 2006;331:219–225.

CHAPTER 26

OPHTHALMIC SURGERY

Jessica Zuleta and Aldo Pavon Canseco

BACKGROUND

In the United States, ambulatory surgery rates have been steadily increasing since the early 1980s. Ophthalmic surgery is a high-volume ambulatory surgery. There were 34.7 million ambulatory surgical visits in 2006 with the leading diagnosis being cataract.[1] The third and fifth most common procedures were extraction of lens (3.1 million) and insertion of prosthetic lens (2.6 million), respectively. However, ophthalmic surgery involves a much broader scope of surgical procedures other than cataract surgery (Table 26.1). Most of these procedures are considered low-risk surgeries customarily performed under either monitored anesthesia care (MAC) or general anesthesia. A comprehensive preoperative assessment evaluates and stratifies risk for perioperative complications. The quality of a preoperative evaluation impacts patient safety, surgical cancellations and delays, prolongation of postoperative stay, unanticipated admission to the hospital or acute care facility, and patient satisfaction.[2,3]

SURGERY-SPECIFIC RISKS

Most ophthalmic surgeries are considered low-risk procedures; however, the perioperative physician needs to be aware of some of the unique risks in this patient population. Although most ophthalmic surgeries are relatively noninvasive and do not incur significant blood loss, hemostasis is of concern under certain conditions. For anesthesia, it is a concern with the administration of local anesthesia utilized to achieve akinesia of the affected eye as an uncontrolled bleeding complication can lead to ocular compartment syndrome and/or irreversible vision loss. For ophthalmologists, oculoplastic surgeries, strabismus repair, and vitreo-retinal surgeries require careful review of the patient's bleeding history and medication profile. Alternatively, the commonly performed cataract surgery is considered a "bloodless" surgery with almost no bleeding risk. Patients undergoing cataract extraction can

Perioperative Medicine: Medical Consultation and Co-Management, First Edition.
Edited by Amir K. Jaffer and Paul J. Grant.
© 2012 Wiley-Blackwell. Published 2012 by John Wiley & Sons, Inc.

TABLE 26.1. Common Ophthalmic Surgeries

Cataract	Oculoplastics
Cornea (includes corneal transplants)	• Chalazion incision and drainage
Refractive surgeries	• Eyelid laceration and biopsy
• LASIK (laser-assisted *in situ* keratomileusis)	• Temporal artery biopsy
• LASEK (laser-assisted subepithelial keratomileusis)	• Lateral tarsorrhaphy
Eye trauma (includes foreign body)	• Ectropion repair
Glaucoma	• Blepharoplasty
Strabismus	• Ptosis repair
Vitreo-retina	• Endoscopic forehead/eyebrow lift
• Posterior segment vitrectomy	• Dacryocystorhinostomy
• Retinal detachment with sclera buckle	• Punctoplasty
• Pars plana lensectomy	• Enucleation
	• Evisceration
	• Exenteration
Endophthalmitis	Optic nerve sheath fenestration

remain on antiplatelet therapies (including aspirin, nonsteroidal anti-inflammatory drugs, and thienopyridines) as well as warfarin during the perioperative period.[4,5]

Another unique perioperative concern for ophthalmic surgery pertains to patients with benign prostatic hypertrophy being treated with alpha-1 receptor antagonists. These patients have been shown to be at increased risk of intraoperative floppy iris syndrome (IFIS). IFIS is characterized by iris muscle prolapse and pupil constriction; both of which lead to a restricted surgical field in ophthalmic surgeries, particularly cataract surgeries. The limitation of surgical access can result in significant complications such as retinal detachment and endophthalmitis. Several studies suggest that the frequency and severity of IFIS are higher in patients taking tamsulosin compared with other alpha-1 receptor antagonists.[6,7] If a patient is noted to be on an alpha-1 receptor antagonist preoperatively, then the surgeon should be engaged in discussion about the patient's medication regimen to ensure special precautions are undertaken to diminish complication rates associated with IFIS. Unfortunately, there is no consensus if discontinuing alpha-1 receptor antagonist therapy or switching to an alternative class of medications several weeks before eye surgery decreases IFIS risk.

PREOPERATIVE ASSESSMENT

During a preoperative evaluation, a patient may be referred for additional testing to further investigate the status of an underlying medical condition if the results will affect perioperative management. Previous studies have shown that eliminating unwarranted preoperative testing prior to cataract surgery has a potential cost saving of $150 million annually.[8,9] Of particular interest is the utility of routine preoperative electrocardiograms. The American College of Cardiology/American Heart Association (ACC/AHA) guidelines do not advocate routine preoperative resting 12-lead electrocardiograms (ECGs) in asymptomatic patients undergoing low-risk surgical procedures.[10] Retrospective studies of low-risk surgeries have shown only a 0.5% difference in cardiovascular death among patients having routine preoperative ECGs compared with those that did not have ECGs.[11] Testing that is unlikely to influence perioperative management may lead to patient harm from unnecessary interventions, surgical delays, and inappropriate use of healthcare resources. Surgical delay for ophthalmology patients translates into delayed visual recuperation.

The most concerning perioperative complication of noncardiac surgery is a cardiac event. Although ophthalmic surgical procedures are considered low cardiac risk, the underlying medical history and health status of the patient needs to be reviewed to identify active cardiac conditions and uncover previously undiagnosed and/or untreated medical conditions that may adversely affect the patient's outcome. Current 2007 ACC/AHA guidelines provide a systematic and evidence-based framework to evaluate and manage patients undergoing noncardiac surgery; this is done by evaluating the patient's clinical risk of a cardiovascular event, the surgery-specific risk, and the patient's self-reported functional exercise capacity. Elective ophthalmic procedures allow sufficient time to address active cardiac conditions prior to surgery. Patients without active cardiac conditions may proceed with their planned ophthalmic procedure barring any decompensated preexisting medical condition.

Additional cardiovascular management issues of concern for ophthalmology surgery are hypertension, presence of a coronary stent, and cardiac rhythm devices (CRDs). Hypertension is known to affect the eye's retina, choroid, and optic nerve. Hypertension, with systolic readings less than 180 mm Hg and diastolic readings less than 110 mm Hg, is not an independent clinical predictor of perioperative cardiac outcome.[12] Values above these ranges are known to increase and potentiate a patient's underlying cardiovascular risk of myocardial ischemia, heart failure, stroke, and kidney disease.[13] Blood pressure levels above the aforementioned values should be controlled prior to elective surgeries to attenuate cardiovascular risk and avoid surgical delays.

A patient with severely uncontrolled stage 2 hypertension and clinical evidence of end-organ damage has significant perioperative morbidity. Preexisting hemodynamic lability can be further aggravated intraoperatively by type of surgery, volume status, depth of anesthesia, and anesthetic agents.[14] Evaluation and management of severe stage 2 hypertension take precedence over elective surgery. If the patient is evaluated preoperatively in a timely manner, then physicians may be able to achieve safe blood pressure control prior to ambulatory surgery. However, if a patient with severe stage 2 hypertension and end-organ damage does not undergo a preoperative evaluation prior to an elective surgery, then the case may be cancelled on the day of surgery. Prescribed antihypertensive medications should be taken as regularly scheduled with a small sip of water the morning of day surgery. Administering oral angiotensin-converting enzyme (ACE) inhibitors and angiotensin receptor blockers (ARBs) the morning of surgery has always been a point of controversy with regard to their tendency to promote refractory intraoperative hypotension upon induction of anesthesia; the general recommendations are to hold these antihypertensives at least 10 h prior to surgery.[14,15] Fortunately, few ophthalmology day surgeries require general anesthesia so the concern with preoperative ACE inhibitors and ARBs is not prominent.

Today, medical device implants are ubiquitous. Of particular importance to ophthalmic surgery are coronary stents and CRDs. In terms of coronary stents, the repercussions of prematurely stopping dual antiplatelet therapy can be catastrophic to the patient. Current guidelines strongly advise against interrupting dual antiplatelet therapy earlier than 6 weeks for bare metal stents and 12 months for drug-eluting stents.[10,16] Ideally, elective ophthalmic surgeries should be postponed until it is safe to temporarily suspend thienopyridines; even then, it is recommended that at least the aspirin therapy be continued perioperatively. For those few patients whose procedure cannot be delayed for the advised time, then dual antiplatelet therapy should be managed in consultation with the patient's cardiologist.

In 2005, 223,425 pacemakers (PMs) and 119,121 implantable cardioverter-defibrillators (ICDs) were implanted in the United States.[17] Therefore, it is of no surprise that a significant number of patients scheduled to undergo ambulatory ophthalmic procedures have some form of CRD. Ophthalmology surgeons occasionally utilize bi- and monopolar electrocautery, which can potentially interfere with CRDs via electromagnetic interference. During an intraoperative ICD device malfunction, patients may display involuntary head movements with disastrous ocular injury. To avoid inadvertent intraoperative CRD malfunctions, preoperative evaluation of these patients should include the following: device identification, patient's underlying rhythm and dependence on device, copy of the latest in-office device interrogation, and presence or absence of minute ventilation sensors that may inadvertently trigger tachycardia by concomitant ECG and respiratory rate monitoring.[18,19] Per ACC/AHA recommendations, the acceptable interval between CRD evaluation and surgical date is 6 months, but an evaluation performed 1–2 weeks prior to surgery may be preferable.

The preoperative evaluation needs to include a thorough bleeding history, which should address bleeding symptoms (using quantitative descriptors), prior hemostatic challenges (focusing on excessive posttraumatic or postsurgical bleeding), family history of bleeding diatheses, and use of antithrombotic or antiplatelet drugs.[20,21] Herbal supplements with antithrombotic or antiplatelet tendencies also need to be identified preoperatively. Patients with identifiable risk factors for perioperative bleeding may be referred for additional coagulation testing and evaluation. These patients may still be eligible for ophthalmic day surgeries, but if therapeutic blood products are needed preoperatively and postoperatively, then arrangements need to be coordinated prior to the ambulatory surgical date.

The presence of an underlying thrombotic condition, as well as any medication used for its treatment, requires careful consideration. These factors serve as a guide in selecting the most judicious course of action in managing antithrombotic therapy for patients undergoing invasive procedures. Most patients undergoing cataract surgery may undergo the procedure without altering their anticoagulation regimen as this is considered a "bloodless" surgery.[4,5] However, for other more invasive eye surgeries such as strabismus repair and oculoplastic surgeries, the regimen will likely need to be modified perioperatively with medications such as aspirin, thienopyridines, and warfarin typically being discontinued. The perioperative management of antithrombotic therapy for patients undergoing elective ophthalmic day surgeries can be coordinated as per the current American College of Chest Physicians (ACCP) practice guidelines.[22] For patient safety, patients on antithrombotic regimens (i.e., warfarin) should have an international normalized ratio (INR) value drawn and reviewed the morning of the procedure.

Medical management of preexisting noncardiac health conditions may also impact operative outcome. Intraoperative respiratory complications are the second most reported adverse events in day surgeries, while postoperative pulmonary complications occur in 6.8% of patients undergoing major noncardiac surgeries.[3] Predictors of perioperative pulmonary events are patient centered and surgery related. Patient-centered characteristics include advanced age, airway disease such as asthma and chronic obstructive pulmonary disease (COPD), smoking, overall health status, and sleep apnea.[23] Surgery-related factors include type and duration of surgery, and type of anesthesia. By their very nature, ophthalmic day surgeries inherently attenuate surgery-related factors associated with increased pulmonary complications. One unique feature of eye surgery is patients with significant cough are at increased risk of ocular injury from involuntary head movement. Therefore, elective ophthalmic procedures in patients with significant cough are usually delayed until the cough has subsided.

Patient risk factors of pulmonary complications are more pronounced in the elderly. They are more likely to have thoracic cage stiffness, decreased lung elasticity, diminished mucociliary clearance, and kyphosis.[24] These age-related traits are further aggravated by concomitant neurologic diseases such as Parkinson's disease, cerebrovascular disease, and neuromuscular disorders. However, airway diseases are not necessarily age related. They may be congenital, environmental (allergies), or smoking related. Well-controlled asthma does not seem to be a risk factor for either intraoperative or postoperative complications.[25] Underlying symptomatic COPD increases the risk of postoperative complications such as wound infections and atrial arrhythmias; this risk can be mitigated by optimizing lung function preoperatively with long-acting inhaled anticholinergics, long-acting beta-agonists, and inhaled corticosteroids.[26]

There is increased medical awareness of the impact sleep-disordered breathing has on overall health. Individuals with obstructive sleep apnea (OSA) have increased rates of coexisting medical diseases including diabetes, hypertension, coronary heart disease, and cardiac arrhythmias.[27] Airway management is also more difficult in OSA patients. Therefore, preoperative evaluation should identify patients at risk for OSA and address associated medical conditions in an effort to minimize potential postoperative complications: airway obstruction, tachyarrhythmias, hypoxemia, atelectasis, ischemia, pneumonia, and prolonged intubation and hospitalizations.[28] Generally, OSA patients are advised to bring their respective noninvasive airway assist devices to the ambulatory surgical center the day of surgery.

Preexisting neurologic diseases or neuromuscular disorders must be evaluated preoperatively to assess the patient's ability to remain supine and relatively motionless during ophthalmic surgeries. For example, an underlying seizure disorder needs to be evaluated in terms of its characteristics, its frequency, and the medication regimen that optimally controls the epileptic condition. Antiepileptic drugs should be continued during the perioperative period. Individuals with Parkinson's disease are usually prescribed L-DOPA and/or dopamine receptor agonists to improve and stabilize motor function. Patients may also be taking monoamine oxide inhibitors to prolong the effect of dopamine on motor function. These medications need to be considered when counseling patients preoperatively. Some medications can only be taken orally while others have short half-lives requiring them to be taken very close to the procedure time to maximally stabilize the patient's underlying movement disorder.[29,30] Abrupt withdrawal of dopamine agonists result in movement disorder decompensation and, potentially, neuroleptic malignant syndrome (NMS).

Dialysis patients present a particular challenge for ambulatory surgery. Patients scheduled for elective ophthalmic surgeries are advised to undergo hemodialysis within 24 h of surgery to minimize fluid overload and electrolyte imbalances that may lead to cardiopulmonary complications intraoperatively or postoperatively. These patients are also at risk for adverse events with medications that are renally excreted. This is taken into consideration by the anesthesiologist when selecting the patient's anesthetic regimen.

Autoimmune and inflammatory diseases necessitate careful preoperative evaluations from both the disease and medication point of view. These patients often have significant systemic manifestations that could impact the anesthetic ultimately chosen for the planned eye surgery. In rheumatoid arthritis, temporomandibular and cervical joint involvement can result in movement limitations that affect airway management. Atlantoaxial subluxation predisposes patients to inadvertent cervical cord compression. Spine deformities associated with osteoporosis and ankylosing spondylitis may result in restrictive lung disease and an inability to be supine for ophthalmic surgeries under MAC. Frequently, these diseases are treated with medications that may impact the perioperative course. For example, long-term steroids can result in hypothalamic–pituitary–adrenal (HPA) axis suppression. Patients prescribed systemic steroid therapy for more than 3 weeks are at risk for HPA suppression. Perioperative glucocorticoid coverage should be equivalent to the body's physiologic response to both anesthesia and surgery-related stress.[31] Relative to other surgeries and invasive procedures, eye surgeries do not physiologically stress patients to a great extent. Patients receiving therapeutic doses of steroids may continue to receive their usual oral daily dose of steroid the morning of surgery or receive hydrocortisone 25 mg intravenously at the time of surgery. Postoperatively, patients should resume their usual scheduled oral steroid regimen. However, patients with primary dysfunction of the HPA axis (Addison's disease and panhypopituitarism) are usually on physiologic replacements doses of corticosteroids preoperatively. These patients always require supplemental adjustment of their glucocorticoid dose to compensate for the surgical stress.[31,32]

Inflammatory arthritis patients are often prescribed disease-modifying drugs such as methotrexate (MTX), hydroxychloroquine, and biologic response modifiers such as tumor necrosis factor (TNF)-alpha inhibitors and rituximab. Current literature supports the continuation of MTX and hydroxychloroquine perioperatively.[33,34] With regard to TNF antagonists, the literature is inconclusive but the cautionary recommendations are to suspend TNF antagonists at least one dosage cycle before surgery, and another dose after surgery until sutures may be removed. For patients on rituximab, the conservative recommendation is to consider delaying elective surgeries until B-cell counts have recovered.[35] If the procedure cannot be delayed without jeopardizing the patient, then previous treatment with rituximab is not a contraindication to surgical procedures. Postoperatively, these patients need close surveillance for infectious complications. The preoperative cautionary measures advised for TNF antagonists and rituximab do not figure as prominently for general ophthalmic surgeries with the exception of oncologic oculoplastic surgery. Oncologic eye surgery patients may also be treated with radiation and/or chemotherapy so they incur a greater risk of postoperative infectious complications. In this context, preoperative management of these medications should be undertaken in consultation with the patient's surgeon and rheumatologist.

Patients with thyroid disease may safely undergo low-risk elective ophthalmic procedures as long as they are reasonably stable on their medication regimen. Clinically stable hypothyroid and hyperthyroid patients are instructed to take their thyroid-related medications preoperatively the morning of surgery and to resume them postoperatively. If it is clinically evident that the patient is symptomatic from his or her thyroid disease, then thyroid hormone levels need to be evaluated preoperatively and his or her medical condition stabilized prior to proceeding with elective procedures.

Diabetic patients constitute a significant portion of the patients that undergo eye surgeries. Current treatment recommendations by the American Association of Clinical Endocrinologists and the American Diabetes Association endorse preprandial serum glucose targets of less than 140 mg/dL and random serum blood glucose levels less than 180 mg/dL for hospitalized patients.[36,37] Most ophthalmic surgeries for diabetic patients are of relatively short duration and scheduled as one of the first surgical cases of the day. The characteristics of these surgical procedures and the type of anesthesia utilized allow for conservative blood glucose management and observation. Rarely do ophthalmic surgeries for diabetic patients require insulin infusions and frequent blood glucose monitoring. Less stringent preoperative fasting blood glucose levels of 180 mg/dL the day of surgery are permissible under these circumstances. In general, grossly uncontrolled hyperglycemia has been linked to poor surgical outcomes and is a relative contraindication for elective ophthalmic procedures.

Patients with strabismus and ptosis are more susceptible to malignant hyperthermia (MH).[38] Therefore, the preoperative evaluation of patients scheduled to undergo strabismus or ptosis surgery should assess for risk of MH. Family history should be reviewed for myopathies and unexplained perioperative deaths. Physical examination should target an evaluation for unexplained muscle wasting, short stature with kyphoscoliosis out of proportion to biological age, and low set ears with craniofacial abnormalities. Preoperative identification of the at-risk patient allows for timely evaluation by an anesthesiologist to plan for an anesthetic agent less likely to trigger MH and close intraoperative monitoring. If the patient, surgery, and anesthetic agent are deemed to be too high risk for MH, then the patient may not be a candidate for ambulatory surgery.

POSTOPERATIVE ASSESSMENT

In addition to the traditional postoperative concerns of ambulatory patients, ophthalmology cases may have unique postprocedure events. One must be mindful of the increased risk of postoperative nausea and vomiting (PONV) associated with stra-bismus patients, sympathetic ophthalmia associated with eye trauma (either surgical or accidental), dysrhythmia and hypotension associated with the trigemino-cardiac reflex, and postoperative orbital compartment syndrome in patients resuming anti-coagulation or antiplatelet agents. Orbital compartment syndrome is considered an ophthalmic emergency as lack of prompt decompression can result in permanent vision loss within 90–120 min.[39] Acute unexplained postoperative vision loss is another ophthalmic emergency. These patients need to be immediately evaluated for the possibility of central retinal artery occlusion, ischemic optic neuropathy, acute angle-closure glaucoma, or retinal detachment. In the acute postoperative period, strabismus patients have an increased incidence of PONV because manipulation of their extraocular muscles triggers the oculogastric reflex. This is analogous to the trigemino-cardioreflex triggered by manipulation of the sensory branches of the trigeminal nerve, which may cause brady-arrhythmias and hypotension.

Ophthalmic procedures utilize topical ophthalmic medications with a variety of aims. It is important to be aware of the potential systemic absorption of these agents. Depending on the ophthalmic agent utilized perioperatively, the patient may display significant side effects such as disorientation, malignant hypertension, hypo-tension, myocardial ischemia and infarction, dysrhythmias, and bronchospasms.[40] Dacryocystorhinostomy (a procedure for nasolacrimal duct dysfunction) tradition-ally utilizes cocaine-infused nasal packing for its vasoconstrictive properties but incurs the risk of malignant hypertension, myocardial ischemia, and ventricular arrhythmias.[41]

DISCHARGE RECOMMENDATIONS

Upon discharge, patients resuming anticoagulation or antiplatelet agents postopera-tively should be counseled about the risk of orbital compartment syndrome. Patients at risk are those recovering from blunt eye trauma, eyelid surgery, and retrobulbar anesthesia. In the subacute postprocedure period, sympathetic ophthalmia is rare but presents as ocular inflammation within 3 months after the eye injury.[42] It involves both the previously injured eye and the contralateral nontraumatized eye. This requires prompt referral for an ophthalmic evaluation and intervention to ensure good visual prognosis.

CONCLUSION

Comprehensive preoperative evaluation and patient-centered management of medical conditions can positively impact a patient's ophthalmic operative course. Although ambulatory surgical patients with complex medical conditions can present a chal-lenge to physicians involved with their perioperative care, the majority of ophthal-mic day surgeries present low surgical risk to patients. Preoperative care based on accepted guidelines and expert opinion help ensure the safest possible perioperative course.

REFERENCES

1. Cullen KA, Hall MJ, Golosinskiy A. Ambulatory surgery in the United States, 2006. *Natl Health Stat Report*. Jan 28 2009;(11):1–25.
2. Fleisher LA, Pasternak LR, Lyles A. A novel index of elevated risk of inpatient hospital admission immediately following outpatient surgery. *Arch Surg*. 2007;142(3):263–268.
3. Shnaider I, Chung F. Outcomes in day surgery. *Curr Opin Anaesthesiol*. 2006;19(6):622–629.
4. Dunn AS, Turpie AG. Perioperative management of patients receiving oral anticoagulants: a systematic review. *Arch Intern Med*. 2003;163(8):901–908.
5. Konstantatos A. Anticoagulation and cataract surgery: a review of the current literature. *Anaesth Intensive Care*. 2001;29(1):11–18.
6. Bell CM, Hatch WV, Fischer HD, et al. Association between tamsulosin and serious ophthalmic adverse events in older men following cataract surgery. *JAMA*. 2009;301(19):1991–1996.
7. Chang DF, Braga-Mele R, Mamalis N, et al. Clinical experience with intraoperative floppy-iris syndrome. Results of the 2008 ASCRS member survey. *J Cataract Refract Surg*. 2008;34(7):1201–1209.
8. Schein OD, Katz J, Bass EB, et al. The value of routine preoperative medical testing before cataract surgery. Study of Medical Testing for Cataract Surgery. *N Engl J Med*. 2000;342(3):168–175.
9. Sweitzer BJ. Preoperative medical testing and preparation for ophthalmic surgery. *Ophthalmol Clin North Am*. 2006;19(2):163–177.
10. Fleisher LA, Beckman JA, Brown KA, et al. ACC/AHA 2007 guidelines on perioperative cardiovascular evaluation and care for noncardiac surgery: executive summary: a report of the American College of Cardiology/American Heart Association Task Force on practice guidelines (writing committee to revise the 2002 guidelines on perioperative cardiovascular evaluation for noncardiac surgery). *J Am Coll Cardiol*. 2007;50(17):1707–1732.
11. Noordzij PG, Boersma E, Bax JJ, et al. Prognostic value of routine preoperative electrocardiography in patients undergoing noncardiac surgery. *Am J Cardiol*. 2006;97(7):1103–1106.
12. Howell SJ, Sear JW, Foex P. Hypertension, hypertensive heart disease and perioperative cardiac risk. *Br J Anaesth*. 2004;92(4):570–583.
13. Chobanian AV, Bakris GL, Black HR, et al. Seventh report of the joint national committee on prevention, detection, evaluation, and treatment of high blood pressure. *Hypertension*. 2003;42(6):1206–1252.
14. Marik PE, Varon J. Perioperative hypertension: a review of current and emerging therapeutic agents. *J Clin Anesth*. 2009;21(3):220–229.
15. Feneck R. Drugs for the perioperative control of hypertension: current issues and future directions. *Drugs*. 2007;67(14):2023–2044.
16. Grines CL, Bonow RO, Casey DE, Jr., et al. Prevention of premature discontinuation of dual antiplatelet therapy in patients with coronary artery stents: a science advisory from the American Heart Association, American College of Cardiology, Society for Cardiovascular Angiography and Interventions, American College of Surgeons, and American Dental Association, with representation from the American College of Physicians. *Circulation*. 2007;115(6):813–818.
17. Mond HG, Irwin M, Ector H, Proclemer A. The world survey of cardiac pacing and cardioverter-defibrillators: calendar year 2005 an International Cardiac Pacing and Electrophysiology Society (ICPES) project. *Pacing Clin Electrophysiol*. 2008;31(9):1202–1212.
18. Zaiden JR, Atlee JL, Belott P, et al. Practice advisory for the perioperative management of patients with cardiac rhythm management devices: pacemakers and implantable cardioverter-defibrillators: a report by the American Society of Anesthesiologists Task Force on Perioperative Management of Patients with Cardiac Rhythm Management Devices. *Anesthesiology*. 2005;103(1):186–198.
19. Stoller GL. Ophthalmic surgery and the implantable cardioverter defibrillator. *Arch Ophthalmol*. 2006;124(1):123–125.
20. Chee YL, Crawford JC, Watson HG, Greaves M. Guidelines on the assessment of bleeding risk prior to surgery or invasive procedures: British Committee for Standards in Haematology. *Br J Haematol*. 2008;140:496–504.
21. Keeling DC, Tait C, Makris M. Guideline on the selection and use of therapeutic products to treat haemophilia and other hereditary bleeding disorders. A United Kingdom Haemophilia Center

Doctors' Organisation (UKHCDO) guideline approved by the British Committee for Standards in Haematology. *Haemophilia*. 2008;14(4):671–684.

22. Douketis JD, Berger PB, Dunn AS et al. The perioperative management of antithrombotic therapy: American College of Chest Physicians Evidence-Based Clinical Practice Guidelines (8th Edition). *Chest*. 2008;133(6 Suppl):299S–339S.

23. Smetana GW, Lawrence VA, Cornell JE. Preoperative pulmonary risk stratification for noncardiothoracic surgery: systematic review for the American College of Physicians. *Ann Intern Med*. 2006;144(8):581–595.

24. Christmas C, Makary MA, Burton JR. Medical considerations in older surgical patients. *J Am Coll Surg*. 2006;203(5):746–751.

25. Silvanus MT, Groeben H, Peters J. Corticosteroids and inhaled salbutamol in patients with reversible airway obstruction markedly decrease the incidence of bronchospasm after tracheal intubation. *Anesthesiology*. 2004;100(5):1052–1057.

26. Qaseem A, Snow V, Shekelle P, et al. Diagnosis and management of stable chronic obstructive pulmonary disease: a clinical practice guideline from the American College of Physicians. *Ann Intern Med*. 2007;147(9):633–638.

27. Caples SM, Gami AS, Somers VK. Obstructive sleep apnea. *Ann Intern Med*. 2005;142(3): 187–197.

28. Hwang D, Shakir N, Limann B, et al. Association of sleep-disordered breathing with postoperative complications. *Chest*. 2008;133(5):1128–1134.

29. Nicholson G, Pereira AC, Hall GM. Parkinson's disease and anaesthesia. *Br J Anaesth*. 2002;89(6):904–916.

30. Kalenka A, Schwarz A. Anaesthesia and Parkinson's disease: how to manage with new therapies? *Curr Opin Anaesthesiol*. 2009;22(3):419–424.

31. Axelrod L. Perioperative management of patients treated with glucocorticoids. *Endocrinol Metab Clin North Am*. 2003;32(2):367–383.

32. Marik PE, Varon J. Requirement of perioperative stress doses of corticosteroids: a systematic review of the literature. *Arch Surg*. 2008;143(12):1222–1226.

33. Loza E, Martinez-Lopez JA, Carmona L. A systematic review on the optimum management of the use of methotrexate in rheumatoid arthritis patients in the perioperative period to minimize perioperative morbidity and maintain disease control. *Clin Exp Rheumatol*. 2009;27(5):856–862.

34. Scanzello CR, Figgie MP, Nestor BJ, Goodman SM. Perioperative management of medications used in the treatment of rheumatoid arthritis. *HSS J*. 2006;2(2):141–147.

35. Mushtaq S, Goodman SM, Scanzello CR. Perioperative management of biologic agents used in treatment of rheumatoid arthritis. *Am J Ther*. 2010;epub Mar 5. PMID: 20216205.

36. Moghissi ES, Korytkowski MT, DiNardo M, et al. American Association of Clinical Endocrinologists and American Diabetes Association consensus statement on inpatient glycemic control. *Diabetes Care*. 2009;32(6):1119–1131.

37. Meneghini LF. Perioperative management of diabetes: translating evidence into practice. *Cleve Clin J Med*. 2009;76(Suppl 4):S53–S59.

38. Marmor M. Malignant hyperthermia. *Surv Ophthalmol*. 1983;28(2):117–127.

39. Lima V, Burt B, Leibovitch I, Prabhakaran V, Goldberg RA, Selva D. Orbital compartment syndrome: the ophthalmic surgical emergency. *Surv Ophthalmol*. 2009;54(4):441–449.

40. Gayer S, Zuleta J. Perioperative management of the elderly undergoing eye surgery. *Clin Geriatr Med*. 2008;24(4):687–700.

41. Meyers EF. Cocaine toxicity during dacryocystorhinostomy. *Arch Ophthalmol*. 1980;98(5):842–843.

42. Damico FM, Kiss S, Young LH. Sympathetic ophthalmia. *Semin Ophthalmol*. 2005;20(3):191–197.

PART IV

COMMON POSTOPERATIVE CONDITIONS

CHAPTER 27

SEPSIS

Lena M. Napolitano

BACKGROUND

Incidence and Outcomes of Sepsis

The incidence of severe sepsis is approximately 300 cases per 100,000 population, which is higher than population-based rates of AIDS, colon and breast cancers, and congestive heart failure. The incidence of severe sepsis is projected to increase by 1.5% per year. Severe sepsis has been associated with high mortality rates ranging from 28% to 50%.[1] More than 750,000 cases of severe sepsis occur in the United States annually with 215,000 deaths. In the United States, more than 500 patients die of severe sepsis daily. The mortality rate associated with severe sepsis is greater than the mortality rates for AIDS and breast cancer, and similar to mortality rates for patients with acute myocardial infarction. It is especially common in the elderly and is likely to increase substantially as the U.S. population ages. Sepsis is a major cause of morbidity and mortality worldwide, and is the leading cause of death in noncoronary (including surgical) ICUs in the United States. Severe sepsis is the 10th leading cause of death overall in the United States. Septicemia was the 10th cause of death overall in the United States in 2007.[2]

Review of the control arms of recent sepsis trials also documents a variable mortality rate of sepsis, dependent on the number of patients enrolled with systemic inflammatory response syndrome (SIRS) and presumed infection, severe sepsis, and septic shock in each trial (Figure 27.1). Variability in sepsis mortality rates in the control arm of these trials is also likely related to variability in treatment of sepsis in the individual institutions.[3]

Epidemiology of Sepsis in Surgical Patients

Sepsis is a common postoperative condition in surgical patients. A study of the Nationwide Inpatient Sample between 2002 and 2006 identified patients with postoperative sepsis after elective surgery. Of 6,512,921 elective surgical cases, 1.21% developed postoperative sepsis. Esophageal, pancreatic, and gastric procedures represented the greatest risk for the development of postoperative sepsis. Thoracic,

Perioperative Medicine: Medical Consultation and Co-Management, First Edition.
Edited by Amir K. Jaffer and Paul J. Grant.
© 2012 Wiley-Blackwell. Published 2012 by John Wiley & Sons, Inc.

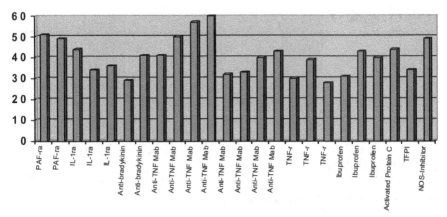

Figure 27.1.   Variability in the mortality rate (percent) of control arms of clinical trials classified according to type of mediator-specific anti-inflammatory agent. See color insert.

adrenal, and hepatic operations accounted for the greatest mortality rates if sepsis developed. Factors associated with the development of postoperative sepsis included race (black, Hispanic), increasing age, and male gender.[4] An additional study of the Nationwide Inpatient Sample from 1997 to 2006 documented that the rate of postoperative severe sepsis increased significantly over the 10-year period, but a concomitant decrease in the in-hospital mortality rate was noted, from 44.4% in 1997 to 34.0% in 2006.[5]

In an analysis of the 1990–2006 data from the Healthcare Cost and Utilization Project (HCUP) inpatient database for the state of New Jersey, the rates of postoperative sepsis (4.24%) and severe sepsis (2.28%) were significantly greater for nonelective than for elective surgery. Interestingly, nonelective surgical procedures had a significant increase in the rates of postoperative sepsis (from 3.74% to 4.51%) and severe sepsis (from 1.79% to 3.15%) over time with the proportion of severe sepsis increasing from 47.7% to 69.9%. The in-hospital mortality rate after nonelective surgery decreased from 37.9% to 29.8%, but no change in mortality was found for elective surgery patients who developed sepsis.[6]

Recent data document that the incidence of sepsis and septic shock exceed those of pulmonary embolism and myocardial infarction.[7] A recent study of general surgery patients in the 2005–2007 National Surgical Quality Improvement Program dataset documented that of 363,897 patients, sepsis occurred in 8350 (2.3%), septic shock in 5977 (1.6%), pulmonary embolism in 1078 (0.3%), and myocardial infarction in 0.2%. The 30-day mortality rate for sepsis was 5.4% and 33.7% for septic shock. Risk factors for increased mortality included age older than 60 years, the need for emergency surgery, and the presence of any comorbidity. These population-based data document the need for early recognition of patients with sepsis and septic shock and the rapid implementation of evidence-based guidelines for sepsis management.

Sepsis: Definitions

Sepsis and septic shock, the systemic response to infection, are the leading causes of morbidity and mortality in surgical patients. Sepsis connotes a clinical syndrome that may occur in any age group, in markedly different patient populations, and in response to a multitude of microbial pathogens from multiple different anatomical sites within the human body. Sepsis may range in severity from mild systemic inflammation without significant clinical consequences to multisystem organ failure in septic shock with an exceedingly high mortality rate.[8]

In 1991, the American College of Chest Physicians and the Society of Critical Care Medicine convened a consensus conference to more accurately define sepsis.[9,10] The term "systemic inflammatory response syndrome" (SIRS) was defined as a clinical response arising from a nonspecific insult such as infection, trauma, thermal injury, or sterile inflammatory processes such as pancreatitis. This clinical response included fever or hypothermia, tachycardia, tachypnea, and leukocytosis or leukopenia (Table 27.1). SIRS is characterized by two or more of these clinical manifestations. "Sepsis" was defined as SIRS with a presumed or confirmed infectious process. Sepsis can progress to "severe sepsis," which was defined as sepsis with organ dysfunction or evidence of hypoperfusion or hypotension. "Septic shock" was defined as sepsis-induced hypotension, persisting despite adequate fluid resuscitation, along with the presence of hypoperfusion abnormalities or organ dysfunction.

TABLE 27.1.   Definitions of Systemic Inflammatory Response Syndrome (SIRS), Sepsis, and Severe Sepsis

Term	Definition
SIRS	A clinical response arising from a nonspecific insult, including ≥ 2 of the following:
	– Temperature $\geq 38°C$ or $\leq 36°C$
	– Heart rate ≥ 90 beats/min
	– Respirations ≥ 20/min
	– White blood cell count $\geq 12,000/mm^3$ or $\leq 4,000/mm^3$ or $>10\%$ neutrophils
Sepsis	SIRS with a presumed or confirmed infectious process
Severe sepsis	Sepsis with ≥ 1 sign of organ failure:
	– Cardiovascular (refractory hypotension)
	– Renal
	– Respiratory
	– Hepatic
	– Hematologic
	– Central nervous system
	– Metabolic acidosis
Septic shock	Sepsis-induced hypotension, despite adequate fluid resuscitation, with presence of perfusion abnormalities

In 2001, an International Sepsis Definitions Conference was convened to review the strengths and weaknesses of the current definitions of sepsis and related conditions, identify ways to improve the current definitions, and identify methodologies for increasing the accuracy, reliability, and/or clinical utility of the diagnosis of sepsis.[11]

A new conceptual framework for understanding sepsis was developed, called the PIRO concept (predisposition, infection, response, and organ dysfunction). PIRO is a classification scheme that could stratify patients on the basis of their predisposing conditions, the nature and extent of the insult (in the case of sepsis, infection), the nature and magnitude of the host response, and the degree of concomitant organ dysfunction (Table 27.2). This has been conceptually modeled from the TNM classification (tumor size, nodal spread, metastases) that has been successfully used in defining treatment and prognostic indicators in clinical oncology. PIRO was introduced as a hypothesis-generating model for future research, and extensive testing will be necessary before it can be considered ready for routine application in clinical practice.

Diagnosis Biomarkers and Diagnostic Tests in Sepsis

The early diagnosis of sepsis, the identification of the origin, adequate therapeutic management, and the monitoring of the disease may help to overcome sepsis-associated mortality, which is unacceptably high and is the third leading cause of death in Western countries. At present, our diagnostic methods in sepsis are insufficient; that is, culture results with antimicrobial susceptibility data take 3–4 days. Furthermore, a definite microbiological diagnosis cannot be made in one-third or more of patients with clinical manifestations of sepsis.[12,13]

Advances in sepsis research will require better markers to delineate more homogenous subsets of patients within a highly heterogenous group of critically ill patients. Molecular techniques and tools for the identification of pathogen-associated molecular patterns (PAMPs) and analysis of danger-associated molecular patterns (DAMPs) will challenge our current diagnostic tests, potentially increasing sensitivity but also dramatically reducing time requirements to identify pathogens and their resistance patterns.[14]

A roundtable meeting on biomarkers in sepsis was held in 2000[15] and in 2005[16] to develop a taxonomy of markers relevant to clinical research in sepsis. A "marker" is a measure that identifies a biological state or that predicts the presence or severity of a pathologic process or disease. More than 100 distinct molecules have been proposed as useful biological markers of sepsis. Virtually all of the putative sepsis markers can be classified as prognostic markers because they identify patient groups at increased risk for mortality. None of these markers (including procalcitonin, interleukin [IL]-6, C-reactive protein) as of yet has shown utility in stratifying patients with respect to therapy (i.e., diagnostic markers) or in titrating that therapy (i.e., response markers). It is clear that further refinements in the definitions and predisposing factors of severe sepsis should improve the understanding and management of severe sepsis and septic shock in the near future.

TABLE 27.2. The PIRO System for Staging Sepsis

Domain	Present	Future	Rationale
Predisposition	Premorbid illness with reduced probability of short-term survival; cultural or religious beliefs, age, sex	Genetic polymorphisms in components of inflammatory response (e.g., TLR, TNF, IL-1, CD14); enhanced understanding of specific interactions between pathogens and host diseases	In the present, premorbid factors impact on the potential attributable morbidity and mortality of an acute insult; deleterious consequences of insult heavily dependent on genetic predisposition (future)
Insult, infection	Culture and sensitivity of infecting pathogens; detection of disease amenable to source control	Assay of microbial products (LPS, mannan, bacterial DNA); gene transcript profiles	Specific therapies directed against inciting insult require demonstration and characterization of that insult
Response	SIRS, other signs of sepsis, shock, CRP	Nonspecific markers of activated inflammation (e.g., PCT or IL-6) or impaired host responsiveness (e.g., HLA-DR); specific detection of target of therapy (e.g., protein C, TNF, PAF)	Both mortality risk and potential to respond to therapy vary with nonspecific measures of disease severity (e.g., shock); specific mediator-targeted therapy is predicated on presence and activity of mediator
Organ dysfunction	Organ dysfunction as number of failing organs or composite score (e.g., MODS, SOFA, LODS, PEMOD, PELOD)	Dynamic measures of cellular response to insult—apoptosis, cytopathic hypoxia, cell stress	Response to preemptive therapy (e.g., targeting microorganism or early mediator) not possible if damage already present; therapies targeting the injurious cellular process require that it be present

TLR, Toll-like receptor; TNF, tumor necrosis factor; IL, interleukin; LPS, lipopolysaccharide; SIRS, systemic inflammatory response syndrome; CRP, C-reactive protein; PCT, procalcitonin; HLA-DR, human leukocyte antigen-Dr; PAF, platelet-activating factor; MODS, multiple organ dysfunction syndrome; SOFA, sepsis-related organ failure assessment; LODS, logistic organ dysfunction system; PEMOD, pediatric multiple organ dysfunction; PELOD, pediatric logistic organ dysfunction.

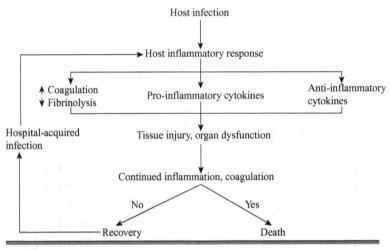

Figure 27.2.   Pathophysiology of severe sepsis. See color insert.

Pathophysiology of Sepsis

With increased understanding of the pathophysiology of sepsis (Figure 27.2), particularly the intricate interplay between activation of coagulation and inflammation, novel therapeutic agents that may improve clinical outcomes are being researched and developed. The prevailing theory has been that sepsis represents an uncontrolled inflammatory response or hyperinflammation manifest as the SIRS. But more recent data document a subsequent state of severe immunosuppression or hypoimmune state in sepsis.[17] We have come to realize that initially, sepsis may be characterized by increases in inflammatory mediators; but as sepsis persists, there is a shift toward an anti-inflammatory immunosuppressive state. The term "compensatory anti-inflammatory response syndrome (CARS)" has been used to define immunologically those patients with sepsis syndromes who are manifesting predominantly a pattern of macrophage deactivation, reduced antigen presentation, and T-cell anergy.

Genetic Variability in Sepsis

Genetic differences may be important markers or determinants of clinical outcomes, including nosocomial infection and severe sepsis.[18] This is a complex area of investigation in humans and relies on identification of particular genetic markers (DNA sequences) and the association with risk for sepsis and ultimate outcome in sepsis. The genetic risk for pneumonia, sepsis, and other serious infections is generally unrecognized or underestimated. Genetic and environmental variables may influence why one patient with infection gets sicker than the next. For example, people may be programmed to respond to infection in different ways; some with aggressive immune responses that may be able to eradicate infection before it manifests itself in physical symptoms, while others may have less aggressive immune systems that allow them to get sick more often. The discovery of various common genetic poly-morphisms in genes that control the inflammatory response has lent credence to this hypothesis, yet discovery of the actual relationship between risks of infection or severe sepsis and individual genotypes will require larger, more rigorously designed studies.

Recent studies of single-nucleotide polymorphisms (SNPs) within the endo-toxin receptor and its signaling system showed an association with the risk of sepsis development. Several candidate genes have been identified as important in the inflammatory response and investigated in case-controlled studies, including the tumor necrosis factor-alpha (TNF-α) and TNF-β genes, positioned next to each other within the cluster of human leukocyte antigen class III genes on chromosome 6. Other candidate genes for sepsis and septic shock include the IL-1 receptor antago-nist gene, the heat shock protein gene, the IL-6 gene, the IL-10 gene, the CD14 gene, the Toll-like receptor (TLR)-4 gene,[19] and the TLR-2 gene, to name a few. There is significant evidence for a genetic susceptibility to development of sepsis and death from sepsis, with candidate genes likely to be involved in the pathogenesis of sepsis, and future potential for targeted therapy of sepsis and septic shock based on genetic variability.[20]

MANAGEMENT

Treatment Strategies in Sepsis

Standard therapy for sepsis and severe sepsis includes source control (i.e., control of the source of the infection), early administration of broad-spectrum systemic antibiotic therapy that is *adequate* (i.e., spectrum of activity appropriate for bacteria causing infection), aggressive fluid resuscitation and hemodynamic support, and nutrition and supportive therapy for other organ dysfunctions, compiled in the evidence-based Surviving Sepsis Campaign guidelines.

Surviving Sepsis Campaign Guidelines and Sepsis Bundles

The Surviving Sepsis Campaign guidelines were initially published in 2004,[21] updated in 2008,[22] and provide evidence-based rationale for each of the recommen-dations. The recommendations of these international evidence-based guidelines have been compiled into two "sepsis bundles" (Table 27.3) to be completed within 6 h (sepsis resuscitation bundle) and 24 h (sepsis management bundle) after the diagno-sis of sepsis is made. A pocket guide for the Surviving Sepsis Campaign 2008 Guidelines is available for clinician use and education.[23]

A number of reports have documented that performance improvement initia-tives using the two sepsis bundles have resulted in significantly improved patient outcomes.[24-26] Results of an international performance improvement program, from January 2005 through March 2008, targeting severe sepsis with use of the bundles was very successful.[27] Data from 15,022 patients at 165 sites documented that com-pliance with the entire sepsis resuscitation bundle increased from 10.9% in the first

TABLE 27.3. Sepsis Bundles: The Goal Is to Perform All Indicated Tasks 100% of the Time within the First 6 h (Sepsis Resuscitation Bundle) or First 24 h (Sepsis Management Bundle) of the Diagnosis of Severe Sepsis

Sepsis resuscitation bundle—(to be started immediately and completed within 6 h)

- Serum lactate measured
- Blood cultures obtained prior to antibiotic administration
- Broad-spectrum antibiotics administered within 3 h for ED admissions and 1 h for non-emergency department ICU admissions
- In the event of hypotension and/or lactate >4 mmol/L:
  - Deliver a minimum of 20 mL/kg of crystalloid (or colloid equivalent)
  - Apply vasopressors for hypotension not responding to initial fluid resuscitation to maintain mean arterial pressure (MAP) ≥65 mm Hg
- In the event of persistent arterial hypotension despite volume resuscitation (septic shock) and/ or initial lactate >4 mmol/L (36 mg/dL):
  - Achieve central venous pressure (CVP) of ≥8 mm Hg
  - Achieve central venous oxygen saturation (ScvO$_2$) of ≥70%.[a]

Sepsis management bundle—(to be started immediately and completed within 24 h)
- Low-dose steroids administered for septic shock in accordance with a standardized ICU policy
- Drotrecogin alfa (activated) administered in accordance with a standardized ICU policy
- Glucose control maintained ≥lower limit of normal, but <150 mg/dL (8.3 mmol/L)
- For mechanically ventilated patients inspiratory plateau pressures maintained <30 cm H$_2$O

[a] Achieving a mixed venous oxygen saturation of 65% is an acceptable alternative.

quarter to 31.3% by the end of 2 years. Similarly, compliance with the entire management bundle started at 18.4% and increased to 36.1% by the end of 2 years. Unadjusted hospital mortality decreased from 37% to 30.8% over 2 years. The adjusted odds ratio (OR) for mortality improved the longer a site was in the campaign, resulting in an adjusted absolute drop of 0.8% per quarter and 5.4% over 2 years. The implementation of the Surviving Sepsis Campaign was associated with sustained, continuous quality improvement in sepsis care.

In an analysis of eight unblinded clinical trials, one randomized and seven with historical controls, sepsis bundles were associated with a consistent and significant increase in survival (OR 1.91; 95% confidence interval [CI] 1.49–2.45; $P < 0.0001$). For all studies reporting such data, there were consistent decreases in time to antibiotics, and increases in the appropriateness of antibiotics. Use of other bundle components changed heterogeneously across the studies, making their impact on survival uncertain.[28]

Components of the Sepsis Resuscitation Bundle (to Be Completed within 6 h)

Antimicrobial Therapy and Source Control Standard therapy for sepsis and severe sepsis includes early administration of empiric broad-spectrum systemic antibiotic and/or antifungal therapy that is *adequate* (i.e., spectrum of activity appropriate for bacteria or fungi causing infection) and "source control" (i.e., control of the source of the infection). Guidance regarding appropriate empiric antimicrobial therapy for patients with abdominal infection[29,30] is available from recent evidence-based guidelines.

Initiation of effective antimicrobial therapy is a critical determinant of survival in severe sepsis and septic shock.[31] A multicenter study ($n = 2731$) in 14 intensive care units in the United States and Canada documented that the risk of death significantly increased with each hour of delay of initiation of antimicrobial therapy. In this study, pneumonia and intra-abdominal infection were the most common sources of sepsis. Only 50% of septic shock patients received effective antimicrobial therapy within 6 h of documented hypotension related to septic shock.[32] The Surviving Sepsis Campaign guidelines recommend the initiation of intravenous broad-spectrum empiric antibiotics within 1 h of sepsis diagnosis, with initiation of early empiric antimicrobial therapy to cover all potential pathogens (Table 27.4). Once clinical culture results return, de-escalation of antimicrobial therapy is warranted, preferably to monotherapy if possible. De-escalation of this therapy from broad-spectrum initial coverage to targeted antimicrobial therapy after results of cultures and susceptibility tests become available is a necessary component of this strategy, in order to minimize unnecessary use of broad-spectrum antibiotics and possibly promote further bacterial resistance.

Source control is very important in surgical patients with sepsis. In patients with intra-abdominal infection, source control may require surgical intervention for the removal of the infected/perforated organ (gallbladder, appendix, colon, small bowel), debridement of infected/necrotic tissue (necrotizing infected pancreatitis, surgical site infection, necrotizing soft tissue infection), or drainage of abscess or infected fluid collection. Interventional radiology techniques are also effective for source control. Throughout the course of treatment of surgical patients with sepsis,

TABLE 27.4. Surviving Sepsis Guidelines Recommendations Regarding Antibiotic Therapy

Antibiotic therapy

♦ Begin intravenous antibiotics as early as possible, and always within the first hour of recognizing severe sepsis(1D) and septic shock.(1B)
♦ Broad-spectrum: one or more agents active against likely bacterial/fungal pathogens and with good penetration into presumed source.(1B)
♦ Reassess antimicrobial regimen daily to optimize efficacy, prevent resistance, avoid toxicity, and minimize cost.(1C)
◊ Consider combination therapy in *Pseudomonas* infections.(2D)
◊ Consider combination empiric therapy in neutropenic patients.(2D)
◊ Combination therapy no more than 3–5 days and de-escalation following susceptibilities.(2D)
♦ Duration of therapy typically limited to 7–10 days; longer if response is slow or there are undrainable foci of infection or immunologic deficiencies.(1D)
♦ Stop antimicrobial therapy if cause is found to be noninfectious.(1D)

From http://www.survivingsepsis.org/SiteCollectionDocuments/2008%20Pocket%20Guides.pdf.

it is important to reevaluate whether "source control" is adequate, particularly for patients with intra-abdominal infections, as postsurgical intra-abdominal abscesses can occur in patients following emergent abdominal surgical procedures.

Fluid Resuscitation Early aggressive fluid resuscitation is a standard component of sepsis therapy and should be the initial step in hemodynamic support of patients with septic shock.[33] The goal of fluid resuscitation in sepsis is restoration of tissue perfusion and normalization of oxidative metabolism.[34] Increasing cardiac output and oxygen delivery is dependent on expansion of blood and plasma volume. Intravascular volume can be repleted through the use of packed red cells, crystalloid solutions, and colloid solutions. Fluid infusion is best initiated with boluses titrated to clinical end points of heart rate, urine output, and blood pressure. Patients who do not respond rapidly to initial fluid boluses or those with poor physiologic reserve should be considered for invasive hemodynamic monitoring.

A more aggressive approach to resuscitation in sepsis (early goal-directed therapy [EGDT] "Rivers protocol,"[35] Figure 27.3) has been shown to improve survival for patients presenting to the emergency department with septic shock in a randomized, controlled, single-institution trial. In-hospital mortality was 30.5% in the group assigned to EGDT, as compared with 46.5% in the group assigned to standard therapy ($P = 0.009$). During the interval from 7 to 72 h, the patients assigned to EGDT had a significantly higher mean central venous oxygen saturation, a lower lactate concentration, a lower base deficit, and a higher pH than the patients assigned to standard therapy ($P \leq 0.02$ for all comparisons). During the same period, mean Acute Physiology and Chronic Health Evaluation (APACHE) II scores were significantly lower, indicating less severe organ dysfunction, in the patients assigned to EGDT than in those assigned to standard therapy (13.0 ± 6.3 vs. 15.9 ± 6.4, $P < 0.001$). EGDT provided significantly improved outcome in patients with severe sepsis and septic shock.

The control group in this study received significantly less fluid in the first 6 h during unblinded treatment in the emergency department, and both central venous pressure (CVP) and mean arterial pressure (MAP) were lower in the control group at 6 h. Later in the ICU, the control group received more fluid resuscitation than the EGDT group, but the adverse effect on survival based on the early differences in fluid resuscitation could not be overcome. Death attributable to sudden cardiovascular collapse but not to multiple organ failure occurred less frequently in the EGDT group. Because of several treatment differences between study groups, it cannot be determined which aspect of the protocol was most crucial in producing this observed effect on survival. Moreover, large beneficial effects of some interventions, such as better fluid resuscitation, could have obscured harmful effects of others. A point not addressed but of equal importance to rapid resuscitation is the need to start antibiotics within 60 min of diagnosing severe sepsis. Approximately 6 h after randomization for severe sepsis or septic shock, 1 in 10 patients in this study had not received antibiotics. Clearly, septic patients are best served by promptly initiating antimicrobial therapy and rapid lifesaving resuscitation based on frequent physiologic measurements.

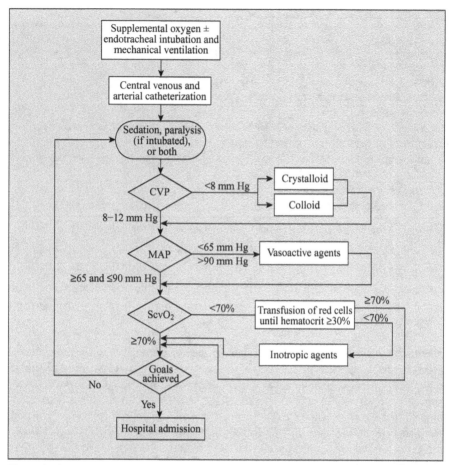

Figure 27.3.   Protocol for early goal-directed therapy (EGDT). From Rivers et al.[35] CVP, central venous pressure; MAP, mean arterial pressure; ScvO$_2$, central venous oxygen saturation. See color insert.

Multiple international randomized controlled trials (RCTs) of EGDT for patients with severe sepsis are under way to validate the findings of the single-center Rivers trial. These include Protocolized Care for Early Septic Shock (ProCESS), Australian Resuscitation in Sepsis Evaluation (ARISE), and Protocolized Management in Sepsis (ProMISe). The ProCESS trial will randomize 1950 patients who present to the emergency department in septic shock to three arms: (1) the EGDT Rivers protocol described above, (2) a simpler less invasive protocol using esophageal Doppler monitor and no blood transfusion, and (3) usual care.[36] The ARISE trial will randomize 1600 patients to EGDT versus standard care and assess 90-day mortality in patients presenting to the emergency department with severe sepsis.[37] The ProMISe trial will randomize 1260 patients to EGDT versus standard care and

TABLE 27.5.   Surviving Sepsis Guidelines Recommendations regarding Vasopressors

Vasopressors

- ◆ Maintain MAP ≥65 mm Hg.(1C)
- ◆ Norepinephrine or dopamine centrally administered is the initial vasopressor of choice.(1C)
- ◆ Epinephrine, phenylephrine, or vasopressin should not be administered as the initial vasopressor in septic shock.(2C)
  - • Vasopressin 0.03 units/min may be subsequently added to norepinephrine with anticipation of an effect equivalent to norepinephrine alone.
- ◊ Use epinephrine as the first alternative agent in septic shock when blood pressure is poorly responsive to norepinephrine or dopamine.(2B)
- ◆ Do not use low-dose dopamine for renal protection.(1A)
- ◆ In patients requiring vasopressors, insert an arterial catheter as soon as practical.(1D)

From http://www.survivingsepsis.org/SiteCollectionDocuments/2008%20Pocket%20Guides.pdf.

assess 90-day mortality in patients presenting to the emergency department with septic shock.[38] Furthermore, an individual patient data meta-analysis will be performed across the three trials.

Hemodynamic Support   If fluid therapy alone fails to restore adequate arterial pressure and organ perfusion, therapy with vasopressors should be initiated. Either norepinephrine or dopamine is the initial vasopressor of choice to correct hypotension in septic shock (Table 27.5). In end-stage vasodilatory shock, it has been documented that the baroreceptor reflex is impaired and vasopressin stores are depleted. Persistent elevation of catecholamines may lead to downregulation of beta-adrenergic receptors, reducing smooth muscle response to catecholamines, and leading to an inability to maintain organ perfusion.

Vasopressin is emerging as a rational therapy for the hemodynamic support of septic shock and vasodilatory shock.[39] Both hemorrhagic and septic shock are associated with a biphasic response in vasopressin levels. In early shock, appropriately high levels of vasopressin are produced to support organ perfusion. As the shock state progresses, plasma vasopressin levels fall for reasons that are not entirely clear. Importantly, vasopressin levels in established septic and vasodilatory shock are low. Several mechanisms for this vasopressin deficiency have been proposed. The potential mechanisms of vasopressin deficiency include (1) depletion of pituitary stores of vasopressin due to excessive baroreceptor firing or exhaustive release in early septic shock, (2) autonomic dysfunction, citing lack of baroreflex-mediated bradycardia after vasopressin infusion as evidence, (3) elevated norepinephrine levels (endogenous or exogenous) that have a central inhibitory effect on vasopressin release, and (4) increased nitric oxide release by vascular endothelium within the posterior pituitary during sepsis that may inhibit vasopressin production.

Vasopressin deficiency may contribute to the refractory hypotension of septic shock, resulting in the continued requirement of vasopressor therapy. In physiologic doses (0.01–0.04 U/min), low-dose vasopressin infusion causes a pressor response in septic shock and sparing of exogenous catecholamines. Vasopressin mediates vasoconstriction via V1-receptors, coupled to phospholipase C, and increases intra-cellular calcium concentration. This action is not impaired during sepsis, and thus vasopressin has been shown effective in reversal of catecholamine-resistant hypoten-sion in septic shock patients. Supplementary vasopressin infusion improved cardio-circulatory function in a number of studies in advanced vasodilatory shock.[40]

The Vasopressin and Septic Shock Trial (VASST) randomized 779 patients in septic shock requiring norepinephrine (5 μg/min) for at least 6 h and at least one organ system dysfunction present for <24 h to vasopressin (0.01–0.03 U/min) versus norepinephrine at higher dose (5–15 μg/min).[41] No difference in 28-day or 90-day mortality was identified. In the prospectively defined stratum of less severe septic shock, the mortality rate was lower in the vasopressin group than in the norepineph-rine group at 28 days (26.5% vs. 35.7%, $P = 0.05$), which persisted to 90-day mor-tality (35.8% vs. 46.1%, $P = 0.04$). In a post hoc analysis of the VASST study, it was identified that the combination of low-dose vasopressin and corticosteroids was associated with decreased mortality and organ dysfunction compared with norepi-nephrine and corticosteroids.[42] Based on the results of studies to date, clinicians should consider the addition of low-dose (up to 0.03 U/min) continuous infusion vasopressin in individual septic shock patients who are adequately resuscitated and still requiring high doses of vasopressors (Table 27.5).

When adequately fluid resuscitated, most septic patients are hyperdynamic, but myocardial contractility, as assessed by ejection fraction, is impaired. In patients with low cardiac output and impaired perfusion despite adequate fluid resuscitation, dobutamine may be considered to increase cardiac output. The Surviving Sepsis Campaign guidelines states the following: "Use dobutamine in patients with myo-cardial dysfunction as supported by elevated cardiac filling pressures and low cardiac output. (1C). Do not increase cardiac index to predetermined supranormal levels (1B)."

Components of the Sepsis Management Bundle (to Be Completed within 24 h)

Low-Dose Steroids   The hypothalamic–pituitary–adrenal axis is a major deter-minant of the host response to stress. During sepsis or acute respiratory distress syndrome, the hypothalamic–pituitary–adrenal axis is rapidly activated through a systemic pathway, that is, by circulating pro-inflammatory cytokines and through the vagus nerve. Subsequently, the adrenal glands release cortisol, a hormone that will likely counteract the inflammatory process and restore cardiovascular homeo-stasis. Both experimental models and studies in humans suggest that inadequate hypothalamic–pituitary–adrenal axis response to stress accounts, at least partly, for the genesis of shock and organ dysfunction in sepsis. But the benefit of corticoste-roids in severe sepsis and septic shock remains controversial. A recent systematic review of 20 clinical trials concluded that low-dose corticosteroid therapy was asso-ciated with reduced mortality, increased shock reversal, and reduced ICU length of stay.[43]

Adrenal insufficiency has been documented in a significant portion of patients with severe sepsis and septic shock. The correct method to diagnosis of adrenal insufficiency in a septic shock patient remains controversial. Traditionally, an adrenocorticotropic hormone (ACTH) (corticotropin) stimulation test is utilized to make the diagnosis of adrenal insufficiency, with a baseline cortisol measurement, followed by the administration of 250 µg of synthetic ACTH, and then repeat plasma cortisol concentrations at 30 and 60 min after ACTH administration. An incremental increase of <9 µg/dL is interpreted as adrenal insufficiency.[44]

In a randomized trial of septic shock patients ($n = 300$) in France by Annane and colleagues, the 7-day treatment with low-dose corticosteroids (200 mg daily of hydrocortisone) significantly reduced mortality without increasing adverse events.[45] Subsequent meta-analyses documented that a 5- to 7-day course of physiologic hydrocortisone doses with subsequent tapering increases survival rate and shock reversal in patients with vasopressor-dependent septic shock.[46]

CORTICUS, the largest trial to date, randomized septic shock patients ($n = 499$) to receive hydrocortisone (50mg q 6 h) or placebo for 5 days with subsequent tapering for a 6-day period.[47] No difference in 28-day all-cause mortality was identified, but earlier shock resolution was confirmed in the steroid group (median time to reverse shock 3.1 vs. 5.7 days, $P = 0.003$). However, it is noted that the patients enrolled in this trial had a lower placebo group mortality (63% in Annane study; 31% in the CORTICUS trial). The Annane study enrolled only patients with vasopressor-dependent septic shock, while the CORTICUS trial enrolled all patients with septic shock. The CORTICUS trial patients were different as well, with more abdominal sepsis and more surgical patients, and less pneumonia patients. The CORTICUS trial documented that 46.7% of patients did not have a response to corticotropin stimulation test, and these patients had a higher mortality rate. CORTICUS was underpowered for the primary outcome measure, death within 28 days in patients who did not respond to corticotropin. Therefore, considerable controversy still remains. An important contribution of the CORTICUS trial was the identification that hospital-based immunoassays are not accurate for cortisol measurements in critically ill patients.[48] Therefore, the current Surviving Sepsis Campaign guidelines recommendations for corticosteroids in septic shock patients are as follows: "We suggest intravenous hydrocortisone be given only to adult septic shock patients after blood pressure is identified to be poorly responsive to fluid resuscitation and vasopressor therapy." Recommendations also state that steroid therapy should no longer be guided by corticotropin stimulation test results (Table 27.6).

Relative adrenal insufficiency and "peripheral glucocorticoid resistance syndrome" are the two main features of the inappropriate hormonal response and provide the grounds for cortisol replacement in sepsis.[49] The administration of modest doses of hydrocortisone in the setting of pressor-dependent septic shock resulted in a significant improvement of hemodynamics and a beneficial effect on survival, *unrelated* to adrenal insufficiency in other studies. It is presumed that these patients have "peripheral glucocorticoid resistance syndrome." Increased cytokines induce glucocorticoid resistance in targeted tissues by altering steroid receptor function. Cytokines also reduce steroid-binding affinity for cortisol. Exogenous administration of pharmacologic low-dose steroids may be sufficient for treatment in this

TABLE 27.6.   Surviving Sepsis Guidelines Recommendations regarding Steroids

Steroids

◊ Consider intravenous hydrocortisone for adult septic shock when hypotension responds poorly to adequate fluid resuscitation and vasopressors.(2C)

◊ ACTH stimulation test is not recommended to identify the subset of adults with septic shock who should receive hydrocortisone.(2B)

◊ Hydrocortisone is preferred to dexamethasone.(2B)

◊ Fludrocortisone (50 μg orally once a day) may be included if an alternative to hydrocortisone is being used, which lacks significant mineralo-corticoid activity. Fludrocortisone is optional if hydrocortisone is used.(2C)

◊ Steroid therapy may be weaned once vasopressors are no longer required.(2D)

♦ Hydrocortisone dose should be ≤300 mg/day.(1A)

♦ Do not use corticosteroids to treat sepsis in the absence of shock unless the patient's endocrine or corticosteroid history warrants it.(1D)

From http://www.survivingsepsis.org/SiteCollectionDocuments/2008%20Pocket%20Guides.pdf.

steroid-resistant state. The adverse effects of steroids relate to increased myopathy and neuropathy.

Recombinant Human Activated Protein C (rhAPC) for Severe Sepsis   Dysregulation of coagulation and inflammation is common in sepsis and is thought to be fundamental to the pathogenesis of multiple organ dysfunction syndrome (MODS). Severe infection and inflammation almost invariably lead to hemostatic abnormalities, ranging from insignificant laboratory changes to severe disseminated intravascular coagulation (DIC). Systemic inflammation results in activation of coagulation, due to tissue factor-mediated thrombin generation, downregulation of physiological anticoagulant mechanisms, and inhibition of fibrinolysis. Increased D-dimers and decreased protein C blood concentrations are common in patients with sepsis and organ dysfunction. Decreased protein C concentrations play an active role in the development of the hypercoagulable state in patients with severe sepsis, and are linked to the development of organ dysfunction and increased mortality.[50] In fact, protein C deficiency was documented in approximately 80% of all severe sepsis patients studied. The conversion of protein C to activated protein C may be impaired during sepsis as a result of the downregulation of thrombomodulin by inflammatory cytokines.

Activated protein C, an endogenous protein that promotes fibrinolysis and inhibits thrombosis and inflammation, is an important modulator of the coagulation and inflammation associated with severe sepsis (Figure 27.4). The properties of activated protein C include (1) antithrombotic activity, by inhibition of thrombin formation and inhibition of Factors V and VIII; (2) profibrinolytic activity, enhancing the body's ability to lyse fibrin, via inhibition of plasminogen-activator-inhibitor-1 (PAI-1); and (3) anti-inflammatory activity, indirectly through reduced thrombin resulting in less TNF and IL-1 production, and via a direct effect on monocytes and endothelial cells through an NFκB mechanism.

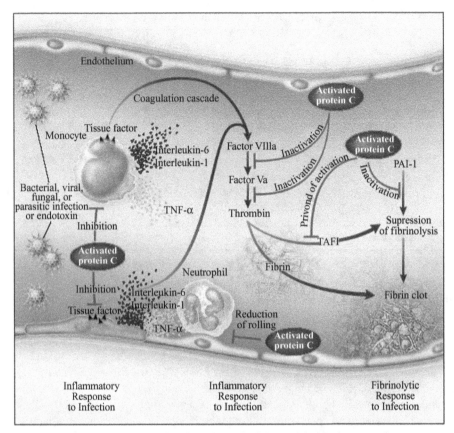

Figure 27.4.   Proposed action of activated protein C in modulating the systemic inflammatory, procoagulant, and fibrinolytic host responses to infection. From Bernard et al.[51] TAFI, thrombin activatable fibrinolysis inhibitor. See color insert.

The administration of a 96-h continuous infusion of drotrecogin alfa (activated) or rhAPC (24 µg/kg/h) in the Recombinant Human Activated Protein C Worldwide Evaluation in Severe Sepsis (PROWESS) trial[51] was associated with a significant reduction in 28-day mortality in patients with severe sepsis (sepsis associated with acute organ dysfunction) who have a high risk of death (assessed by APACHE II score). Patients with an APACHE II score ≥25 that received rhAPC had reduced mortality (31%, relative risk [RR] 0.71, CI 0.59–0.85) compared with 44% mortality in the placebo patients, reflecting a 13% absolute mortality difference. This survival advantage in septic patients who were randomized to rhAPC treatment was confirmed to persist for 1 year after conclusion of the PROWESS trial.[52]

Analysis of protein C levels in patients from the PROWESS trial demonstrated that severe protein C deficiency was associated with increased odds of death at 28 days as compared with subjects without protein C deficiency. Furthermore, increased protein C levels were associated with better outcome. Two additional analyses of the PROWESS trial[53,54] documented significant improvements in organ function measured by sepsis-related organ failure assessment (SOFA) scores for 28 days, and significantly faster resolution of cardiovascular ($P = 0.009$) and respiratory ($P = 0.009$) dysfunction and significantly slower onset of hematologic organ dysfunction ($P = 0.041$) compared with placebo patients.

No efficacy of rhAPC was demonstrated in septic patients with low risk of death or pediatric septic patients. The Drotrecogin Alfa (Activated) for Adults with Severe Sepsis and Low Risk of Death (ADDRESS) was a placebo-controlled double-blind multicenter RCT of rhAPC in septic patients with a low risk of death (APACHE <25 in the United States or single organ failure in Europe).[55] Overall 28-day mortality was not significantly different with rhAPC compared with placebo (18.5% vs. 17.0%, respectively; $P = 0.34$). The Researching Severe Sepsis and Organ Dysfunction in Children: A Global Perspective (RESOLVE) was an open-label placebo-controlled trial in pediatric patients.[56] Compared with placebo, rhAPC did not alter the primary end point of composite time to complete organ failure resolution (CTCOFR) score (6% vs. 6%; $P = 0.72$) nor did it improve 28-day mortality (17.5% vs. 17.2%, respectively; $P = 0.93$). Additional data from the Extended Evaluation of rhAPC in Treatment of Severe Sepsis (ENHANCE) trial,[57] a single-arm, open-label trial of rhAPC in 2434 adult patients in 25 countries at 361 sites confirmed a similar mortality rate (25.3%) as PROWESS, but a higher bleeding rate (1–3% higher). ENHANCE patients treated within 0–24 h from their first sepsis-induced organ dysfunction had lower observed mortality than those treated after 24 h (22.9% vs. 27.4%; $P = 0.01$). In a recently completed clinical trial (PROWESS-SHOCK[58,59]), rhAPC failed to show a survival benefit for patients with severe sepsis and septic shock. The PROWESS-SHOCK trial included 1680 patients randomized to rhAPC vs. placebo, and no significant difference in 28-day all-cause mortality was identified (rhAPC 26.4% vs. placebo 24.2%, RR 1.09, 95% confidence interval 0.92–1.28, $p = 0.31$). The mortality rate in the placebo cohort was markedly lower (24.2%) compared with the mortality in the placebo cohort of the initial PROWESS trial (44%), documenting significant improvement in outcomes of septic shock patients over the last decade. The risk of severe bleeding events was 1.2% in the rhAPC arm and 1.0% in the placebo arm, suggesting there was no increased harm. Based on the results of the PROWESS-SHOCK trial, the FDA notified healthcare professionals that on October 25, 2011, a worldwide voluntary market withdrawal of rhAPC was to occur.[60] The European Medicine Agency provided similar guidance.[61] An editorial recently concluded that "more sophisticated selection of patients seems key if we are to most wisely test agents designed to manipulate the septic host response."[62]

The Surviving Sepsis Campaign guidelines state that "Consider rhAPC in adult patients with sepsis-induced organ dysfunction with clinical assessment of high risk of death (typically APACHE II ≥25 or multiple organ failure) if there are no contraindications. (2B; 2C for postoperative patients). Adult patients with severe sepsis and low risk of death (e.g, APACHE II <20 or one organ failure) should not receive rhAPC (1A)."

Insulin and Glycemic Control Hyperglycemia and insulin resistance are common in critically ill patients, even without prior history of diabetes. A pivotal study[63] in surgical ICU patients ($n = 1548$) showed that mortality is significantly reduced by maintenance of normoglycemia using intensive insulin therapy (maintenance of blood glucose between 80 and 110 mg/dL) compared with conventional treatment (insulin infusion only if blood glucose >215 mg/dL and maintenance of glucose between 180 and 200 mg/dL). Intensive insulin therapy reduced mortality from 8.0% to 4.6% ($P < 0.04$). The greatest reduction in mortality involved deaths due to MODS with a proven septic focus. Intensive insulin therapy also reduced overall in-hospital mortality by 34%, bloodstream infections by 46%, and acute renal failure requiring dialysis or hemofiltration by 50%. A subsequent analysis of this study cohort[64] determined that the lowered blood glucose level rather than the insulin dose was related to reduced mortality ($P < 0.0001$), critical illness polyneuropathy ($P < 0.0001$), bacteremia ($P = 0.02$), and inflammation ($P = 0.0006$) but not to prevention of acute renal failure, for which the insulin dose was an independent determinant ($P = 0.03$). As compared with normoglycemia, an intermediate blood glucose level (110–150 mg/dL) was associated with worse outcome. Metabolic control, as reflected by normoglycemia, rather than the infused insulin dose, was related to the beneficial effects of intensive insulin therapy in these surgical critical care patients. In a prospective, randomized trial in medical ICU patients ($n = 1200$), intensive insulin therapy significantly reduced morbidity but not mortality.[65] Interestingly, among 767 patients who stayed in the ICU for 3 or more days, in-hospital mortality in the intensive insulin therapy patients was reduced from 52.5% to 43% ($P = 0.0009$) and morbidity was also reduced. Glycemic control therefore emerged as a strategy for prevention of septic complications in critically ill patients.

More recently, a number of prospective randomized clinical trials investigating the role of intensive insulin therapy in critically ill patients have been completed. The Glucontrol study[66] documented a lack of clinical benefit of intensive insulin therapy, and there was an associated increased incidence of hypoglycemia. The VISEP study examined intensive insulin therapy and pentastarch resuscitation in severe sepsis and documented that the use of intensive insulin therapy placed critically ill patient with sepsis at increased risk for serious adverse events related to hypoglycemia.[67] The rate of severe hypoglycemia (glucose level, <40 mg/dL) was higher in the intensive therapy group than in the conventional therapy group (17.0% vs. 4.1%, $P < 0.001$), as was the rate of serious adverse events (10.9% vs. 5.2%, $P = 0.01$). Both of these trials were stopped early for safety reasons related to hypoglycemia.

The largest international clinical trial (NICE-SUGAR) in critically ill patients ($n = 6104$) randomized patients to intensive (target blood glucose range of 81–108 mg/dL) or conventional (target blood glucose <180 mg/dL) blood glucose control. Intensive glucose control increased mortality among adults in the ICU: a blood glucose target of 180 mg or less per deciliter resulted in lower mortality than did a target of 81–108 mg/dL (24.9% vs. 27.5%, OR for intensive control 1.14, 95% CI 1.02–1.28, $P = 0.02$). The treatment effect did not differ significantly between operative (surgical) patients and nonoperative (medical) patients (OR for death in the intensive control group, 1.31 and 1.07, respectively; $P = 0.10$). Severe hypoglycemia (blood glucose level, <40 mg/dL) was reported in 6.8% of the intensive control group and 0.5% of the conventional control group ($P < 0.001$).[68]

Based on these results, the current Surviving Sepsis Campaign guidelines recommend the use of intravenous insulin to maintain glycemic control (blood glucose <150 mg/dL) using a validated protocol, and provision of a glucose calorie

TABLE 27.7.   Surviving Sepsis Guidelines Recommendations regarding Glucose Control

Glucose control

- Use intravenous (IV) insulin to control hyperglycemia in patients with severe sepsis following stabilization in the ICU.[1B]
- ◊ Aim to keep blood glucose Ω8.3 mmol/L (150 mg/dL) using a validated protocol for insulin dose adjustment.[2C]
- Provide a glucose calorie source and monitor blood glucose values every 1–2 h (4 h when stable) in patients receiving IV insulin.[1C]
- Interpret with caution low glucose levels obtained with point of care testing, as these techniques may overestimate arterial blood or plasma glucose values.[1B]

From http://www.survivingsepsis.org/SiteCollectionDocuments/2008%20Pocket%20Guides.pdf.

source (Table 27.7). It should be noted, however, that a recent meta-analysis including the NICE-SUGAR study data documented that surgical patients may benefit from intensive insulin therapy (RR 0.63, 95% CI 0.44–0.91).[69]

CONCLUSION

Sepsis is a common postoperative condition in surgical patients, and is associated with high mortality rates. It is important to differentiate "severe sepsis" (defined as sepsis with organ dysfunction or evidence of hypoperfusion or hypotension) with reported mortality rates of approximately 30% and "septic shock" (defined as sepsis-induced hypotension, persisting despite adequate fluid resuscitation, along with the presence of hypoperfusion abnormalities or organ dysfunction) requiring continuous infusion vasopressors with reported higher mortality rates ranging from 45% to 70%. Early aggressive and definitive management of severe sepsis and septic shock is associated with improved outcomes. The Surviving Sepsis Campaign guidelines provide evidence-based recommendations for sepsis care and advocate treatment including early aggressive fluid resuscitation, intravenous broad-spectrum antibiotic/antifungal administration within 1 h of diagnosis, adequate source control and organ support, vasopressors, glycemic control, and consideration of the use of steroids and recombinant activated protein C in patients with high risk of death. Clinicians should be familiar with the sepsis resuscitation bundle and the sepsis management bundle to guide early sepsis management in these patients.

REFERENCES

1. Angus DC, Linde-Zwirble WT, Lidicker J, Clermont G, Carcillo J, Pinsky MR. Epidemiology of severe sepsis in the United States: analysis of incidence, outcome, and associated costs of care. *Crit Care Med* Jul 2001;29(7):1303–1310.
2. Xu J, Kochanek KD, Murphy SL, Te Jada-Vera B. Deaths: Final data for 2007. *National Vital Statistics Reports*. May 20, 2010;58(19):1–136.

3. Natanson C, Esposito CJ, Banks SM. The sirens' song of confirmatory sepsis trials: selection bias and sampling error. Editorial. *Crit Care Med.* 1998;26:1927–1931.
4. Vogel TR, Dombrovskiy VY, Carson JL, Graham AM, Lowry SF. Postoperative sepsis in the United States. *Ann Surg.* Jun 21 2010;252(6):1065–1071.
5. Bateman BT, Schmidt U, Berman MF, Bittner EA. Temporal trends in the epidemiology of severe postoperative sepsis after elective surgery: a large, nationwide sample. *Anesthesiology.* Apr 2010;112(4):917–925.
6. Vogel TR, Dombrovskiy VY, Lowry SF. Trends in postoperative sepsis: are we improving outcomes? *Surg Infect (Larchmt).* Feb 2009;10(1):71–78.
7. Moore LJ, Moore FA, Todd SR, et al. Sepsis in general surgery: the 2005–2007 National Surgical Quality Improvement Program (NSQIP) perspective. *Arch Surg.* Jul 2010;145(7):695–700.
8. Opal SM. Severe sepsis and septic shock: defining the clinical problem. *Scand J Infect Dis* 2003;35(9):529–534.
9. Bone RC, Balk RA, Cerra FB, et al. American College of Chest Physicians/Society of Critical Care Medicine Consensus Conference: definitions for sepsis and organ failure and guidelines for use of innovative therapies in sepsis. *Chest.* 1992;101:1644–1655.
10. American College of Chest Physicians/Society of Critical Care Medicine Consensus Conference: definitions for sepsis and organ failure and guidelines for the use of innovative therapies in sepsis. *Crit Care Med.* 1992;20:864–874.
11. Levy MM, Fink MP, Marshall JC et al. 2001 SCCM/ESICM/ACCP/ATS/SIS International Sepsis Definitions Conference. *Crit Care Med.* 2003;31:1250–1256.
12. Sands KE, Bates DW, Lanken PN, et al. Epidemiology of sepsis syndrome in 8 academic medical centers. *JAMA.* 1997;278:234–240.
13. Vincent J-L, Sakr Y, Sprung CL, et al. Sepsis in European intensive care units: results of the SOAP study. *Crit Care Med.* 2006;34:344–353.
14. Claus RA, Otto GP, Deigner HP, Bauer M. Approaching clinical reality: markers for monitoring inflammation and sepsis. *Curr Mol Med.* Mar 2010;10(2):227–235.
15. Marshall JC, Vincent JL, Fink MP, Cook DJ, Rubenfeld G, Foster D, Fisher CJ, Faist E, Reinhart K. Measures, markers and mediators: toward a staging system for clinical sepsis. A report of the Fifth Toronto Sepsis Roundtable, Toronto, Ontario, Canada, October 25–26, 2000. *Crit Care Med.* 2003;31:1560–1567.
16. Marshall JC, Reinhart K, for the International Sepsis Forum. Biomarkers of sepsis. *Crit Care Med.* 2009;27:2290–2298.
17. Hotchkiss RS, Karl IE. The pathophysiology and treatment of sepsis. *N Engl J Med.* 2003;348(2):138–150.
18. Tabrizi AR, Zehnbauer BA, Freeman BD, Buchman TG. Genetic markers in sepsis. *J Am Coll Surg.* 2001;192(1):106–117.
19. Kumpf O, Giamarellos-Bourboulis EJ, Koch A, et al. Influence of genetic variations in TLR2 and TIRAP/Mal on the course of sepsis and pneumonia and cytokine release: an observational study in three cohorts. *Crit Care.* 2010;14(3):R103.
20. Holmes CL, Russell JA, Walley KR. Genetic polymorphisms in sepsis and septic shock: role in prognosis and potential for therapy. *Chest* Sep 2003;124(3):1103–1115.
21. Dellinger RP, Carlet JM, Masur H et al. Surviving Sepsis Campaign guidelines for management of severe sepsis and septic shock. *Crit Care Med.* 2004;32:858–873.
22. Surviving Sepsis Campaign. International guidelines for management of severe sepsis and septic shock. *Crit Care Med.* Jan 2008;36(1):296–327.
23. Willson J, Bion J. SSC authors guidelines for management of severe sepsis and septic shock. Available at http://www.survivingsepsis.org/SiteCollectionDocuments/2008%20Pocket%20Guides.pdf.
24. Ferrer R, Artigas A, Levy MM, et al.; Edusepsis Study Group. Improvement process of care and outcome after a multicenter severe sepsis educational program in Spain. *JAMA.* May 21 2008;299(19):2294–2303.
25. Lefrant JY, Muller L, Raillard A, et al. Reduction of the severe sepsis or septic shock-associated mortality by reinforcement of the recommendations bundle: a multicenter study. *Ann Fr Anesth Reanim.* Jul 13 2010;29(9):621–628.

26. Gao F, Melody T, Daniels DF, et al. The impact of compliance with 6-hour and 24-hour sepsis bundles on hospital mortality in patients with severe sepsis: a prospective observational study. *Crit Care*. 2005;9:R764–R770.

27. Levy MM, Dellinger RP, Townsend SR, et al. The Surviving Sepsis Campaign: results of an international guideline-based performance improvement program targeting severe sepsis. *Crit Care Med*. Feb 2010;38(2):367–374.

28. Barochia AV, Cui X, Vitberg D, et al. Bundled care for septic shock: an analysis of clinical trials. *Crit Care Med*. Feb 2010;38(2):668–678.

29. Solomkin JS, Mazuski JE, Bradley JS, et al. Diagnosis and management of complicated intra-abdominal infection in adults and children: guidelines by the Surgical Infection Society and the Infectious Diseases Society of America. *Surg Infect (Larchmt)*. Feb 2010;11(1):79–109.

30. Solomkin JS, Mazuski JE, Bradley JS, et al. Diagnosis and management of complicated intra-abdominal infection in adults and children: guidelines by the Surgical Infection Society and the Infectious Diseases Society of America. *Clin Infect Dis*. Jan 15 2010;50(2):133–164.

31. Kumar A, Ellis P, Arabi Y, et al.; Cooperative Antimicrobial Therapy of Septic Shock Database Research Group. Initiation of inappropriate antimicrobial therapy results in a 5-fold reduction of survival in human septic shock. *Chest*. Nov 2009;136(5):1237–1248.

32. Kumar A, Roberts D, Wood KE, et al. Duration of hypotension before initiation of effective antimicrobial therapy is the critical determinant of survival in human septic shock. *Crit Care Med*. 2006;34:1589–1596.

33. Hollenberg SM, Ahrens TS, Annane D, et al. Practice parameters for hemodynamic support of sepsis in adult patients: 2004 update. *Crit Care Med*. 2004;32:1928–1948.

34. Rivers EP, Jaehne AK, Eichhorn-Wharry L, et al. Fluid therapy in septic shock. *Curr Opin Crit Care*. Aug 2010;16(4):297–308.

35. Rivers E, Nguyen B, Havstad S, Ressler J, Muzzin A, Knoblich B, Peterson E, Tomlanovich M; Early Goal-Directed Therapy Collaborative Group. Early goal-directed therapy in the treatment of severe sepsis and septic shock. *N Engl J Med* Nov 8 2001;345(19):1368–1377.

36. ProCESS study. Available at https://crisma.upmc.com/processtrial/index.asp; http://clinicaltrials.gov/ct2/show/NCT00510835.

37. ARISE-RCT. Available at http://www.anzicrc.monash.org/process.html; http://clinicaltrials.gov/ct2/show/NCT00975793.

38. ProMISe (Protocolized Management in Sepsis). Available at http://www.icnarc.org; https://www.icnarc.org/documents/ProMISe%20Information%20Sheet.pdf.

39. Holmes CL, Walley KR. Arginine vasopressin in the treatment of vasodilatory septic shock. *Best Pract Res Clin Anaesthesiol*. Jun 2008;22(2):175–186.

40. Russell JA. Vasopressin in septic shock. *Crit Care Med*. Sep 2007;35(9 Suppl):S609–S615.

41. Russell JA, Walley KR, Singer J, et al. Vasopressin versus norepinephrine infusion in patients with septic shock. *N Engl J Med*. Feb 28 2008;358(9):877–887.

42. Russell JA, Walley KR, Gordon AC, et al. Interaction of vasopressin infusion, corticosteroid treatment, and mortality of septic shock. *Crit Care Med*. Mar 2009;37(3):811–818.

43. Annane D, Bellissant E, Bollaert PE, et al. Corticosteroids in the treatment of severe sepsis and septic shock in adults: a systematic review. *JAMA*. Jun 10 2009;301(22):2362–2375.

44. Marik PE, Pastores SM, Annane D, et al.; American College of Critical Care Medicine. Recommendations for the diagnosis and management of corticosteroid insufficiency in critically ill adult patients: consensus statements from an international task force by the American College of Critical Care Medicine. *Crit Care Med*. Jun 2008;36(6):1937–1949.

45. Annane D, Sebille V, Charpentier C, et al. Effect of treatment with low doses of hydrocortisone and fludrocortisone on mortality in patients with septic shock. *JAMA*. 2002;288:862–971.

46. Minneci PC, Deans KJ, Banks SM, et al. Meta-analysis: the effect of steroids on survival and shock during sepsis depends on the dose. *Ann Inter Med*. 2004;141:47–56.

47. Sprung C, Annane D, Keh D, et al.; CORTICUS Study Group. Hydrocortisone therapy for patients with septic shock. *N Engl J Med*. Jan 10 2008;358(2):111–124.

48. Sprung CL, Goodman S, Weiss YG. Steroid therapy of septic shock. *Crit Care Clin*. Oct 2009;25(4):825–834.

49. Annane D. Glucocorticoids in the treatment of severe sepsis and septic shock. *Curr Opin Crit Care*. Oct 2005;11(5):449–453.
50. Shorr AF, Bernard GR, Dhainaut JF, et al. Protein C concentrations in severe sepsis: an early directional change in plasma levels predicts outcome. *Crit Care*. Jun 2006;10(3):R92.
51. Bernard GR, Vincent JL, Laterre PF, et al. Efficacy and safety of recombinant human activated protein C for severe sepsis. *N Engl J Med*. 2001;344:699–709.
52. Angus DC, Laterre PF, Helterbrand J, et al.; PROWESS Investigators. The effect of drotrecogin alfa (activated) on long-term survival after severe sepsis. *Crit Care Med*. Nov 2004;32(11):2199–2206.
53. Vincent JL, Angus DC, Artigas A, et al. Effects of drotrecogin alfa (activated) on organ dysfunction in the PROWESS trial. *Crit Care Med*. Mar 2003;31(3):834–840.
54. Dhainaut JF, Laterre PF, Janes JM, et al. Drotrecogin alfa (activated) in the treatment of severe sepsis patients with multiple organ dysfunction: data from the PROWESS trial. *Intensive Care Med*. Jun 2003;29(6):894–903.
55. Abraham E, Laterre PF, Garg R, et al. Drotrecogin alfa (activated) for adults with severe sepsis and a low risk of death. *N Engl J Med* 2005;353(13):1332–1341.
56. Nadel S, Goldstein B, Williams MD, et al. Drotrecogin alfa (activated) in children with severe sepsis: a multicentre phase III randomised controlled trial. *Lancet* 2007;369(9564):836–843.
57. Vincent JL, Bernard GR, Beale R, et al. Drotrecogin alfa (activated) treatment in severe sepsis from the global open-label trial ENHANCE: further evidence for survival and safety and implications for early treatment. *Crit Care Med*. Oct 2005;33(10):2266–2277.
58. Eliezer S, deFigueiredo LF, Colombari F. Prowess-Shock Trial: A protocol overview and perspectives. *Shock*. 2010;34(7):48–53.
59. Philip S. Barie. "All in" for a huge pot: The PROWESS-SHOCK Trial for refractory septic shock. *Surgical Infections*. October 2007;8(5):491–494.
60. http://www.fda.gov/Drugs/DrugSafety/DrugSafetyPodcasts/ucm277212.htm.
61. http://www.ema.europa.eu/ema/index.jsp?curl=pages/news_and_events/news/2011/10/news_detail_001373.jsp&mid=WC0b01ac058004d5c1&murl=menus/news_and_events/news_and_events.jsp.
62. Angus DC. Drotrecogin alfa (activated) . . . a sad final fizzle to a roller-coaster party. *Crit Care*. Feb 6, 2012;16(1):107.
63. Van Den Berghe G, Wouters P, Weekers F, et al. Intensive insulin therapy in critically ill patients. *N Engl J Med*. 2001;345:1359–1367.
64. Van Den Berghe G, Wouters PJ, Bouillon R, Weekers F, Verwaest C, Schetz M, Vlasselaers D, Ferdinande P, Lauwers P. Outcome benefit of intensive insulin therapy in the critically ill: insulin dose versus glycemic control. *Crit Care Med*. 2003;31:359–366.
65. Van Den Berghe G, Wilmer A, Hermans G, et al. Intensive insulin therapy in the medical ICU. *N Engl J Med*. Feb 2006;354(5):449–461.
66. Preiser JC, Devos P, Ruiz-Santana S, et al. A prospective randomized multicenter controlled trial on tight glucose control by intensive insulin therapy in adult intensive care units: the Glucontrol study. *Intensive Care Med*. Oct 2009;35(10):1738–1748.
67. Brunkhorst FM, Engel C, Bloos F, et al.; German Competence Network Sepsis (SepNet). Intensive insulin therapy and pentastarch resuscitation in severe sepsis. *N Engl J Med*. Jan 10 2008;358(2):125–139.
68. NICE-SUGAR Study Investigators; Finfer S, Chittock DR, Su SY, et al. Intensive versus conventional glucose control in critically ill patients. *N Engl J Med*. Mar 26 2009;360(13):1283–1297.
69. Griesdale DE, de Souze RJ, van Dam RM, et al. Intensive insulin therapy and mortality among critically ill patients: a meta-analysis including NICE-SUGAR study data. *EMAJ*. Apr 14 2009;180(8):821–827.

CHAPTER 28

POSTOPERATIVE CARDIAC COMPLICATIONS

Efren C. Manjarrez, Karen F. Mauck, and Steven L. Cohn

INTRODUCTION

Approximately 100 million adults undergo noncardiac surgery annually worldwide. Of these, about 900,000 will experience major cardiac complications after surgery, resulting in prolonged hospitalizations and increased short- and long-term mortality.[1,2] Advances in preoperative risk assessment, surgical and anesthetic techniques, and improved medical therapies have decreased the frequency of cardiovascular complications associated with noncardiac surgery. Despite these advances, cardiovascular complications remain the most common and most treatable consequences of noncardiac surgery.[3] This chapter will review the most common postoperative cardiovascular complications including myocardial ischemia/myocardial infarction (MI), arrhythmias, and congestive heart failure (CHF).

MYOCARDIAL ISCHEMIA/MI

Background

The reported incidence of postoperative myocardial ischemia and infarction after noncardiac surgery varies considerably based on how ischemia and infarction are defined (electrocardiogram [ECG] changes, increase in serum cardiac enzymes, etc.), the surveillance method used to identify ischemia (clinical symptoms, continuous cardiac monitoring, serial cardiac enzyme measurement, intermittent ECGs, etc.), and the patient population measured (high-risk patient, high-risk surgical procedure, etc.). Perioperative MI has been reported to occur in approximately 1% of general surgical procedures, and up to 3.2% of vascular surgical procedures[4]; however, this likely underestimates the true incidence of MI. Indeed, one study of high-risk patients undergoing noncardiac surgery, where myocardial ischemia was determined by biomarkers combined with either postoperative ECG changes or one

Perioperative Medicine: Medical Consultation and Co-Management, First Edition.
Edited by Amir K. Jaffer and Paul J. Grant.
© 2012 Wiley-Blackwell. Published 2012 by John Wiley & Sons, Inc.

of three clinical symptoms consistent with MI (chest pain, dyspnea, or requirement for hemodynamic support), the incidence of MI was 2.8–19% based on different criterion levels of troponin or creatine phosphokinase-MB (CPK-MB) used.[5]

Patients who experience perioperative MI after noncardiac surgery have a hospital mortality rate of 15–25%. Nonfatal perioperative MI is a risk factor for cardiovascular death and nonfatal MI for 6 months following surgery. Furthermore, patients who suffer cardiac arrest after noncardiac surgery have a hospital mortality of 65%, and survivors are at increased risk for cardiac death during the 5 years following surgery.[1,6] Risk stratification, risk reduction strategies, close postoperative surveillance, and early identification and treatment can significantly reduce the morbidity and mortality associated with postoperative myocardial ischemia and MI.

Pathophysiology

The mechanisms underlying perioperative MI and myocardial ischemia are not well understood. Plaque rupture with platelet aggregation is an etiology in nonoperative patients as well as postoperative MI. However, evidence suggests that other hemodynamic mechanisms that occur in the perioperative setting contribute to a mismatch between myocardial oxygen supply and demand, which is unrelated to plaque rupture. This prolonged mismatch can also cause myocardial injury, and it is likely responsible for about half of all postoperative MIs.[7]

Prevention Strategies

There are two major strategies to reduce the incidence of postoperative ischemic cardiac complications: medication management and prophylactic coronary revascularization. The American College of Cardiology/American Heart Association Guidelines for Perioperative Cardiovascular Evaluation and Care for Noncardiac Surgery (ACC/AHA Guidelines)[3] tend to favor medication management over revascularization in all but a small subset of the highest-risk patients because the evidence supporting an invasive approach has failed to show improved cardiac outcomes in the perioperative setting. Aggressive medical therapy avoids the short-term risk associated with coronary artery bypass and the dilemma associated with the management of antiplatelet therapy after percutaneous coronary intervention (PCI) and the timing of surgery. However, controversy remains as studies investigating perioperative beta-blockers have yielded conflicting results, and the data on perioperative alpha-2 adrenergic agonists are inconclusive at present.

Medication Management Beta-blockers have been shown to effectively reduce postoperative cardiovascular death, MI, and cardiac arrest in high-risk patients. However, this benefit can be offset by an increased risk of stroke and total mortality when high-dose, long-acting beta-blockers are started on the day of surgery without appropriate dose titration.[8] Although there is no clear practice standard with respect to the use of beta-blockers in the perioperative period, the ACC/AHA Guidelines[3] suggest the following:

- *Class I.* Beta-blockers should be continued in patients already taking them for stable angina, hypertension, and/or arrhythmias.
- *Class IIa.* Beta-blockers titrated to heart rate and blood pressure are
  - probably recommended for vascular surgery patients with known coronary artery disease (CAD) or ischemia on preoperative testing;
  - reasonable for patients undergoing vascular surgery with more than one of the following clinical risk factors: history of ischemic heart disease, compensated or prior heart failure, cerebrovascular disease, diabetes mellitus, or serum creatinine ≥2 mg/dL;
  - reasonable for patients undergoing intermediate-risk surgery who have CAD or more than one of the above clinical risk factors.
- *Class IIb.* The usefulness of beta-blockers is uncertain for patients undergoing intermediate-risk or vascular surgery who have only a single risk factor in the absence of CAD or for vascular surgery patients with no clinical risk factors.
- *Class III.* Beta-blockers should not be given to patients with absolute contra-indications to them. Routine administration of high-dose beta-blockers in the absence of dose titration is not useful and may be harmful to patients not currently taking beta-blockers who are undergoing noncardiac surgery.

If perioperative beta-blockers are to be employed, they should be initiated well before the planned procedure with careful dose titration to achieve adequate heart rate control while avoiding frank bradycardia or hypotension.

Recently, attention has been focused on the role of HMG-CoA reductase inhibitors (statins) for their potential of reducing adverse perioperative cardiac events. Statins have been shown to have beneficial effects in the nonsurgical setting due to both lipid-lowering effects and pleiotropic effects. It is thought that the anti-inflammatory and plaque-stabilizing effects of statins may prevent perioperative MIs. The data regarding perioperative statins are still emerging, which will help guide practice in the future. Currently, the ACC/AHA Guidelines recommend continuing statins in patients who are currently taking them despite the pharmaceutical manufacturers' recommendations to the contrary. Additionally, for those patients undergoing vascular surgery, initiating a statin drug perioperatively may be reasonable. However, there is less evidence to support the practice of initiating statins in the perioperative period for those patients who have one or more clinical risk factors who are undergoing an intermediate surgical risk procedure.[3]

Alpha-2 adrenergic agonists, when administered perioperatively, have been shown to reduce myocardial ischemia during the intraoperative and postoperative period. Small studies using clonidine have demonstrated reduced perioperative ischemia but not MI, and one study showed improved 30-day and 2-year survival.[9] A recent systematic review provides encouraging evidence that alpha-2 adrenergic agonists may reduce cardiac risk, especially during vascular surgery. However, results were driven by a drug not available in the United States (mivazerol), and the data remain insufficient to make firm conclusions about their efficacy and safety.[10] The Evaluating Perioperative Ischemia Reduction by Clonidine (EPIC) trial is currently under way and hopes to determine if the addition of clonidine to chronic beta-blockers will reduce mortality and cardiac morbidity among intermediate-to-high-risk patients undergoing noncardiac surgery. Additionally, the Perioperative Ischemic Evaluation-2 (POISE-2) trial is also under way and will evaluate the efficacy and safety of clonidine with or without aspirin in noncardiac surgery. The ACC/AHA Guidelines recommend that alpha-2 agonists be considered for patients with known CAD, or have at least one clinical risk factor, who are undergoing noncardiac surgery. This recommendation, however, is specific for perioperative control of hypertension, and not for the purpose of cardiac risk reduction.[3]

Coronary Revascularization Prophylactic coronary revascularization with either coronary artery bypass grafting (CABG) or PCI before noncardiac surgery is only useful in the following subset of patients:

- preoperative acute ST-segment elevation MI,
- non-ST-segment elevation MI,
- high-risk unstable angina,
- stable angina in combination with significant left main CAD,
- three- or two-vessel disease with significant proximal left anterior descending stenosis and either an ejection fraction <50% or ischemia during noninvasive testing.

For patients with stable CAD, however, routine prophylactic coronary revascularization is not recommended prior to noncardiac surgery. The benefits of preoperative coronary revascularization are not well established for patients with reversible ischemia identified on preoperative testing but do not meet the above criteria. In this case, clinicians should consult a cardiologist for an individualized approach.

The ACC/AHA Guidelines make recommendations regarding the timing of noncardiac surgery after preoperative coronary revascularization to decrease the risk of stent thrombosis. They recommend continuing dual antiplatelet therapy after PCI and postponing all nonemergent surgery for at least

- 2 weeks after balloon angioplasty without stent placement,
- 1 month after CABG,
- 4–6 weeks after PCI with bare metal stent placement,
- 1 year after PCI with drug-eluting stent placement.

If surgery is necessary before these time frames and dual antiplatelet therapy cannot be continued, they recommend proceeding with aspirin therapy if possible.[3]

Postoperative Assessment

Perioperative MI most often occurs in the first 48 hours after surgery, with 44% occurring on the evening of surgery, 34% on postoperative day 1, 16% on postoperative day 2, and only 6% on or after postoperative day 3. Ischemia often develops immediately after surgery at a time when sympathetic discharge, increased blood pressure, and tachycardia often occur.[11] Unlike the usual symptoms that occur with myocardial ischemia in the nonoperative setting, most postoperative MIs are silent.[12–14] Indeed, Devereaux et al. reported that only 14% of patients experiencing a perioperative MI will have chest pain and only 53% will have a clinical sign or symptom that may trigger a physician to consider an MI.[1] The usual sequence of events is as follows: an increase in heart rate to 90–100 beats per minute followed by ST-segment depression on ECG, then elevation of cardiac enzymes. Findings associated with postoperative MI include heart failure, arrhythmia, hypotension, and confusion.

Although the data supporting an optimal strategy for surveillance of perioperative MI are limited, the ACC/AHA Guidelines[15] make the following recommendations:

- Surveillance in patients without documented CAD should be restricted to those that develop perioperative signs of cardiovascular dysfunction.
- For patients with documented or suspected CAD, intermediate or high clinical risk, and undergoing intermediate-to-high surgical risk procedures, the following cost-effective management is suggested: obtain a baseline ECG, repeat immediately post-op, then on post-op days 1 and 2. Measurement of cardiac specific troponins should be limited to those patients who develop ECG changes or symptoms suggestive of an acute coronary syndrome.

Although some experts advocate the use of continuous postoperative ECG monitoring with ST-wave trend analysis and measurement of troponins as surveillance measures in asymptomatic patients who are at high risk of postoperative cardiac events (i.e., vascular surgery patients), the utility and cost-effectiveness of this practice is not well established.

Medical Management

There are no randomized controlled trials addressing the medical management of postoperative MI. Postoperative MIs are classified as either non-ST-elevation MI (NSTEMI) or ST-elevation MI (STEMI). The management of perioperative MI is complicated by the increased risk of bleeding in the postoperative patient, especially when thrombolytics, antiplatelet agents, and antithrombotic agents are considered. Potential algorithms to help direct the management of NSTEMI and STEMI in the perioperative period are illustrated in Figures 28.1 and 28.2.[16]

Patients who sustain a perioperative MI should have an evaluation of left ventricular function performed before hospital discharge, and standard postinfarction medical therapy should be prescribed. After an appropriate delay from the time of infarction, the use of pharmacologic stress or exercise testing for risk stratification can help determine which patients might benefit from coronary revascularization. Aggressive management of ongoing angina, heart failure, hypertension, diabetes, and tobacco use is warranted. Additionally, it is important to communicate with the patient's primary care provider at the time of discharge to ensure a safe transition of care for these high-risk patients.

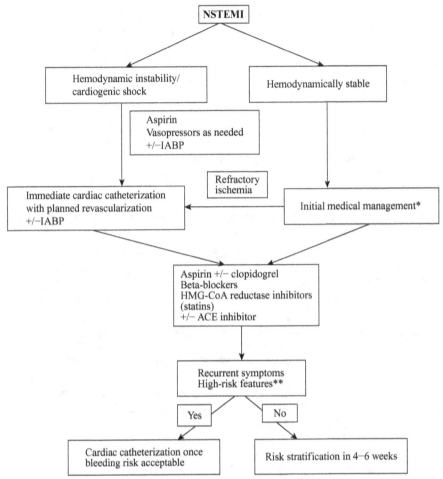

Figure 28.1.   Suggested algorithm for the management of perioperative non-ST-elevation MI (NSTEMI). *Initial medical management includes morphine sulfate, oxygen, nitroglycerin, and aspirin with or without unfractionated heparin if bleeding risk is acceptable. **High-risk features include major arrhythmias (ventricular tachycardia, ventricular fibrillation), dynamic ST-segment depression in multiple leads, an ECG pattern that precludes the assessment of ST-segment changes, evidence of severe CHF, or left ventricular dysfunction. Refractory ischemia is ischemia unresponsive to medical management. IABP, intra-aortic balloon pump; ACE, angiotensin-converting enzyme. From Adesanya et al.,[16] p. 589. Reproduced with permission.

ARRHYTHMIAS

Background

Cardiac arrhythmias are common in the postoperative period and are associated with significant morbidity, mortality, and prolonged hospitalization.[17] There is a considerable body of literature describing perioperative arrhythmias in cardiothoracic surgery

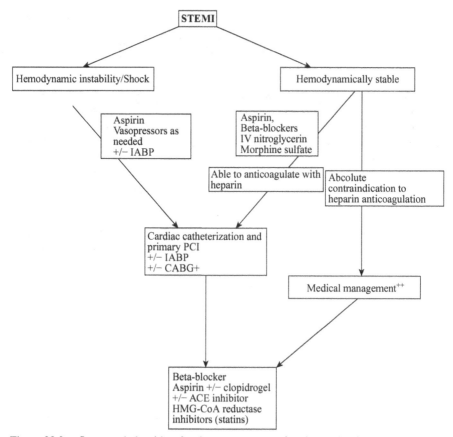

Figure 28.2.   Suggested algorithm for the management of perioperative ST-elevation MI (STEMI). [+]Clopidogrel should not be administered if coronary artery bypass grafting (CABG) is planned within 5 days. [++]Medical management includes morphine sulfate, oxygen, nitroglycerin, and aspirin. IABP, intra-aortic balloon pump; PCI, percutaneous coronary intervention; ACE, angiotensin-converting enzyme. From Adesanya et al.,[16] p. 589. Reproduced with permission.

patients. However, only a few studies exist in the noncardiac surgery population. Supraventricular arrhythmias are significantly more common than ventricular arrhythmias in the postoperative setting, affecting nearly 1 million elderly Americans each year who undergo cardiac or noncardiac surgery. Supraventricular arrhythmias have been reported in 8% of patients undergoing noncardiac surgery (2% intraoperatively and 6% postoperatively), with most occurring within the first 3–5 days after surgery.[17,18] By far, the most common supraventricular arrhythmias in the perioperative setting are atrial fibrillation (AF) and atrial flutter, representing 63% of all perioperative supraventricular arrhythmias in one study.[19] Few studies have reported on ventricular arrhythmias after noncardiac surgery. Forrest et al. reported a 6.3% incidence of perioperative ventricular arrhythmias in 17,201 patients undergoing both cardiac and noncardiac surgeries. However, the incidence of significant ventricular arrhythmias requiring treatment was only 1%.[20]

Pathophysiology

The pathophysiology of cardiac arrhythmias in the postoperative setting is complex, and several factors likely contribute including patient-related factors, metabolic derangements, and medication-related effects. Arrhythmias are more likely to occur in patients with underlying structural heart disease such as patients with a history of ischemic heart disease, MI, valvular heart disease, congenital heart disease, cardiomyopathy, sick sinus or long QT syndrome, or with Wolff–Parkinson–White syndrome.[21] Transient disturbances in the perioperative period may also contribute, such as[21,22]

- surgical stress (increased catecholamines attributed to surgery leads to increased sympathetic tone, volume fluctuations, inflammatory response, and a hypercoagulable state);
- electrolyte and metabolic imbalances;
- hypoxia;
- hypercarbia;
- anxiety/pain;
- cardiac ischemia;
- cardiac rhythm device malfunction;
- drug effects;
- increased vagal activity from laryngoscopy, endotrachial intubation, or surgical stimulation.

Prevention Strategies

Postoperative arrhythmias can be classified into bradyarrhythmias and tachyarrhythmias. Tachyarrhythmias can be further subclassified into ventricular and supraventricular origin. In general, the first line of defense for preventing all types of arrhythmias in the perioperative setting is to prevent and aggressively manage the transient disturbances listed above. Also, it is important that patients taking beta-blockers for hypertension, CAD, or arrhythmias do not have them discontinued in the perioperative setting.

Bradycardias and Heart Block Bradycardias associated with sinus node dysfunction (sinus bradycardia, sinus pause, sinoatrial block, and sinus arrest) often result from increased vagal tone due to spinal or epidural anesthesia, laryngoscopy, surgical stimulation, or the effect of drugs on the sinus node.[22] These disturbances are often transient and only require treatment if the patient is symptomatic or has evidence of compromised perfusion. In patients with known sinus node dysfunction, consideration should be given to inserting a temporary pacemaker prior to the surgical procedure.

Heart block is commonly due to fibrosis of the conducting system. Preexisting conduction system disease is a risk factor for the development of complete heart block in the perioperative setting. Transient complete heart block can also be seen in the setting of myocardial ischemia. The best prevention strategy is to have a high index of suspicion in patients at risk and plan accordingly by arranging telemetry monitoring and having temporary pacing available postoperatively.

Ventricular Arrhythmias Ventricular arrhythmias are uncommon after noncardiac surgery. They are most often seen in the setting of postoperative MI in patients with underlying structural heart disease,[23] in patients with ECG evidence of myocardial ischemia, history of CHF, and cigarette smoking. Additionally, patients with preoperative arrhythmias are more likely to have intraoperative or postoperative ventricular arrhythmias.[24] Fortunately, most ventricular arrhythmias seen in the postoperative setting (i.e., nonsustained ventricular tachycardia [VT] or multiple ventricular ectopic beats) are not associated with significant symptoms and occur in patients with structurally normal hearts, and therefore, treatment is likely not necessary. However, for those patients with underlying structural heart disease, asymptomatic ventricular arrhythmias can be predictive of more malignant arrhythmias and steps should be taken to reverse precipitating factors (i.e., ischemia and electrolyte abnormalities) and prevention strategies with beta-blockade can be considered. The data on the effectiveness of beta-blockade for the prevention of ventricular arrhythmias after noncardiac surgery are sparse, but beta-blockers could be considered on an individual patient basis if no contraindications exist. It should be noted, however, that it is not standard practice to initiate beta-blockers prior to noncardiac surgery for the sole purpose of preventing perioperative ventricular arrhythmias. Statins have also been studied for their potential anti-arrhythmic effects. Most of these data, however, is observational and not in the perioperative setting.[25]

Torsades de pointes is a specific type of ventricular arrhythmia associated with QT interval prolongation. Most often this is due to an acquired prolongation of the QT interval by drugs and electrolyte disturbances, especially hypomagnesemia and hypokalemia. Administration of QT-prolonging drugs to hospitalized patients may be more likely to cause Torsades de pointes compared with administering the same drug in the outpatient setting. This is likely due to other risk factors (or transient imbalances mentioned earlier) that occur in hospitalized patients, which increases their proarrhythmic response.[26] There are many drugs that have been associated with Torsades—an updated list can be found on http://www.qtdrugs.org. The best preventive measure is to avoid using drugs that prolong the QT interval and to monitor the QT interval closely when at-risk drugs are necessary.

Supraventricular Arrhythmias Supraventricular arrhythmias can be divided into atrial tachycardias, atrioventricular nodal reentrant tachycardias, accessory pathway reentrant tachycardias, AF, and atrial flutter. Of these, AF/atrial flutter and ectopic supraventricular tachyarrhythmias (SVTs) are the most common in the perioperative setting. The ratio of SVT to AF is 2:1 intraoperatively, whereas postoperatively, the ratio is 1:2.[27]

The most consistent risk factor for perioperative atrial arrhythmias is age greater than 60 years. Advanced age is associated with degenerative and inflammatory modifications in atrial anatomy (i.e., dilatation, fibrosis), which causes alterations in atrial electrophysiological properties (shortness of effective refractory period, dispersion of refractoriness and conduction, abnormal automaticity, and anisotropic conduction) that act as potential substrates for postoperative atrial arrhythmias.[28] Other risk factors for postoperative atrial arrhythmias are male gender, CHF, history of supraventricular arrhythmias, significant valvular disease, premature atrial complexes on preoperative ECG, American Society of Anesthesiologists (ASA) Class III or IV, history of asthma, and type of surgical procedure.[17] There is a greater incidence of postoperative atrial arrhythmias in patients who undergo thoracic (20%) or cardiac surgery (30% for CABG and up to 65% for valvular surgery) compared with other major surgeries. This suggests that the amount of surgical trauma to the atria and autonomic innervation system plays a significant role.[27] As potential preventive strategies, beta-blockers, amiodarone, sotalol, digoxin, procainamide, propafenone, calcium channel blockers, corticosteroids, intravenous magnesium, statins, and atrial pacing have been studied in cardiac surgery patients. Unfortunately, there have been few studies in the noncardiac surgery patient population. Although it makes intuitive sense that the medications used to prevent AF in cardiac surgery patients may potentially be efficacious in noncardiac surgery patients, bear in mind that the risk-to-benefit ratio is likely higher in the noncardiac surgery patient because the incidence of postoperative AF is lower. After a limited review of the literature, Sedrakyan et al. concluded that calcium channel blockers and beta-blockers are effective in reducing postoperative atrial arrhythmias after noncardiac surgery. However, they recommended that the use of these agents be individualized because of associated increased adverse events.[29] Two observational studies have reported that statins were highly protective against perioperative atrial arrhythmias in patients undergoing vascular and thoracic surgical procedures[30,31]; however, there are no data from randomized trials at this time to support the use of statins for the purpose of preventing postoperative AF after noncardiac surgery.

Postoperative Assessment

The presence of an arrhythmia perioperatively should prompt the clinician to search for potential etiologies such as myocardial ischemia/MI, pulmonary disease, drug toxicity, infection, hypoxia, hypotension, or other metabolic derangements.[32] Second, the clinician needs to determine the urgency of treatment. The ACC does not define a specific duration of postoperative monitoring for arrhythmia in its guidelines. Clinicians are left to apply recommendations for ischemia surveillance with ST-segment monitoring. There is good evidence (Class IIa) from the ACC Guidelines to support intraoperative and postoperative ST-segment monitoring for patients with known CAD undergoing vascular surgery in order to diagnose perioperative myocardial ischemia. Equivocal evidence exists on using ST-segment monitoring perioperatively for patients with single or multiple risk factors for CAD undergoing noncardiac surgery.[32]

About 85% of the supraventricular arrhythmias revert to sinus rhythm during hospitalization with treatment. This means that up to 15% leave the hospital with AF and an increased risk of stroke.[19,27,33,34]

Medical Management

Initial diagnosis is key, since the treatment approach depends on the etiology and mechanism. If the arrhythmia is symptomatic, causes loss of consciousness, or leads to hemodynamic instability, acute management is indicated perioperatively.

Bradycardias   Bradycardias may arise from sinus node dysfunction or heart block. Sinus node dysfunction may manifest as sinus bradycardia, sinus pause, sinoatrial block, or sinus arrest. Perioperatively, these may be due to increased vagal tone from spinal or epidural anesthesia, laryngoscopy, or surgical intervention. Acute management can be summarized as follows[22]:

- If the bradycardia is transient and without hemodynamic compromise, then no treatment is indicated.
- If the bradycardia is sustained or results in hemodynamic compromise, then acute treatment with atropine or ephedrine is indicated. Rarely, transcutaneous pacing is indicated.
- With transient heart block, clinicians should have a high index of suspicion for perioperative MI as the etiology.
- High-grade second-degree or third-degree atrioventricular (AV) block require insertion of a pacemaker. If these high-grade heart blocks persist beyond 7 days postoperatively, then a permanent pacemaker is indicated.

Tachycardias   Sustained (>30 s) ventricular arrhythmias that cause symptoms and require immediate treatment are rare in the perioperative setting. VT (particularly nonsustained VT) after noncardiac surgery is not associated with adverse long-term outcomes in patients without known ischemia, MI, or cardiomyopathy. Therefore, expectant treatment is all that is required.[23] Acute management can be summarized as follows[22]:

- Sustained unstable VT should be treated with rapid defibrillation and epinephrine or vasopressin according to Advanced Cardiac Life Support guidelines.
- Stable monomorphic VT should be treated with amiodarone acutely, then call a cardiologist for further management.
- Polymorphic VT, clinicians should have a high index of suspicion for acute MI, defibrillate and start amiodarone as above for monomorphic VT.
- Torsades de pointes, begin empiric treatment immediately with magnesium. After administering magnesium, review the patient's medication profile to look for agents known to cause QT prolongation.
- After stabilizing the VT, evaluate the patient for perioperative MI, hypoxia, and electrolyte disturbance.

In supraventricular arrhythmias, the arrhythmia crosses the AV node. As such, agents that affect AV nodal conduction are good treatment options[22,35]:

- SVT responds well to adenosine, but beta-blockers or calcium blockers may work as well.

Regarding postoperative AF, the ACC has published guidelines that address prevention and treatment.[36] They are summarized as follows:

Class I

- Unless contraindicated, treatment with an oral beta-blocker to prevent postoperative AF in cardiac surgery patients is recommended.
- Treatment with AV nodal blocking agents is recommended to achieve rate control for patients with postoperative AF.

Class IIa

- Preoperative amiodarone probably reduces postoperative AF in cardiac surgery patients.
- Ibutilide or direct-current cardioversion is reasonable to restore sinus rhythm.
- Anti-arrhythmic medications are a reasonable option for recurrent or refractory postoperative AF.
- Antithrombotic agents may be administered postoperatively as one would do so in nonsurgical patients.

Class III

- Prophylactic sotalol may be considered for patients at risk of developing AF after cardiac surgery.

Since the potential for thromboembolism develops in the first 24–48 hours after arrhythmia onset, clinicians should attempt to restore sinus rhythm as early as possible. The American College of Chest Physicians has published guidelines regarding anticoagulation in postoperative AF after cardiac surgery[37]:

- If AF lasts longer than 48 hours, then anticoagulation with a vitamin K antagonist such as warfarin to reach a target international normalized ratio (INR) of 2.5 (range 2–3).
- Anticoagulation should be continued for up to 4 weeks after restoration and maintenance of sinus rhythm.

CHF

Background

CHF is not only a risk factor for perioperative morbidity and mortality but is also an important postoperative cardiac complication, occurring in approximately 6% of noncardiac surgery cases.[2,38] Most studies focus on ischemia as the most important perioperative cardiac outcome; however, Medicare beneficiaries with heart failure were found to have an increased 30-day postoperative mortality and hospital readmission rate compared with CAD and control patients.[39] The odds ratio of short-term postoperative death and hospital readmission after major noncardiac surgery in heart failure patients was significantly more than patients with coronary disease.[40]

Pathophysiology

There are many potential causes of CHF in the perioperative setting including myocardial ischemia and MI, hypertension, valvular or pericardial disease, and cardiomyopathy. The most common cause of postoperative CHF, however, is due to a primary myocardial abnormality—either left ventricular systolic dysfunction or left ventricular diastolic dysfunction. Recent evidence suggests increased 30-day mortality among vascular surgery patients with asymptomatic diastolic dysfunction. Diastolic dysfunction results in left ventricular hypertrophy or dilatation. During surgery, increased catecholamines result in vasoconstriction and hemodynamic stress. The addition of intravenous fluids may also contribute to a diastolic dysfunction heart failure exacerbation. Diastolic dysfunction at baseline results in decreased coronary perfusion, so the addition of surgical stresses may lead to an increased risk of perioperative myocardial damage.[41]

Postoperative heart failure often manifests or worsens during two periods in the postoperative setting: (1) immediately after surgery, due to the length of surgery, myocardial ischemia, or iatrogenic fluid overload; and (2) on postoperative days 2–3 when third-spaced fluids begin to be reabsorbed intravascularly.

Prevention Strategies

Medical optimization of CHF patients preoperatively according to the ACC Guidelines is crucial. Although CHF has shown to be an independent clinical predictor of perioperative cardiovascular events,[42] the data are not undisputed. A retrospective review of patients with stable CHF undergoing noncardiac surgery demonstrated no increase in perioperative mortality,[43] suggesting that optimizing these patients preoperatively improves outcomes.[42]

The ACC recommends the following Class I measures for medication management to optimize the patient with structural heart disease with prior or current signs or symptoms of heart failure[44]:

- Diuretics and salt restriction are indicated for patients with current or prior symptoms of heart failure and reduced left ventricular ejection fraction (LVEF).
- Angiotensin-converting enzyme (ACE) inhibitors are recommended for all patients with current or prior symptoms of heart failure and reduced LVEF unless otherwise contraindicated.
- Use of beta-blockers proven to reduce mortality (bisoprolol, carvedilol, or sustained release metoprolol).

- Angiotensin II receptor blockers (ARBs) are recommended in patients with current or prior symptoms of heart failure and reduced LVEF who are ACE inhibitor intolerant.
- Addition of an aldosterone antagonist for selected patients with moderately severe-to-severe symptoms of heart failure that can be monitored for preserved renal function and normal potassium concentration.
- The combination of hydralazine and nitrates is recommended to improve outcomes for African–American patients, with moderate-to-severe symptoms on optimal therapy with ACE inhibitors, beta-blockers, and diuretics.

There is a paucity of data and hence a lack of best practices to direct management of heart failure perioperatively. Thus, the following is a list of concerns clinicians will face when prescribing medications perioperatively for the patient with heart failure:

- *Diuretics.* Clinicians should be cautious to avoid overdiuresis as this may exacerbate intraoperative hypotension, a precipitant to poor cardiac outcomes. Our recommendation is to consider withholding these agents on the day of surgery and consider restarting these agents postoperatively when the patient is tolerating oral intake.[45]
- *ACE Inhibitors.* Patients treated with ACE inhibitors are prone to hypotension with induction and maintenance of general anesthesia. However, despite multiple case reports, no firm guidelines exist regarding the management of these agents. We suggest withholding these agents on the day of surgery, particularly if blood pressure is running low preoperatively.
- *Beta-Blockers.* When titrated over time to a stable dose, beta-blockers have shown to be beneficial for perioperative cardiac risk reduction. Furthermore, if beta-blockers are used to treat concurrent hypertension, coronary disease, or arrhythmias, the ACC recommends continuing these agents as sudden withdrawal can be harmful. It is our strong recommendation to continue stable doses of beta-blockers perioperatively.
- *ARBs.* These agents have a longer duration of action than ACE inhibitors and are associated with more resistant hypotension during anesthetic induction. We recommend discontinuing ARBs at least 24 h prior to surgery to avoid intraoperative hypotension.[46]

Postoperative Assessment

Right heart catheterization is not recommended perioperatively as it results in as much harm as benefit.[45,47] B-type natriuretic peptide (BNP) measurement may be of value for perioperative risk stratification and predicting cardiac outcomes. However, until further data from large prospective trials are available, it is not the current standard of care to measure BNP or the N-terminal (NT)-proBNP for perioperative risk stratification purposes. Patients with heart failure due to diastolic dysfunction merit special attention because of their susceptibility to be intolerant of fluid shifts.

In a recent retrospective study, these patients were found to have a higher hospital length of stay and 30-day readmission rate after elective noncardiac surgery.[43]

Medical Management

In general, the perioperative management of CHF should be directed toward the presumed cause (i.e., volume overload, significant valvular dysfunction, diastolic dysfunction, and ischemia).[45] However, clinicians are best advised to follow the 2009 ACC/AHA Guidelines on the diagnosis and management of heart failure by using beta-blockers, ACE inhibitors/ARBs, and combinations of hydralazine with nitrates for patients who meet the criteria for each agent.[44] Diuretics (loop and aldosterone antagonists) should be held the morning of surgery and restarted postoperatively when the patient resumes oral intake.[44]

Perioperative use of statins has been associated with decreased perioperative cardiac complications, including exacerbations of CHF.[30] Use of a continuous insulin infusion for tight perioperative glucose control showed a nonstatistically significant reduction in perioperative CHF.[48] Levosimendan, a calcium sensitizing agent and inotrope, has been shown in some studies to enhance cardiac performance perioperatively[49]; however, long-term data are still lacking, and this agent is currently not available in the United States.

The 2007 ACC/AHA Guidelines comment on the unique difficulties posed by hypertrophic cardiomyopathy. Decreased blood volume, decreased systemic vascular resistance, and increased venous capacitance may result in decreased left ventricular volume and therefore increased outflow tract obstruction. Decreased filling pressures may decrease stroke volume due to decreased compliance of the hypertrophied ventricle. While beta-blockers are helpful for the treatment of hypertrophic cardiomyopathy, beta-adrenergic agonists should be avoided because they decrease diastolic filling and may increase obstructive physiology.[32]

A recent retrospective study concluded that ambulatory patients with clinically stable heart failure who were managed at an academic medical center did not have increased perioperative mortality rates after elective major noncardiac surgery compared with control subjects. However, they were more likely than patients without heart failure to have a longer hospital length of stay and higher rates of hospital readmission. Preoperatively, most of these patients were on beta-blockers, statins, aspirin, and ACE inhibitors, further emphasizing the importance of medically optimizing the heart failure patient preoperatively.[43]

CONCLUSION

Cardiovascular complications after noncardiac surgery are common and are associated with an increased risk of perioperative morbidity and mortality. Herein, we have outlined a management approach to the most common cardiovascular complications including myocardial ischemia/MI, arrhythmias, and CHF, based on the best available evidence, guidelines, and expert opinion.

REFERENCES

1. Devereaux PJ, Goldman L, Cook DJ, Gilbert K, Leslie K, Guyatt GH. Perioperative cardiac events in patients undergoing noncardiac surgery: a review of the magnitude of the problem, the pathophysiology of the events and methods to estimate and communicate risk. *CMAJ*. Sep 13 2005;173(6): 627–634.
2. Mangano DT, Browner WS, Hollenberg M, Li J, Tateo IM. Long-term cardiac prognosis following noncardiac surgery. The Study of Perioperative Ischemia Research Group. *JAMA*. Jul 8 1992;268(2): 233–239.
3. Fleisher LA, Beckman JA, Brown KA, et al. 2009 ACCF/AHA focused update on perioperative beta blockade incorporated into the ACC/AHA 2007 guidelines on perioperative cardiovascular evaluation and care for noncardiac surgery. *J Am Coll Cardiol*. Nov 24 2009;54(22):e13–e118.
4. Mangano DT, Goldman L. Preoperative assessment of patients with known or suspected coronary disease. *N Engl J Med*. Dec 28 1995;333(26):1750–1756.
5. Martinez EA, Nass CM, Jermyn RM, et al. Intermittent cardiac troponin-I screening is an effective means of surveillance for a perioperative myocardial infarction. *J Cardiothorac Vasc Anesth*. 2005;19:577–582.
6. Badner NH, Knill RL, Brown JE, Novick TV, Gelb AW. Myocardial infarction after noncardiac surgery. *Anesthesiology*. Mar 1998;88(3):572–578.
7. Landesberg G. The pathophysiology of perioperative myocardial infarction: facts and perspectives. *J Cardiothorac Vasc Anesth*. Feb 2003;17(1):90–100.
8. Devereaux PJ, Yang H, Yusuf S, et al. Effects of extended-release metoprolol succinate in patients undergoing non-cardiac surgery (POISE trial): a randomised controlled trial. *Lancet*. May 31 2008;371(9627):1839–1847.
9. Wallace AW, Galindez D, Salahieh A, et al. Effect of clonidine on cardiovascular morbidity and mortality after noncardiac surgery. *Anesthesiology*. Aug 2004;101(2):284–293.
10. Wijeysundera DN, Bender JS, Beattie WS. Alpha-2 adrenergic agonists for the prevention of cardiac complications among patients undergoing surgery. *Cochrane Database Syst Rev (Online)*. 2009;(4): CD004126.
11. Landesberg G, Luria MH, Cotev S, et al. Importance of long-duration postoperative ST-segment depression in cardiac morbidity after vascular surgery. *Lancet*. Mar 20 1993;341(8847):715–719.
12. Landesberg G, Mosseri M, Zahger D, et al. Myocardial infarction after vascular surgery: the role of prolonged stress-induced, ST depression-type ischemia. *J Am Coll Cardiol*. Jun 1 2001;37(7): 1839–1845.
13. McCann RL, Clements FM. Silent myocardial ischemia in patients undergoing peripheral vascular surgery: incidence and association with perioperative cardiac morbidity and mortality. *J Vasc Surg*. Apr 1989;9(4):583–587.
14. Ouyang P, Gerstenblith G, Furman WR, Golueke PJ, Gottlieb SO. Frequency and significance of early postoperative silent myocardial ischemia in patients having peripheral vascular surgery. *Am J Cardiol*. Nov 15 1989;64(18):1113–1116.
15. Fleischmann KE, Beckman JA, Buller CE, et al. 2009 ACCF/AHA focused update on perioperative beta blockade. *J Am Coll Cardiol*. Nov 24 2009;54(22):2102–2128.
16. Adesanya AO, de Lemos JA, Greilich NB, Whitten CW. Management of perioperative myocardial infarction in noncardiac surgical patients. *Chest*. Aug 2006;130(2):584–596.
17. Polanczyk CA, Goldman L, Marcantonio ER, Orav EJ, Lee TH. Supraventricular arrhythmia in patients having noncardiac surgery: clinical correlates and effect on length of stay. *Ann Intern Med*. Aug 15 1998;129(4):279–285.
18. Walsh SR, Oates JE, Anderson JA, Blair SD, Makin CA, Walsh CJ. Postoperative arrhythmias in colorectal surgical patients: incidence and clinical correlates. *Colorectal Dis*. Mar 2006;8(3): 212–216.
19. Goldman L. Supraventricular tachyarrhythmias in hospitalized adults after surgery. Clinical correlates in patients over 40 years of age after major noncardiac surgery. *Chest*. Apr 1978;73(4):450–454.
20. Forrest JB, Rehder K, Cahalan MK, Goldsmith CH. Multicenter study of general anesthesia. III. Predictors of severe perioperative adverse outcomes. *Anesthesiology*. Jan 1992;76(1):3–15.

21. Atlee JL. Perioperative cardiac dysrhythmias: diagnosis and management. *Anesthesiology.* Jun 1997;86(6):1397–1424.
22. Heintz KM, Hollenberg SM. Perioperative cardiac issues: postoperative arrhythmias. *Surg Clin North Am.* Dec 2005;85(6):1103–1114, viii.
23. Mahla E, Rotman B, Rehak P, et al. Perioperative ventricular dysrhythmias in patients with structural heart disease undergoing noncardiac surgery. *Anesth Analg.* Jan 1998;86(1):16–21.
24. O'Kelly B, Browner WS, Massie B, Tubau J, Ngo L, Mangano DT. Ventricular arrhythmias in patients undergoing noncardiac surgery. The Study of Perioperative Ischemia Research Group. *JAMA.* Jul 8 1992;268(2):217–221.
25. Abuissa H, O'Keefe JH, Bybee KA. Statins as anti-arrhythmics: a systematic review part II: effects on risk of ventricular arrhythmias. *Clin Cardiol.* Oct 2009;32(10):549–552.
26. Drew BJ, Ackerman MJ, Funk M, et al. Prevention of Torsade de pointes in hospital settings: a scientific statement from the American Heart Association and the American College of Cardiology Foundation. *Circulation.* Mar 2, 2010;121(8):1047–1060.
27. Amar D. Perioperative atrial tachyarrhythmias. *Anesthesiology.* Dec 2002;97(6):1618–1623.
28. Hadi HA, Mahmeed WA, Suwaidi JA, Ellahham S. Pleiotropic effects of statins in atrial fibrillation patients: the evidence. *Vasc Health Risk Manag.* 2009;5(3):533–551.
29. Sedrakyan A, Treasure T, Browne J, Krumholz H, Sharpin C, van der Meulen J. Pharmacologic prophylaxis for postoperative atrial tachyarrhythmia in general thoracic surgery: evidence from randomized clinical trials. *J Thorac Cardiovasc Surg.* May 2005;129(5):997–1005.
30. O'Neil-Callahan K, Katsimaglis G, Tepper MR, et al. Statins decrease perioperative cardiac complications in patients undergoing noncardiac vascular surgery: the Statins for Risk Reduction in Surgery (StaRRS) study. *J Am Coll Cardiol.* Feb 1 2005;45(3):336–342.
31. Amar D, Zhang H, Heerdt PM, Park B, Fleisher M, Thaler HT. Statin use is associated with a reduction in atrial fibrillation after noncardiac thoracic surgery independent of C-reactive protein. *Chest.* Nov 2005;128(5):3421–3427.
32. Fleisher LA, Beckman JA, Brown KA, et al. ACC/AHA 2007 guidelines on perioperative cardiovascular evaluation and care for noncardiac surgery: a report of the American College of Cardiology/American Heart Association Task Force on Practice Guidelines (Writing Committee to Revise the 2002 Guidelines on Perioperative Cardiovascular Evaluation for Noncardiac Surgery). *J Am Coll Cardiol.* Oct 23 2007;50(17):e159–e241.
33. Lee JK, Klein GJ, Krahn AD, et al. Rate-control versus conversion strategy in postoperative atrial fibrillation: a prospective, randomized pilot study. *Am Heart J.* Dec 2000;140(6):871–877.
34. Amar D. Postoperative atrial fibrillation. *Heart Dis.* Mar–Apr 2002;4(2):117–123.
35. Amar D. Prevention and management of perioperative arrhythmias in the thoracic surgical population. *Anesthesiol Clin.* Jun 2008;26(2):325–335, vii.
36. Fuster V, Ryden LE, Cannom DS, et al. ACC/AHA/ESC 2006 guidelines for the management of patients with atrial fibrillation: a report of the American College of Cardiology/American Heart Association Task Force on practice guidelines and the European Society of Cardiology Committee for Practice Guidelines (Writing Committee to Revise the 2001 Guidelines for the Management of Patients with Atrial Fibrillation). *Circulation.* Aug 15 2006;114(7):e257–e354.
37. Singer DE, Albers GW, Dalen JE, et al. Antithrombotic therapy in atrial fibrillation: American College of Chest Physicians Evidence-Based Clinical Practice Guidelines (8th Edition). *Chest.* Jun 2008;133(6 Suppl):546S–592S.
38. Charlson M, Peterson J, Szatrowski TP, MacKenzie R, Gold J. Long-term prognosis after perioperative cardiac complications. *J Clin Epidemiol.* Dec 1994;47(12):1389–1400.
39. Hernandez AF, Whellan DJ, Stroud S, Sun JL, O'Connor CM, Jollis JG. Outcomes in heart failure patients after major noncardiac surgery. *J Am Coll Cardiol.* Oct 6 2004;44(7):1446–1453.
40. Hammill BG, Curtis LH, Bennett-Guerrero E, et al. Impact of heart failure on patients undergoing major noncardiac surgery. *Anesthesiology.* Apr 2008;108(4):559–567.
41. Flu WJ, van Kuijk JP, Hoeks SE, et al. Prognostic implications of asymptomatic left ventricular dysfunction in patients undergoing vascular surgery. *Anesthesiology.* Jun 2010;112(6):1316–1324.
42. Lee TH, Marcantonio ER, Mangione CM, et al. Derivation and prospective validation of a simple index for prediction of cardiac risk of major noncardiac surgery. *Circulation.* Sep 7 1999;100(10):1043–1049.

43. Xu-Cai YO, Brotman DJ, Phillips CO, et al. Outcomes of patients with stable heart failure undergoing elective noncardiac surgery. *Mayo Clin Proc.* Mar 2008;83(3):280–288.

44. Hunt SA, Abraham WT, Chin MH, et al. 2009 focused update incorporated into the ACC/AHA 2005 guidelines for the diagnosis and management of heart failure in adults a report of the American College of Cardiology Foundation/American Heart Association Task Force on Practice Guidelines developed in collaboration with the International Society for Heart and Lung Transplantation. *J Am Coll Cardiol.* Apr 14 2009;53(15):e1–e90.

45. Auerbach A, Goldman L. Assessing and reducing the cardiac risk of noncardiac surgery. *Circulation.* Mar 14 2006;113(10):1361–1376.

46. Groban L, Butterworth J. Perioperative management of chronic heart failure. *Anesth Analg.* Sep 2006;103(3):557–575.

47. Polanczyk CA, Rohde LE, Goldman L, et al. Right heart catheterization and cardiac complications in patients undergoing noncardiac surgery: an observational study. *JAMA.* Jul 18 2001;286(3): 309–314.

48. Subramaniam B, Panzica PJ, Novack V, et al. Continuous perioperative insulin infusion decreases major cardiovascular events in patients undergoing vascular surgery: a prospective, randomized trial. *Anesthesiology.* May 2009;110(5):970–977.

49. Katsaragakis S, Kapralou A, Markogiannakis H, et al. Preoperative levosimendan in heart failure patients undergoing noncardiac surgery. *Neth J Med.* Apr 2008;66(4):154–159.

CHAPTER 29

POSTOPERATIVE NAUSEA AND VOMITING

Tina P. Le and Tong J. Gan

BACKGROUND

Postoperative nausea and vomiting (PONV) is one of the most common complaints following surgery, and without antiemetic prophylaxis, it occurs in over 30% of surgeries under general anesthesia, and can be as high as 70–80% in certain high-risk populations.[1] While generally nonfatal and self-limited, PONV may lead to rare but serious medical consequences, including dehydration and electrolyte imbalance, venous hypertension, bleeding, hematoma formation, suture dehiscence, esophageal rupture, and aspiration. Furthermore, PONV has a profound impact on patient satisfaction, quality of life, and estimated healthcare costs as a result of delayed discharge, prolonged nursing care, and unanticipated hospital admissions.

Nausea and vomiting due to surgery may also occur beyond the immediate postoperative period. Even patients who experience no PONV immediately after surgery may later develop postdischarge nausea and vomiting (PDNV). Surveys of patients following ambulatory surgery have found the rate of PDNV to range between approximately 20% and 50%, resulting in increased difficulty in performing activities of daily living and longer recovery times before resuming normal activity.[2]

PATHOPHYSIOLOGY

The central coordinating site for nausea and vomiting is located in an ill-defined area of the lateral reticular formation in the brain stem (Figure 29.1).[3] This "vomiting center," as it is traditionally called, is not so much a discrete center of emetic activity as it is a "central pattern generator" (CPG) that sets off a specific sequence of neuronal activities throughout the medulla to result in vomiting.[4] Multiple inputs may arrive from areas such as the higher cortical centers, cerebellum, vestibular apparatus, vagal, and glossopharyngeal nerve afferents to trigger the complex motor response of emesis; direct electrical stimulation of the CPG also causes emesis.[5]

Perioperative Medicine: Medical Consultation and Co-Management, First Edition.
Edited by Amir K. Jaffer and Paul J. Grant.
© 2012 Wiley-Blackwell. Published 2012 by John Wiley & Sons, Inc.

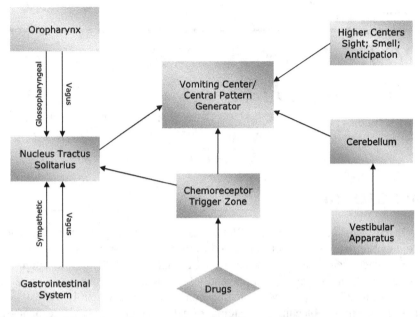

Figure 29.1. Mechanism of nausea and vomiting. See color insert.

A particularly important afferent is the chemoreceptor trigger zone (CTZ), which is located at the base of the fourth ventricle in the area postrema, outside the blood–brain barrier, and plays a role in detecting emetogenic agents in the blood and cerebrospinal fluid (CSF).[6] Although direct electrical stimulation of the CTZ does not cause vomiting, the CTZ communicates with the adjacent nucleus tractus solitarius (NTS), which in turn projects into the CPG.[7] Signals between these anatomical areas are mediated through a variety of neurotransmitter receptor systems via one or more associated receptors, such as serotonin 5-HT_3, dopamine D_2, histamine H_1, muscarinic cholinergic, and neurokinin NK_1.[8]

RISK FACTORS FOR PONV AND PDNV

A variety of surgical, anesthetic, and patient factors have been investigated as predictors of patient risk for PONV, the most significant of which are listed in Table 29.1. A simplified scoring system by Apfel and colleagues identifies four highly predictive risk factors for PONV: female gender, history of motion sickness or PONV, nonsmoker, and use of perioperative opioids.[9] Similarly, the postoperative vomiting in children (POVOC) score identifies four independent pediatric risk factors: duration of surgery ≥ 30 min, age ≥ 3 years, strabismus surgery, and a positive history of postoperative vomiting (POV) in the child or POV/PONV in close relatives (mother, father, or siblings).[10] Other adult and pediatric studies have identified duration of anesthesia longer than 30 min, general anesthesia with volatile anesthetics, use of

TABLE 29.1.   Risk Factors for Postoperative Nausea and Vomiting (PONV) and
Postdischarge Nausea and Vomiting (PDNV)

Patient factors	Anesthetic factors	Surgical factors
Female	Use of perioperative opioids	Duration of surgery
Nonsmoker	Use of volatile anesthetics	Type of surgery, including:
History of motion sickness or previous PONV	Nitrous oxide	Abdominal
		Ear, nose, and throat
Family history of motion sickness or PONV (pediatric)		Gynecological
		Laparoscopic
		Ophthalmologic
Age ≥ 3 (pediatric)		Orthopedic
		Plastic
		Strabismus (pediatric)

nitrous oxide, administration of intraoperative and postoperative opioids, and type of surgery as independent predictors of PONV.[11] The few studies attempting to identify specific PDNV risk factors have found them to be similar to those typically associated with PONV.[12]

PREVENTION STRATEGIES

After determining the patient's overall risk for PONV, the anesthesia technique should be tailored to minimize the patient's baseline risk. Figure 29.2 shows a variety of anesthetic approaches appropriate for patients at various levels of PONV risk.

PROPHYLACTIC ANTIEMETIC MEDICATIONS

In comparing various antiemetics and the evidence for or against them, it is helpful to determine the number needed to treat (NNT), or the number of patients that must be exposed to a particular intervention in order for one patient to benefit over receiving placebo or no treatment. Similarly, the number needed to harm (NNH) is an estimate of the frequency of drug-related adverse effects. A list of common antiemetics, typical dosages, and NNT is listed in Table 29.2.

Serotonin Antagonists

Originally used to prevent chemotherapy-induced nausea and vomiting, serotonin antagonists have become one of the cornerstones of PONV prophylaxis and therapy. Serotonin is found in high levels in the enterochromaffin cells of the gastrointestinal (GI) tract, as well as in the central nervous system (CNS), and may be released to stimulate either the vagal afferent neurons or the CTZ to activate the vomiting

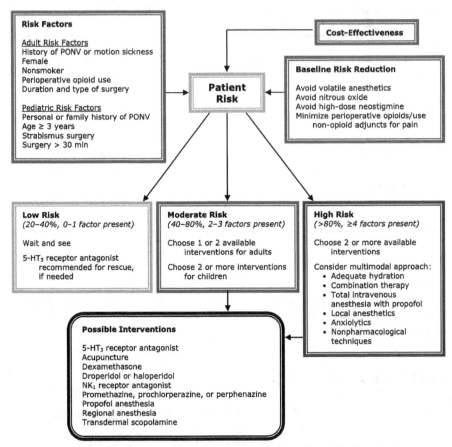

Figure 29.2.   Antiemetic management strategies based on patient risk. See color insert.

center.[13] The 5-HT$_3$ subtype of serotonin receptor appears largely in the NTS, area postrema, and the dorsal motor nucleus of the vagus nerve, all of which play significant roles in coordinating the vomiting reflex.[14] The 5-HT$_3$ receptor antagonists (5-HT$_3$ RAs), which include ondansetron, granisetron, dolasetron, ramosetron, tropisetron, and most recently, palonosetron, act by inhibiting the action of serotonin in 5-HT$_3$ receptor-rich areas of the brain.

Ondansetron (Zofran), granisetron (Kytril), dolasetron (Anzemet), and palonosetron (Aloxi) are all approved for use in PONV by the U.S. Food and Drug Administration (FDA) (ramosetron and tropisetron are not available in the United States). Side effects are usually short-term and of mild-to-moderate intensity, with the most common being headache, dizziness, constipation, and diarrhea.[15] Most available data suggest that 5-HT$_3$ RAs are most effective when administered at the end of surgery, but at least one study has suggested that dolasetron may be administered around the time of induction of anesthesia, with little effect on efficacy.[16]

Despite minor differences in optimal dosing and duration of action, all of the 5-HT$_3$ RAs are comparably effective for treating PONV.[15] Ondansetron is the pro-

TABLE 29.2. Number Needed to Treat (NNT) for Common Prophylactic Antiemetic Regimens (Complete References as Cited)

Agent or strategies	Nausea	Vomiting	PONV
Ondansetron 4 mg IV[13]	4.6	6.4	4.4
Dexamethasone 8 mg IV or 10 mg PO (adults)[14]	Early 5.0 Late 4.3	Early 3.6 Late 4.3	
Dexamethasone 1–1.5 mg/kg IV (children)[14]		Early 10 Late 3.1	
Transdermal scopolamine 1.5 mg patch[15]	4.3	5.6	3.8
Droperidol 0.625–1.25 mg IV	5	7	
Haloperidol 0.5–4 mg IM/IV[16]	3.2–4.5	3.9–5.1	
Metoclopramide[17]	No significant effect	Early 9.1 Late 10	
Propofol infusion[18]	8.6 (postdischarge 12.5)	11.2 (postdischarge 10.3)	
Acupuncture[19]	11 (30% baseline risk) 5 (70% baseline risk)	11 (30% baseline risk) 5 (70% baseline risk)	

PONV, postoperative nausea and vomiting.

totypical 5-HT$_3$ RA, and at the 4-mg dose, it has an NNT of about 4.6 for the prevention of vomiting, 6.4 for the prevention of nausea, and 4.4 for the prevention of both in the first 48 h postoperatively.[17] For PONV prophylaxis using 5-HT$_3$ RAs, the Society for Ambulatory Anesthesia (SAMBA) guidelines recommend doses of 4 mg IV for ondansetron, 0.35–1.5 mg IV (5–20 μg/kg) for granisetron, and 12.5 mg IV for dolasetron.[11]

Palonosetron is the newest 5-HT$_3$ RA and has recently been approved in the United States for PONV. For PONV prophylaxis, the recommended dose of palonosetron is 0.075 mg IV.[18] Palonosetron exhibits features not observed in other drugs of its class, namely high affinity and positive cooperativity in binding to its receptor, allosteric binding, and promotion of receptor internalization.[19] Thus, palonosetron has a relatively long half-life that may confer an antiemetic effect for several days after administration, which could be useful in minimizing PDNV following ambulatory surgery. However, further studies are necessary to confirm any advantage over other serotonin antagonists.

Few studies have examined 5-HT$_3$ RAs for the prevention of PDNV. Although ondansetron 4 mg has been shown in at least one study to reduce PDNV, the NNT was 12.9 for nausea and 13.6 for vomiting.[20] Ondansetron is available as an orally disintegrating tablet (ODT), and some studies suggest that providing adult and pediatric patients with the ODT before discharge may be particularly helpful in

reducing the incidence of PDNV at home.[21,22] Ondansetron, granisetron, and dolasetron are available as intravenous medications or oral tablets; palonosetron is currently only available as an intravenous medication.

Steroids

The mechanism of antiemetic activity for dexamethasone has not been fully eluci-
dated, but it is believed that corticosteroids act centrally to inhibit prostaglandin
synthesis or to control endorphin release. Dexamethasone may also be particularly
effective when used in combination with 5-HT$_3$ RAs, as it may (1) reduce levels of
serotonin by depleting its precursor tryptophan, (2) prevent release of serotonin in
the gut, and (3) sensitize the 5-HT$_3$ receptor to other antiemetics.[23]

Dexamethasone is most effective for PONV prophylaxis when administered
at induction rather than at the end of surgery.[24] It has been found to significantly
reduce PONV compared with placebo, with the incidences of headache and dizziness
being similar between the two groups.[25] The NNT is 7.1 for the prevention of early
vomiting in adults and children, and 3.8 for the prevention of late vomiting.[23] The
recommended prophylactic dose of dexamethasone 4–5 mg IV at induction appears
to be as effective as ondansetron 4 mg IV in preventing PONV.[11]

Cholinergic Antagonists

The anticholinergic agents act by blocking muscarinic cholinergic emetic receptors
in the cerebral cortex and the pons.[26] The most common anticholinergic used for
PONV prophylaxis is the transdermal scopolamine (TDS) patch, designed to release
1.5 mg of scopolamine over 3 days. Premedication with TDS appears to be as effective as ondansetron or droperidol in the prevention of both early and late PONV/
PDNV.[27] Although TDS has an NNT of 5.6 for the prevention of POV, the NNH is
5.6 for visual disturbances, 12.5 for dry mouth, and 50 for dizziness.[28] Thus, the
high rate of anticholinergic side effects of scopolamine may limit its use as a stand-
alone antiemetic agent.

Scopolamine may be most useful in combination with other antiemetics. The
preoperative TDS patch along with intraoperative ondansetron has been found to
reduce the incidence of PONV compared with ondansetron alone.[29,30] The incidence
of adverse effects, including anticholinergic effects, does not appear to be statistically different between the two groups, while patient satisfaction in the TDS group
has reportedly been significantly higher. Thus, scopolamine might be a safe and
effective adjunct in the management of PONV, especially when used in combination
with ondansetron.

Dopamine Antagonists

The dopamine RAs act at the D2 receptors in the CTZ and area postrema to suppress
nausea and vomiting. There are three types of dopamine antagonists commonly used
as antiemetics: butyrophenones, phenothiazines, and benzamides.

Butyrophenones In addition to their strong D2 receptor antagonism, the butyrophenones are α-blockers, contributing to their adverse effects of sedation and extrapyramidal symptoms, although the latter are rare at the low doses given for PONV.[31] The two primary antiemetic agents in this group are haloperidol and droperidol.

The clinical efficacy of droperidol 0.625–1.25 mg IV before the end of surgery has been well established, and until recently, it had been widely viewed as a safe and cost-effective antiemetic.[32] However, in 2001, the FDA issued a "black box" warning for droperidol, citing reports of severe cardiac arrhythmias and rare cases of sudden cardiac death associated with its use.[33] Although many experts and anesthesia providers believe that the warning was not justified and continue to use droperidol, its use has declined in recent years, due to both the warning and an FDA recommendation that all elective surgery patients receiving droperidol be placed on continuous electrocardiographic monitoring for 2–3 h following administration.

Accordingly, there has been an increased interest in the antiemetic properties of haloperidol. Traditionally used as an antipsychotic, haloperidol has a faster onset of antiemetic action and has a longer half-life than droperidol, but its effect does not last as long, most likely because it has a weaker binding affinity than droperidol for the D2 receptors in the CTZ and area postrema.[31] A few small studies have suggested that haloperidol, either alone or in combination with ondansetron, is effective for the prevention of early PONV, with an NNT of 3.2–5.1 and no observed QTc prolongation.[34–37] However, additional studies are necessary to determine the optimal dosing, timing, and safety profile of haloperidol for PONV.

Phenothiazines The phenothiazines, which include promethazine, chlorpromazine, and prochlorperazine, are some of the most commonly used antiemetics worldwide. However, their use has fallen out of favor due to their high incidence of adverse effects, such as sedation, restlessness, diarrhea, agitation, CNS depression, and more rarely, extrapyramidal effects, hypotension, neuroleptic syndrome, and supraventricular tachycardia.[8] Promethazine 12.5–25 mg IV given at the induction of surgery and prochlorperazine 5–10 mg IV given at the end of surgery have both been shown to have antiemetic efficacy when combined with ondansetron.[11] Promethazine 6.25 mg, a dose low enough to limit most adverse effects, may be more effective than ondansetron for treating PONV in patients who have failed previous ondansetron prophylaxis.[38] However, strong data are lacking and phenothiazines are currently not recommended as first-line antiemetic agents.

Benzamides The most commonly used antiemetic in this group is metoclopramide, a procainimide derivative that blocks D2 receptors both centrally at the CTZ and area postrema, and peripherally in the GI tract.[31] The most common clinical dose is 10 mg IV. Although there is no significant antinausea effect with metoclopramide, it does have an NNT of 9.1 to prevent vomiting in adults in the early postoperative period, and an NNT of 10 to prevent late vomiting in the same population.[39] However, given the overall lack of evidence demonstrating antiemetic efficacy, metoclopramide is not recommended for PONV at this time.

Propofol

The mechanism of antiemetic activity of propofol is unclear, but it has been found that maintenance with a propofol infusion results in a decreased incidence of PONV and PDNV over inhaled anesthetics, with an NNT of 8.6 and 11.2 for postoperative nausea (PON) and POV, respectively, and an NNT of 12.5 and 10.3 for postdischarge nausea and vomiting, respectively.[40] However, economic analyses have suggested that routine use of total intravenous anesthesia (TIVA) for PONV prophylaxis is generally not cost-effective.[41] In addition, a small study found that while there were no significant differences in early PONV outcomes between patients given dolasetron prophylaxis and those given propofol-based TIVA, PDNV was significantly more common for patients in the TIVA group.[42] As a result, the effects of TIVA may be too short-lived to offer protection against PDNV, and it may not be optimal as a sole agent for PONV prophylaxis. Nevertheless, propofol-based TIVA is a reasonable option for high-risk patients as part of a multimodal management strategy, particularly because propofol is now available in a less costly generic formulation (see the section "Combination Therapy and Multimodal Management").

Neurokinin-1 Antagonists

The neurokinin-1 receptor antagonists (NK_1 RAs) are a new class of antiemetic drugs that competitively inhibit the binding of substance P, a neuropeptide released from enterochromaffin cells.[43] Substance P plays an important role in emesis as a ligand for NK_1 receptors, which are located in the GI tract and the area postrema.[8] The NK_1 RAs are believed to suppress nausea and vomiting by acting centrally or peripherally to block neurotransmission between the NTS or the vagal terminals of the gut and the CPG.[44,45]

Aprepitant (Emend) was the first FDA-approved NK_1 RA. Preoperative aprepitant 40 and 125 mg orally have been found to be equivalent to preoperative ondansetron 4 mg IV in terms of complete response (no emesis or rescue antiemetics needed in 24 h) rates, nausea control, and use of rescue antiemetics.[46] Aprepitant may also be superior to ondansetron for prevention of vomiting in the first 24 and 48 h, with lower peak nausea scores in patients receiving either dose of aprepitant.[47] Because the 125-mg dose has been observed to be similar or even slightly less effective than the lower dose, the recommended and approved dose for PONV prophylaxis is 40 mg preoperatively.

NK_1 RAs are safe and well tolerated, with the most common side effects being asthenia, diarrhea, dizziness, and hiccups.[48] The NK_1 RAs offer many potential benefits for the management of PONV, especially as an alternative to patients who have failed treatment or prophylaxis with antiemetics in other classes. Aprepitant has the added benefit of availability in both an oral and an intravenous form (fosaprepitant), the latter of which may be useful for established PONV,[49] although clinical trials with the intravenous formulation have not been conducted in the PONV setting.

NONPHARMACOLOGICAL PROPHYLACTIC ANTIEMETIC TECHNIQUES

Of the nonpharmacological treatments for PONV, acupuncture is one of the most well studied. It may work by activating A-β and A-δ fibers to influence neurotransmission in the dorsal horn or other centers, influence the release of endogenous opioids, or inhibit gastric acid secretion and normalize gastric dysrrhythmia.[50]

Most studies have examined the use of the acupuncture point pericardial 6 (P6), located 4 cm proximal from the wrist crease between the tendons of the palmaris longus and flexor carpi radialis muscles. Acupoint stimulation of P6 has been demonstrated to be effective in the prevention of PONV, with few side effects.[51] In patients with a baseline risk of PONV of 30% (the estimated overall incidence of PONV), the NNT for acupuncture is about 11 for both nausea and vomiting. At a baseline risk of 70% (estimate for high-risk populations), the NNT is about 5 for both nausea and vomiting.

There are a number of comparable variations on traditional acupuncture, including acupressure and acupressure wristbands, acustimulation using transcutaneous electrical stimulation, acupuncture injections, and electroacupuncture.[50] These techniques may be of particular benefit as an adjunct to antiemetic drugs in the ambulatory setting, since many of them can be performed rapidly and do not require special training. The risk of adverse events is about 0.1%, with the most common side effects being mild, such as fainting, exacerbation of symptoms, and lost or forgotten needle.[52]

COMBINATION THERAPY AND MULTIMODAL MANAGEMENT

Because no single antiemetic agent is completely effective in preventing or treating PONV, combination therapy using multiple agents is particularly appealing. Ondansetron 4 mg IV, dexamethasone 4 mg IV, and droperidol 1.25 mg IV are equally effective as single agents for the prevention of PONV.[1] They are generally well tolerated and have comparable safety profiles, even when used in combination.[53] Each drug acts independently, such that combinations of any two or three of them will reduce the risk of PONV in an additive manner. Thus, therapy using at least one of these three drugs is recommended for patients at moderate risk for PONV.[11]

For patients at high risk of PONV, combination antiemetic therapy can be used in conjunction with other pharmacological and nonpharmacological techniques. This approach is often labeled "multimodal management" or "balanced antiemesis," as it combines multiple therapeutic options to maximize antiemetic efficacy. A multimodal approach may include preoperative anxiolysis, aggressive hydration, supplemental oxygen, droperidol and dexamethasone at induction, ondansetron at the end of surgery, TIVA with propofol and remifentanil, and/or ketorolac, with avoidance of volatile anesthetics, nitrous oxide, or neuromuscular blockade. While patient satisfaction scores are similar or only slightly higher for multimodal approaches than for antiemetic monotherapy, multimodal approaches do appear to be slightly superior to monotherapy in achieving higher rates of complete response.[54,55]

POST-OP ASSESSMENT

Postoperative evaluation should include asking the patient about nausea, and if present, the severity of nausea based on a verbal description, numerical scale (0–10), or visual analogue scale. There are no definitive guidelines for the assessment of PONV, but all patients should at least be assessed for nausea on admission to and discharge from the postanesthesia care unit (PACU), and more frequently as necessary (e.g., high-risk patients, patients receiving opioids or antiemetics).[56] Since some patients experience late (6–24 h after surgery) or delayed (more than 24 h after surgery) PONV, it is appropriate to ask patients about nausea during those periods as well, especially after potential emetogenic triggers, such as patient transport, initiation of oral nutrition or solid foods, or beginning ambulation after surgery. For patients with only a brief hospital stay following surgery, counseling on the prevention and management of PDNV prior to discharge should be encouraged.

MEDICAL MANAGEMENT OF ESTABLISHED PONV

Before initiating rescue antiemetic drugs, other factors that may contribute to PONV should be considered and addressed, including pain, concomitant use of opioids or other medications, inadequate hydration, environmental factors (e.g., auditory, olfactory, or psychological stimuli), or mechanical reasons (e.g., blood in the throat, abdominal obstruction, etc.). Pain should be treated with appropriate analgesics as needed, and opioids should not be withheld purely out of concern for PONV risk. However, if opioid-induced PONV is suspected, nonsteroidal anti-inflammatory drugs (NSAIDs) or other non-opiate adjuncts may be preferable. Hypotension may also increase the risk of PONV by releasing emetogenic chemicals and decreasing blood flow to the emetogenic areas of the brain; thus, intravenous hydration (up to 20 mL/kg) and replacement of intraoperative blood loss may be necessary.[31]

In general, patients who have not previously received antiemetic prophylaxis should be given a 5-HT$_3$ RA, while patients who have already received prophylaxis should be given a rescue antiemetic from a different treatment class than the prophylactic drug.[11] The NNT of 5-HT$_3$ RAs for established PONV is about 4–5.[57] Treatment doses of 5-HT$_3$ RAs for established PONV are usually smaller than those needed for prophylaxis: ondansetron 1 mg, dolasetron 12.5 mg (similar to the recommended prophylactic dose), and granisetron 0.1 mg. Although ondansetron 1 mg has been shown to be as effective as ondansetron 4 mg for antiemetic rescue, most clinicians tend to use the standard prophylactic dose (i.e., ondansetron 4 mg) in practice.

In patients who received a 5-HT$_3$ RA for prophylaxis, no further benefit is achieved from repeat doses within 6 h after the initial dose.[58] In such cases, alternatives to 5-HT$_3$ RAs are recommended and include dexamethasone 4 mg, droperidol

0.625 mg, or promethazine 6.25–12.5 mg, although dexamethasone and TDS are not recommended for emetic episodes, which occur more than 6 h postoperatively, due to their longer duration of action.[11]

Rescue therapy for PDNV has not been well studied. Ondansetron (ODT), promethazine or prochlorperazine (oral or suppository), and TDS have been recommended for outpatient use following discharge.[56,59] The choice of rescue is generally left to the discretion of the clinician and should take into account factors such as what, if any, antiemetic therapies were given prior to discharge, the patient's preferred route of administration, and which antiemetics have worked for the patient in the past.

SUMMARY

Management of PONV begins with risk assessment and baseline risk reduction, followed by consideration of antiemetic prophylaxis, and if necessary, rescue treatment. In patients at increased risk for PONV, combination therapy or a multimodal approach is recommended. Effective management of PONV and PDNV are necessary to prevent negative medical consequences, maximize patient satisfaction and return to normal activity, and minimize healthcare costs.

REFERENCES

1. Apfel CC, et al. A factorial trial of six interventions for the prevention of postoperative nausea and vomiting. *N Engl J Med*. 2004;350(24):2441–2451.
2. Wu CL, et al. Systematic review and analysis of postdischarge symptoms after outpatient surgery. *Anesthesiology*. 2002;96(4):994–1003.
3. Wang SC, Borison HL. The vomiting center; a critical experimental analysis. *Arch Neurol Psychiatry*. 1950;63(6):928–941.
4. Hornby PJ. Central neurocircuitry associated with emesis. *Am J Med*. 2001;111(Suppl 8A):106S–112S.
5. Watcha MF, White PF. Postoperative nausea and vomiting. Its etiology, treatment, and prevention. *Anesthesiology*. 1992;77(1):162–184.
6. Borison HL. Area postrema: chemoreceptor circumventricular organ of the medulla oblongata. *Prog Neurobiol*. 1989;32(5):351–390.
7. Leslie RA. Neuroactive substances in the dorsal vagal complex of the medulla oblongata: nucleus of the tractus solitarius, area postrema, and dorsal motor nucleus of the vagus. *Neurochem Int*. 1985;7:191–211.
8. Gan TJ. Mechanisms underlying postoperative nausea and vomiting and neurotransmitter receptor antagonist-based pharmacotherapy. *CNS Drugs*. 2007;21(10):813–833.
9. Apfel CC, et al. A simplified risk score for predicting postoperative nausea and vomiting: conclusions from cross-validations between two centers. *Anesthesiology*. 1999;91(3):693–700.
10. Eberhart LH, et al. The development and validation of a risk score to predict the probability of postoperative vomiting in pediatric patients. *Anesth Analg*. 2004;99(6):1630–1637.
11. Gan TJ, et al. Society for Ambulatory Anesthesia guidelines for the management of postoperative nausea and vomiting. *Anesth Analg*. 2007;105(6):1615–1628.
12. Mattila K, et al. Postdischarge symptoms after ambulatory surgery: first-week incidence, intensity, and risk factors. *Anesth Analg*. 2005;101(6):1643–1650.
13. Scuderi PE. Pharmacology of antiemetics. *Int Anesthesiol Clin*. 2003;41(4):41–66.

14. Barnes NM, et al. The 5-HT3 receptor—the relationship between structure and function. *Neurophar-macology.* 2009;56(1):273–284.
15. Gan TJ. Selective serotonin 5-HT3 receptor antagonists for postoperative nausea and vomiting: are they all the same? *CNS Drugs.* 2005;19(3):225–238.
16. Chen X, et al. The effect of timing of dolasetron administration on its efficacy as a prophylactic antiemetic in the ambulatory setting. *Anesth Analg.* 2001;93(4):906–911.
17. Tramer MR, et al. Efficacy, dose-response, and safety of ondansetron in prevention of postoperative nausea and vomiting: a quantitative systematic review of randomized placebo-controlled trials. *Anesthesiology.* 1997;87(6):1277–1289.
18. Candiotti KA, et al. A randomized, double-blind study to evaluate the efficacy and safety of three different doses of palonosetron versus placebo for preventing postoperative nausea and vomiting. *Anesth Analg.* 2008;107(2):445–451.
19. Kloth DD. New pharmacologic findings for the treatment of PONV and PDNV. *Am J Health Syst Pharm.* 2009;66(1 Suppl 1):S11–S18.
20. Gupta A, et al. Does the routine prophylactic use of antiemetics affect the incidence of postdischarge nausea and vomiting following ambulatory surgery?: a systematic review of randomized controlled trials. *Anesthesiology.* 2003;99(2):488–495.
21. Davis PJ, et al. The effects of oral ondansetron disintegrating tablets for prevention of at-home emesis in pediatric patients after ear-nose-throat surgery. *Anesth Analg.* 2008;106(4):1117–1121.
22. Gan TJ, Franiak R, Reeves J. Ondansetron orally disintegrating tablet versus placebo for the preven-tion of postdischarge nausea and vomiting after ambulatory surgery. *Anesth Analg.* 2002;94(5):1199–1200.
23. Henzi I, Walder B, Tramer MR. Dexamethasone for the prevention of postoperative nausea and vomiting: a quantitative systematic review. *Anesth Analg.* 2000;90(1):186–194.
24. Wang JJ, et al. The effect of timing of dexamethasone administration on its efficacy as a prophylactic antiemetic for postoperative nausea and vomiting. *Anesth Analg.* 2000;91(1):136–139.
25. Karanicolas PJ, et al. The impact of prophylactic dexamethasone on nausea and vomiting after lapa-roscopic cholecystectomy: a systematic review and meta-analysis. *Ann Surg.* 2008;248(5):751–762.
26. McCarthy BG, Peroutka SJ. Differentiation of muscarinic cholinergic receptor subtypes in human cortex and pons: implications for anti-motion sickness therapy. *Aviat Space Environ Med.* 1988;59(1):63–66.
27. White PF, et al. Transdermal scopolamine: an alternative to ondansetron and droperidol for the prevention of postoperative and postdischarge emetic symptoms. *Anesth Analg.* 2007;104(1):92–96.
28. Kranke P, et al. The efficacy and safety of transdermal scopolamine for the prevention of postopera-tive nausea and vomiting: a quantitative systematic review. *Anesth Analg.* 2002;95(1):133–143.
29. Sah N, et al. Transdermal scopolamine patch in addition to ondansetron for postoperative nausea and vomiting prophylaxis in patients undergoing ambulatory cosmetic surgery. *J Clin Anesth.* 2009;21(4):249–252.
30. Gan TJ, et al. A randomized, double-blind, multicenter trial comparing transdermal scopolamine plus ondansetron to ondansetron alone for the prevention of postoperative nausea and vomiting in the outpatient setting. *Anesth Analg.* 2009;108(5):1498–1504.
31. Kovac AL. Prevention and treatment of postoperative nausea and vomiting. *Drugs.* 2000;59(2):213–243.
32. McKeage K, Simpson D, Wagstaff AJ. Intravenous droperidol: a review of its use in the management of postoperative nausea and vomiting. *Drugs.* 2006;66(16):2123–2147.
33. White PF. Droperidol: a cost-effective antiemetic for over thirty years. *Anesth Analg.* 2002;95(4):789–790.
34. Buttner M, et al. Is low-dose haloperidol a useful antiemetic?: a meta-analysis of published and unpublished randomized trials. *Anesthesiology.* 2004;101(6):1454–1463.
35. Aouad MT, et al. Haloperidol vs. ondansetron for the prevention of postoperative nausea and vomiting following gynaecological surgery. *Eur J Anaesthesiol.* 2007;24(2):171–178.
36. Grecu L, et al. Haloperidol plus ondansetron versus ondansetron alone for prophylaxis of postopera-tive nausea and vomiting. *Anesth Analg.* 2008;106(5):1410–1413.

37. Rosow CE, et al. Haloperidol versus ondansetron for prophylaxis of postoperative nausea and vomiting. *Anesth Analg.* 2008;106(5):1407–1409.

38. Habib AS, et al. A comparison of ondansetron with promethazine for treating postoperative nausea and vomiting in patients who received prophylaxis with ondansetron: a retrospective database analysis. *Anesth Analg.* 2007;104(3):548–551.

39. Henzi I, Walder B, Tramer MR. Metoclopramide in the prevention of postoperative nausea and vomiting: a quantitative systematic review of randomized, placebo-controlled studies. *Br J Anaesth.* 1999;83(5):761–771.

40. Gupta A, et al. Comparison of recovery profile after ambulatory anesthesia with propofol, isoflurane, sevoflurane and desflurane: a systematic review. *Anesth Analg.* 2004;98(3):632–641.

41. Visser K, et al. Randomized controlled trial of total intravenous anesthesia with propofol versus inhalation anesthesia with isoflurane-nitrous oxide: postoperative nausea with vomiting and economic analysis. *Anesthesiology.* 2001;95(3):616–626.

42. White H, et al. Randomized comparison of two anti-emetic strategies in high-risk patients undergoing day-case gynaecological surgery. *Br J Anaesth.* 2007;98(4):470–476.

43. Apfel CC, Malhotra A, Leslie JB. The role of neurokinin-1 receptor antagonists for the management of postoperative nausea and vomiting. *Curr Opin Anaesthesiol.* 2008;21(4):427–432.

44. Saito R, Takano Y, Kamiya HO. Roles of substance P and NK(1) receptor in the brainstem in the development of emesis. *J Pharmacol Sci.* 2003;91(2):87–94.

45. Minami M, et al. Antiemetic effects of sendide, a peptide tachykinin NK1 receptor antagonist, in the ferret. *Eur J Pharmacol.* 1998;363(1):49–55.

46. Gan TJ, et al. A randomized, double-blind comparison of the NK1 antagonist, aprepitant, versus ondansetron for the prevention of postoperative nausea and vomiting. *Anesth Analg.* 2007;104(5): 1082–1089.

47. Diemunsch P, et al. Single-dose aprepitant vs. ondansetron for the prevention of postoperative nausea and vomiting: a randomized, double-blind phase III trial in patients undergoing open abdominal surgery. *Br J Anaesth.* 2007;99(2):202–211.

48. Poli-Bigelli S, et al. Addition of the neurokinin 1 receptor antagonist aprepitant to standard antiemetic therapy improves control of chemotherapy-induced nausea and vomiting. Results from a randomized, double-blind, placebo-controlled trial in Latin America. *Cancer.* 2003;97(12):3090–3098.

49. Diemunsch P, Joshi G, Brichant JF. Neurokinin-1 receptor antagonists in the prevention of postoperative nausea and vomiting. *Br J Anaesth.* 2009;103(1):7–13.

50. Rowbotham DJ. Recent advances in the non-pharmacological management of postoperative nausea and vomiting. *Br J Anaesth.* 2005;95(1):77–81.

51. Lee A, Fan LT. Stimulation of the wrist acupuncture point P6 for preventing postoperative nausea and vomiting. *Cochrane Database Syst Rev.* 2009;(2):CD003281.

52. White A, et al. Adverse events following acupuncture: prospective survey of 32,000 consultations with doctors and physiotherapists. *BMJ.* 2001;323(7311):485–486.

53. Leslie JB, Gan TJ. Meta-analysis of the safety of 5-HT3 antagonists with dexamethasone or droperidol for prevention of PONV. *Ann Pharmacother.* 2006;40(5):856–872.

54. Scuderi PE, et al. Multimodal antiemetic management prevents early postoperative vomiting after outpatient laparoscopy. *Anesth Analg.* 2000;91(6):1408–1414.

55. Habib AS, et al. A randomized comparison of a multimodal management strategy versus combination antiemetics for the prevention of postoperative nausea and vomiting. *Anesth Analg.* 2004;99(1):77–81.

56. American Society of Perianesthesia Nurses PONV/PDNV Strategic Work Team. ASPAN'S evidence-based clinical practice guideline for the prevention and/or management of PONV/PDNV. *J Perianesth Nurs.* 2006;21(4):230–250.

57. Kazemi-Kjellberg F, Henzi I, Tramer MR. Treatment of established postoperative nausea and vomiting: a quantitative systematic review. *BMC Anesthesiol.* 2001;1(1):2.

58. Kovac AL, et al. Efficacy of repeat intravenous dosing of ondansetron in controlling postoperative nausea and vomiting: a randomized, double-blind, placebo-controlled multicenter trial. *J Clin Anesth.* 1999;11(6):453–459.

59. Golembiewski J, Tokumaru S. Pharmacological prophylaxis and management of adult postoperative/postdischarge nausea and vomiting. *J Perianesth Nurs.* 2006;21(6):385–397.

CHAPTER 30

DELIRIUM

Dimitriy Levin and Jeffrey J. Glasheen

BACKGROUND

Delirium is an acute confusional state that commonly causes morbidity and mortality in hospitalized patients. In susceptible populations, it can be triggered by physiologic stress such as acute illness or surgery. Incidence of delirium has been reported to be as high as 73.5% after surgery and 87% in the intensive care unit (ICU).[1,2] Consequences include increased hospital length of stay, inability to return home after hospitalization, increased costs, poor surgical outcomes, and increased mortality.[1,3] Management of delirium consists of identifying at-risk populations, proactively controlling modifiable risk factors, and promptly recognizing and treating delirium once it develops.

PATHOPHYSIOLOGY

The pathophysiology of delirium remains poorly understood. The leading theories focus on disruption of normal neurotransmitter function and inflammation. Anticholinergic and dopaminergic drugs are well-documented precipitants of delirium, and perturbations in most other neurotransmitters have been implicated as well.[1] Inflammatory cytokines such as interleukin (IL)-1, -2, and -6; tumor necrosis factor-alpha (TNF-α); and interferon alter neurotransmission and increase permeability of the blood–brain barrier.[1] Furthermore, IL-1, IL-6, and TNF-α activate monocyte- and macrophage-derived microglial cells in the brain, which cause neuroinflammation and neurodegeneration that persist far past the inciting event, possibly explaining the sometimes lingering course of delirium.[4] Interestingly, pro-inflammatory activity of microglial cells appears to be under cholinergic control, so cholinergic depletion seen with older age and certain drugs may exacerbate delirium by both direct disruption of neurotransmission and increased inflammation.[4] Finally, sedatives such as propofol are known to induce long-lasting changes in the thalamus, which is also responsible for processing sensory information and may contribute to the

Perioperative Medicine: Medical Consultation and Co-Management, First Edition.
Edited by Amir K. Jaffer and Paul J. Grant.
© 2012 Wiley-Blackwell. Published 2012 by John Wiley & Sons, Inc.

hyperaroused state frequently seen in delirium.[5] Gas anesthetics such as isoflurane and desflurane increase brain levels of amyloid β-peptide, which interferes with the normal function of acetylcholine receptors in a manner that some researchers postulate may be similar to the mechanism of Alzheimer's disease.[6]

PREVENTION STRATEGIES

Development of delirium is typically multifactorial. It begins with a susceptible subject who receives one or more insults that precipitate the acute confusional state. Delirium risk factors can be categorized by whether or not they can be modified, and potentially prevented, by the medical care team (Table 30.1).

TABLE 30.1. Postoperative Delirium Risk Factors[1-3,7,26]

Nonmodifiable risk factors
Demographics:
Male sex
Older age[3]
Age 50–59, incidence 22%
Age 60–69, incidence 42%
Age 70–79, incidence 72%
Age 80–89, incidence 92%
Cognitive:
Dementia or cognitive impairment (Mini-Mental State Examination <24/30, Mini-Cog 0–2)[7]
History of delirium
Depression
Physiologic and nutritional:
Poor functional status, low Barthel Index, Timed Get Up and Go Test >20 s
History of falls (≥1 in the past 6 months)
Malnutrition
Alcohol abuse
Comorbidities:
Multiple coexisting medical illnesses or comorbidities, high Charlson Index
American Society of Anesthesiologists (ASA) status 3–4
Infection
Chronic renal or hepatic disease
History of stroke or other neurologic disease
Fracture or trauma
HIV infection
Advanced, severe, or terminal illness, Acute Physiology and Chronic Health Evaluation score >16

TABLE 30.1. *Continued*

Modifiable risk factors

Cognitive:
  Disturbance of day–night and sleep–wake cycles
Sensory impairment:
  Visual impairment (<20/70 corrected)
  Hearing impairment
  Tethers (restraints, indwelling urinary catheters, telemetry, oxygen, drains)
Toxic–metabolic:
  Dehydration (BUN/Cr > 18)
  Electrolyte abnormalities
  Hypoxemia
  Polypharmacy
  Anticholinergic and psychotropic drugs
Perioperative:
  Intraoperative hypotension
  Need for blood transfusions
  Depth of anesthesia
  Uncontrolled pain
  Constipation
  Urinary retention

BUN, blood urea nitrogen.

Nonmodifiable Risks

The daunting list of nonmodifiable risk factors for delirium can be condensed into the general concepts of frailty, disability, and comorbidity. Calculating scores, such as the Acute Physiology and Chronic Health Evaluation (APACHE) for acute illness, the Barthel Index for functional impairment, and the Charlson Index for comorbidities, is not always feasible in daily clinical practice. Instead, the assessment should begin with a careful history, with more risk factors causing a greater concern for delirium and prompting closer attention to the modifiable risks.

The most helpful additional screen is the Mini-Cog[7] (Table 30.2). It was studied in a prospective cohort of 132 general medical inpatients aged 65 and older without delirium. Patients in the study were deemed to be at high risk for developing delirium in the hospital based on the presence of cognitive impairment, age 80 or older, or any two of the following: presence of functional impairment, visual or hearing impairment, or critical comorbid illness. The study excluded patients in coma, those experiencing alcohol or drug withdrawal or intoxication, and those with an inpatient length of stay less than 72 h. Presence of delirium was assessed twice daily using the confusion assessment method (CAM, summarized in Table 30.3 and discussed in detail below). Overall, 83% of enrolled subjects did not have known

TABLE 30.2.   Mini-Cog Score[7]

---

1. Name three unrelated words and ask patient to repeat them back.

2. Have the patient draw a clock with hands at "ten past eleven o'clock."

3. Ask the patient to recall the three words.

Scoring:

One point for each recalled word (3 points possible)

Two points for correct clock with numbers 1–12 present in correct order and direction, evenly spaced in the circle, and with hands at 10 and 2 indicating "ten past eleven o'clock." Error in any element results in incorrect clock and 0 points.

Mini-Cog score 0–2 indicates a fivefold risk of developing inpatient delirium.

TABLE 30.3.   Confusion Assessment Method (CAM)[17]

---

1. Acute onset and fluctuating course

2. Inattention

3. Disorganized thinking

4. Altered level of consciousness

Presence of features 1 *and* 2 plus either 3 *or* 4 is 94% sensitive and 89% specific for delirium.

baseline dementia or cognitive impairment. Delirium developed in 15% of the study cohort during the hospitalization, and in the multivariate analysis, a Mini-Cog score of 0–2 was a significant predictor of in-hospital delirium (odds ratio [OR] 5.24, 95% confidence interval [CI] 1.50–18.31, $P < 0.01$). The Mini-Cog remained a significant predictor of delirium even after excluding patients with known history of dementia or cognitive impairment (OR 3.96, 95% CI 1.11–14.20, $P < 0.03$).

Modifiable Risks

The prevention of perioperative delirium focuses on modifiable cognitive, sensory, and pharmacologic risk factors.

Cognitive Risk Factors

Sleep disruption and deprivation are common in hospitalized patients. Research in ICU patients has mechanistically linked sleep deprivation with delirium due to the development of neurotransmitter imbalances.[8] Since most sleep medications can increase risk of delirium, the emphasis should be on nonpharmacologic interventions. Attention should be paid to maintaining normal day–night cycles by using bright natural light and stimulating environments that discourage naps during the day, and dark, quiet rooms with the television turned off at night. Nighttime vital signs and lab draws should be minimized to avoid disruptions in sleep. Decaffeinated tea and warm milk can be used to aid with the onset of sleep. If a medication must be prescribed, trazodone 25–50 mg orally is considered one of the safest agents due to its low anticholinergic activity, although there is a dearth of high-quality data to support its use.[1,9]

Sensory Impairment

Sensory impairment can contribute to delirium by causing disorientation and anxiety. The key intervention is to ensure that patients are using their assistive devices such as eyeglasses, hearing aids, and dentures, at all times to maintain maximum awareness and familiarity with the environment. Along the same lines, tethers such as physical restraints, oxygen tubing, indwelling urinary catheters, sequential compression devices, telemetry, and drains should be discontinued as soon as possible. In addition to contributing to disorientation, they also increase the risk of falls.

Pharmacologic Risk Factors

Medications represent one of the greatest modifiable delirium risks. Anticholinergic and psychotropic substances can both directly alter neurotransmission in the brain and negatively impact cognition, arousal, and sensory awareness (Table 30.4). Although the general recommendation is that these medications are avoided in at-risk patients, the reality is often complicated by medical necessity (e.g., with opioids, especially since uncontrolled pain is also a delirium risk), risk of withdrawal, and the fact that many commonly used medications have some anticholinergic activity (e.g., amoxicillin, cephalexin, digoxin, furosemide, and levofloxacin).[9]

Intraoperative Risk Factors

While several intraoperative factors have been associated with the development of postoperative delirium (Table 30.1), the most controllable one is the type of anesthesia. In a Cochrane review, regional anesthesia was associated with a significant decrease in postoperative delirium compared with general anesthesia in hip fracture patients (9.4% vs. 19.2%, relative risk 0.50, 95% CI 0.26–0.95).[10] The importance of depth of sedation was also demonstrated in a double-blind randomized controlled trial of patients 65 and older undergoing hip fracture repair surgery.[5] The trial

TABLE 30.4. High-Risk Medications in Patients Predisposed to Delirium[1,9,27]

Antidepressants (amitriptylene, doxepin, paroxetine, nortriptyline)
Antihistamines (diphenhydramine, hydroxyzine, promethazine)
Anticholinergics (atropine, dicyclomine, scopolamine)
Antipsychotics
Benzodiazepines
Opioids, especially meperidine, and tramadol
Other hypnotics (chloral hydrate, zolpidem)
Urinary incontinence agents (oxybutynin, tolterodine)
Other medications on the Beers list of potentially inappropriate medications for older adults[28]

screened for delirium using the CAM and excluded patients with Mini-Mental State Examination (MMSE) scores of <15. All 114 patients received spinal anesthesia and propofol sedation titrated to Bispectral Index (BIS) of 50 in the deep sedation group and 80 or higher in the light sedation group. The light sedation group experienced considerably less postoperative delirium than the deep sedation group (19% vs. 40%, $P = 0.02$).

Prophylactic Therapy

There is a dearth of high-quality studies of interventions to prevent delirium.[11] A randomized placebo-controlled trial of acetylcholinesterase inhibitor donepezil 5 mg daily for 14 days before and after elective knee and hip arthroplasty in 80 patients aged 50 and older showed no difference in incidence or duration of delirium.[12] Furthermore, a randomized double-blind, placebo-controlled trial of cholinesterase inhibitor rivastigmine 1.5 mg three times daily started the night before surgery and continued for 6 days after elective cardiac surgery with cardiopulmonary bypass in 120 patients aged 65 or older, demonstrated no benefit in decreasing incidence or duration of delirium.[13] Finally, a randomized placebo-controlled trial of typical antipsychotic haloperidol 0.5 mg three times daily started before surgery and continued for 3 days postoperatively in 430 hip surgery patients aged 70 and older, showed no difference in the incidence of postoperative delirium.[14] However, when delirium developed in the haloperidol group, it had a lower severity and shorter duration (5.4 vs. 11.8 days, $P < 0.001$), and patients also experienced a shorter hospital length of stay (17.1 vs. 22.6 days, $P < 0.01$). No extrapyramidal side effects were seen in the haloperidol group.

In contrast, benefit was demonstrated in a randomized, double-blind, placebo-controlled trial of a single dose of atypical antipsychotic risperidone 1 mg oral disintegrating tablet given in the ICU following elective cardiac surgery with cardiopulmonary bypass in 126 patients aged 40 or older.[15] The presence of delirium was assessed twice daily using the CAM. The risperidone group had a significantly lower incidence of delirium (11.1% vs. 31.7%, $P = 0.009$). The authors did not report extrapyramidal side effects.

A blinded, randomized, controlled trial of 126 patients aged 65 and older undergoing hip fracture surgery compared proactive geriatric consultation with "usual care" by orthopedics with as-needed medicine or geriatrics consultation.[16] Geriatrics consultation using 10 structured modules, each with two to five interventions, took place preoperatively or within 24 h of surgery, and daily thereafter. The modules focused on adequate oxygen delivery to the central nervous system, fluid and electrolyte balance, treatment of severe pain, elimination of unnecessary medications, regulation of bowel and bladder function, adequate nutritional intake, early mobilization and rehabilitation, prevention and early detection and treatment of major postoperative complications, appropriate environmental stimuli, and treatment of agitated delirium. The presence of delirium was assessed using the CAM. The intervention resulted in a significant decrease in the incidence of delirium (32% vs. 50%, $P = 0.04$), although the duration of delirium and the hospital length of stay were unchanged. Because the study group received multiple interventions as part of the protocol, it is impossible to determine the individual elements that were beneficial for the prevention of delirium. Of note, a similar structured geriatrics intervention with attention to geriatric medical problems, orientation, cognition, sensory and mobility issues, pain, sleep, fluid and food intake, and patient, family, and nursing staff education, as well as titration of haloperidol and/or lorazepam for symptoms, was used in both placebo and intervention groups in the negative haloperidol trial noted above, which may explain lack of added benefit from scheduled prophylactic haloperidol.

Recommendations

Prevention of delirium begins with recognizing high-risk patients through careful history taking and Mini-Cog assessment. Modifiable cognitive, sensory, and pharmacologic risk factors can then be addressed. Literature on prevention of postoperative delirium is limited. The benefit of a proactive geriatric intervention likely stems from expert management of modifiable delirium risk factors and published protocols can be labor intensive. The use of antipsychotics to decrease the incidence, duration, and severity of delirium is promising, but more data are needed before an unequivocal endorsement can be made. The recommendations are further tempered by the U.S. Food and Drug Administration Black Box Warning on increased mortality associated with antipsychotic use in elderly patients with dementia.

POST-OP ASSESSMENT

Prompt recognition of delirium is essential to decrease the likelihood of a prolonged and severe course and the resultant complications. The most widely used evaluation tool is the CAM, which is easy to perform and has excellent characteristics with sensitivity of 94% and specificity of 89% when used as part of a formal cognitive assessment.[17] CAM examines four cardinal features of delirium: (1) acute onset and fluctuating course, (2) inattention, (3) disorganized thinking, and (4) altered level of consciousness (Table 30.3). Diagnosis of delirium requires the presence of features 1 and 2 and either 3 or 4.

Acute Onset and Fluctuating Course

Determination of this feature may require interviews with the patient's family members or care providers to ascertain whether the mental status is changed from baseline and if the alteration is rapid in onset and fluctuating. This stands in contrast with more gradual and generally irreversible decline seen in dementia. While a rapid decline in cognition can also be seen in multi-infarct dementia, it is not accompanied by a waxing and waning clinical course.

Inattention

This can be clinically observed as poor attention span, distractibility, perseveration, or inability to engage the patient in a meaningful conversation. For example, the patient may be fixated on television and have difficulty shifting attention to a new task. Patients may also appear dazed and disconnected from their environment. As a more objective test, the patient can be asked to count backward from 20. Whereas a demented patient will usually at least generate a string of numbers, the inattentive delirious patient may forget the task altogether and stop or switch from numbers to words.

Disorganized Thinking

This commonly presents as rambling or disorganized speech with illogical flow of ideas and rapid switching of topics. Patients may offer nonsensical answers to posed questions. An objective way to screen for disorganized thinking is with asking a simple question such as "what is a log made of?" or "will a stone float on water?" More involved questions, such as the meaning of proverbs, tend to be less helpful due to concurrent issues with inattention and baseline cognitive dysfunction.

Altered Level of Consciousness

This may present as hyperactive or hypoactive delirium. In the hyperactive state, the patient is hypervigilant, agitated, easily startled, and overly sensitive to environmental stimuli. In the hypoactive state, the patient may appear lethargic or drowsy and slow to respond even if they are easily aroused. The same patient may alternate between hyperactive and hypoactive states.

It is worth reiterating that the CAM diagnostic accuracy as a rapid bedside assessment is lower than in formal studies where it was used alongside other tools such as the MMSE. Clinical judgment should always be used to avoid missing subtle and atypically presenting delirium.

MEDICAL MANAGEMENT

The mainstay of delirium treatment is continuation of preventive measures with good sleep and day–night cycle hygiene; use of assistive devices; elimination of tethers; addressing pain, oxygenation, hydration, and electrolyte imbalances; and a careful review of medications, including the "as-needed" and one-time orders, for potential culprits (Table 30.5). In addition, acute reversible causes of delirium such as urinary retention, constipation, and infection should be investigated.

Managing Pain

Undertreated postoperative pain is a risk factor for delirium. In a prospective cohort of 541 patients with hip fracture and without delirium, very low doses of opioids (less than 10 mg/day of parenteral morphine equivalents) were associated with a 5.4-fold relative risk of developing delirium.[18] In the same study, cognitively intact patients had a ninefold relative risk of delirium if they reported an episode of severe pain at rest in the preceding 48 h. In a cohort of 86 patients older than 50 undergoing

TABLE 30.5. Treatment of Delirium

Nonpharmacologic

Implement delirium prevention strategies with attention to assistive devices and sleep–wake cycles

Reorientation with sitter or family in the room

Activity vest

Review medication list, including one-time and "as-needed" orders

Check for electrolyte abnormalities and evidence of infection

Treat dehydration, electrolyte derangements, and acute medical illness

Treat pain with scheduled non-opioid regimens (acetaminophen, COX-2 inhibitors), preferentially use oral opioids

Minimize tethers and avoid restraints

Pharmacologic

Low-dose antipsychotics:

Haloperidol 0.25–1 mg orally or IV scheduled two to three times a day or every 4–6 h if needed

Risperidone 0.5 mg orally one to two times a day

Quetiapine 12.5–25 mg one to two times a day (sedating, avoid morning/daytime doses if possible)

Lorazepam 0.25–1 mg orally or IV every 4 h if needed, only if contraindication to antipsychotics or patient is in alcohol/sedative withdrawal

major elective noncardiac surgery, higher levels of pain at rest were associated with a 1.2-fold relative risk of delirium.[19] The risk of delirium was not affected by pain with movement or by the average total daily dose of opioids.

Although uncontrolled pain can be a precipitant of delirium, so too can the opioids used to treat it. Opioid-sparing analgesia with scheduled acetaminophen and cyclooxygenase-2 (COX-2) inhibitors, if renal function allows, should be instituted when possible. Morphine, fentanyl, and hydromorphone appear to be equivalent in terms of delirium risk, while meperidine stands out as having the highest risk of delirium.[20] Tramadol does not appear to be safer than opioids. The risk of delirium is not affected by epidural compared with intravenous delivery of opioids.[20] In contrast, a prospective observational study of 333 patients aged 65 and older undergoing major elective noncardiac surgery found that patients using only oral opioids were significantly less likely to develop delirium than those using intravenous patient-controlled anesthesia. This finding remained true even after adjustment for severity of pain (OR 0.4, 95% CI 0.2–0.7).[21]

Managing Agitation

While antipsychotics are commonly used for the treatment of agitated delirium, nonpharmacologic management is the preferred first-line therapy due to adverse effects of these drugs, including paradoxical agitation, extrapyramidal symptoms, hypotension, cardiac dysrhythmias, and QT interval prolongation. Physical restraints can worsen agitation and result in patient self-injury. Instead, attempts should be made to reorient the patient several times a day, introduce familiar environmental cues such as family members, offer a sitter to help with orientation, and provide an activity vest (also known as a distraction vest) whose zippers, laces, and snaps can distract the patient from picking at their IVs and indwelling urinary catheters.

There is a scarcity of high-quality studies on the pharmacologic treatment of delirium, although both typical and atypical antipsychotics appear to be effective. As noted earlier, prophylactic haloperidol 0.5 mg three times daily decreases both severity and duration of delirium in orthopedic surgery patients.[14] In a Cochrane analysis, neither risperidone nor olanzapine was superior to low-dose (less than 3 mg/day) haloperidol, and there was no difference in adverse effects.[22] However, haloperidol at greater than 4.5 mg/day has been associated with increased extrapyramidal symptoms compared with olanzapine. Quetiapine has garnered some interest because it is sedating and has a low rate of extrapyramidal side effects. In a double-blind, randomized, placebo-controlled trial, 36 ICU patients received quetiapine 50 mg twice daily, titrated to a maximum dose of 200 mg twice daily if needed.[23] The quetiapine group experienced less agitation and faster resolution of delirium. The study group also required less haloperidol and less fentanyl, the latter not surprising given the sedating properties of quetiapine. No statistically significant difference in adverse events was noted in this underpowered pilot study. The acetylcholinesterase inhibitor donepezil has not been shown to be effective in the treatment of delirium,[24] while the cholinesterase inhibitor rivastigmine is a focus of ongoing research with small pilot trials showing inconclusive findings to date.

Benzodiazepines are generally not recommended for the treatment of delirium because they can increase both severity and duration of symptoms.[25] However, they can be a useful tool in patients with contraindications to antipsychotic therapy due to extrapyramidal side effects, neuroleptic malignant syndrome, parkinsonism, or QTc prolongation over 450 ms.

Recommendations

Nonpharmacologic therapy is the mainstay of delirium treatment (Table 30.5). If pharmacologic therapy needs to be instituted, it should be started at low scheduled or as-needed doses with gradual titration. The agent of choice is haloperidol due to the greatest experience and scientific evidence supporting its efficacy. It is worth noting that despite common use in clinical practice, intravenous haloperidol is not approved by the U.S. Food and Drug Administration. The IV formulation has the advantage of fewer extrapyramidal side effects but greater risk of cardiac dysrhythmias.[25] Atypical antipsychotics have not shown superiority in the medical literature and their lower risk of extrapyramidal side effects is offset by parkinsonism (risperidone) and sedation (olanzapine, quetiapine). Although sedation may be helpful in restoring sleep–wake cycles, it can also increase the incidence of confusion. If a benzodiazepine must be used, lorazepam is the agent of choice due to its relatively short duration of action and lack of active metabolites.

SUMMARY

Delirium is a common cause of increased morbidity and mortality in hospitalized patients, and it is frequently seen in the perioperative setting. Prevention requires early identification of at-risk patients and attentive medical management to minimize the modifiable triggers. Tools such as the CAM have good accuracy in detecting delirium once it develops, and efficacious nonpharmacologic and pharmacologic treatments exist.

REFERENCES

1. Inouye SK. Delirium in older persons. *N Engl J Med.* 2006;354:1157–1165.
2. Dasgupta M, Dumbrell AC. Preoperative risk assessment for delirium after noncardiac surgery: a systematic review. *J Am Geriatr Soc.* 2006;54:1578–1589.
3. Robinson TN, Raeburn CD, Tran ZV, Angels EM, Brenner LA, Moss M. Postoperative delirium in the elderly: risk factors and outcomes. *Ann Surg.* 2009;249:173–178.
4. Van Gool WA, Van De Beek D, Eikelenboom P. Systemic infection and delirium: when cytokines and acetylcholine collide. *Lancet.* 2010;375:773–775.
5. Sieber FE, Zakriya KJ, Gottschalk A, et al. Sedation depth during spinal anesthesia and the development of postoperative delirium in elderly patients undergoing hip fracture repair. *Mayo Clin Proc.* 2010;85:18–26.
6. Fodale V, Santamaria LB, Schifilliti D, Mandal PK. Anaesthetics and postoperative cognitive dysfunction: a pathological mechanism mimicking Alzheimer's disease. *Anaesthesia.* 2010;65:388–395.
7. Alagiakrishnan K, Marrie T, Rolfson D, et al. Simple cognitive testing (Mini-Cog) predicts in-hospital delirium in the elderly. *J Am Geriatr Soc.* 2007;55:314–316.
8. Figueroa-Ramos MI, Arroyo-Novoa CM, Lee KA, Padilla G, Puntillo KA. Sleep and delirium in ICU patients: a review of mechanisms and manifestations. *Intensive Care Med.* 2009;35:781–795.
9. Chew ML, Mulsant BH, Pollock BG, et al. Anticholinergic activity of 107 medications commonly used by older adults. *J Am Geriatr Soc.* 2008;56:1333–1341.
10. Parker MJ, Handoll HHG, Griffiths R. Anaesthesia for hip fracture surgery in adults. *Cochrane Database Syst Rev.* 2004;(4):CD000521.
11. Siddiqi N, Holt R, Britton AM, Holmes J. Interventions for preventing delirium in hospitalised patients. *Cochrane Database Syst Rev.* 2007;(2):CD005563.
12. Liptzin B, Laki A, Garb JL, Fingeroth R, Krushnell R. Donepezil in the prevention and treatment of post-surgical delirium. *Am J Geriatr Psychiatry.* 2005;13:1100–1106.
13. Gamberini M, Bolliger D, Lurati Buse GA, et al. Rivastigmine for the prevention of postoperative delirium in elderly patients undergoing elective cardiac surgery—a randomized controlled trial. *Crit Care Med.* 2009;37:1762–1768.
14. Kalisvaart KJ, De Jonghe JFM, Bogaards MJ, et al. Haloperidol prophylaxis for elderly hip-surgery patients at risk for delirium: a randomized placebo-controlled study. *J Am Geriatr Soc.* 2005;53:1658–1666.
15. Prakanrattana U, Prapaitrakool S. Efficacy of risperidone for prevention of postoperative delirium in cardiac surgery. *Anaesth Intensive Care.* 2007;35:714–719.
16. Marcantonio ER, Flacker JM, Wright RJ, Resnick NM. Reducing delirium after hip fracture: a randomized trial. *J Am Geriatr Soc.* 2001;49:516–522.
17. Wei LA, Fearing MA, Sternberg EJ, Inouye SK. The confusion assessment method (CAM): a systematic review of current usage. *J Am Geriatr Soc.* 2008;56:823–830.
18. Morrison RS, Magaziner J, Gilbert M, et al. Relationship between pain and opioid analgesics on the development of delirium following hip fracture. *J Gerontol.* 2003;58A:76–81.
19. Lynch EP, Lazor MA, Gellis JE, Orav J, Goldman L, Marcantonio ER. The impact of postoperative pain on the development of postoperative delirium. *Anesth Analg.* 1998;86:781–785.

20. Fong HK, Sands LP, Leung JM. The role of postoperative analgesia in delirium and cognitive decline in elderly patients: a systematic review. *Anesth Analg.* 2006;102:1255–1266.

21. Vaurio LE, Sands LP, Wang Y, Mullen EA, Leung JM. Postoperative delirium: the importance of pain and pain management. *Anesth Analg.* 2006;102:1267–1273.

22. Lonergan E, Britton AM, Luxenberg J. Antipsychotics for delirium. *Cochrane Databse Syst Rev.* 2007;(2):CD005594.

23. Devlin JW, Roberts RJ, Fong JJ, et al. Efficacy and safety of quetiapine in critically ill patients with delirium: a prospective, multicenter, randomized, double-blind, placebo-controlled pilot study. *Crit Care Med.* 2010;38:419–426.

24. Overshott R, Karim S, Burns A. Cholinesterase inhibitors for delirium. *Cochrane Database Syst Rev.* 2008;(1):CD005317.

25. Attard A, Ranjith G, Taylor D. Delirium and its treatment. *CNS Drugs.* 2008;22:631–644.

26. Brouquet A, Cudennec T, Benoist S, et al. Impaired mobility, ASA status and administration of tramadol are risk factors for postoperative delirium in patients aged 75 years or more after major abdominal surgery. *Ann Surg.* 2010;251:759–765.

27. Sieber FE. Postoperative delirium in the elderly surgical patient. *Anesthesiol Clin.* 2009;27: 451–464.

28. Fick DM, Cooper JW, Wade WE, Waller JL, Maclean JR, Beers MH. Updating the Beers criteria for potentially inappropriate medication use in older adults. *Arch Intern Med.* 2003;163:2716–2724.

CHAPTER 31

POSTOPERATIVE FEVER

James C. Pile

BACKGROUND

Although the reported incidence of fever after surgery varies both by the surgical population studied as well with the definition of fever, an elevated temperature is clearly one of the most common sequelae of a wide variety of surgeries. Experienced surgeons and medical consultants have long understood that in many instances, fever in the postoperative setting will prove to be self-limited and have little diagnostic or prognostic importance; however, postoperative fever may be associated with infection or another defined process, and on occasion may herald a life-threatening complication. Unfortunately, fever suffers not only from a lack of specificity in the postoperative milieu, but also from poor sensitivity, as some investigators have found that half or more of individuals with postsurgical infection will fail to mount a febrile response.[1-3]

Considerable misunderstanding continues to shroud this topic, despite the emergence of a wealth of evidence over the past 25 years. This chapter will examine the evidence surrounding postoperative fever, as well as acknowledge remaining questions and controversies.

PATHOPHYSIOLOGY

Fever is best considered a regulated elevation of body temperature, in which a raised central set point leads to "intentional" increased heat generation through some combination of shivering/muscle contraction, peripheral vasoconstriction, and increased metabolism in brown adipose tissue.[4] In contrast, life-threatening hyperthermic states such as heat stroke and malignant hyperthermia involve dysregulation of thermogenesis, with heat generation bypassing usual regulatory controls and leading to core temperatures of >41.0°C, levels seldom if ever encountered with true fever.[5] Conceptually, fever may be understood as the result of the release of multiple cytokines (interleukin-1 [IL-1], interleukin-6 [IL-6], tumor necrosis factor-α, interferon-γ) as a final common pathway in response to a variety of insults, which include infection, tissue trauma, and burns. These so-called "endogenous pyrogens" appear

Perioperative Medicine: Medical Consultation and Co-Management, First Edition.
Edited by Amir K. Jaffer and Paul J. Grant.
© 2012 Wiley-Blackwell. Published 2012 by John Wiley & Sons, Inc.

to act in concert on the preoptic area of the brain located in and near the hypothalamus, leading to prostaglandin release and culminating in fever. Although widely held, this sequence of events is almost certainly overly simplistic, and the entire topic of thermoregulation remains relatively poorly understood.[5]

Normal human temperature has been widely considered to be 98.6°F/37.0°C since Wunderlich's work published in 1868. More recent evidence suggests that mean body temperature is probably closer to 36.8°C, with substantial diurnal variation. Mackowiak and colleagues found in a study of 140 healthy individuals that the upper limit of normal temperature (i.e., 99th percentile) appeared to be 37.7°C in the late afternoon, and thus proposed that any temperature ≥37.8°C be considered a fever.[6] Despite these fairly convincing data, most physicians continue to adhere to Wunderlich's time-honored cutoff of ≥38.0°C as indicative of fever. It should be recognized that any definition of fever represents a somewhat arbitrary balance of sensitivity and specificity.[7]

No consensus exists regarding the definition of postoperative fever, although many authors have selected a temperature of ≥38.0°C on two occasions several hours apart, with some utilizing a more rigorous definition of ≥38.5°C. Multiple investigators have confirmed the importance of IL-6 as an apparent mediator of postoperative fever, while IL-1 and tumor necrosis factor-α have not been clearly linked to fever in this situation.[8–11] Wortel and colleagues as well as Frank and colleagues have shown that the extent of surgery appears to correlate with release of IL-6, as well as demonstrated a high degree of correlation between IL-6 production and the magnitude of fever: in other words, the larger the surgery, the greater the amount of IL-6 production, with an attendant increased likelihood of fever.[8,9] More recent work suggests that IL-6 production and postoperative fever are also determined in part by genetic predisposition.[10]

POSTOPERATIVE ASSESSMENT

Generations of surgeons have recognized that cryptic fever is commonly encountered shortly after many procedures, and that in most cases it is relatively brief in duration and benign. Probably as a result of the desire for clear attribution of these fevers to a defined cause, countless surgical and medical house officers have been taught that the most common etiology of fever occurring in the early postoperative period is atelectasis, despite a paucity of evidence to support this. Engoren debunked this putative association in an elegant 1995 study, demonstrating a clear inverse relationship between fever and atelectasis early in the postoperative period in patients undergoing open heart surgery.[12] This was recently substantiated by another study of post-coronary artery bypass grafting patients, in which lung expansion maneuvers after surgery were found to markedly reduce atelectasis, but to have no effect on postoperative fever.[13]

Abundant evidence now exists for the causation of most early, self-limited fever after surgery by direct tissue trauma with attendant release of pyrogenic cytokines, particularly IL-6 as discussed above. This appears to explain why larger surgeries with a greater extent of tissue damage are more likely to lead to fever, a

TABLE 31.1.   Serious/Life-Threatening Causes of Postoperative Fever

Adrenal crisis

Pulmonary embolism

Peritoneal soilage

Alcohol/benzodiazepine withdrawal

Bacterial meningitis (after neurosurgical procedures)

Clostridial/group A streptococcal myonecrosis

Toxic shock syndrome

Septicemia (bacterial or fungal)

Malignant hyperthermia

Fat embolism

phenomenon demonstrated in a study by Frank and colleagues. In their series, patients with major vascular procedures were more likely to develop postoperative fever than those undergoing abdominal surgeries, who in turn had higher postoperative temperatures than those having carotid endarterectomy, a procedure involving relatively little tissue trauma.[9] This has been corroborated by studies showing significantly greater risk of fever with hysterectomy performed via abdominal compared with vaginal approach, or cholecystectomy done in open fashion versus laparoscopically.[14,15]

Unfortunately, no single litmus test exists to differentiate the majority of postoperative fevers with a benign and self-limited course from those with a definable cause, but timing of fever onset is typically very helpful in this regard. Garibaldi and colleagues showed in a 1985 landmark study of 871 general surgical patients that the large majority of fevers occurring on postoperative day 1 proved to be unexplained, with virtually all of these resolving by postoperative day 4, while those fevers beginning 5 or more days after surgery typically proved to have an infectious etiology.[16] A wide variety of investigators have since confirmed that early postoperative fever (i.e., beginning in the first 2 days after surgery) is highly likely to be noninfectious, and in fact not to have a definable cause, while fevers appearing 3–4 days or more after surgery are increasingly likely to have a discrete cause, which in the majority of cases will prove to be infectious.[1,17–20] While most patients who develop fever in the early postoperative time frame do not require extensive investigation, no surgical patient with fever should be dismissed without a thoughtful evaluation based on history and physical examination. Potentially life-threatening conditions presenting with fever may occur at any time after surgery, and while most of these are not common, all need to be considered in the correct setting (Table 31.1).

SPECIFIC CAUSES OF POSTOPERATIVE FEVER

Infectious

Surgical Site Infection   Surgical site infections, either superficial or deep, are important causes of fever in the postoperative period. Surgical site infections are uncommon in the first several days after a procedure, with Garibaldi and colleagues reporting a peak incidence approximately 1 week after surgery.[16] Superficial (wound) infections are usually clinically apparent, while deeper infections (e.g., intra-abdominal abscesses) are frequently more challenging to diagnose, especially since the reliability of the physical examination may be compromised as a result of the surgery itself. One uncommon but important exception to the general rule that the appearance of surgical site infection tends to lag the surgical procedure by several days or more is that of wound myonecrosis, resulting from either group A strepto-coccal or clostridial infections. Infections caused by these organisms tend to be fulminant, uniformly require urgent surgical intervention with antibiotics playing an adjunctive role, and may occur within hours of surgery.

Urinary Tract Infection   Urinary tract infection rivals surgical site infection as the most common infectious etiology of postoperative fever in many studies, and is typically seen in patients exposed to urinary catheters perioperatively. Recent trends toward elimination of urinary catheters in hospitalized patients except when these are truly necessary should help to reduce the future incidence of urinary tract infec-tions in the postoperative setting. Undoubtedly, some instances of urinary tract infection diagnosed in the febrile postoperative patient actually represent coincident asymptomatic bacteriuria, rather than reflecting true causation. Unfortunately, this is frequently difficult or impossible to resolve, and points out the need for restraint in ordering urinalyses and urine cultures in the early postoperative period.[21,22]

Pneumonia   Pneumonia is a less common cause of postoperative fever than surgi-cal site infection or urinary tract infection, but is nonetheless seen with some fre-quency in this setting, particularly in patients who have required intubation after surgery or have other risk factors for postoperative pulmonary complications (surgery in proximity to the diaphragm, chronic obstructive pulmonary disease, etc.). The diagnosis of pneumonia in ventilated patients is notoriously challenging to make as a variety of other entities including atelectasis, congestive heart failure, pulmonary hemorrhage, and adult respiratory distress syndrome may present with similar mani-festations, and clinical acumen plays an important role in avoiding the overuse of broad-spectrum antibiotics in this situation.[23,24]

Clostridium difficile *Infection*   Infection with *C. difficile*, typically character-ized by diarrhea, abdominal pain, and frequently fever and leukocytosis, has long been recognized as a potential complication of surgery, and has become both increas-ingly common as well as more virulent in recent years due to emergence of the NAP1/BI clonal strain. A recent review of postsurgical *C. difficile* infection in Quebec found that of 98 affected patients, 40 had received only short prophylactic courses of antibiotics prior to onset of symptoms.[25] Avoidance of unnecessary anti-biotics after surgery is an important principle of antimicrobial stewardship, but the vast majority of patients hospitalized after surgery has received antibiotic prophylaxis, and *C. difficile* infection should be considered as a potential etiology of fever in this setting, even in the absence of diarrhea.

Other Infections   Cholecystitis is occasionally encountered in the postoperative setting, and may be either acalculous or calculous, with the former typically seen in patients who are older, more debilitated, and/or on prolonged bowel rest. The diagnosis may be challenging to make in patients with recent abdominal surgery, as typical signs and symptoms may be masked.[26] Ultrasound of the right upper quadrant will usually suffice to confirm the presence of cholecystitis in this setting. Toxic shock syndrome caused by either *Staphylococcus aureus* or group A *Streptococcus* is unusual after surgery, but has been reported after a wide variety of procedures, is typically abrupt in onset, and frequently life threatening in severity.[27,28] Central catheter-associated bloodstream infection has traditionally been a significant cause of postsurgical fever, although the increasing adoption of optimal insertion and care technique of these devices has made vascular catheter-related infections unusual in many institutions.[29] Sinusitis is probably a less common cause of fever after surgery than often believed, but nevertheless may cause symptomatic disease in the patient with prolonged nagogastric or nasotracheal intubation. Computed tomography (CT) of the sinuses has a high degree of sensitivity but rather poor specificity in confirmation of postoperative sinusitis. Transfusion-related infections manifesting as febrile illness may be seen after surgery, most commonly caused by cytomegalovirus. Typically, these patients will develop fever after hospital discharge, although they may manifest with cryptic fever as inpatients when hospitalization is complicated and prolonged.

Noninfectious Etiologies

Venous Thromboembolism (VTE)   VTE (i.e., deep venous thrombosis and pulmonary embolism) is a frequent concomitant of major surgery. In particular, major orthopedic procedures involving the lower extremities, oncologic, and trauma surgeries are complicated by significant rates of VTE events, even with appropriate prophylaxis. Although literature specifically linking VTE to fever is surprisingly scant, available evidence does support the impression of most experienced clinicians that thromboembolism may be responsible for fever. Stein and colleagues convincingly demonstrated that pulmonary embolism may cause fever, finding in a subanalysis of the PIOPED study that 43/211 (20%) of patients with angiographically proven pulmonary embolism had fever with no other apparent source. Contrary to popular belief, pulmonary infarction or hemorrhage did not appear to be necessary for the development of fever, and importantly almost all fevers were low grade, with only 5 of 43 patients manifesting a temperature higher than 38.8°C.[30] Evidence supporting the role of isolated deep venous thrombosis as a cause of fever is less robust; although taken in aggregate, these data do modestly support this relationship.[31–33]

Gout Acute exacerbation of crystal-associated arthropathy, particularly gout, is a reasonably common cause of fever after surgery, but its recognition in this situation is often delayed, which may have negative implications for a rapid response to therapy. Craig and colleagues found that 45 of 302 patients with a history of gout experienced exacerbations early after surgery, with most attacks involving the knee or ankle, and most patients manifesting associated fever.[34] In a more recent series, Kang and associates found that gout patients not receiving prophylaxis in the perioperative setting were at clearly elevated risk of developing an acute attack after surgery, underscoring the need to continue prophylactic medication through the perioperative period.[35,36]

Drug Reaction Febrile reactions to medications constitute an important cause of fever after surgery. The frequency of drug-related fever is not well understood, in part because of an absence of well-defined criteria for this diagnosis. Although virtually any medication may lead to fever, certain classes of medications have a particular predilection to do so, including beta-lactam and sulfa-based antibiotics and anti-epileptic drugs, especially phenytoin and carbamazepime. Drug fever does not present in any characteristic manner, contrary to popular belief, and although peripheral eosinophilia and/or rash may be helpful clues, they are seldom present. Although fever is reported to persist for a week or longer after discontinuation of the offending agent, in the author's experience, most patients will defervesce with considerably more alacrity.

Malignant Hyperthermia Malignant hyperthermia is a rare but a life-threatening condition associated with an autosomal-dominant genetic predisposition, and triggered by exposure to inhalational anesthetic agents, with or without succinylcholine. Signs and symptoms include hypercarbia, tachycardia, muscular rigidity, hyperthermia that may be extremely high, and in severe cases multiorgan failure. Although most cases are recognized intraoperatively, a recent review of 286 patients found that the maximum temperature occurred up to 14 h after surgical induction.[37] Thus, occasional cases of malignant hyperthermia are recognized in the postanesthesia care unit or even later. Dantrolene is the treatment of choice.

Drug Withdrawal Patients dependent on alcohol or benzodiazepines are at high risk for withdrawal states when these drugs are abruptly discontinued, such as after surgery. Typical symptoms include tremulousness and agitation frequently progressing to delirium, tachycardia, elevated blood pressure, and fever that is generally low grade but may occasionally be much higher. An accurate history of both alcohol and benzodiazepine use is critically important at the time of preoperative assessment, but as this may not be available when evaluating a febrile, delirious patient after surgery, a high index of suspicion for withdrawal states is essential, and may be lifesaving.

Adrenal Insufficiency Patients with significant chronic exposure to corticosteroid administration may manifest signs of distress when these are not continued perioperatively, including refractory hypotension, fever, abdominal symptoms, and delirium. Rarely, individuals with previously undiagnosed adrenal insufficiency may manifest evidence of adrenal crisis triggered by the stress of a surgical procedure. While general agreement exists that patients chronically receiving steroids should at least continue their usual dose perioperatively, the issue of "stress dose" supplementation of steroids at the time of surgery is highly controversial, with current data insufficient to allow definite recommendations.[38]

Other Noninfectious Etiologies A variety of other noninfectious entities may present with fever. Hematomas are underappreciated as such, but appear to be a relatively common cause of fever and leukocytosis after surgery, both of which may be quite persistent.[39] Transfusion of blood products may cause febrile reactions, and although most often seen at the time of transfusion, fever may be delayed. Serotonin syndrome should be considered in the appropriate setting, given the increasing use of medications predisposing to its development, particularly psychotropics and linezolid. The possibility of fat embolism needs to be entertained in the patient who has undergone long bone fracture and/or repair, and classically presents with fever, respiratory distress, petechial rash, and confusion. A summary of representative causes of postoperative fever, both infectious and noninfectious in nature, is presented in Table 31.2.

TABLE 31.2. Causes of Postoperative Fever

Infectious	Noninfectious
Surgical site infection	Surgical tissue trauma related (most common)
Urinary tract infection	Pulmonary embolism
Pneumonia	Deep venous thrombosis
Clostridium difficile infection	Gout
Catheter-associated bacteremia	Transfusion reaction
Cholecystitis	Drug reaction
Sinusitis	Adrenal insufficiency
Mediastinitis	Pancreatitis
Fungal infection (esp. *Candida*)	Postpericardiotomy syndrome
Cytomegalovirus (posttransfusion)	Retained surgical sponge
Intra-abdominal abscess	Thrombotic thrombocytopenic purpura (TTP)
Septic thrombophlebitis	Hematoma
Parotitis	Malignant hyperthermia
Bowel perforation	Alcohol withdrawal
Bowel anastomotic leak	Aspiration pneumonitis
Toxic shock syndrome	Serotonin syndrome
Postneurosurgical meningitis	Fat embolism
Endocarditis (nosocomial)	Antimicrobial-impregnated surgical mesh
	Hyperthyroidism
	Stroke/central fever
	Myocardial infarction
	Transplant rejection

INVESTIGATION OF THE PATIENT WITH POSTOPERATIVE FEVER

While the self-limited nature of most early postoperative fever sometimes results in the assumption that this phenomenon may be safely ignored, the fact that serious complications can and do present with fever even soon after surgery mandates that all patients with postoperative fever receive a thoughtful evaluation. On the other hand, the fact that the large majority of patients who develop fever in the first 48 h after surgery will not prove to have a clearly definable responsible process suggests that a simple, "less-is-more" approach is typically appropriate when assessing these patients. In most situations, a careful history and focused physical examination will suffice to reassure the clinician that all is well, or, conversely, to persuade him or her that further investigation is necessary. Essential elements of the history include careful elucidation of the past medical history, including history of gout, medications and medication allergies, alcohol and other drug use; details of the surgery itself, which are often best provided directly by the surgeon; receipt of blood products; and any complaints of cough, shortness of breath, chest pain, diarrhea, joint pain, dysuria, flank pain, and so on. The nursing staff and family members are often able to provide valuable information, particularly when the patient's ability to give a clear history is impaired. Physical examination should focus on the lungs and heart, abdomen, skin looking for any evidence of rash, joints, careful inspection of the surgical wound(s), and all current or recent intravenous catheter sites. In most cases of early postoperative fever, if the evaluation just described fails to suggest a more serious process, no further laboratory or imaging studies are indicated. The time-honored approach of reflexively ordering a "fever workup" consisting of some combination of blood cultures, urinalysis, urine culture, and chest radiograph cannot be condoned, and in fact de la Torre and colleagues tellingly found that on their postoperative gynecology service at an academic medical center, 55% of patients who received laboratory or radiology "investigation" of fever by a resident physician did so without being seen by the resident.[40] The lack of utility of blood cultures when obtained in the investigation of postoperative fever, particularly when fever occurs early, has been well described. Fanning and colleagues found that 0/77 blood cultures drawn in the investigation of fever after major gynecologic surgery yielded a pathogen, Swisher and colleagues found that 0/60 blood cultures in patients who developed fever after hysterectomy were positive, and Bindelglass and Pellegrino found no positive results in 100 total joint replacement patients who had blood cultures drawn to assess postoperative fever.[41-43] When higher-risk cohorts have been examined, blood cultures remain low yield. Claridge and associates as well as Kiragu and colleagues have reported that even in the intensive care unit setting, blood cultures were of essentially no utility when obtained soon after surgery, while an older study found that 85% of patients with serious postlaparotomy abdominal infections had negative blood cultures.[44-46]

Having said the above, the appearance of fever after the initial two to three postoperative days is progressively more likely to signal an infectious or other serious etiology, and the yield of additional investigation rises significantly. In particular, a CT scan of the abdomen and pelvis can be invaluable in the diagnosis of infectious complications after abdominal or pelvic surgery, and should be considered fairly early for persistent fever or other signs of potential infection in this situation.[19] Considerable interest exists in the use of novel markers such as procalcitonin to identify the subset of febrile postoperative patients with an infectious etiology, but at the time of this writing, these do not yet appear to have a clear clinical role.[47]

PREVENTION STRATEGIES

In view of the fact that most postoperative fever is directly related to surgical tissue trauma and self-limited, no preventive strategy is practical in the majority of cases. When fever is due to a defined complication after surgery, its appearance often serves as a valuable clue to the diagnosis, and so in these cases, preventing fever per se is not necessarily beneficial. Avoiding surgical complications associated with fever is desirable, however. Optimal deployment of prophylactic antibiotics, including use of the correct agent(s) administered at the appropriate time, in conjunction with other measures including intraoperative normothermia and clipping rather than shaving hair preoperatively, will help to minimize surgical site infections, while avoiding unnecessary antibiotics will decrease the incidence of *C. difficile* infections. The removal of urinary catheters as soon as feasible, continuation of prophylactic gout medications at the time of surgery, using best VTE prevention practices, avoiding inadvertent discontinuation of chronic corticosteroid administration, and early recognition of patients at risk for alcohol withdrawal will all help to decrease the incidence of febrile complications of surgery.

MEDICAL MANAGEMENT

The role of medical management in postoperative fever consists largely of attempting to identify and treat those patients with a definable complication causing the fever, and of expectant management of those who do not. Although treatment of fever with antipyretic medications (and sometimes active cooling measures such as cooling blankets) has been widely employed for both surgical and medical patients for decades, the wisdom of this strategy is questionable. Both older as well as more recent data suggest that fever is associated with improved survival in serious infections, as demonstrated in large retrospective trials of bloodstream infections, both surgical and nonsurgical.[48–50] A recent trial by Schulman and colleagues randomized febrile trauma patients in a surgical intensive care unit to either aggressive fever treatment or permissive management in which fever was not treated unless it exceeded 40°C. Although only 82 patients were randomized, the study was halted at the time of interim analysis when a trend toward greater mortality approaching statistical significance was found in the treatment group.[51]

Although these data do not distinguish whether fever is truly protective in the setting of serious infection or merely an epiphenomenon of a more robust immune response, they do suggest caution in treating most instances of postoperative fever until higher-quality prospective data are available. When the metabolic cost of fever appears likely to be excessively high (e.g., the patient with severe cardiac disease) antipyretic therapy may well be appropriate, but in most other situations probably has no role.

CONCLUSION

Postoperative fever is one of the most common surgical complications, and although the causes are myriad and potentially dangerous, most cases prove to be self-limited, and presumably arise on the basis of pyrogenic cytokines released by the trauma of surgery itself. The cornerstone of evaluation is a meticulous history and physical examination, and most fevers occurring shortly after surgery do not require additional investigation. Although interest persists in the development of a biomarker to serve as a definitive indicator of infection in the patient with postoperative fever, careful evaluation with currently available methods is sufficient to make a diagnosis in the vast majority of cases with a discrete etiology.

REFERENCES

1. Galicier C, Richet H. A prospective study of postoperative fever in a general surgery department. *Infect Control.* 1985;6:487–490.
2. Crabtree TD, Pelletier SJ, Antevil JL, Gleason TG, Pruett TL, Sawyer RG. Cohort study of fever and leukocytosis as diagnostic and prognostic indicators in infected surgical patients. *World J Surg.* 2001;25:739–744.
3. Shackelford DP, Hoffman MK, Davies MF, Kaminski PF. Predictive value for infection of febrile morbidity after vaginal surgery. *Obstet Gynecol.* 1999;93:928–931.
4. Mackowiak PA. Concepts of fever. *Arch Intern Med.* 1998;158:1870–1881.
5. Mackowiak PA. Temperature regulation and the pathogenesis of fever. In: *Principles and Practice of Infectious Diseases*, 7th edition, Mandell GL, Bennett JE, Dolin R (eds.), p. 765. Philadelphia: Churchill Livingston Elsevier; 2010.
6. Mackowiak PA, Wasserman SS, Levine MM. A critical appraisal of 98.6°F, the upper limit of the normal body temperature, and other legacies of Carl Reinhold August Wunderlich. *JAMA.* 1992;268:1578–1580.
7. Pile JC, Weed HG. Fever. In: *Perioperative Medicine: Just the Facts*, Cohn SL, Smetana GW, Weed HG (eds.), p. 275. New York: McGraw-Hill; 2006.
8. Wortel CH, van Deventer SJH, Aarden LA, et al. Interleukin-6 mediates host defense responses induced by abdominal surgery. *Surgery.* 1993;114:564–570.
9. Frank SM, Kluger MJ, Kunkel SL. Elevated thermostatic setpoint in postoperative patients. *Anesthesiology.* 2000;93:1426–1431.
10. Mitchell JD, Grocott HP, Phillips-Bute B, Mathew JP, Newman MF, Bar-Yosef S. Cytokine secretion after cardiac surgery and its relationship to postoperative fever. *Cytokine.* 2007;38:37–42.
11. Andres BM, Taub DD, Gurkan I, Wenz JF. Postoperative fever after total knee arthroplasty: the role of cytokines. *Clin Orthop Relat Res.* 2003;415:221–231.
12. Engoren M. Lack of association between atelectasis and fever. *Chest.* 1995;107:81–84.
13. Westerdahl E, Lindmark B, Eriksson T, Friberg O, Hedensteirna G, Tenling A. Deep-breathing exercises reduce atelectasis and improve pulmonary function after coronary artery bypass surgery. *Chest.* 2005;128:3482–3488.
14. Peipert JF, Weitzen S, Cruickshank C, Story E, Ethridge D, Lapane K. Risk factors for febrile morbidity after hysterectomy. *Obstet Gynecol.* 2004;103:86–91.

15. Dauleh MI, Rahman S, Townell NH. Open versus laparoscopic cholecystectomy: a comparison of postoperative temperature. *J R Coll Surg Edinb*. 1995;40:116–118.
16. Garibaldi RA, Brodine S, Matsumiya S, Coleman M. Evidence for the non-infectious etiology of early postoperative fever. *Infect Control*. 1985;6:273–277.
17. Shaw JA, Chung R. Febrile response after knee and hip arthroplasty. *Clin Orthop Relat Res*. 1999;367:181–189.
18. Ward DT, Hansen EN, Takemoto SK, Bozic KJ. Cost and effectiveness of postoperative fever diagnostic evaluation in total joint arthroplasty patients. *J Arthroplasty*. April 2010;25(3):e25.
19. da Luz Moreira A, Vogel JD, Kaladay MF, Hammel J, Fazio VW. Fever evaluations after colorectal surgery: identification of risk factors that increase yield and decrease cost. *Dis Colon Rectum*. 2008;51:508–513.
20. Mellors JW, Kelly JJ, Gusberg RJ, Horwitz SM, Horwitz RI. A simple index to estimate the likelihood of bacterial infection in patients developing fever after abdominal surgery. *Am Surg*. 1988;54:558–564.
21. Nicolle LE, Bradley S, Colgan R, Rice JC, Schaeffer A, Hooton TM. Infectious Diseases Society of America guidelines for the diagnosis and treatment of asymptomatic bacteriuria in adults. *Clin Infect Dis*. 2005;40:643–654.
22. Hooton TM, Bradley SF, Cardenas DD, et al. Diagnosis, prevention, and treatment of catheter-associated urinary tract infections in adults: 2009 international clinical practice guidelines from the Infectious Diseases Society of America. *Clin Infect Dis*. 2010;50:625–663.
23. O'Grady NP, Barie PS, Bartlett JG, et al. Guidelines for evaluation of new fever in critically ill adult patients: 2008 update from the American College of Critical Care Medicine and the Infectious Diseases Society of America. *Crit Care Med*. 2008;36:1330–1349.
24. Singh N, Falestiny MN, Rogers P, et al. Pulmonary infiltrates in the surgical ICU: prospective assessment of predictors of etiology and mortality. *Chest*. 1998;114:1129–1136.
25. Carignan A, Allard C, Pepin J, Cossette B, Nault V, Valiquette L. Risk of *Clostridium difficile* infection after perioperative antibacterial prophylaxis before and during an outbreak of infection due to a hypervirulent strain. *Clin Infect Dis*. 2008;46:1838–1843.
26. Fabian TC, Hickerson WL, Mangiante EC. Posttraumatic and postoperative acute cholecystitis. *Am Surg*. 1986;52:188–192.
27. Bartlett P, Reingold AL, Graham DR. Toxic shock syndrome associated with surgical wound infections. *JAMA*. 1982;247:1448–1450.
28. de Moya MA, Del Carmen MG, Allain RM, Hirschberg RE, Shepard JO, Kradin RL. Case 33-2009: a 35-year-old woman with fever, abdominal pain, and hypotension after cesarean section. *N Engl J Med*. 2009;361:1689–1697.
29. Pronovost P, Needham D, Berenholtz S, et al. An intervention to decrease catheter-related bloodstream infections in the ICU. *N Engl J Med*. 2006;355:2725–2732.
30. Stein PD, Afzal A, Henry JW, Villareal CG. Fever in acute pulmonary embolism. *Chest*. 2000;117:39–42.
31. Appleberg M. The value of the postoperative temperature chart as an aid to the diagnosis of deep vein thrombosis. *S Afr Med J*. 1976;50:2149–2150.
32. Faris IB, Rosengarten DS, Dudley HAF. Temperature-chart analysis in the diagnosis of postoperative deep-vein thrombosis. *Lancet*. 1972;2(7781):775–776.
33. Rickford CRK, Negus D. The early detection of postoperative deep vein thrombosis: an assessment of Doppler ultrasound, physical examination and the temperature chart. *Br J Surg*. 1975;62:182–185.
34. Craig MH, Poole GV. Postsurgical gout. *Am Surg*. 1995;61:56–59.
35. Kang EH, Lee EY, Lee YJ, Lee EB. Clinical features and risk factors of postsurgical gout. *Ann Rheum Dis*. 2008;67:1271–1275.
36. Mandel BF, Edwards NL, Sundy JS, Simkin PA, Pile JC. Preventing and treating acute gout attacks across the clinical spectrum: a roundtable discussion. *Cleve Clin J Med*. 2010;77(Suppl 2):S2–25.
37. Larach MG, Gronert GA, Allen GC, Brandom BW, Lehman EB. Clinical presentation, treatment, and complications of malignant hyperthermia in North America from 1987 to 2006. *Anesth Analg*. 2010;110:498–507.
38. Marik PE, Varon J. Requirement of perioperative stress doses of corticosteroids: a systematic review of the literature. *Arch Surg*. 2008;143:1222–1226.

39. Hausmann MJ, Kachko L, Basok A, Schnaider A, Yom-Tov G, Shefer A. Prolonged fever following kidney biopsy: a case report. *Int Urol Nephrol.* 2009;41:423–425.
40. de la Torre SH, Mandel L, Goff BA. Evaluation of postoperative fever: usefulness and cost-effectiveness of routine workup. *Am J Obstet Gynecol.* 2003;188:1642–1647.
41. Fanning J, Neuhoff RA, Brewer JE, Castaneda T, Marcotte MP, Jacobson RL. Frequency and yield of postoperative fever evaluation. *Infect Dis Obstet Gynecol.* 1998;6:252–255.
42. Swisher ED, Kahleifeh B, Pohl JF. Blood cultures in febrile patients after hysterectomy: cost effectiveness. *J Reprod Med.* 1997;42:547–550.
43. Bindelglass DF, Pellegrino J. The role of blood cultures in the acute evaluation of postoperative fever in arthroplasty patients. *J Arthroplasty.* 2007;22:701–702.
44. Claridge JA, Golob JE, Fadlalla AMA, Malangoni MA, Blatnik J, Yowler CJ. Fever and leukocytosis in critically ill trauma patients: it is not the blood. *Am Surg.* 2009;75:405–410.
45. Kiragu AW, Zier J, Cornfield DN. Utility of blood cultures in postoperative pediatric intensive care unit patients. *Pediatr Crit Care Med.* 2009;10:364–368.
46. Le Gall JR, Fagniez PL, Meakins J, Brun Buisson C, Trunet P, Carlet J. Diagnostic features of early high post-laparotomy fever: a prospective study of 100 patients. *Br J Surg.* 1982;69:452–455.
47. Hunziker A, Hugle T, Schuchardt K, et al. The value of serum procalcitonin level for differentiation of infectious from noninfectious causes of fever after orthopaedic surgery. *J Bone Joint Surg Am.* 2010;92:138–148.
48. Bryant RE, Hood AF, Hood CE, Koenig MG. Factors affecting mortality of gram-negative rod bacteremia. *Arch Intern Med.* 1971;127:120–128.
49. Mackowiak PA, Browne RH, Southern PM, Smith JW. Polymicrobial sepsis: an analysis of 184 cases using log linear models. *Am J Med Sci.* 1980;280:73–80.
50. Swenson BR, Hedrick TL, Popovsky K, Pruett TL, Sawyer RG. Is fever protective in surgical patients with bloodstream infection? *J Am Coll Surg.* 2007;204:815–823.
51. Schulman CI, Namias N, Doherty J, et al. The effect of antipyretic therapy upon outcomes in critically ill patients: a randomized, prospective study. *Surg Infect (Larchmt).* 2005;6:369–375.

CHAPTER 32

VENOUS THROMBOEMBOLISM

Darrell W. Harrington and Katayoun Mostafaie

BACKGROUND/EPIDEMIOLOGY

Venous thromboembolism (VTE), including deep vein thrombosis (DVT) and pulmonary embolism (PE), remains one the most common preventable perioperative complications. In the absence of effective prophylactic regimens, rates of VTE range from 15% to 20% in hospitalized medical patients to as high as 80% in high-risk patients undergoing elective major surgery. The annual incidence of VTE has been estimated at approximately 100 per 100,000 persons, and PE is responsible for at least 200,000 deaths annually in the United States alone.[1] The true incidence of perioperative VTE is unknown as many events go undiagnosed and occur postdischarge. In a large prospective study, 74% of all VTEs occurred in the outpatient setting with 23% of such patients undergoing a recent surgery.[2] The vague presentation and resulting delay or misdiagnosis of this important postoperative complication leads to increasing morbidity and mortality.

Unfortunately, acute PE is often lethal and over 10% of symptomatic patients die within the first hour of onset of symptoms. Despite the resolution of the majority of PE within the first 30 days, up to 5% may go on to develop chronic pulmonary hypertension during the first 2 years following the inciting event. Chronic venous insufficiency develops in approximately 40% of patients diagnosed with DVT and is strongly associated with the development of post-thrombotic syndrome.

The risk of postoperative VTE varies from patient to patient depending on a variety of procedure-specific and patient-specific risk factors. Although some postoperative patients may still suffer new symptomatic events even with the administration of perioperative VTE prophylaxis, the use of evidence-based VTE prophylaxis remains the most effective strategy for reducing the burden of VTE in the population.

Appreciation of the burden of VTE in the perioperative period, appropriate prophylaxis, and timely treatment are critical in the management of surgical patients.

Perioperative Medicine: Medical Consultation and Co-Management, First Edition.
Edited by Amir K. Jaffer and Paul J. Grant.
© 2012 Wiley-Blackwell. Published 2012 by John Wiley & Sons, Inc.

PATHOPHYSIOLOGY

During the last decade, the basic science and pathophysiology of VTE has grown tremendously. The identification of circulating tissue factor and the role of specific binding ligands produced and expressed in various diseases continues to evolve. However, Virchow's triad has endured over 150 years and offer clear rationale for the most important risk factors associated with VTE. Each factor (hypercoagulability, injured endothelium and stasis) alone or in combination explain the pathophysiological context of the perioperative patient and VTE. Risk can be described as *predisposing* and *exposing* factors. Predisposing factors are those patient-specific factors present at baseline and are independent of the planned procedure and perioperative period (i.e., advanced age, heart failure, malignancy). Exposing risk factors can be defined as those factors more directly related to the perioperative setting such as the surgery itself, anesthesia, immobility, and severe infection. Ultimately, trauma to vessels leads to endothelial injury and resulting aggregation of platelets. Subsequently activation of the procoagulant cascade and suppression of fibrinolytic pathways provide for fibrin deposition and the formation of thrombus. Furthermore, supine positioning, indwelling catheters, ICU stay, postoperative infection, anemia, and venous pooling of blood due to the anesthetic agents also contribute to the risk of perioperative VTE. The dynamic interplay between both predisposing and exposing risk factors define the VTE risk in an individual patient.

It is well known that most DVT starts in the lower extremity; however, 10% is associated with the upper extremity and is usually associated with indwelling catheters, trauma, or anatomical lesions. Early studies have demonstrated asymptomatic thrombus development during the early surgical period. However, most symptomatic events occur postoperative often after hospital discharge. Recurrent VTE after adequate treatment varies according to the patient risk. Patients with reversible or transient risk factors have a 5-year recurrent VTE risk of 10% compared with approximately 30% in patients without a known etiology. Patients with symptomatic VTE and hypercoagulable states are at much higher risk for recurrent VTE and are often prescribed extended anticoagulant therapy.

Patients undergoing surgery for malignancy are at especially high risk for VTE as they often possess multiple risk factors for VTE including the primary cancer site, advanced age, history of VTE, active chemotherapy, indwelling catheters, use of erythropoiesis-stimulating agents, and poor functional status.

PREVENTION

Perioperative VTE leads to substantial inpatient costs, morbidity, and mortality.

The most important and effective strategy for managing VTE are those that focus on the active prevention of VTE in the at-risk patient.

Risk Assessment

In order for risk stratification to be successful, it should be simple and evidence based. Recently, two risk assessment models (RAMs) have been validated in single-center populations.[3,4] However, many of such models are not widely incorporated into clinical practice as they are often viewed as too cumbersome or criticized as not adequately validated.

It is expected that each hospitalized patient is assessed for VTE risk. One of the methods of risk assessment is to evaluate risk in each patient based on their individual predisposing factors and the risk associated with their procedure. The patient-specific risk factors for DVT and PE are listed in Table 32.1.[5] Such risk factors are used in combination with the surgical procedure to stratify VTE risk in individual patients. The American College of Chest Physicians (ACCP) evidence-based guideline stratifies VTE risk based on the procedure as well as patient-specific risk factors into three categories—low risk, moderate risk, and high risk. In the absence of appropriate prophylaxis, the rate of proximal DVT and PE is <1% and <0.01% in low-risk, 2–4% and 0.1–0.4% in moderate-risk, and 4–8% and 0.4–1% in high-risk patients, respectively.[5] Although intuitive and widely adopted, there is little evidence to validate this approach. Alternatively, VTE risk may be assigned to groups of patients based on the overall risk to the target population as it relates to the procedure itself.

Prevention Strategies

An ideal prophylactic method for VTE should be safe and effective when compared with placebo or active approaches. In addition, the treatment modality should also be easily administered; have good compliance by patients, nurses, and physicians; and be cost-effective. Although early ambulation of postoperative patients may intuitively decrease risk of DVT, it has not been rigorously tested. In addition, this is not always possible and should not be used as the sole strategy in patients at moderate-to-high risk for VTE. A variety of methods have been used to prevent VTE and include both mechanical and pharmacological therapy strategies, as well as placement of prophylactic inferior vena cava (IVC) filters. Table 32.2 outlines the current ACCP recommendations for VTE prophylaxis in patients undergoing surgery.[5]

Mechanical Thromboprophylaxis Specific mechanical methods are graduated compression stockings (GCSs), intermittent pneumatic compression (IPC) devices, and the venous foot pump. All of the mentioned devices increase venous flow and decrease stasis. In addition, none of these methods increase the risk of bleeding in the postoperative patient. Overall, mechanical prophylaxis is not as efficacious in preventing DVT as anticoagulant thromboprophylaxis. The ACCP guideline provides a strong recommendation against the use of mechanical methods of thromboprophylaxis unless there is a contraindication to the recommended pharmacological strategy and to introduce pharmacological preventive strategies as soon as possible

TABLE 32.1. Risk Factors for VTE

Surgery requiring more than 30 min of anesthesia
    Trauma
    Orthopedic surgery especially hip fracture, hip and knee replacement, knee arthroscopy
    Gynecology, general and urological surgery especially for cancer
    Fracture of pelvis, femur, or tibia

Cancer and chemotherapy

Prolonged immobilization, nursing home confinement

Venous compression

History of VTE

Increasing age (>40 years)

Pregnancy and the postpartum period

Estrogen-containing oral contraceptives or hormonal replacement

Selective estrogen receptor modulators

Erythropoiesis-stimulating agents

Acute medical illness (i.e., MI, severe infection, stroke, heart failure, COPD)

Inflammatory bowel disease

Nephrotic syndrome

Myeloproliferative disorder

Paroxysmal nocturnal hemoglobinuria

Cigarette smoking

Obesity

Long-haul air travel

Central venous catheterization

Inherited or acquired thrombophilia

    Antithrombin deficiency
    Protein C or S deficiency
    Prothrombin G20210A mutation
    Factor V Leiden
    Anticardiolipin antibody syndrome

Lupus anticoagulant

VTE, venous thromboembolism; COPD, chronic obstructive pulmonary disease; MI, myocardial infarction. Adapted from Geerts et al.[5]

TABLE 32.2. ACCP Recommendations for Thromboprophylaxis Based on Risk (Alternative)

Level of risk	DVT risk without prophylaxis	Thromboprophylaxis	Level of evidence
Low risk	<10%	Early ambulation	Grade 1A
Moderate risk	10–40%		
General surgery		LMWH, LDUH,[a] fondaparinux	Grade 1A
Gyn surgery			
– Minor		Early ambulation	Grade 1A
– Laparoscopic		Early ambulation	Grade 1B
– Major surgery		LMWH, LDUH	Grade 1A
– Gyn/onc surgery		LMWH, LDUH[a]	Grade 1A
Urological surgery			
– Transurethral		Early ambulation	Grade 1A
		LDUH, LMWH	Grade 1B
		Fondaparinux	Grade 1C
– Major urological		Early ambulation	Grade 1C
		LMWH, LDUH TID, fondaparinux	Grade 1C
Vascular surgery			
Bariatric surgery			
High risk	40–80%		
Major trauma		LMWH	Grade 1A
TKR, THR		LMWH, fondaparinux, warfarin	Grade 1A
HFS		Fondaparinux, LMWH, warfarin, LDUH	Grades 1A–1B
Neurosurgery		IPC	Grade 1A
Spinal cord injury		LMWH	Grade 1B

[a] The dose of LDUH for higher-risk patients undergoing cancer operations or major surgery is recommended three times per day.
Grade system:
I = There is strong certainty regarding the magnitude of benefit and risks, burden, and cost.
II = There is less certainty regarding the magnitude of benefit and risks, burden, and cost.
A. There is high-quality evidence to support the recommendation.
B. There is moderate-quality evidence to support the recommendation.
C. There is low-quality evidence to support the recommendation.
LDUH, low-dose unfractionated heparin; LMWH, low-molecular-weight heparin; IPC, intermittent pneumatic compression; TKR, total knee replacement; THR, total hip replacement; HFS, hip fracture surgery; TID, three times daily.
Adapted from Geerts et al.[5]

postoperatively. This recommendation is based on methodological flaws in many trials, the lack of uniformity or standardization of the devices, and most importantly poor compliance by both patients and providers. Furthermore, increasing data confirm that the efficacy of mechanical devices is directly associated with compliance and duration of use of device within a 24-h period. Therefore, mechanical methods of thromboprophylaxis should be used primarily in patients at high risk for bleeding, or as an adjunct to pharmacological thromboprophylaxis.

Pharmacological Thromboprophylaxis Aspirin is not considered an effective thromboprophylaxis agent in surgical patients. Although listed as a strategy in the American Association of Orthopedic Surgery (AAOS) guideline, the AAOS only recommend use of aspirin in patients with lower risk for VTE or in those with increased risk of bleeding.[7] Low-dose unfractionated heparin (LDUH) is inexpensive; however, given its short half-life, it requires two to three injections per day. The risk of heparin-induced thrombocytopenia (HIT) is also a concern and can be as high as 5%. Another inexpensive option is warfarin, which is orally administered. However, use of warfarin requires international normalized ratio (INR) monitoring and based on pharmacokinetic properties exhibits a delay in the onset of action. Patients on warfarin alone lack prophylaxis for several days and are at increased risk of DVT during this period. Therefore, warfarin should not be used alone as thromboprophylaxis in high-risk patients. Low-molecular-weight heparins (LMWHs) administered subcutaneously one to two times per day are another option for prophylaxis. LMWHs are more expensive than LDUH; yet, they are associated with less incidence of HIT. Fondaparinux is an inhibitor of factor X and can be administered once daily due to its long half-life. Certain LMWHs such as enoxaparin can be used in patients with a creatinine clearance of <30 mL/min, but the dose of medication needs to be adjusted. Fondaparinux on the other hand is contraindicated in patients with creatinine clearances of <30 mL/min.

New Anticoagulants During the last few years, several novel anticoagulants have emerged in the management of VTE. Three agents—apixaban and rivaroxaban (oral direct factor Xa inhibitors) and dabigatran (an oral direct thrombin inhibitor)––show promise in the prevention of VTE. Phase III trials particularly in patients undergoing major orthopedic surgery have confirmed that these agents are equal to or superior in efficacy compared with standard prophylactic regimens. These agents also exhibit a good overall safety profile including hepatoxicity in the setting of a clinical trial. Currently, only dabigatran is U.S. Food and Drug Administration (FDA) approved for use in patients with chronic atrial fibrillation. Only routine use in clinical practice will ensure their role in a broad spectrum of patients with comorbidities and other unmeasurable risk. However, these target-specific oral anticoagulants with predictable pharmacologic properties will likely add to the antithrombotic regimens available to manage VTE particularly when considering outpatient prophylaxis regimens after high-risk general and orthopedic surgery.

Timing and Duration of Thromboprophylaxis Optimally, prophylaxis should begin as soon as the patient develops a risk for VTE. DVT may begin as soon as patient is immobilized or during the operation itself. However, the physician should always weigh both risk and benefit when considering when to initiate thromboprophylaxis perioperatively. Furthermore, the timing of initiation postoperatively pharmacological thromboprophylaxis should also be determined based on the type of the surgery and risk of bleeding complications.

The optimal duration of VTE prophylaxis in surgical patients has not yet been established. Most studies evaluating the efficacy of pharmacological prophylaxis in a surgical population provided treatment for 7–14 days. It should be noted, however, that the average length of hospital stay in surgical patients at risk of VTE is approximately 3–7 days. Therefore, it may be necessary to continue prophylaxis beyond discharge in some patients. For the majority of surgical patients, duration of prophylaxis is limited to the hospital stay. However, it is recommended that patients undergoing total hip replacement (THR), total knee replacement (TKR), and hip fracture surgery (HFS) receive at least 10 days of prophylaxis. In addition, extension of the thromboprophylaxis beyond 10 days and up to 35 days postoperatively confers additional benefit especially in patients with THR and HFS.[8] In addition, for patients undergoing major abdominal or pelvic surgery for cancer, prolonged prophylaxis for up to 4 weeks should be considered (see Table 32.3).[6]

Neuraxial Blockade   Timing of the anticoagulant for prophylaxis may also require coordination with the anesthesiologist as there is additional bleeding risk associated with neuraxial blockade.

The actual incidence of neurologic dysfunction resulting form hemorrhagic complication associated with neuraxial blockade is unknown but may be as high as

TABLE 32.3.   2008 ACCP VTE Prophylaxis Recommendations

General surgery
- Patients <40 years without additional risk factors or those undergoing minor surgery do not require specific thromboprophylaxis (grade 1A)
- Benign disease: LMWH, LDUH (two to three times daily), or fondaparinux (daily) (grade 1A)
- Malignant disease: LMWH, LDUH (three times daily), or fondaparinux (daily) (grade 1A). Multiple risk factors for venous thromboembolism: LMWH, LDUH, or fondaparinux + mechanical methods (grade 1C)
- High risk for bleeding: mechanical methods until the bleeding risk improves (grade 1A), following which pharmacologic methods should be considered (grade 1C)

Vascular surgery
- Major procedures with risk factors for DVT: LMWH, LDUH, or fondaparinux (grade 1C)

Gynecologic surgery
- Laparoscopic procedures with risk factors for DVT: LMWH, LDUH, +/− IPC, or GCS (grade 1C)
- Major procedures: LMWH, LDUH,[a] or fondaparinux (grade 1A)

Urologic surgery
- Major, open procedures: LMWH, LDUH, or fondaparinux (grade 1A)
- High risk for bleeding: mechanical methods until the bleeding risk improves (grade 1A), following which pharmacologic methods should be considered (grade 1C)

Laparoscopic surgery
- With additional risk factors (i.e., previous VTE): LMWH, LDUH, +/− IPC, or GCS (grade 1C)

Bariatric surgery
- LMWH, LDUH, or fondaparinux +/− IPC (grade 1C)

(Continued)

TABLE 32.3. *Continued*

Thoracic surgery
- Major procedures: LMWH, LDUH, or fondaparinux (grade 1C)
- High risk for bleeding: properly fitted GCS and/or IPC (grade 1C)

Coronary artery bypass surgery
- LMWH, LDUH +/– IPC, or GCS (grade 1C)
- High risk for bleeding: properly fitted GCS and/or IPC (grade 1C)

Elective hip/knee replacement surgery
- LMWH started 12 h before or 12–24 h after the procedure, or start with a half dose 4–6 h after surgery, with a full dose the next day; *or*
- Fondaparinux 2.5 mg SC started 6–24 h after surgery; *or*
- Adjusted dose vitamin K antagonist, starting 1 day before the surgery with a target INR of 2–3.0 (grade 1A)
- Pharmacologic therapy continued for a minimum of 10 days (up to 35 days in hip replacement) after surgery (grade 1A)
- High-risk bleeding: optimal use of VFP or IPC (grade 1A)

Hip fracture surgery
- Same as above; *or*
- LMWH or LDUH, started at the time of admission if surgery delayed (grade 1C)

Knee arthroscopy
- Patients with additional risk factors for VTE should receive LMWH (grade 1B)

Elective spine surgery
- Patients with a high risk for deep DVT or PE should receive postoperative LDUH, LMWH +/– GCS, IPC

Isolated, distal-to-the-knee surgery
- No specific therapy

Neurosurgery
- Major procedures: postoperative LMWH or LDUH +/– GCS or IPC (grade 2B)

Trauma/burns/spinal cord injury
- For all patients LMWH, when safe to use (grade 1A)
- Bleeding complications: mechanical methods with GCS or IPC (grade 1B); duplex surveillance only in patients at high risk for DVT (grade 1C)

---

[a] The dose of LDUH for higher risk patients undergoing cancer operations or major surgery is recommended three times per day.

Grade system:

I = There is strong certainty regarding the magnitude of benefit and risks, burden, and cost.

II = There is less certainty regarding the magnitude of benefit and risks, burden, and cost.

A. There is high-quality evidence to support the recommendation.

B. There is moderate-quality evidence to support the recommendation.

C. There is low-quality evidence to support the recommendation.

LDUH, low-dose unfractionated heparin; LMWH, low-molecular-weight heparin; IPC, intermittent pneumatic compression; SC, subcutaneous; VFP, venous foot pump.

Adapted from Geerts et al.[5]

1 in 3000. Patients receiving pharmacologic prophylaxis for VTE are at increased risk of spinal hematoma when undergoing spinal or epidural anesthesia based on the anesthetic technique used, patient factors, and dose of anticoagulant. Special precautions are to be taken with the timing of the prophylactic medication and the needle placement and removal of epidural catheters. The American Society of Regional Anesthesia and Pain Medicine Evidence-Based Guideline details proposed management guidelines to reduce the risk (Table 32.4).[9]

POSTOPERATIVE ASSESSMENT

Clinical Presentation of VTE

The signs and symptoms of both DVT and PE are notoriously unreliable. Such nonspecific presentations may result in delay of diagnosis and subsequent initiation of antithrombotic therapy thereby blunting effective reduction of morbidity and mortality. In addition, VTE in the postoperative setting most commonly presents after discharge in the outpatient setting following elective surgery. Furthermore, diagnosing VTE in the perioperative setting is complex as there is a paucity of data regarding test characteristics in the surgical patients.

Diagnosing DVT

The diagnosis of DVT has eluded clinicians for centuries as the presenting features vary from subtle aching to frank erythema and pain. While the gold standard for the confirmation of DVT has been contrast venography, this test is seldom performed. In addition, unnecessary testing may lead to unnecessary cost as well as exposure to the potential risk of unnecessary therapy. Ultrasound is now routinely ordered in patients suspected of DVT; however, the sensitivity and specificity of the test dictate that its result is interpreted in the context of the patients' likelihood of having the disease. Accordingly, the best outcomes are associated with the incorporation of clinical prediction rules with the results of objective test to best determine not only application of cost-effective strategies but also optimize clinical outcomes.

Compression Ultrasound for Suspected DVT   Venous compression ultrasonography (CUS) is currently the most widely utilized noninvasive test for suspected DVT. CUS has a sensitivity of 97% and a specificity of 98% for proximal DVT, which is present in 85% of patients with symptomatic DVT. However, in the remaining 15%, the DVT is confined to the calf veins with less reliable CUS results. Approximately 25% of patients with isolated calf DVT will propagate more proximally within a week, and thus, serial noninvasives may prove beneficial in the highly suspect patient. Most recently, comprehensive CUS has emerged as a noninvasive modality to maximize the accuracy. In a 3-month follow-up study in patients with initial negative comprehensive CUS, the incidence of symptomatic DVT was 0.8%.[10] Due to significant variation in expertise, this technique must be more broadly studied before incorporation into routine practice. Other limitations of CUS include poor visualization of deep

TABLE 32.4.   Neuraxial Anesthesia in the Patient Receiving Anticoagulant Therapy

Intervention	Neuraxial anesthesia guideline	Grade
Heparin 5,000 units subQ BID	No contraindication.	1C
Heparin >10,000 subQ daily (i.e., TID dosing schedule)	Unclear if increased risk of spinal hematoma. Evaluate risks/benefits on individual basis.	2C
Epidural catheter in place >4 days	Check platelet count prior to removing catheter (HIT)	1C
Intraoperative heparin use	Ensure no preexisting coagulopathy.	
	Delay heparin 1 h after instrumentation.	
	Remove catheter 2–4 h after heparin dose; wait 1 h to restart heparin.	
	Monitor post-op and use minimal amounts of local anesthetic to increase early detection of hematoma.	
	No data to support mandatory case cancellation if bloody or difficult placement occurs. Discuss on case-by-case basis with surgeon.	
Traumatic/bloody placement	Do not delay surgery but first dose LMWH should be delayed 24 h post-op.	2C
Pre-op LMWH	Prophylactic dose: wait 10–12 h before needle placement.	1C
	High dose (i.e., enoxaparin 1 mg/kg q12h or 1.5 mg/kg qday): delay needle placement at least 24 h.	1C
	LMWH 2 h pre-op—recommend against neuraxial technique.	1A
Post-op LMWH	Twice daily dosing: first dose >24 h post-op. Remove indwelling catheters 2 h prior to first dose.	1C
	Once daily dosing: first dose 6–8 h post-op. Subsequent dose 24 h after first dose. Indwelling catheters are OK but must be removed 10–12 h after last dose and redosing should not occur until 2 h after catheter removal.	1C
Discontinuation of chronic warfarin	Stop 4–5 days preprocedure, normalize INR.	1B
Removal of epidural catheters with warfarin thromboprophylaxis	Ensure INR <1.5. Continue neurologic assessment for 24 h.	2C
Epidural removal with INR between 1.5–3.0	Review record to ensure no other hemostasis altering medications being taken. Neurological assessment prior to removal and continue until INR stable.	1C
Removal of epidural with INR >3	Warfarin dose should be held or reduced. No definitive recommendation to facilitate catheter removal.	2C
NSAIDs	No specific concerns for performance of block or removal of catheters.	1A
NSAIDs + concurrent oral anticoagulants, UFH, or LMWH	Neuraxial technique *not* recommended.	2C
Ticlopidine	Stop 14 days prior to neuraxial block.	1C
Clopidogrel	Stop 7 days prior to neuraxial block.	1C

LMWH, low-molecular-weight heparin; HIT, heparin-induced thrombocytopenia; UFH, unfractionated heparin; NSAIDs, nonsteroidal anti-inflammatory drugs; TID, three times daily; BID, twice daily.
Adapted from Horlocker et al.[9]

iliac and pelvic veins. Given the increased risk associated with venography, computed tomography (CT) and magnetic resonance venography have become alternative modalities when more proximal structures are poorly visualized.

D-Dimer Testing in DVT   D-dimer is a plasma protein produced as a by-product fibrin cleavage by plasmin. Levels are elevated in the presence of acute VTE, and therefore, D-dimer may be useful as a sensitive test to rule out acute VTE. However, D-dimer elevation is nonspecific and may be elevated by other conditions including sepsis, advanced age, surgery, pregnancy, and malignancy. Therefore, D-dimer use in the acute hospital setting may have limited utility as the presence of both comorbidities and increased prevalence of VTE in the inpatient setting undermine the predictive value of the D-dimer. In addition, diagnostic performance varies among D-dimer assays, and therefore, it is important to know the assay utilized before incorporation into the diagnostic management strategy for VTE. A recent systematic review of 12 management studies found a 3-month incidence of VTE of 0.4% in low-to-moderate pretest probability (PTP) and a normal highly sensitive D-dimer result.[11] Thus, a negative D-dimer may not only allow the provider to forego the use of additional diagnostic test, but also prevent unnecessary exposure to anticoagulant therapy. In addition, D-dimer testing should not routinely be used as a diagnostic tool in symptomatic patients with a high likelihood of DVT. Thus, D-dimer should be reserved for patients presenting as outpatients setting and not those who present to the hospital with acute signs and symptoms of VTE.

Clinical Prediction Rules for DVT   Bayes' theorem dictates that the likelihood of disease influences the interpretation of an imperfect test. While subjective clinical assessment is often used to judge likelihood of disease in a given patient, clinical prediction rules utilize standardized variables derived from patient cohorts with a suspected condition. Wells' criteria are the most widely utilized and validated clinical prediction tool for VTE and include both risk factors and clinical findings. Table 32.5 details the prediction rule and includes nine variables with 1 point assigned to each. As it is recognized that empirical physician assessment remains important to fine-tune the PTP and estimate of DVT, 2 points are subtracted from the Wells' score if an alternative diagnosis is felt to be as likely or more likely than DVT. Patients with low (score < 1), moderate (score 1–2), and high (score ≥ 3) PTP of DVT have been shown prospectively to have a prevalence of DVT of 3%, 17%, and 75%, respectively, when used alone. When evaluated systematically over multiple populations, the prevalence of DVT is 5%, 17%, and 53%, respectively. Of note, growing evidence supports the use of a dichotomized Wells' score of unlikely (≤1) or likely (≥2) in the management of DVT.[12]

Diagnostic Algorithms   Understanding the utility of the clinical history, physical exam and noninvasive test may help clinicians to provide more consistent and cost-effective management of the patient with DVT. Figure 32.1 outlines the diagnostic algorithm for DVT and begins with an estimate of PTP.[13] Use of D-dimer in the management strategy is dictated by the specific assay available. It should be noted that in the patient presenting with recurrent DVT symptoms that CUS and even

TABLE 32.5.   Simplified Clinical Model for Assessment of DVT[a]

Clinical parameter score	Score
Active cancer (treatment ongoing, or within 6 months or palliative)	+1
Paralysis or recent plaster immobilization of the lower extremities	+1
Recently bedridden for >3 days or major surgery <4 weeks	+1
Localized tenderness along the distribution of the deep venous system	+1
Entire leg swelling	+1
Calf swelling >3 cm compared with the asymptomatic leg	+1
Pitting edema (greater in the symptomatic leg)	+1
Previous DVT documented	+1
Collateral superficial veins (nonvaricose)	+1
Alternative diagnosis (as likely or greater than that of DVT)	−2

[a] Probability of DVT is "likely" if total score ≥2, probability for DVT is "unlikely" if total score is ≤1. Alternatively (original model), <1 is low probability, 1 or 2 is moderate probability, and high is >2.
DVT, deep vein thrombosis.
Adapted from Wells et al.[12]

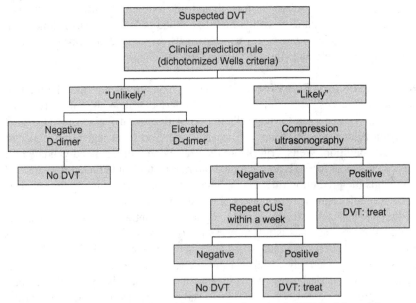

Figure 32.1.   Management algorithm for deep vein thrombosis (DVT). Adapted from Wells.[13] CUS, compression ultrasonography.

venography may be unreliable. Although preliminary data are promising, the utilization of D-dimer in the management of recurrent DVT is still unclear.

Diagnosing PE

Clinical signs and symptoms of PE are vague, and as a result, suspicion for PE in many patients is based on nonspecific chest and respiratory complaints. The PIOPED

II investigators most recently found that while 75% of patients diagnosed with PE had dyspnea, approximately 52% were tachypnic, only 20% were tachycardic, and 44% had a cough.[14] In addition, many patients with PE have no lower extremity symptoms, and in as many as 30% of patients, no etiology or risk factor can be identified. No constellation of clinical signs or symptoms is specific or sensitive enough to reliably rule in or out the diagnosis of PE. Equally important is the limitation of objective examinations such as electrocardiogram (ECG), chest X-ray, and arterial blood gas. Such test even when abnormal rarely provide the diagnostic accuracy to alone or in combination confirm or remove suspicion of the disease. For example, the classic "$S_1Q_3T_3$" changes strongly suggestive of PE are found in less than 10% of patients diagnosed with PE and are also found in many other cardiac and pulmonary disorders. Therefore, the significant risk of morbidity and mortality of PE require that clinicians utilize evidence-based strategies to diagnose PE.

Diagnostic Imaging for PE Pulmonary angiography is regarded as the gold standard test for the diagnosis of PE and is invasive and accompanied by significant expense. Even the setting of a negative pulmonary angiogram, as many as 1.6% of patients may develop PE during a 1-year follow-up with most in the first month. A normal ventilation–perfusion scan essentially rules out PE, and a high-probability scan rules in PE. However, a large proportion of these studies remain nondiagnostic and dictate additional investigation in which the incidence of PE in this population varies from 10% to 30%. Therefore, the ventilation–perfusion lung scan has largely been replaced by computer tomographic pulmonary angiography (CTPA). However, early single-slice CTPA was unable to detect subsegmental arteries sufficiently. The sensitivity and specificity of CTPA single-detector scanners were most recently evaluated in 627 consecutive patients and found to be 69% and 84%, respectively.[15] Because of fear of missing PE, management strategies have been incorporated with the use of CTPA. Multidetector CT with its improved resolution and speed, as well as three-dimensional reconstruction, makes CTPA an attractive noninvasive test for patients with symptomatic PE and has largely supplanted single-detector scanners. The PIOPED investigators published the results of a large prospective management study demonstrating a much better sensitivity and specificity of 83% and 96%, respectively.[14] Unfortunately, multidetector scanners may be too good, and now questions regarding the false detection of PE or the potential detection of clinically irrelevant embolism are important considerations requiring further investigation and follow-up.

D-Dimer Testing in PE Use of a D-dimer test to exclude PE is well established, and its utility is dependent on both the clinical PTP of PE and the sensitivity of the D-dimer test employed. Although the negative predicative value is the most important characteristic of the D-dimer assay, it should not be without clinical assessment of the likelihood for PE (i.e., PTP) and also lacks sufficient specificity to be used to confirm the suspicion of PE. Like DVT, the population in which the test is utilized strongly influences its utility. Therefore, highly sensitive D-dimers with likelihood ratio of 0.06–0.09 may still be inadequate to exclude the diagnosis of PE in the immediate postoperative setting especially in extreme elderly patients (>80 years of age) and in the critically ill patient. Even with the above exceptions, a single, rapid, highly sensitive D-dimer test, if negative (i.e., 500 μg/L), can safely exclude PE in the majority of patients with a "nonhigh" clinical PTP of PE. All patients suspected of PE with a positive D-dimer test must undergo further diagnostic testing.

CUS for Suspected PE Most experts agree that symptomatic VTE represents only a fraction of the disease and that many patients have subclinical disease, which may go undetected. Historically, venographic studies of the lower extremities are positive in over 85% of patients with proven PE. Abnormal CUS can be demonstrated in up to 30% of patients with proven PE—although many of such patients had none or vague lower extremity symptoms. Accordingly, CUS is still incorporated into the management strategies for PE especially when there are discordant clinical likelihood and imaging results. Results of the PIOPED II study demonstrated that a negative CTPA was inadequate to rule out VTE in patients with a high clinical PTP of PE, making it necessary for patients to undergo further testing.[14] Likewise, in patients with a low clinical PTP of PE and a positive CTPA, confirmation of VTE with additional test may be required. However, the PIOPED II investigators allowed the use of both single-detector and multidetector CTPA. Multidetector CTPA is now the most widely utilized imaging modality for PE. There are now multiple large prospective management studies that demonstrate that fewer than 1.5% of patients with a negative multidetector CTPA will have an abnormal CUS, making routine use of CUS cost-ineffective. However, there may be utility for CUS in a patient presenting with concomitant leg symptoms, thus avoiding unnecessary radiation exposure, if only single-detector CTPA is available, or if a VQ scan is used as the imaging modality and there is a nondiagnostic result (see Figure 32.2).

Clinical Prediction Rules for PE While physician gestalt and diagnostic impression have proven value, it is difficult to generalize such empiric and subjective strategy. Several clinical prediction rules have been described to assess the probability of PE using clinical findings. The most widely applied model was developed by Wells.[16] The original Wells model utilized seven clinical variables (Table 32.6) and categorized patients into three levels of probability for PE (low, moderate, or high). Most recently, this model has been simplified, and patients are now risk-stratified into two groups: "likely" (Wells score > 4) or "unlikely" (Wells score ≤ 4). This dichotomized model has subsequently been validated to reliably stratify patients suspected of PE. The revised Geneva rule has also been utilized in the evaluation of patients with suspected PE and utilizes nine clinical variables without the use of arterial blood gas and the reliance on empiric clinical judgment.[17] The Geneva rule has been primarily validated in the emergency room setting and performs comparatively with the Wells model.

Diagnostic Algorithms Evaluation of patients with suspected PE is most effectively guided by adherence to evidence-based strategies that incorporate clinical assessment, D-dimer testing, and imaging modalities. Furthermore, it is important not only to diagnose PE, but to consider prognostic information when considering treatment strategies. Figure 32.2 shows an evidence-based diagnostic algorithm using a multidetector CTPA as the imaging modality.[18] It is important to remember

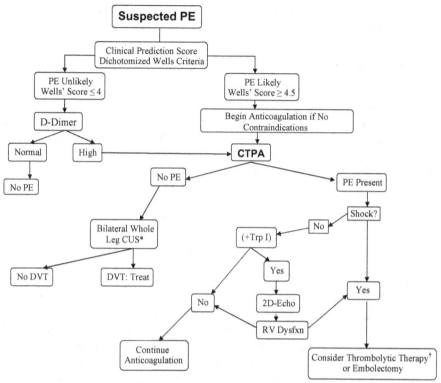

Figure 32.2.   Management algorithm for pulmonary embolism (PE). Adapted from Piazza and Goldhaber.[18] *Bilateral compression ultrasonography (CUS) indicated if only a single-detector computer tomographic pulmonary angiography (CTPA) is available. Good quality multidetector CTPA adequately rules out clinically significant PE. †Thrombolytic therapy should only be considered in the absence of contraindications. DVT, deep vein thrombosis; RV Dysfxn, right ventricular dysfunction; Trp I, troponin I.

TABLE 32.6.   Clinical Model for the Assessment of Pulmonary Embolism Risk[a]

Clinical characteristic	Score
Previous pulmonary embolism or deep vein thrombosis	+1.5
Heart rate greater than 100 beats per minute	+1.5
Recent surgery or immobilization (within the last 30 days)	+1.5
Clinical signs of deep vein thrombosis	+3
Alternative diagnosis less likely than pulmonary embolism	+3
Hemoptysis	+1
Cancer (treated within the last 6 months or palliative)	+1

[a] Probability of PE is "likely" if total score >4, and probability is "unlikely" if ≤4. Alternatively, <2 is low probability, 2–6 is moderate, and >6 is high probability.
From Wells et al.[16]

that in the absence of contraindications, treatment should not be delayed in patients with a "likely" clinical probability while the diagnostic strategy evolves.

Management of VTE

The most effective management of VTE is the prevention of VTE with the appropriate use of prophylactic therapy. However, even with appropriate prophylaxis some surgical patients will develop VTE. Unless, patients are at unusual high risk or have prolonged inpatient stays, most patients with symptomatic VTE will present after discharge in the outpatient setting with no contraindications to therapeutic anticoagulants. Anticoagulants remain mainstay of treatment for VTE and decrease the risk of thrombus propagation while the endogenous fibrinolytic system strives to reduce the clot burden. Given the significant risk of morbidity and mortality early in the clinical course of PE, it is important to initiate anticoagulant therapy as soon as possible—even if confirmatory test are pending in a high-risk patient. However, in the immediate postoperative period, patients may be at increased risk of bleeding, and thus, initiation of anticoagulation may be delayed and alternative strategies such as IVC filter employed.

The 2008 ACCP guidelines outline treatment strategies for symptomatic VTE, which include recommendations for acute management and secondary prevention.[19] The ACCP guideline grades each recommendation based on both strength and quality of the evidence. Implementation of the ACCP recommendations requires a thorough understanding of both the risk and benefits for each patient especially in the perioperative setting. It is important to recognize that the ACCP considers reduction in both VTE-related morbidity and mortality as significant outcomes. Table 32.7 summarizes the most important recommendations related to the initial management and secondary prevention of VTE.[20] Most patients presenting with uncomplicated DVT and PE may be managed using a combination of a short-term parenteral anticoagulant and oral vitamin K antagonist started simultaneously and continued for the duration of treatment. Recommendations for duration of treatment are based on the type and location of the thrombus, the presence of transient identifiable risk factors and cancer. Most uncomplicated events occurring after surgery in the absence of cancer can be treated with 3 months of anticoagulation. Other guidelines have also been recently published and include the American College of Physician/ American Academy of Family Physician guideline, the European Society of Cardiology, and the National Comprehensive Cancer Network, and reflect the growing interest in evidence-based management of VTE.[21–23]

Special Management Considerations   Table 32.8 summarizes the important considerations in the management of VTE including the role of IVC filters, thrombolytic therapy, catheter-based extraction, pulmonary embolectomy, use of anticoagulants in renal insufficiency, outpatient management of VTE, and prevention of post-thrombotic syndrome.[19] Notably, considerable controversy still exist over the management of PE when there is evidence of right ventricular dysfunction seen on echocardiogram. Furthermore, biomarkers such as troponin I and T, as well as brain natriuretic peptide, have been shown to predict right ventricular dysfunction and

TABLE 32.7. 2008 ACCP Recommendations for Initial Treatment and Secondary Prevention of VTE

Initial treatment	Specific treatment regimen[a]	Grade
SC LMWH	Enoxaparin: 1 mg/kg every 12 h or 1.5 mg/kg once daily; dalteparin: 200 IU/kg once daily (can be administered as outpatient)	1A
Intravenous UFH	Get baseline aPTT, PT, and platelet count; if normal, proceed with weight-based heparin infusion protocol. aPTT monitored every 4–6 h and adjust per normogram. Monitor platelet count for HIT every 3–4 days.	1A
Fixed-dose SC-UFH	Initial dose of 333 U/kg, followed by a fixed dose of 250 U/kg every 12 h (can be administered as outpatient).	1A
SC fondaparinux	Weight-based regimen: 5 mg (body weight <50 kg), 7.5 mg (body weight 50–100 kg), or 10 mg (body weight >100 kg) once daily.	1A
Vitamin K antagonist (VKA)	Should be initiated on first day of treatment to a target INR of 2.5. Usual initial dose of 5 mg.	1A
IVC filter	Indicated when anticoagulation is contraindicated.	1C

Scenario	Duration	
First episode and transient risk factor	3 months	1A
Isolated calf vein thrombosis	3 months	1A
Unprovoked thrombosis	At least 3 months	1A
Unprovoked with low risk of bleeding	Consider long term (≥12 months)	1A
Cancer-related thrombosis	LMWH for 3–6 months then LMWH or VKA until cancer resolved.	1A,1C
Recurrent thrombosis	Indefinite	2A

[a] Specific dose regimens not included in the ACCP guideline. A minimum of a 5-day overlap of warfarin and the chosen parenteral agent is recommended.
LMWH, low-molecular-weight heparin; HIT, heparin-induced thrombocytopenia; UFH, unfractionated heparin; SC, subcutaneous; INR, international normalized ratio; PT, prothrombin time; aPTT, activated partial thromboplastin time; IVC, inferior vena cava.
Adapted from Kearon et al.[20]

complications in patients with PE in the absence of shock. Although, some observational data suggest reduction in recurrence, this benefit was offset by a significantly increased risk of bleeding. Furthermore, large prospective registries have failed to show mortality benefit in hemodynamically stable patients with PE receiving thrombolytic therapy. Therefore, routine use of thrombolytic therapy in PE patients who are hemodynamically stable with evidence of right ventricular dysfunction is not recommended.

TABLE 32.8. Special Management Considerations for Venous Thromboembolism

Topic	2008 ACCP Recommendation	Grade
Initial choice of anticoagulant	In patients with acute DVT or nonmassive PE, LMWH is recommended over IV UFH.	1A
[a]Systemic thrombolytic therapy	In DVT, systemic thrombolysis can be used in selected patients when catheter-directed therapy is not available.	2C
	In massive PE with hemodynamic compromise, systemic thrombolysis is recommended.	1B
	In patients with PE without hypotension and low risk of bleeding systemic thrombolysis is recommended.	2B
[a]Catheter-directed thrombolysis (thrombolysis would be contraindicated within 14 days of surgery)	In selected patients with extensive acute DVT (i.e., ileofemoral DVT, symptoms for <14 days) and local expertise is available.	2B
Renal insufficiency	Renal function should be considered when making decisions about the use and/or dose of LMWH, fondaparinux, and other antithrombotic agents that are cleared by the kidney, especially in patients with diabetes mellitus, the elderly, and those with a high risk of bleeding. Dose adjustment or an alternative agent should be selected.	1A
Inferior vena cava filter	Recommend against insertion of an inferior vena cava filter for most patients with DVT or PE.	1A
	In patients with DVT and PE, if anticoagulant therapy is not possible because of risk of bleeding inferior vena cava filter insertion is recommended. A conventional course of anticoagulant therapy should be started once the bleeding resolves and the filter removed if possible.	1C
Pulmonary embolectomy and catheter-based extraction	In carefully selected patients who are unable to receive thrombolytic therapy because of bleeding risk and whose critical status does not allow time for systemic thrombolytic therapy to be effective and where expertise if available.	2C
Treatment of upper extremity DVT (UEDVT)	For most patients with UEDVT, we recommend similar treatment as described for lower extremity DVT. For most patients, catheter-directed or systemic thrombolytic therapy is not recommended.	1C
Prevention of PTS	For patients with symptomatic DVT of the lower extremity, use of elastic compression stocking with an ankle pressure gradient of 30–40 mm Hg if feasible.	1A

[a] Thrombolytic therapy should be considered only after weighing the risk of bleeding in the individual patient.
DVT, deep vein thrombosis; PE, pulmonary embolism; LMWH, low-molecular-weight heparin; UFH, unfractionated heparin; PTS, post-thrombotic syndrome.
Adapted from Hirsh et al.[19]

It is also important to note that systemic thrombolysis would be a contraindication within 14 days of surgery and sometimes up to 4 weeks later in the case of major neurosurgery.

Use of IVC filter should be limited to patients with documented thrombosis who have an absolute contraindication to anticoagulation. Due to high complication rates associated with such devices, they should be removed as soon as risk of bleeding is reduced and anticoagulation should be resumed.

Quality Indicators

Prevention of postoperative VTE has been described as one of the most cost-effective and evidence-based strategies to reduce inhospital death. The length of hospitalization is also increased when surgery is complicated by postoperative VTE. Adherence to recommended prophylaxis strategies in the surgical patient is an important quality measure and is now publicly reported as a metric of hospital performance. The Joint Commission and the Centers for Medicare and Medicaid Services have also identified the elimination of hospital-acquired VTE as a critical patient safety issue. Multiple clinical trials have demonstrated the effectiveness of VTE prophylaxis. In addition, a recent study has directly linked adherence with VTE prophylaxis with the incidence of hospital-acquired VTE.[4] The ACCP strongly recommends that every hospital have a formal, active strategy and written policy that addresses VTE prevention. A recent analysis of a large study evaluating the use of guideline prophylaxis described thromboprophylaxis practices in 81 U.S. hospitals.[24] The investigators found that although similar proportion of patients were at risk, adherence to recommended thromboprophylaxis guidelines varied from 45% to 84%. Additionally, higher rates of adherence were strongly associated with the presence of a hospital-wide VTE prophylaxis protocol. Current quality measures related to VTE include adherence to recommended guidelines, anticoagulation related bleeding, and incidence of postoperative VTE. In addition, it is expected that there is appropriate communication between the inpatient and outpatient provider at the time of discharge when a patient is treated with therapeutic anticoagulants. Providers must also emphasize the important risk associated with anticoagulant therapy.

SUMMARY

VTE remains as one of the most important preventable postoperative complications. Risk factors for VTE are well established, and a variety of tools are available to identify at-risk patients. Safe and effective evidence-based strategies for VTE prevention are widely available. However, the balance of risk and benefit of prophylaxis must be considered in each patient to optimize outcome. The 2008 ACCP guidelines provide strong recommendations for type and duration of prophylaxis regimens for patients undergoing major surgery. However, current data suggest that suboptimal use of VTE prophylaxis is still prevalent and will result in the development of symptomatic VTE in the postoperative setting. Recognition of VTE in the postoperative setting may be difficult. Together, the use of clinical prediction rules, D-dimer, and diagnostic imaging can reliably identify patients requiring treatment. Anticoagulation remains the mainstay of therapy for VTE in the postoperative setting.

REFERENCES

1. Hortlander KT, Mannino DM, Leeper KV. Pulmonary embolism mortality in the United States, 1979–1998: an analysis using multiple-cause mortality data. *Arch Intern Med.* 2003;163:1711–1717.
2. Spencer FA, Lessard D, Emery C, Reed G, Goldberg RJ. Venous thromboembolism in the outpatient setting. *Arch Intern Med.* 2007;167:1471–1475.
3. Bahl V, Hu HM, Henke PK, Wakefield TW, Campbell DA, Caprini JA. A validation study of a retrospective venous thromboembolism risk scoring method. *Ann Surg.* 2010;251:344–350.
4. Maynard GA, Morris TA, Jenkins IH, Stone S, Lee J, Renvall M, Fink E, Schoenhaus R. Optimizing prevention of hospital-acquired venous thromboembolism (VTE): prospective validation of a VTE risk assessment model. *J Hosp Med.* 2010;5:10–18.
5. Geerts WH, Bergqvist D, Pineo GF, et al. American College of Chest Physicians. Prevention of venous thromboembolism: American College of Chest Physicians evidence-based clinical practice guidelines (8th edition). *Chest.* 2008;133(6 Suppl):381S–453S.
6. Lyman GH, Khorana AA, Falanga A, et al. American Society of Clinical Oncology guideline: recommendations for venous thromboembolism prophylaxis and treatment in patients with cancer. *J Clin Oncol.* 2007;25:5490–5505.
7. Johanson NA, Lachiewicz PF, Lieberman JR, et al. AAOS clinical practice guideline summary: prevention of pulmonary embolism in patients undergoing total knee and hip arthroplasty. *J Am Acad Orthop Surg.* 2009;17:183–196.
8. Hull RD, Pineo GF, Stein PD, et al. Extended out-of-hospital low-molecular-weight heparin prophylaxis against deep venous thrombosis in patients after elective hip arthroplasty: a systematic review. *Ann Intern Med.* Nov 20 2001;135(10):858–869.
9. Horlocker TT, Wedel DJ, Rowlingson JC, et al. Regional anesthesia in the patient receiving antithrombotic or thrombolytic therapy: American Society of Regional Anesthesia and Pain Medicine Evidence-Based Guidelines (Third Edition). *Reg Anesth Pain Med.* 2010;35(1):64–101.
10. Stevens SM, Elliott CG, Chan KJ, et al. Withholding anticoagulation after a negative result on duplex ultrasonography for suspected symptomatic deep venous thrombosis. *Ann Intern Med.* 2004;140:985–991.
11. Rathbun SW, Whitsett RL, Raskob GE. Negative D-dimer result to exclude recurrent deep venous thrombosis: a management trial. *Ann Intern Med.* 2004;141:839–845.
12. Wells PS, Hirsh J, Anderson DR, et al. A simple clinical model for the diagnosis of deep vein thrombosis combined with impedance plethysmography: potential for an improvement in the diagnostic process. *J Thromb Haemost.* 1998;243(1):1888–1896.
13. Wells PS. Integrated strategies for the diagnosis of venous thromboembolism. *J Thromb Haemost.* 2007;5:41–50.
14. Stein PD, Fowler SE, Goodma LR, et al. Multidector computed tomography for acute pulmonary embolism. *N Engl J Med.* 2006;354:2317–2327.
15. Van Strijen MJ, Monye W, Kieft GJ, et al. Accuracy of single-detector spiral CT in the diagnosis of pulmonary embolism: a prospective multicenter cohort study of consecutive patients with abnormal perfusion scintigraphy. *J Thromb Haemost.* 2005;3:17–25.
16. Wells PS, Anderson DR, Rodger MA, et al. Derivation of a simple clinical model to categorize patients probability of pulmonary embolism: increasing the models utility with the SimpliRED D-dimer. *Thromb Haemost.* 2000;83:416–420.
17. Wicki J, Perrier A, Perneger TV, et al. Predicting adverse outcome in patients with acute pulmonary embolism: a risk score. *Thromb Haemost.* 2000;84:548–552.
18. Piazza G, Goldhaber SZ. Acute pulmonary embolism: part II: treatment and prophylaxis. *Circulation.* 2006;114:e28–e32 and e42–e47.

19. Hirsh J, Guyatt G, Albers GW, Harrington R, Schunemann HJ; the American College of Chest Physicians. Antithrombotic and thrombolytic therapy: American College of Chest Physicians evidence-based clinical practice guidelines (8th edition). *Chest.* Jun 2008;133(6 Suppl):71S–105S.

20. Kearon C, Kahn SR, Agnelli G, et al.; American College of Chest Physicians. Antithrombotic therapy for venous thromboembolic disease. American College of Chest Phsycians Evidence-Based Clinical Practice Guidelines (8th Edition). *Chest.* 2008;133:454S–545S.

21. Snow V, Qaseem A, Barry P, et al.; American College of Physicians, American Academy of Family Physicians Panel on Deep Venous Thrombosis Pulmonary Embolism. Management of venous thromboembolism: a clinical practice guideline from the American College of Physicians and the American Academy of Family Physicians. *Ann Intern Med.* 2007;146:204–210.

22. Torbicki A, Perrier A, Kostantinides S, et al. Task force for the diagnosis and management of acute pulmonary embolism of the European Society of Cardiology (ESC). *Eur Heart J.* 2008;29:2276–2315.

23. National Comprehensive Cancer Network (NCCN). Venous thromboembolic disease in cancer patients: practice guidelines in Oncology V.1, 2009. Available at http://www.nccn.org/professionals/physician_gls/f_guidelines.asp#vte. Accessed October 2010.

24. Cohen AT, Tapson VF, Bergmann JF, et al. Venous thromboembolism risk and prophylaxis in the acute hospital care setting (ENDORSE study). *Lancet.* 2008;371:387–394.

CHAPTER 33

SURGICAL SITE INFECTIONS
Emily K. Shuman and Carol E. Chenoweth

BACKGROUND

Introduction

Surgical site infection (SSI) occurs in 2–5% of patients undergoing inpatient surgery in the United States with an estimated 500,000 cases occurring each year.[1] Each SSI is associated with an additional 7–10 days of postoperative hospitalization, and patients with SSI have a risk of death that is 2–11 times greater than operative patients without SSI.[1] The attributable cost of each SSI ranges from $3000 to $29,000, and overall costs related to SSIs account for nearly $10 billion in healthcare expenditures each year.[1,2]

Definitions

SSIs are typically classified as superficial incisional, deep incisional, or organ/space infections. The National Healthcare Safety Network (NHSN) definitions for each of these types of SSI are outlined in Table 33.1.[3] These definitions are used routinely for surveillance of SSIs. Infections must occur within 30 days after the surgical procedure to be classified as SSIs, or within 1 year if there is an implanted device (e.g., prosthetic joint) in place and the infection appears to be related to the procedure. In addition, the definition of SSI is met if a patient is diagnosed by a surgeon or other attending physician as having an SSI.

Several frameworks exist to stratify the risk of SSI. The first of these is the classification of surgical wounds, which divides surgical wounds into four categories based on the amount of microbial contamination.[4] The four classes of surgical wounds are as follows:

1. *Clean.* A clean surgical procedure is elective, is primarily (rather than secondarily) closed, encounters no inflammation, and experiences no lapse in technique. There is no entry into the gastrointestinal or respiratory tracts (except in the case of appendectomy or cholecystectomy in the absence of inflammation). Genitourinary or biliary procedures may be considered clean if the urine or bile is sterile.

Perioperative Medicine: Medical Consultation and Co-Management, First Edition.
Edited by Amir K. Jaffer and Paul J. Grant.
© 2012 Wiley-Blackwell. Published 2012 by John Wiley & Sons, Inc.

TABLE 33.1. Definitions of Surgical Site Infection (SSI) from the National Healthcare Safety Network[3]

Type of SSI	Definition
Superficial incisional	Infection involves only skin and subcutaneous tissue of incision and must have at least one of the following: • Purulent drainage from incision • Organisms isolated from aseptically obtained culture of fluid or tissue from incision • At least one of the following signs or symptoms: pain or tenderness, localized swelling, redness, or heat, and superficial incision is deliberately opened (must have positive culture or no culture obtained)
Deep incisional	Infection involves deep soft tissues (e.g., muscle and fascia) and must have at least one of the following: • Purulent drainage from incision but not organ/space component of surgical site • Deep incision spontaneously dehisces or is deliberately opened (must have positive culture or no culture obtained) with at least one of the following signs or symptoms: fever ($>38°C$) or localized pain or tenderness • An abscess is found by direct examination, during reopening of wound or reoperation, or by histopathologic or radiologic examination
Organ/space	Infection involves any part of the body (excluding skin, subcutaneous tissue, muscle, and fascia) opened during the operative procedure, and must have at least one of the following: • Purulent drainage from a drain placed into the organ/space • Organisms isolated from aseptically obtained culture of fluid/tissue in organ/space • An abscess is found by direct examination, during reopening of wound or reoperation, or by histopathologic or radiologic examination

2. *Clean-Contaminated.* A surgical procedure with minor lapse in technique is classified as clean-contaminated. Clean-contaminated procedures include entry into the gastrointestinal or respiratory tracts without major spillage, or entry into the genitourinary or biliary tracts in the presence of infection.

3. *Contaminated.* A surgical procedure with major lapse in technique, acute inflammation without purulent material, spillage from the gastrointestinal tract, or involving a fresh traumatic wound from a relatively clean source is classified as contaminated.

4. *Dirty.* This category includes any surgical procedure where there is purulent material, a perforated viscus, or a traumatic wound that is older or from a more contaminated source.

In order to create a risk stratification system that provides additional information, the basic risk index was developed.[5] This risk index takes into account three separate variables, each of which is assigned 1 point, with a possible score of 0–3. Wound class is accounted for, with a point assigned for contaminated or dirty cases. The American Society of Anesthesiology physical status index is also used, with a preoperative assessment score of 3, 4, or 5 (indicating more than mild systemic disease) assigned 1 point. Finally, operative duration >75th percentile for the surgical procedure being performed is assigned 1 point. Application of the basic risk index is described further in the section on risk factors.

PATHOPHYSIOLOGY

Pathogenesis

Most SSIs are caused by microbial contamination of surgical wounds with endogenous flora present at the surgical site. However, Burke found in 1963 that 100% of clean surgical wounds contained bacteria at the end of an operation, but only 4% became infected.[4] Animal studies have demonstrated that the risk of SSI is related to the bacterial inoculum, but that there is no bacterial inoculum resulting in either zero or 100% risk of infection.[4] Therefore, in addition to microbial inoculum, virulence of the microorganism(s), patient-related factors, and procedure-related factors also affect susceptibility to infection. Although microbial contamination of the surgical wound is the most common route of infection, it is also possible for a surgical site to become infected via secondary spread (e.g., bloodstream infection) from an infection at a distant site. This is particularly the case when a patient undergoes placement of an implanted device.[6]

Epidemiology

Etiology   The microbial etiology of SSIs depends primarily on the type of surgical procedure and operative site. Responsible pathogens typically originate from the patient's own endogenous flora. The most commonly isolated pathogens are *Staphylococcus aureus* (30%) and coagulase-negative staphylococci (CoNS) (14%), which are common skin colonizers.[7] Other frequently isolated pathogens include enterococci (11%), *Escherichia coli* (10%), other enteric gram-negative bacilli (8%), and *Candida* species (2%), which are endogenous microorganisms typically associated with SSIs after surgical procedures involving entry of the gastrointestinal or genitourinary tracts. Such infections are often polymicrobial. Common pathogens involved in SSIs based on type of surgical procedure are outlined in Table 33.2.[6,7]

The proportion of SSIs due to multidrug-resistant organisms is increasing, likely as a result of patient-related factors (e.g., immunosuppression) as well as increasing use of broad-spectrum antimicrobials.[6] According to the most recent data from the NHSN, 49% of *S. aureus* isolates from SSIs were methicillin resistant, 20% of enterococci were vancomycin resistant, and 23% of *E. coli* were fluoroquinolone resistant.[7]

TABLE 33.2. Common Pathogens Involved in Surgical Site Infections Based on the Type of Surgical Procedure[6,7]

Type of surgical procedure	Common pathogens
Placement of graft, prosthesis, or implant	*Staphylococcus aureus*, CoNS
Cardiac	*S. aureus*, CoNS
Vascular	*S. aureus*, CoNS, gram-negative bacilli
Breast	*S. aureus*, CoNS
Neurosurgery	*S. aureus*, CoNS
Orthopedic	*S. aureus*, CoNS, gram-negative bacilli
Noncardiac thoracic	*S. aureus*, CoNS, streptococci, gram-negative bacilli
Ophthalmic	*S. aureus*, CoNS, streptococci, gram-negative bacilli
Head and neck	*S. aureus*, streptococci, oropharyngeal anaerobes, gram-negative bacilli
Gastroduodenal	Gram-negative bacilli, streptococci, oropharyngeal anaerobes
Other abdominal (including appendectomy, hepatobiliary, and colorectal)	Gram-negative bacilli, enterococci, anaerobes, *Candida* species
Obstetric or gynecologic	*S. aureus*, CoNS, enterococci, group B streptococci, gram-negative bacilli, anaerobes
Urologic	Gram-negative bacilli, enterococci

CoNS, coagulase-negative staphylococci.

Risk Factors Risk factors for SSI include procedure-related factors and patient-related factors (Table 33.3). Important procedure-related factors are wound class, operative duration, and other factors that impact microbial contamination of surgical wounds. In a historical series, SSI rates were found to correlate with wound class, with rates of 1.4–2.1% for clean wounds, 2.8–10.8% for clean-contaminated wounds, 6.4–16.3% for contaminated wounds, and 7.1–40% for dirty wounds.[4] Prolonged operative duration (specifically, >75th percentile for the surgical procedure being performed) is also a risk factor for SSI, although the exact reason for this is not entirely understood. Proposed mechanisms include hypothermia, dessication of tissues, and increased exposure of the wound to microbes.[4,8] It is also possible that prolonged operative duration is a surrogate for other important factors such as complexity of the surgical procedure.[4]

Poor operative technique is typically considered a risk factor for SSI. Poor hemostasis and receipt of blood transfusion each increase the risk of SSI.[9,10] In addition, use of drains to evacuate fluid from surgical sites increases the risk of SSI.[11] Glove puncture and other episodes of contamination of the sterile field also raise the SSI rate.[4] Evidence that preoperative hand scrubbing by surgical staff impacts the risk of SSI is lacking, but one study showed a higher risk of SSI in vascular surgery patients when surgical staff scrubbed with plain soap rather than povidone-iodine

TABLE 33.3.   Risk Factors for Surgical Site Infection[4,6,8,10,11,13–18,20–24]

Patient-related risk factors	Procedure-related risk factors
Age	Wound class (higher risk with contaminated or dirty wounds)
Diabetes	Prolonged operative duration
Obesity	Poor hemostasis
Smoking	Need for blood transfusion
Use of immunosuppressive medications	Use of drains
Infection at another site at the time of surgery	Improper preoperative hand scrubbing by surgical staff
Preoperative colonization with multidrug-resistant organisms	Inadequate preparation of surgical site with antiseptic solution
	Hair removal at surgical site, especially using razor
	Improper sterilization of surgical instruments
	Inadequate perioperative antimicrobial prophylaxis
	Perioperative hypothermia

solution.[12] Inadequate preparation of the surgical site with an antiseptic solution is also a risk factor for SSI.[1,13] In addition, any hair removal at the surgical site, especially using a razor, increases the risk of SSI.[14] Improper sterilization of surgical instruments raises the risk of SSI.[1,13] Inadequate perioperative antimicrobial prophylaxis is associated with increased risk of SSI.[9] Finally, perioperative hypothermia may predispose to SSI after colorectal surgery, presumably due to resulting vasoconstriction with poor subcutaneous oxygen tension.[8]

Important patient-related factors affecting the risk of SSI include those that are modifiable and those that are not. The most important nonmodifiable patient-related risk factor is age, but the relationship between age and risk of SSI is not straightforward. One study found that age >60 years was an independent risk factor for all infections, but not specifically for SSI, after noncolorectal abdominal surgery.[15] However, another study demonstrated that patients over 70 years of age were not at increased risk for postoperative infections, but that their risk of mortality from infection was much higher.[16] Another recent study found that the risk of SSI increased by 1.1% per year between ages 17 and 65, but that the risk of SSI actually decreased after age 65.[17] This was thought to be related to better health of those individuals who survive past age 65, as well as perhaps more selective choice of older surgical candidates by physicians.

Modifiable patient-related risk factors include diabetes, obesity, smoking, and use of immunosuppressive medications. Dronge et al. found that having a preoperative hemoglobin A1c of <7% decreased the risk of postoperative infectious complications.[18] In the shorter term, tight control of blood glucose after cardiac surgical procedures has been shown to reduce the risk of SSI.[19] Obesity has been identified as an independent predictor of SSI after a wide variety of surgical procedures.[20]

Proposed mechanisms for this association include presence of comorbidities (e.g., diabetes), suboptimal tissue oxygen tension, and reduced tissue concentrations of antimicrobials. A recent study of patients undergoing general and vascular surgery found that smoking is also an independent risk factor for SSI.[21] Use of immunosuppressive medications increases the risk for many types of infections and is therefore thought to be an important risk factor for SSI.[1] Finally, patients who have an active infection at a location other than the surgical site are at increased risk for SSI.[6]

The basic risk index is currently the most widely used attempt to quantify the risk of SSI.[4,5] Overall SSI rates based on the basic risk index are as follows: 1.5% for 0 points, 2.9% for 1 point, 6.8% for 2 points, and 13% for 4 points.[5] SSI rates for selected surgical procedures based on basic risk index are listed in Table 33.4. Other systems have recently been developed to quantify the risk of SSI.[21]

In addition to procedure-related and patient-related factors, virulence of microbial pathogens also impacts the risk of SSI.[6] Some pathogens, such as *S. aureus* and group A streptococci, are considered to be particularly virulent due to their ability to produce toxins and induce significant tissue damage. Other pathogens, such as

TABLE 33.4. Rates of Surgical Site Infection (SSI) for Selected Inpatient Surgical Procedures Based on Basic Risk Index Category[42]

	Rate of SSI[a] by basic risk index category			
Type of surgical procedure	0	1	2	3
Abdominal aortic aneurysm repair	2.1		6.5	
Limb amputation	1.3		3	
Appendectomy	1.2		3.5	
Bile duct, liver, or pancreatic surgery	8		13.7	
Breast surgery	1	3	6.4	
Cardiac surgery	1.1		1.9	
Cholecystectomy	0.2	0.6	1.7	
Colon surgery	4	5.6	7	9.5
Craniotomy	2.2		4.7	
Spinal fusion	0.7	1.8	4.2	
Open reduction of fracture	1.1	1.8	3.4	
Herniorraphy	0.7	2.4	5.3	
Hip prosthesis	0.7	1.4	2.4	
Abdominal hysterectomy	1.1	2.2	4	
Knee prosthesis	0.6	1	1.6	
Prostate surgery	0.9		2.9	
Peripheral vascular bypass surgery	2.9		7	
Rectal surgery	3.5	8	26.7	
Ventricular shunt	4		5.9	

[a] Per 100 surgical procedures. SSI rates for adjacent risk index groupings that were not significantly different are grouped together.

enterococci and CoNS, are relatively avirulent, as they require fairly high inoculums in order to produce infection and typically lack significant virulence factors. However, the increasing prevalence of multidrug resistance among microbial pathogens responsible for SSI impacts virulence as well. In certain settings, colonization with multidrug-resistant organisms has become an important risk factor for the development of SSI. For example, preoperative colonization with methicillin-resistant *S. aureus* (MRSA), which is most commonly found in the anterior nares, has been found to increase the risk of SSI after cardiac and orthopedic procedures.[22,23] Patients colonized with vancomycin-resistant enterococci (VRE) prior to liver transplantation were more likely to develop peritonitis postoperatively.[22–24]

Transmission

As noted previously, most SSIs develop as a result of direct contamination of the surgical site with microorganisms. These microorganisms most often come from the patient's own endogenous flora on the skin or other operative sites (e.g., bowel). However, it is also possible that microorganisms may be introduced into the surgical site via contaminated surgical instruments or by surgical staff. Holes in surgical gloves can result in contamination of surgical wounds, resulting in SSI.[4] In addition, infections have been transmitted by surgical staff who did not have direct contact with the surgical site (e.g., anesthesiologists, circulating nurses), likely due to aerosolization of infecting or colonizing microorganisms such as *S. aureus* (including MRSA) and group A streptococci. It is also possible for SSIs to arise secondarily as a result of an infection at a different site.[4] For example, an implanted device may be seeded in the setting of a bloodstream infection.

Acquisition of multidrug-resistant organisms, which increases the risk of SSI in certain settings, occurs for a variety of reasons. These microorganisms are often transmitted from person to person in healthcare settings via the hands of healthcare personnel due to inadequate hand hygiene.[25] Exposure to healthcare settings and to antimicrobials are common risk factors for the acquisition of multidrug-resistant organisms. Other common risk factors include severe underlying disease and use of indwelling devices such as central lines and urinary catheters.

PREVENTION STRATEGIES

Strategies for prevention of SSIs are targeted at known risk factors for SSI and thus address both procedure-related and patient-related issues. Also important are strategies to address multidrug-resistant organisms in healthcare settings. Several guidelines for prevention of SSIs and management of multidrug-resistant organisms are available.[1,13,25] Important prevention strategies are outlined in Table 33.5.

Procedure-related prevention strategies primarily focus on reducing the microbial inoculum and preventing contamination of the surgical site by surgical staff, instruments, and the environment. In preparation for surgery, hair removal should not be performed unless necessary, and if necessary, should be performed with clippers rather than a razor.[1,13] Most importantly, the skin around the incision

TABLE 33.5.   Strategies for Prevention of Surgical Site Infections[1,13]

Patient-related strategies	Procedure-related strategies
For diabetic patients, reduce hemoglobin A1c to <7% preoperatively	No hair removal, or use clippers (not razor)
Maintain blood glucose <200 mg/dL for the first 2 days after cardiac surgery	Wash and clean skin around incision site using appropriate antiseptic solution
Increase dose of perioperative antimicrobials for obese patients	Administer appropriate antimicrobial prophylaxis when indicated; first dose should be given within 1 h prior to incision; should be stopped within 24 h after procedure (except for cardiac surgery)Preoperative surgical hand scrubbing or use of alcohol-based surgical hand rub by surgical team members
Encourage smoking cessation within 30 days prior to surgery	
Avoid use of immunosuppressive medications in the perioperative period if possible	
Consider preoperative screening for and decolonization for *S. aureus* and/or MRSA in high-risk populations	Preoperative sterilization of surgical equipment according to published guidelines
	Reduce environmental contamination of operating room (ventilation, disinfection, minimizing traffic)
	Minimize surgical duration as much as possible
	Maintain perioperative normothermia in all surgical patients

site should be washed and cleaned with an appropriate antiseptic agent.[1,13] In addition to preparation of the surgical site, preoperative bathing or showering with antiseptics has been evaluated in several studies. While showering with chlorhexidine solution was found to be superior to not showering, there was no benefit in studies where chlorhexidine was compared with plain soap.[26] Showering with antiseptics preoperatively is not routinely recommended in the current guidelines, but this strategy is being used increasingly for the prevention of SSIs in high-risk patients.[1]

In addition to preoperative cleansing of the surgical site, use of antimicrobial prophylaxis is another essential strategy for the prevention of SSI, and timing of antimicrobial administration is very important. Antimicrobial prophylaxis should be administered when appropriate within 1 h prior to incision to maximize tissue concentration.[1,13] Antimicrobial prophylaxis should be stopped within 24 h after surgery, except in the case of cardiac surgery, when it should be stopped within 48 h. The choice of antimicrobial agent(s) typically depends on the type of surgical procedure and expected pathogens (Table 33.2). Multiple guidelines exist regarding perioperative antimicrobial prophylaxis and have been synthesized by Bratzler and Houck.[27]

In order to prevent the contamination of the surgical site by surgical staff, surgical team members should perform hand scrubbing with an appropriate antiseptic agent for 2–5 min preoperatively, or should use an alcohol-based surgical hand rub.[1,13] Surgical equipment should be sterilized preoperatively according to published guidelines.[13] To reduce environmental contamination of the operating room, appropriate ventilation should be maintained, surfaces should be cleaned using an appropriate disinfectant, and traffic should be minimized.[1,13] Standard principles of asepsis should be maintained intraoperatively, and surgical duration should be minimized as much as possible.[1,13] Maintenance of perioperative normothermia is now recommended for all surgical patients, although this issue remains somewhat controversial.[1,8,28]

Several preventive strategies address those patient-related factors that are modifiable. For diabetic patients, it is recommended that hemoglobin A1c levels be reduced to <7% preoperatively if possible.[1,18] Perioperative blood glucose control is also important, and maintenance of blood glucose <200 mg/dL for the first 2 days after cardiac surgery is now recommended.[19,28] For obese patients, increasing the dose of perioperative antimicrobials is recommended to ensure adequate tissue penetration.[27] Smoking cessation is recommended within 30 days prior to surgical procedures.[1,13] No formal recommendations exist regarding use of immunosuppressive medications in the perioperative period, but these should be avoided if possible.[1]

Strategies also exist to prevent SSI due to multidrug-resistant organisms. There are general guidelines for the prevention of transmission of multidrug-resistant organisms in healthcare settings, and these should be followed in the perioperative setting as well.[25,29] Measures to prevent transmission of multidrug-resistant organisms during the perioperative period include appropriate use of contact precautions, scheduling patients known to be colonized or infected at the end of the day to avoid cross-transmission, and appropriate disinfection of equipment and environmental surfaces.[29]

In the case of *S. aureus*, which is commonly multidrug resistant, multiple studies have examined the effectiveness of preoperative decolonization of carriers in reducing the risk of SSI. Decolonization is usually achieved with topical mupirocin applied to the anterior nares and/or showering with chlorhexidine solution, typically for 5 days prior to surgery. The results of randomized trials examining this issue have been mixed, but several nonrandomized trials have demonstrated that preoperative decolonization reduces the risk of SSI after cardiac and orthopedic surgery.[30–34] Currently, preoperative screening and decolonization for *S. aureus* or MRSA are not routinely recommended, but may be considered in high-risk patients.[1]

Prevention of SSIs has recently become an area of focus for multiple organizations. The Centers for Medicare and Medicaid Services (CMS) established the Surgical Infection Prevention Collaborative, which focuses primarily on the appropriate use of perioperative antimicrobial prophylaxis. Hospitals that implemented the recommended performance measures noted a reduction in their rates of SSI.[28] The Surgical Care Improvement Project, an extension of the Surgical Infection Prevention Collaborative, focuses on several additional performance measures for the prevention of SSI: proper hair removal, blood glucose control after cardiac surgery, and maintenance of perioperative normothermia for all surgical patients. Medicare payments to hospitals are linked to compliance with these quality measures, and, more recently, CMS denies payment to hospitals for healthcare-associated infections that are deemed preventable, including mediastinitis after coronary artery bypass grafting.[35] The Joint Commission has developed the National Patient Safety Goals, one of which calls for hospitals to implement evidence-based measures for the prevention of SSIs.[36] This program also calls for continuous monitoring of compliance with preventive measures, as well as surveillance of SSI rates to determine if such measures are effective.

POSTOPERATIVE ASSESSMENT

Postoperatively, patients should be monitored closely for the development of SSI. While the definitions of SSI outlined in Table 33.1 are surveillance definitions, they are also useful clinically, as they detail specific signs and symptoms that would be expected in the setting of SSI.[3] SSIs may manifest in different ways, depending on the type of surgical procedure and depth of the infection. Superficial and deep incisional SSIs typically present with erythema, swelling, and pain at the surgical site. Purulent drainage and spontaneous opening of the wound often occur. In deep incisional SSI, an abscess may form, and systemic signs of infection such as fever and leukocytosis may be present. Necrotizing soft tissue infection may occur occasionally.[37] In the case of organ/space SSI, such as mediastinitis after cardiac surgery, systemic signs of infection are common, and concomitant bloodstream infection occurs frequently.[38] Radiologic examination, particularly with computed tomography (CT), is an important diagnostic modality to identify fluid or gas in tissues that may be indicative of organ/space SSI.

Some SSIs may present more subtly, especially those involving implants or prosthetic devices. For example, early (within 3 months postoperatively) prosthetic joint infection often presents with typical signs of SSI, but delayed-onset (3–24 months) and late-onset (>24 months) infection more often present with persistent joint pain with or without loosening of the prosthesis.[39] This makes prosthetic joint infection very difficult to distinguish from other causes of prosthesis failure, and often the diagnosis of infection is only made on joint aspiration or reoperation when pathogens are identified from culture. Similarly, patients with ventricular shunt infection may have no symptoms or may present with subtle symptoms indicative of increased intracranial pressure, such as headache.[40] Note that infection of an implant or prosthesis can occur at any time, not just within 1 year of the surgical procedure as indicated by the surveillance definition of SSI. Therefore, continued careful monitoring is required both by surgeons and other clinicians, particularly primary care physicians.

In addition to clinical monitoring of individual patients for SSI in the postoperative setting, healthcare facilities should perform routine active surveillance to determine facility-wide rates of SSI.[1] Typically, surveillance is directed toward high-risk, high-volume procedures (e.g., coronary artery bypass grafting) and may be accomplished by manual medical record review or automated data systems. Surveillance is often based on culture data, with positive cultures obtained from postoperative patients prompting further medical record review. SSI rates are typically calculated by dividing the number of infections per 100 surgical procedures. Feedback regarding SSI rates should be provided to hospital administration and individual surgeons. Continuous monitoring of rates helps to assess performance compared with national benchmarks and identify areas for improvement.

MEDICAL MANAGEMENT

For superficial and deep incisional infections, it is often adequate to simply open the wound and to perform cleansing and dressing changes two to three times daily.[37] Sharp debridement of infected or devitalized tissue may be necessary, and wound-suctioning devices may assist with healing. Antimicrobial therapy is generally indicated only when there is surrounding cellulitis. Empiric antimicrobial therapy should be directed toward the expected pathogens based on type of surgical procedure (Table 33.2). Cultures should be obtained whenever possible with modification of antimicrobial therapy based on results. If infection with *S. aureus* is suspected, an antimicrobial agent with activity against MRSA should be considered in high-risk patients and in healthcare settings where there is a high prevalence of MRSA.

For organ/space infections, a combination of surgical and medical therapy is generally required.[37] Percutaneous drainage may be performed if infection is localized (e.g., discrete abscess), but surgical drainage is typically necessary in the case of more diffuse infection (e.g., peritonitis, mediastinitis). Again, empiric antimicrobial therapy should be directed toward the anticipated pathogens (Table 33.2), and cultures should be obtained to help guide therapy. Empiric antimicrobial therapy with activity against multidrug-resistant organisms should be considered in select patients (e.g., MRSA after cardiac surgery, VRE after liver transplantation). Complicated organ/space infections often require prolonged intravenous or oral antimicrobial therapy. Response to therapy is typically monitored clinically, and imaging modalities such as CT may be used to document resolution of abscesses. Consultation with a physician specializing in infectious diseases can be helpful in managing patients with complicated organ/space infections.

When an SSI involves a prosthesis, implant, or graft, it is necessary to remove the implanted device in order to adequately treat the infection. Microorganisms typically form biofilms on these devices, which are not adequately penetrated by antimicrobials. Therefore, surgical removal of the device should be performed whenever feasible. For example, for prosthetic joint infection, the preferred approach is a two-stage exchange with removal of the prosthesis and implantation of a temporary spacer, followed by reimplantation of a prosthesis after the patient has completed a course of appropriate antimicrobial therapy.[41] However, for patients who are poor surgical candidates, or who prefer not to undergo further surgical procedures, attempts can be made to salvage an infected implanted device. This approach typically involves surgical removal of as much infected material as possible followed by prolonged suppressive antimicrobial therapy to prevent relapse of clinically apparent infection. As with organ/space infections, management of complicated infections involving implanted devices should also be done in conjunction with a specialist in infectious diseases.

CONCLUSIONS

SSI is a frequent complication of surgical procedures and is associated with significant morbidity, mortality, and excess cost. Important risk factors for SSI include features of the surgical procedure that increase the risk of microbial contamination, as well as patient-related factors that increase susceptibility to infection. Essential strategies for the prevention of SSI include preoperative cleansing of the surgical site, administration of appropriate perioperative antimicrobial prophylaxis, and modification of patient-related risk factors whenever possible. Patients should be monitored closely in the postoperative setting for development of SSI. Management of SSI depends on the type of infection and should be based on culture results whenever possible.

REFERENCES

1. Anderson DJ, Kaye KS, Classen D, et al. Strategies to prevent surgical site infections in acute care hospitals. *Infect Control Hosp Epidemiol.* 2008;29(Suppl 1):S51–S61.
2. Wong ES. Surgical site infections. In: *Hospital Epidemiology and Infection Control*, 3rd edition, Mayhall CG (ed.), pp. 287–310. Baltimore, MD: Lippincott, Williams, and Wilkins; 2004.
3. Horan TC, Andrus M, Dudeck MA. CDC/NHSN surveillance definition of healthcare-associated infection and criteria for specific types of infections in the acute care setting. *Am J Infect Control.* 2008;36:309–332.
4. Dellinger EP, Ehrenkranz NJ, Jarvis WR. Surgical site infections. In: *Bennett and Brachman's Hospital Infections*, 5th edition, Jarvis WR (ed.), pp. 583–598. Philadelphia: Lippincott, Williams, and Wilkins; 2007.
5. Culver DH, Horan T, Gaynes RP. Surgical wound infection rates by wound class, operative procedure, and patient risk index: National Nosocomial Infections Surveillance System. *Am J Med.* 1991;91:S152–S157.
6. Owens CD, Stoessel K. Surgical site infections: epidemiology, microbiology and prevention. *J Hosp Infect.* 2008;70:3–10.
7. Hidron AI, Edwards JR, Patel J, et al. Antimicrobial-resistant pathogens associated with healthcare-associated infections: annual summary of data reported to the National Healthcare Safety Network at the Centers for Disease Control and Prevention, 2006–2007. *Infect Control Hosp Epidemiol.* 2008;29:996–1011.
8. Kurz A, Sessler DI, Lenhardt R. Perioperative normothermia to reduce the incidence of surgical-wound infection and shorten hospitalization. Study of the wound infection and temperature group. *N Engl J Med.* 1996;334:1209–1215.
9. Polk HCJ, Lopez-Mayor JR. Postoperative wound infection: a prospective study of determinant factors and prevention. *Surgery.* 1969;66:97–103.
10. Ford CD, Van Moorleghem G, Menlove RL. Blood transfusions and postoperative wound infection. *Surgery.* 1993;113:603–607.
11. Magee C, Rodeheaver GT, Golden GT, Fox J, Edgerton MT, Edlich RF. Potentiation of wound infections by surgical drains. *Am J Surg.* 1976;131:547–549.
12. Grinbaum RS, de Mendonca JS, Cardo DM. An outbreak of handscrubbing-related surgical site infections in vascular surgical procedures. *Infect Control Hosp Epidemiol.* 1995;16:198–202.
13. Mangram AJ, Horan TC, Pearson ML, Silver LC, Jarvis WR. Guideline for prevention of surgical site infection, 1999. Hospital Infection Control Practices Advisory Committee. *Infect Control Hosp Epidemiol.* 1999;20:250–278.
14. Alexander JW, Fischer JE, Boyajian M, Palmquist J, Morris MJ. Influence of hair-removal methods on wound infections. *Arch Surg.* 1983;118:347–352.

15. Pessaux P, Msika S, Atalla D, Hay JM, Flamant Y. Risk factors for postoperative infectious complications in noncolorectal abdominal surgery: a multivariate analysis based on a prospective multicenter study of 4718 patients. *Arch Surg.* 2003;138:314–324.

16. Raymond DP, Pelletier SJ, Crabtree TD, Schulman AM, Pruett TL, Sawyer RG. Surgical infection and the aging population. *Am Surg.* 2001;67:827–832.

17. Kaye KS, Schmit K, Pieper C, et al. The effect of increasing age on the risk of surgical site infection. *J Infect Dis.* 2005;191:1056–1062.

18. Dronge AS, Perkal MF, Kancir S, Concato J, Aslan M, Rosenthal RA. Long-term glycemic control and postoperative infectious complications. *Arch Surg.* 2006;141:375–380.

19. Furnary AP, Zerr KJ, Grunkemeier GL, Starr A. Continuous intravenous insulin infusion reduces the incidence of deep sternal wound infection in diabetic patients after cardiac surgical procedures. *Ann Thorac Surg.* 1999;67:352–360.

20. Anaya DA, Dellinger EP. The obese surgical patient: a susceptible host for infection. *Surg Infect (Larchmt).* 2006;7:473–480.

21. Neumayer L, Hosokawa P, Itani K, El-Tamer M, Henderson WG, Khuri SF. Multivariable predictors of postoperative surgical site infection after general and vascular surgery: results from the patient safety in surgery study. *J Am Coll Surg.* Jun 2007;204(6):1178–1187.

22. Munoz P, Hortal J, Giannella M, et al. Nasal carriage of *S. aureus* increases the risk of surgical site infection after major heart surgery. *J Hosp Infect.* Jan 2008;68(1):25–31.

23. Yano K, Minoda Y, Sakawa A, et al. Positive nasal culture of methicillin-resistant *Staphylococcus aureus* (MRSA) is a risk factor for surgical site infection in orthopedics. *Acta Orthop.* Aug 2009;80(4): 486–490.

24. McNeil SA, Malani PN, Chenoweth CE, et al. Vancomycin-resistant enterococcal colonization and infection in liver transplant candidates and recipients: a prospective surveillance study. *Clin Infect Dis.* Jan 15 2006;42(2):195–203.

25. Siegel JD, Rhinehart E, Jackson M, Chiarello L. Management of multidrug-resistant organisms in healthcare settings, 2006. *Am J Infect Control.* 2006;35:S165–S193.

26. Webster J, Osborne S. Preoperative bathing or showering with skin antiseptics to prevent surgical site infection. *Cochrane Database Syst Rev.* 2007;(18):CD004985.

27. Bratzler DW, Houck PM. Antimicrobial prophylaxis for surgery: an advisory statement from the National Surgical Infection Prevention Project. *Clin Infect Dis.* 2004;38:1706–1715.

28. Bratzler DW, Hunt DR. The surgical infection prevention and surgical care improvement projects: national initiatives to improve outcomes for patients having surgery. *Clin Infect Dis.* 2006;43:322–330.

29. Grota PG. Perioperative management of multidrug-resistant organisms in healthcare settings. *AORN J.* 2007;86:361–368.

30. Bode LG, Kluytmans JA, Wertheim HF, et al. Preventing surgical-site infections in nasal carriers of *Staphylococcus aureus*. *N Engl J Med.* Jan 7 2010;362(1):9–17.

31. Harbarth S, Fankhauser C, Schrenzel J, et al. Universal screening for methicillin-resistant *Staphylococcus aureus* at hospital admission and nosocomial infection in surgical patients. *JAMA.* Mar 12 2008;299(10):1149–1157.

32. Kallen AJ, Wilson CT, Larson RJ. Perioperative intranasal mupirocin for the prevention of surgical-site infections: systematic review of the literature and meta-analysis. *Infect Control Hosp Epidemiol.* Dec 2005;26(12):916–922.

33. Perl TM, Cullen JJ, Wenzel RP, et al. Intranasal mupirocin to prevent postoperative *Staphylococcus aureus* infections. *N Engl J Med.* Jun 13 2002;346(24):1871–1877.

34. Nicholson MR, Huesman LA. Controlling the usage of intranasal mupirocin does impact the rate of *Staphylococcus aureus* deep sternal wound infections in cardiac surgery patients. *Am J Infect Control.* Feb 2006;34(1):44–48.

35. Rosenthal MB. Nonpayment for performance? Medicare's new reimbursement rule. *N Engl J Med.* Oct 18 2007;357(16):1573–1575.

36. Joint Commission. Approved: 2010 National Patient Safety Goals. Some changes effective immediately. *Jt Comm Perspect.* 2009;29:20–31.

37. Anaya DA, Dellinger EP. Surgical infections and choice of antibiotics. In: *Sabiston Textbook of Surgery*, 18th edition, Townsend CM (ed.). Philadelphia: Saunders Elsevier; 2007.

38. Bor DH, Rose RM, Modlin JF, Weintraub R, Friedland GH. Mediastinitis after cardiovascular surgery. *Rev Infect Dis.* 1983;5:885–897.

39. Zimmerli W, Trampuz A, Ochsner PE. Prosthetic-joint infections. *N Engl J Med.* Oct 14 2004;351(16): 1645–1654.

40. Conen A, Walti LN, Merlo A, Fluckiger U, Battegay M, Trampuz A. Characteristics and treatment outcome of cerebrospinal fluid shunt-associated infections in adults: a retrospective analysis over an 11-year period. *Clin Infect Dis.* Jul 1 2008;47(1):73–82.

41. Bejon P, Berendt A, Atkins BL, et al. Two-stage revision for prosthetic joint infection: predictors of outcome and the role of reimplantation microbiology. *J Antimicrob Chemother.* Jan 6 2010;65(3): 569–575.

42. Edwards JR, Peterson KD, Banerjee S, et al. National Healthcare Safety Network (NHSN) report: data summary for 2006 through 2008, issued December 2009. *Am J Infect Control.* 2009;37:783–805.

CHAPTER 34

POSTOPERATIVE KIDNEY INJURY

Charuhas V. Thakar

BACKGROUND

Acute kidney injury (AKI, previously known as acute renal failure) is a serious morbidity occurring during acute care hospitalizations, which independently contributes to greater length of stay, higher costs of care, and increased risk of death.[1-3] There is gathering evidence to suggest that AKI during hospitalization increases the risk of progressive kidney failure and is associated with poor long-term survival.[4] Although there is a wide range in the reported frequency of AKI due to the variability in its definition, the incidence of AKI usually depends on the clinical setting in which it occurs. It is generally observed in 5–7.5% in all acute care hospitalizations, but accounts for up to 20% of admissions to intensive care units (ICU). Of all the cases of AKI during hospitalization, approximately 35–40% are related to operative settings and the majority of these cases occur in the ICU setting.[2,3]

Of all the surgical settings, much of our knowledge on the epidemiology of AKI is derived from patients undergoing cardiac or vascular surgery, with a minority of studies examining noncardiovascular surgical settings. With limited treatment options, prevention of AKI and amelioration of its severity remain important cornerstones of improving patient outcomes. The purpose of the present chapter is to discuss the epidemiology, risk factors, prevention strategies, management, and outcomes of AKI during the perioperative period in both cardiovascular and noncardiovascular surgical settings.

DEFINITION AND INCIDENCE OF PERIOPERATIVE AKI

Definition

Acute Kidney Injury Network (AKIN), a consensus panel representing national and international societies of nephrology, critical care, and anesthesiology, recently proposed standardized definitions of AKI.[5,6] According to this definition and

Perioperative Medicine: Medical Consultation and Co-Management, First Edition.
Edited by Amir K. Jaffer and Paul J. Grant.
© 2012 Wiley-Blackwell. Published 2012 by John Wiley & Sons, Inc.

TABLE 34.1.   Acute Kidney Injury Network (AKIN) Staging System for Severity of AKI[5]

Stage	Creatinine (Cr) increase	Urine output (UOP)
1	Increased Cr 0.3 mg/dL or 1.5- to 2.0-fold of baseline	UOP <0.5 mL/kg/h for >6 h
2	Cr increase of greater than two- to threefold of baseline	UOP <0.5 mL/kg/h for >12 h
3	Cr increase greater than threefold of baseline (or Cr >4 mg/dL with 0.5 mg/dL acute increase). AKI requiring dialysis.	UOP <0.3 mL/kg/h for 24 h or anuria for 12 h

AKI, acute kidney injury.

classification system (Table 34.1), AKI was considered to be present when an abrupt reduction in kidney function resulted in an absolute increase in serum creatinine of more than or equal to 0.3 mg/dL, a percentage increase in serum creatinine of more than or equal to 50% (1.5-fold increase from baseline), or a reduction in urine output (documented oliguria of less than 0.5 mL/kg/h for more than 6 h). AKI was further classified into three stages (arbitrarily) based on the severity of kidney injury, as indicated by degree of rise of serum creatinine.

Cardiovascular Surgery

Much of the discussion in this section is derived from studies that were published before the development of these standard criteria. When defined as requirement of dialysis during the postoperative period (Stage III AKI), the incidence of AKI after cardiac surgery is <5%.[7–9] Expectedly, the incidence of milder degrees of kidney injury, typically defined as a 0.3 mg/dL increase in serum creatinine or a 50% drop in estimated glomerular filtration rate (GFR) (analogous Stage I or II AKI), is higher and occurs in 10–20% of cardiac surgery patients.[10–12]

In the setting of cardiac transplantation, the incidence of AKI is higher than nontransplant cardiac surgery.[13,14] In a single-center study involving over 750 cardiac transplants, the incidence of AKI requiring dialysis was 6%; by historical comparisons, this incidence was about three- to fourfold higher compared with nontransplant cardiac surgery performed during the same time period at the same institution.[15]

The incidence of AKI after abdominal aortic aneurysm (AAA) repair depends on the surgical technique, and the anatomical location of the aneurysm. For example, AKI occurs in 10–15% of patients undergoing open AAA repair, and the rate is slightly lower in those undergoing endovascular repair.[16] In contrast, thoracic or thoraco-abdominal aortic aneurysm surgery is associated with a 25% incidence of milder AKI (defined as a 30% increase in serum creatinine during the postoperative period), or an 8% incidence of severe AKI requiring dialysis.[17,18]

Noncardiovascular Surgery

Noncardiovascular surgical settings have been less extensively studied compared with cardiovascular surgery. When studied in patients undergoing noncardiac surgery

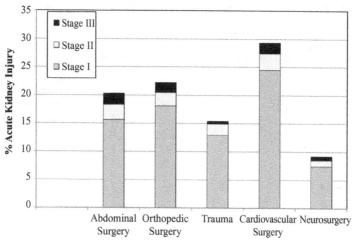

Figure 34.1.   Incidence and severity of acute kidney injury (AKI) in critically ill patients in surgical settings. Primary surgical admission diagnosis categories to ICU; adapted from Thakar et al.[2]

with normal preoperative renal function, the incidence of postoperative AKI was less than 1%,[19] with AKI defined as an absolute level of estimated GFR less than 50 mL/min during the postoperative period (representing a 40% reduction from preoperative levels). Gastric bypass surgery for morbid obesity represents a relatively unique clinical setting and is associated with an 8.5% incidence of postoperative AKI, defined as either a 50% increase in serum creatinine or dialysis requirement.[20]

Similar to cardiac transplantation, the incidence of AKI is also high in other nonrenal solid organ transplant settings; liver transplantation is associated with an 8–17% frequency of severe AKI requiring dialysis during the immediate postoperative period.[21–24]

Summary

Although the reported incidence of AKI varies based on the definition used, there is sufficient information to indicate that clinical settings play an important role in this variability (Figure 34.1). Generally, cardiovascular surgeries and solid organ transplant settings are more commonly associated with AKI than noncardiovascular surgeries. It is very plausible that the differences in preoperative risk factors or intraoperative events associated with each surgical setting are responsible for the variation in the incidence or severity of AKI.

PREOPERATIVE RISK FACTORS

AKI after any surgical procedure is usually a result of a combination of factors including preoperative comorbid diseases, the type of surgical procedure, and

TABLE 34.2.   Preoperative and Intraoperative Risk Factors of Acute Kidney Injury after Cardiovascular Surgery

Preoperative risk factors	Intraoperative risk factors
Age	Bypass time
Female gender	Valve surgery
Diabetes mellitus/hyperglycemia	CABG + valve procedure
COPD	Blood transfusions
CHF	Cross-clamp time
LV function <40%	Vasopressor use
Intra-aortic balloon pump	
Prior cardiac surgery	
Emergency surgery	
Left main disease >70%	
PVD	
Renal dysfunction	

COPD, chronic obstructive pulmonary disease; CHF, congestive heart failure; LV, left ventricular; PVD, peripheral vascular disease; CABG, coronary artery bypass grafting.

complications during the immediate postoperative course. This section will review the role of preoperative risk assessment of AKI.

Cardiovascular Surgery

Several studies have identified risk factors of AKI after cardiac surgery.[10,25–28] The risk of AKI is influenced by demographic factors, preoperative comorbid diseases, and type of surgical procedure. As shown in Table 34.2, demographic characteristics such as female gender and older age predict AKI. Insulin-requiring diabetes, peripheral vascular disease, congestive heart failure (CHF), and chronic obstructive pulmonary disease (COPD) are some of the comorbid diseases that are consistently associated with postoperative AKI. Preoperative level of renal function is one of the most important determinants of postoperative AKI after cardiac surgery. The method of assessment of preoperative renal function may influence the magnitude of the AKI risk; for example, estimation of GFR or creatinine clearance may provide a more precise ascertainment of baseline renal function than serum creatinine alone. Nevertheless, the qualitative relationship between preoperative renal function and postoperative AKI remains the same. Certain risk factors of AKI are unique to the cardiac surgical setting. For example, left main coronary artery stenosis of >70%, history of prior cardiac surgery, emergency surgery, and preoperative use of intra-aortic balloon pump (IABP) are associated with an increased risk of postoperative AKI. Among types of cardiac surgery, coronary artery bypass grafting (CABG) is associated with the lowest risk of AKI, compared with valve surgery, combined CABG and valve procedures, or other cardiac surgeries (e.g., septal defect repair, pericardial surgeries).[10]

Predicting postoperative AKI risk is both a clinical and a research tool. Accurate assessment of the risk of AKI allows in an informed decision-making process for the healthcare provider and the patient, by raising the awareness of potential risks of kidney injury and its associated consequences. The predictive tools can also be used for anticipating resource utilization, or comparing outcomes across healthcare systems. Most importantly, identification of high-risk patients provides an opportunity to optimize preoperative care, and potentially modify outcomes. Furthermore, cardiovascular surgical settings represent a unique "clinical model" to translate recent advances in diagnosis and early treatment of AKI. Because the renal insult can be anticipated, predicting AKI in this setting offers the promise to discover and validate novel diagnostic strategies as well as facilitate therapeutic interventions early in the course of the disease.

Chertow and colleagues were among the first to develop a preoperative renal risk stratification algorithm based on the VA Coronary Artery Surgery Study.[25] Patients, predominantly males, were stratified by dichotomous variables of comorbid disease burden to estimate the probability of postoperative AKI requiring dialysis (area under the receiver operating characteristic [ROC] curve = 0.72). To improve on the clinical utility of risk assessment, Thakar et al. examined over 30,000 cardiac surgeries performed at the Cleveland Clinic Foundation over a 10-year period. By incorporating a graded severity of multiple risk factors, a clinical AKI score was developed and internally validated with an improved predictive accuracy over prior analyses (Figure 34.2).[29] One of the objectives of this score was to incorporate factors that would allow for preoperative risk assessment, and to categorize patients

Risk Factor	Score
Female	1
CHF	1
LVEF < 35%	1
Pre-op IABP	2
COPD	1
IDDM	1
Prior Surgery	1
Emergency Surgery	2
Surgery Type: Valve Only	1
CABG + Valve	2
Other	2
Pre-op Creatinine: 1.2 to < 2.1 mg/dL	2
2.1 mg/dL or Greater	5

Score Group	AKI Dialysis
0–2	0.4%
3–5	2%
6–8	8%
9–13	21%

Figure 34.2.   Clinical score to predict AKI requiring dialysis (AKI-D) after cardiac surgery. Adapted from Thakar et al.[29] CHF, congestive heart failure LVEF, left ventricular ejection fraction; IDDM, insulin-dependent diabetes mellitus.

with a lower- and higher-than-average risk of AKI requiring dialysis after cardiac surgery. There are several other algorithms that have since assessed the probability of postoperative AKI.[26,30–32] Candela-Toha et al. externally validated and compared the performance of two clinical AKI scores published by Thakar et al. (Cleveland Clinic cohort) and Wijeysundera et al. (Toronto cohort) and found the ROC values to be 0.86 and 0.82, respectively.[33] Of note, most of these algorithms predict AKI requiring dialysis during the postoperative period. Palomba et al., on the other hand, included all patients with either a 50% rise in serum creatinine or a creatinine level above 2.0 mg/dL in their definition of AKI along with dialysis requirement.[32] The score yielded a good accuracy (ROC = 0.84) but was derived on a relatively smaller sample size within a single center.

Preoperative risk factors for AKI after cardiac transplantation are subtly different than nontransplant settings. Insulin-requiring diabetes, preoperative renal dysfunction, and a longer cold ischemia time of the solid organ were associated with an increased risk of AKI. In contrast, higher preoperative albumin was associated with lower risk of postoperative AKI requiring dialysis.[13,15,34]

Noncardiovascular Surgery

In noncardiac surgery, a different set of risk factors for AKI have been identified. Patients undergoing gastric bypass surgery present a unique comorbidity profile, which includes a high prevalence of diabetes, hypertension, hyperlipidemia, and osteoarthritis. Thus, these patients are commonly prescribed drug classes including angiotensin-converting enzyme inhibitors (ACE-I) or angiotensin receptor blockers (ARBs), diuretics, and nonsteroidal anti-inflammatory agents. In a single-center study, which examined over 300 gastric bypass surgeries, factors associated with an increased risk of postoperative AKI included higher body mass index (BMI), hyperlipidemia, and preoperative use of ACE-I/ARB agents.[20]

Kheterpal et al. developed a preoperative renal risk index in noncardiovascular surgeries, and identified the following independent risk factors for postoperative AKI: older age, emergency surgery, liver disease, high BMI, high-risk surgery, peripheral vascular disease, and COPD.[19] Higher risk scores were associated with a greater frequency of AKI, which ranged between 0.3% and 4.5%, depending on the risk category (Table 34.3).

In liver transplantation, Cabezuelo et al. studied 184 consecutive patients and defined AKI as a persistent rise in creatinine of 50% or more.[21] Serum albumin <3.2 g/dL and preoperative renal dysfunction was independently associated with postoperative AKI, and these findings have been confirmed by other investigators.[22]

Summary

Similar to the observations regarding incidence or severity of AKI, the surgical setting plays an important role in determining the set of preoperative risk factors that are associated with the risk of postoperative AKI. Comorbid disease burdens of cardiovascular conditions (e.g., CHF, reduced ejection fraction, severity of coronary artery disease) are important determinants of AKI in patients undergoing cardiovas-

TABLE 34.3. Risk Factors and Frequency of AKI after Noncardiovascular Surgery

Risk factors	Risk class	AKI frequency (%)
Age > 59	Class I (0 risk factors)	0.3
BMI > 32	Class II (1 risk factor)	0.5
Emergency surgery	Class III (2 risk factors)	1.3
High-risk surgery	Class IV (≥3 risk factors)	4.3
Peripheral vascular disease		
Liver disease		
COPD		

AKI, acute kidney injury; BMI, body mass index; COPD, chronic obstructive pulmonary disease.
Adapted from Kheterpal et al.[19]

cular surgeries. Type of surgical procedures also influences risk of AKI, and the details about intraoperative events will be discussed in the subsequent section. Across all types of surgeries, however, older age and level of preoperative renal function show a consistent association with postoperative AKI. These subtle yet clinically relevant variations in patient risk factors makes a strong case for providing multidisciplinary, patient-centered care in order to reduce postoperative renal morbidity.

INTRAOPERATIVE RISK FACTORS

Intraoperative factors are difficult to quantify in observational studies and may serve as surrogate for other unmeasured dynamic events during the surgical procedure. In cardiac surgery, intraoperative risk factors for postoperative AKI include use of IABP, hypothermic circulatory arrest, low-output syndrome, low urine output or vasopressor requirement during cardiopulmonary bypass (CPB), and number of blood transfusions during surgery.[28,35] One candidate risk factor, which is consistently linked with AKI, is the exposure to a CPB circuit along with its duration. In patients undergoing on-pump surgery, the risk of AKI increases beyond a threshold of 100–120 min on bypass machine. There is a plausible explanation; first, exposure to CPB circuit promotes a pro-inflammatory state, which may be deleterious to renal perfusion and function.[36] Additionally, evidence suggests that lack of pulsatile blood flow can impair renal perfusion, despite relative preservation of mean arterial pressure.[36,37] Thus, reducing the duration of exposure, or performing off-pump bypass surgery, has gained recent interest as a potentially modifiable risk factor for AKI. Several observational and randomized studies have compared renal outcomes in patients undergoing on-pump versus off-pump procedures. Nigwekar et al. performed a systematic review and meta-analysis of 22 studies (27,806 patients) that have reported renal outcomes, and compared exposure with CPB.[38] Overall, off-pump surgery was associated with a 43% reduction in the risk of postoperative AKI compared with on-pump surgery (odds ratio: 0.57, 95% confidence interval [CI]: 0.43–0.76). The authors caution that the definitions of AKI were variable and that the randomized controlled studies were relatively smaller. But it is reasonable to propose that given a high-risk preoperative profile for AKI, if feasible, off-pump surgery should be considered as a potential option to reduce the AKI risk.

Intraoperative factors during vascular surgery, including repair of AAA, have been studied for their association with AKI. Duration of renal ischemia (clamp time), and intraoperative hypotension are two primary determinants of postoperative AKI in this setting. Observational studies also indicate that newer techniques, such as endovascular aneurysm repair, may be associated with a lower risk of AKI than an open surgical approach.[16]

Incorporating the effect of intraoperative risk factors contributes in improving the accuracy of predictive models, as demonstrated by Kheterpal and colleagues in the setting of noncardiac surgery. For example, the area under the curve (AUC) of their risk index improved from 0.77 to 0.79 after incorporating the effect of intra-operative risk factors such as use of a vasopressor infusion, number of vasopressor bolus doses administered, and the administration of furosemide or mannitol.[19]

Summary

Diverse intraoperative events are associated with AKI. Certain risk factors, such as exposure to a CPB circuit or number of blood transfusions, may have a different pathophysiological basis for inducing kidney injury than others, such as clamp time or intraoperative hypotension. Identification of potentially modifiable risk factors such as duration or exposure to CPB can be used to minimize renal morbidity, particularly in patients that are at a greater risk of AKI. Taken together, preoperative risk assessment and a detailed review of intraoperative events should complement a provider's ability to predict postoperative risk of renal morbidity.

POSTOPERATIVE ASSESSMENT

Events during the immediate postoperative period also influence renal function. The literature in this regard is more difficult to interpret due to the lack of clear temporality between nonrenal events and AKI. In cardiac surgery, Slogoff et al. reported postoperative blood loss or transfusions, postoperative myocardial infarction, and need for emergent reoperation were associated with new renal dysfunction.[35] In the setting of cardiac transplant, Boyle et al. examined the timing of dialysis initiation with respect to the diagnosis of sepsis or other nonrenal complications such as cardiac failure. The majority of cases of AKI requiring dialysis (approximately 60%) were preceded by other nonrenal serious complications.[15] In liver transplant settings, dopamine use, liver graft dysfunction, surgical reoperation, and postoperative infection were significantly associated with AKI.[21] Regardless of the unclear cause-and-effect relationship between AKI and other nonrenal complications during the postoperative period, it is well recognized that the higher number of organ system failures directly contributes to increased mortality. Hence, patients who suffer from AKI and other nonrenal complications should be considered high risk for a poor hospital outcome, and may need a higher intensity of perioperative care.

EARLY DIAGNOSIS OF POSTOPERATIVE AKI: ROLE OF NOVEL BIOMARKERS

Serum creatinine remains the prevalent standard of care to measure changes in GFR. The use of serum creatinine has its limitations; for example, the creatinine level may be influenced by a variety of factors such as volume, catabolic state, or drugs in an inherently "nonsteady" state, particularly in critically ill patients. The search for the ideal biomarker has been the driving force behind the rapidly advancing field related to early ischemic injury.[39,40] Interleukin-18 (IL-18) and neutrophil gelatinase-associated lipocalin (NGAL) are two such biomarkers that have been tested in clinical settings including cardiac surgery. Evidence suggests that these are promising biomarkers (measurable in both urine and serum) for rapid and early detection of kidney injury among cardiac surgery patients.[41-43] Both NGAL levels and IL-18 levels in urine increased between 2 and 10 h after CPB in those patients who went on to develop AKI at 48 h. Although NGAL may be a very sensitive marker of tubular damage, IL-18 elevation may be more specific to ischemic tubular injury, and this may distinguish between patients with prerenal azotemia versus tissue injury. Cystatin C is another marker that has been studied in acute care settings, including cardiac surgery.[44-47] This substance is measured in the serum and is shown to provide a much more precise measure of GFR in a relatively nonsteady state. Additionally, elevation of cystatin C in response to a sudden decline in GFR is more rapid than the kinetics of serum creatinine, and this may allow for earlier determination of AKI. As of 2010, there are several clinical trials in the process of conducting validation studies for markers of AKI. Simultaneous advances have to be made in improving the technology of performing these sophisticated assays in a rapid, reproducible, and cost-effective manner.

Summary

Serum or urinary biomarkers may provide a more sensitive and specific assessment of renal parenchymal injury, including its severity, compared with surrogate measures of GFR. Additionally, these markers may allow for assessment of tissue damage in very early phases of renal injury, which would prove to be a major improvement over existing standards of care. It can be hypothesized that an accurate prediction of early kidney injury, along with preprocedure risk assessment, can facilitate novel interventions and modification of existing therapies in a timely manner.

PREVENTION AND TREATMENT OF AKI

Hemodynamic Agents and Diuretics

Multiple vasoactive agents such as "low-dose" dopamine,[48,49] fenoldopam,[50] or theophylline[51] have been used in the treatment of postoperative AKI, without any conclusive benefits in ameliorating kidney injury. Recombinant human atrial natriuretic peptide (ANP) was examined in a randomized study involving 61 patients with normal preoperative renal function who suffered postoperative cardiogenic shock requiring inotropic and vasoactive support. Infusion of ANP (50 ng/kg/min) enhanced renal excretory function, decreased the probability for dialysis, and improved dialysis-free survival in acute ischemic renal dysfunction after complicated cardiac surgery.[52]

Other randomized controlled trials (RCTs) involving natriuretic peptide administration in solid organ transplantation have shown inconsistent effects for renal end points. Nigwekar et al. (American Society of Nephrology, 2009, Abstract) performed a systematic review and meta-analysis of seven RCTs (three liver transplantation trials, three renal transplantation trials, and one heart transplantation trial) involving 238 participants. Pooled analysis showed reduction in AKI requiring dialysis in the natriuretic peptide group (risk ratio: 0.60, 95% CI 0.37–0.98) and reduction in the duration of dialysis requirement (–44.0 h, 95% CI –60.5 to –27.5 h).

ACE-I/ARB agents are commonly prescribed for coexisting conditions such as hypertension, cardiac failure, or chronic kidney disease. These agents are expected to change the renal autoregulatory mechanisms and induce intrarenal hemodynamic changes. Thus, there is potential that ACE-I/ARB therapy in the setting of acute perturbations to systemic circulation, as seen during anesthesia or surgical procedures, may have adverse influence over renal function. Thakar et al. demonstrated that in patients undergoing gastric bypass surgery, preoperative use of ACE-I/ARB was associated with a twofold increase in the risk of postoperative AKI, independent of other comorbid conditions or treatments.[20] ACE-I/ARB use in cardiac surgery has yielded conflicting reports. Arora et al. showed that preoperative use of ACE-I/ARB was associated with a 27% greater risk of postoperative AKI; but the overall incidence of AKI in this cohort was much higher (over 40%) than historical comparisons limiting the generalizability of their findings.[53] In contrast, Benedetto et al. showed that the incidence of AKI was 6.4% in patients receiving preoperative ACE-I/ARB compared with 12.2% in those who did not.[54] These divergent reports highlight the fact that larger prospective randomized controlled investigations are warranted before making any conclusive therapeutic recommendations.

Diuretic use, with a rationale that it may reduce oxygen consumption and limit tubular obstruction, has also been a matter of controversy in AKI treatment. In the setting of cardiac surgery, a double-blind, randomized, controlled trial involving 126 patients demonstrated that use of furosemide was associated with a higher rate of renal impairment, defined as 0.5 mg/dL increase in serum creatinine over baseline.[55] Similar results have been confirmed by other studies, suggesting that diuretic use, as an intervention to treat kidney injury after cardiac surgery, should be avoided.[56]

Cytoprotective Therapy

Pro-inflammatory cytokines have been extensively studied as mediators of ischemia-reperfusion injury in experimental models of AKI. Their role in patients undergoing cardiac surgery is of particular interest due to the potential stimulation of inflammatory mediators upon exposure to extracorporeal circuit. Use of therapeutic agents to interfere with these mediators, however, has been less than promising in terms of reducing risk of AKI after cardiac surgery. Steroids and N-acetylcysteine (NAC) have both been examined in cardiac surgery patients without any conclusive benefits.

Although NAC treatment prior to intravenous contrast administration has demonstrated a decreased risk of AKI, these observations have not translated to the perioperative setting. There have been at least 10 randomized trials testing NAC use in cardiac surgery. Neither the individual trials nor a recent meta-analysis of the pooled data showed any benefits of NAC in reducing postoperative AKI.[57–61]

Intensive glucose control achieved by insulin infusion is now a common practice in ICU patients, particularly in the setting of major surgery.[62] A post hoc analysis of the initial randomized studies indicated that the risk of AKI was lower in patients with tighter blood sugar control.[63] This beneficial effect was restricted to surgical ICU settings, which included cardiothoracic surgery. Whether glucose control modifies outcome in AKI remains to be examined.

There are limited data to examine the role of HMG-CoA reductase inhibitors (statins) as treatment of postoperative AKI. In a recent single-center study examining 3000 cardiac surgery patients, preoperative use of statins was associated with a 40% reduction in the risk of postoperative AKI requiring dialysis in patients undergoing CABG.[64] This benefit was not observed in valve surgeries or combined CABG and valve procedures. Similar to the experience in ACE-I/ARB use, a therapeutic recommendation cannot be made due to lack of prospective studies.

Studies have also evaluated the role of intravenous bicarbonate infusion, along with ascorbic acid treatment, on the risk of postoperative AKI after cardiac surgery. The results remain inconclusive regarding clear benefits of these therapies in reducing the risk of AKI.[65]

Extracorporeal Therapies

Dialysis has not been shown to reduce perioperative AKI; however, it can treat the associated metabolic complications such as acidosis, hyperkalemia, and hypervolemia, which may otherwise be associated with poor outcomes. For instance, after ruptured aortic aneurysm repair, renal support with dialysis may actually reduce operative 30-day mortality rates in patients that develop loss of renal function.[66] As many as 75% of these survivors may regain kidney function and become independent of dialysis.

Renal replacement therapy is used intraoperatively during liver transplantation. Townsend et al. recently reported their experiences with intraoperative continuous renal replacement therapy (CRRT) in orthotopic liver transplantation.[67] CRRT was used in 6.4% of liver transplant recipients, and was initiated for standard indications such as azotemia, hyperkalemia, acidosis, and hypervolemia, in addition to indications unique to liver transplantation such as need for significant transfusion, lactic acidosis, hypernatremia, and hyponatremia. The majority of cases were on CRRT more than 50% of the operative time. Given the fluid, electrolyte, and acid/base abnormalities associated with liver transplantation, CRRT can be a potentially useful tool in managing these patients.

Summary

Information regarding prevention and treatment of AKI in the perioperative setting is largely derived from cardiac surgery data. Diuretic therapy as a modality to prevent or treat AKI should be avoided. Natriuretic peptides may have a role in certain subgroups of patients. Insulin therapy is the only cytoprotective treatment that has shown some benefit in reducing AKI risk. Based on the present evidence strategies that may be beneficial in the prevention or treatment of contrast nephropathy (e.g., NAC or bicarbonate use) cannot be extrapolated to the perioperative setting. Drugs associated with worse renal outcomes could be avoided (ACE-I/ARB), unless absolute indications exist. Overall, the current evidence about pharmacotherapy during the perioperative period does not support any clear therapeutic benefit. However, very few interventions have been tested as adequately powered prospective clinical trials.

OUTCOMES IN AKI

Cardiovascular Surgery

Although the overall mortality rates after cardiac surgery are low (2–5%), the crude mortality rate among patients who develop AKI can be as high as 60% and account for almost half of the overall hospital deaths during the postoperative period. AKI is an independent risk factor for postoperative death, and the risk of mortality is proportional to the severity of kidney injury. Thus, kidney injury can be viewed as a distinct therapeutic target with its prevention and/or treatment expected to offer a survival benefit.[68]

AKI requiring dialysis is associated with a sevenfold increased risk of death during the perioperative period.[69] It is increasingly recognized that even milder degrees of kidney injury, measured as small increments in creatinine (or a decline in calculated GFR), are associated with an increased risk of death during the postoperative period.[11,12] In these reports, mortality rates in patients with a 30% decline in GFR were 4–6%, whereas in those patients with a 50% drop in GFR were 15%. In contrast, mortality rates in patients without any elevation in serum creatinine were <1%. Furthermore, the level of preexisting renal dysfunction modifies the relationship between postoperative kidney injury and mortality.[11]

There are relatively limited data examining long-term outcomes or renal recovery in AKI after cardiac surgery. In one study, Loef et al. reported that AKI after cardiac surgery was associated with twice the risk of death at 100 months as compared with those without AKI.[70] Although the majority of AKI patients who were alive at the time of hospital discharge experienced an improvement in their renal function, renal recovery did not have a lasting benefit.[70] This observation raises several interesting questions: (1) Could there be permanent tissue damage with long-term consequences despite the GFR returning to "baseline" immediately after the ischemic insult? (2) Could we be masking residual tissue damage by using a relatively insensitive marker of GFR such as creatinine measurement? (3) Could there be other organ–system interactions that are missed by measurement of GFR alone?

There has been improvement in hospital mortality associated with postoperative AKI over time. As reported by Thakar and colleagues, although the incidence of AKI after cardiac surgery has increased, mortality in AKI requiring dialysis showed a 20% reduction over the last decade, in addition to a 44% reduction in mortality associated with milder AKI.[71] It can be speculated that changes in the practice and technology of dialysis over the past decade may have contributed to these trends, along with improvements in delivery of postoperative care in surgical ICUs. However, such factors are very difficult to quantify in a retrospective study design.

Noncardiovascular Surgery

During postoperative period, the association between AKI and increased hospital mortality is also evident in the noncardiac surgical setting. In a retrospective study of 15,000 patients without preexisting renal dysfunction who underwent noncardiovascular surgery, the 30-day, 60-day, and 1-year mortality increased from 2.7% to 15%, 5.1% to 17%, and 15% to 31%, respectively, in patients who developed AKI compared with those without AKI.[19]

After surgery for AAA, patients who require renal replacement therapy experience mortality rates from 53% to 75%.[72,73] Even temporary worsening of renal function during the post-operative period after AAA repair is associated with a higher short-term and long-term mortality.[74]

Patients who develop AKI after with solid organ transplantation are also associated with similar mortality rates as observed in nontransplant setting; this may bear additional significance given the fact that it impacts patient survival as well as an allograft. Furthermore, in those who survive, postoperative AKI after nonrenal solid organ transplantation is associated with elevated risk of chronic renal failure during long-term follow-up.[15,24,67]

Summary

AKI during the postoperative period continues to be a serious morbidity, with devastating consequences during the immediate postoperative period as well as long-term follow-up. There is little doubt that preventing kidney injury or ameliorating its severity will translate into a survival benefit and improved long-term outcomes. Targeted therapeutic interventions and dialytic support have been met with a limited degree of success to modify outcome. However, over the past several decades, advances in the delivery of care have led to a steady improvement in mortality rates associated with AKI. Sufficient information exists to allow risk stratification to estimate the probability of postoperative AKI. This evidence should translate into delivery of better perioperative care, particularly in high-risk individuals. A schematic of a conceptual model for goals of perioperative renal care is illustrated in Figure 34.3. The magnitude of the problem, and the unique set of patient characteristics, calls for a multidisciplinary approach for the perioperative management of renal complications. A coordinated care model with participation from nephrologists, anesthesiologists, surgeons, and internists/hospitalists is necessary to achieve the desired change in improving patient outcomes. Such initiatives are also necessary for future clinical trials that can translate novel strategies of AKI diagnosis and treatment into clinical practice.

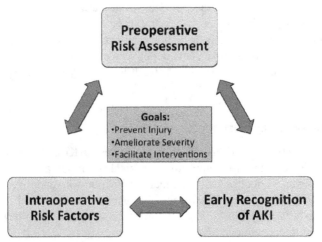

Figure 34.3. Conceptual model for perioperative renal care.

REFERENCES

1. Chertow GM, Burdick E, Honour M, Bonventre JV, Bates DW. Acute kidney injury, mortality, length of stay, and costs in hospitalized patients. *J Am Soc Nephrol*. Nov 2005;16(11):3365–3370.
2. Thakar CV, Christianson A, Freyberg R, Almenoff P, Render ML. Incidence and outcomes of acute kidney injury in intensive care units: a Veterans Administration study. *Crit Care Med*. 2009;37(9): 2552–2558.
3. Uchino S, Kellum JA, Bellomo R, et al. Acute renal failure in critically ill patients: a multinational, multicenter study. *JAMA*. August 17 2005;294(7):813–818.
4. Coca SG, Yusuf B, Shlipak MG, Garg AX, Parikh CR. Long-term risk of mortality and other adverse outcomes after acute kidney injury: a systematic review and meta-analysis. *Am J Kidney Dis*. Jun 2009;53(6):961–973.
5. Mehta RL, Kellum JA, Shah SV, et al. Acute Kidney Injury Network: report of an initiative to improve outcomes in acute kidney injury. *Crit Care*. Mar 1 2007;11(2):R31.
6. Molitoris BA, Levin A, Warnock DG, et al. Improving outcomes from acute kidney injury. *J Am Soc Nephrol*. Jul 2007;18(7):1992–1994.
7. Conlon PJ, Stafford-Smith M, White WD, et al. Acute renal failure following cardiac surgery. *Nephrol Dial Transplant*. 1999;14(5):1158–1162.
8. Mangano CM, Diamondstone LS, Ramsay JG, Aggarwal A, Herskowitz A, Mangano DT. Renal dysfunction after myocardial revascularization: risk factors, adverse outcomes, and hospital resource utilization. The Multicenter Study of Perioperative Ischemia Research Group. *Ann Intern Med*. 1998;128(3):194–203.
9. Abel RM, Buckley MJ, Austen WG, Barnett GO, Beck CH, Jr., Fischer JE. Etiology, incidence, and prognosis of renal failure following cardiac operations. Results of a prospective analysis of 500 consecutive patients. *J Thorac Cardiovasc Surg*. 1976;71(3):323–333.
10. Thakar CV, Liangos O, Yared JP, et al. ARF after open-heart surgery: influence of gender and race. *Am J Kidney Dis*. 2003;41(4):742–751.
11. Thakar CV, Worley S, Arrigain S, Yared J-P, Paganini EP. Influence of renal dysfunction on mortality after cardiac surgery: modifying effect of preoperative renal function. *Kidney Int*. Mar 1 2005;67(3): 1112–1119.
12. Lassnigg A, Schmidlin D, Mouhieddine M, et al. Minimal changes of serum creatinine predict prognosis in patients after cardiothoracic surgery: a prospective cohort study. *J Am Soc Nephrol*. Jun 1 2004;15(6):1597–1605.

13. Greenberg A. Renal failure in cardiac transplantation. *Cardiovasc Clin.* 1990;20(2):189–198.

14. Cruz DN, Perazella MA. Acute renal failure after cardiac transplantation: a case report and review of the literature. *Yale J Biol Med.* Sep–Oct 1996;69(5):461–468.

15. Boyle JM, Moualla S, Arrigain S, et al. Risks and outcomes of acute kidney injury requiring dialysis after cardiac transplantation. *Am J Kidney Dis.* Nov 2006;48(5):787–796.

16. Wald R, Waikar SS, Liangos O, Pereira BJ, Chertow GM, Jaber BL. Acute renal failure after endovascular vs. open repair of abdominal aortic aneurysm. *J Vasc Surg.* Mar 2006;43(3):460–466; discussion 466.

17. Godet G, Fleron MH, Vicaut E, et al. Risk factors for acute postoperative renal failure in thoracic or thoracoabdominal aortic surgery: a prospective study. *Anesth Analg.* Dec 1997;85(6):1227–1232.

18. Prinssen M, Verhoeven EL, Buth J, et al. A randomized trial comparing conventional and endovascular repair of abdominal aortic aneurysms. *N Engl J Med.* Oct 14 2004;351(16):1607–1618.

19. Kheterpal S, Tremper KK, Englesbe MJ, et al. Predictors of postoperative acute renal failure after noncardiac surgery in patients with previously normal renal function. *Anesthesiology.* Dec 2007; 107(6):892–902.

20. Thakar CV, Kharat V, Blanck S, Leonard AC. Acute kidney injury after gastric bypass surgery. *Clin J Am Soc Nephrol.* May 2007;2(3):426–430.

21. Cabezuelo JB, Ramirez P, Rios A, et al. Risk factors of acute renal failure after liver transplantation. *Kidney Int.* Mar 2006;69(6):1073–1080.

22. Yalavarthy R, Edelstein CL, Teitelbaum I. Acute renal failure and chronic kidney disease following liver transplantation. *Hemodial Int.* Oct 2007;11(Suppl 3):S7–12.

23. McCauley J, Van Thiel DH, Starzl TE, Puschett JB. Acute and chronic renal failure in liver transplantation. *Nephron.* 1990;55(2):121–128.

24. Ojo AO, Held PJ, Port FK, et al. Chronic renal failure after transplantation of a nonrenal organ. *N Engl J Med.* Oct 4 2003;349(10):931–940.

25. Chertow GM, Lazarus JM, Christiansen CL, et al. Preoperative renal risk stratification. *Circulation.* 1997;95(4):878–884.

26. Fortescue EB, Bates DW, Chertow GM. Predicting acute renal failure after coronary bypass surgery: cross-validation of two risk-stratification algorithms. *Kidney Int.* 2000;57(6):2594–2602.

27. Mangos GJ, Brown MA, Chan WY, Horton D, Trew P, Whitworth JA. Acute renal failure following cardiac surgery: incidence, outcomes and risk factors. *Aust N Z J Med.* 1995;25(4):284–289.

28. Zanardo G, Michielon P, Paccagnella A, et al. Acute renal failure in the patient undergoing cardiac operation. Prevalence, mortality rate, and main risk factors. *J Thorac Cardiovasc Surg.* 1994;107(6): 1489–1495.

29. Thakar CV, Arrigain S, Worley S, Yared J-P, Paganini EP. A clinical score to predict acute renal failure after cardiac surgery. *J Am Soc Nephrol.* Jan 1 2005;16(1):162–168.

30. Mehta RH, Grab JD, O'Brien SM, et al. Bedside tool for predicting the risk of postoperative dialysis in patients undergoing cardiac surgery. *Circulation.* Nov 21 2006;114(21):2208–2216; quiz 2208.

31. Wijeysundera DN, Karkouti K, Dupuis JY, et al. Derivation and validation of a simplified predictive index for renal replacement therapy after cardiac surgery. *JAMA.* Apr 25 2007;297(16):1801–1809.

32. Palomba H, de Castro I, Neto AL, Lage S, Yu L. Acute kidney injury prediction following elective cardiac surgery: AKICS score. *Kidney Int.* Sep 2007;72(5):624–631.

33. Candela-Toha A, Elias-Martin E, Abraira V, et al. Predicting acute renal failure after cardiac surgery: external validation of two new clinical scores. *Clin J Am Soc Nephrol.* Sep 2008;3(5):1260–1265.

34. Ishani A, Erturk S, Hertz MI, Matas AJ, Savik K, Rosenberg ME. Predictors of renal function following lung or heart-lung transplantation. *Kidney Int.* Jul 2002;61(6):2228–2234.

35. Slogoff S, Reul GJ, Keats AS, et al. Role of perfusion pressure and flow in major organ dysfunction after cardiopulmonary bypass. *Ann Thorac Surg.* Dec 1990;50(6):911–918.

36. Sezai A, Shiono M, Orime Y, et al. Major organ function under mechanical support: comparative studies of pulsatile and nonpulsatile circulation. *Artif Organs.* Mar 1999;23(3):280–285.

37. Orime Y, Shiono M, Hata H, et al. Cytokine and endothelial damage in pulsatile and nonpulsatile cardiopulmonary bypass. *Artif Organs.* Jun 1999;23(6):508–512.

38. Nigwekar SU, Kandula P, Hix JK, Thakar CV. Off-pump coronary artery bypass surgery and acute kidney injury: a meta-analysis of randomized and observational studies. *Am J Kidney Dis.* Sep 2009;54(3):413–423.

39. Hewitt SM, Dear J, Star RA. Discovery of protein biomarkers for renal diseases. *J Am Soc Nephrol.* Jul 1 2004;15(7):1677–1689.
40. Coca SG, Yalavarthy R, Concato J, Parikh CR. Biomarkers for the diagnosis and risk stratification of acute kidney injury: a systematic review. *Kidney Int.* May 2008;73(9):1008–1016.
41. Parikh CR, Jani A, Mishra J, et al. Urine NGAL and IL-18 are predictive biomarkers for delayed graft function following kidney transplantation. *Am J Transplant.* Jul 2006;6(7):1639–1645.
42. Parikh CR, Mishra J, Thiessen-Philbrook H, et al. Urinary IL-18 is an early predictive biomarker of acute kidney injury after cardiac surgery. *Kidney Int.* 2006;70(1):199–203.
43. Mishra J, Dent C, Tarabishi R, et al. Neutrophil gelatinase-associated lipocalin (NGAL) as a biomarker for acute renal injury after cardiac surgery. *Lancet.* Apr 2–8 2005;365(9466):1231–1238.
44. Dagher PC, Herget-Rosenthal S, Ruehm SG, et al. Newly developed techniques to study and diagnose acute renal failure. *J Am Soc Nephrol.* Aug 2003;14(8):2188–2198.
45. Herget-Rosenthal S, Feldkamp T, Volbracht L, Kribben A. Measurement of urinary cystatin C by particle-enhanced nephelometric immunoassay: precision, interferences, stability and reference range. *Ann Clin Biochem.* Mar 2004;41(Pt 2):111–118.
46. Herget-Rosenthal S, Marggraf G, Husing J, et al. Early detection of acute renal failure by serum cystatin C. *Kidney Int.* Sep 2004;66(3):1115–1122.
47. Herget-Rosenthal S, Trabold S, Pietruck F, Holtmann M, Philipp T, Kribben A. Cystatin C: efficacy as screening test for reduced glomerular filtration rate. *Am J Nephrol.* Mar–Apr 2000;20(2):97–102.
48. Tang AT, El-Gamel A, Keevil B, Yonan N, Deiraniya AK. The effect of "renal-dose" dopamine on renal tubular function following cardiac surgery: assessed by measuring retinol binding protein (RBP). *Eur J Cardiothorac Surg.* May 1999;15(5):717–721; discussion 721–712.
49. Woo EB, Tang AT, El-Gamel A, et al. Dopamine therapy for patients at risk of renal dysfunction following cardiac surgery: science or fiction? *Eur J Cardiothorac Surg.* Jul 2002;22(1):106–111.
50. Stone GW, McCullough PA, Tumlin JA, et al. Fenoldopam mesylate for the prevention of contrast-induced nephropathy: a randomized controlled trial. *JAMA.* Nov 5 2003;290(17):2284–2291.
51. Kramer BK, Preuner J, Ebenburger A, et al. Lack of renoprotective effect of theophylline during aortocoronary bypass surgery. *Nephrol Dial Transplant.* May 2002;17(5):910–915.
52. Sward K, Valsson F, Odencrants P, Samuelsson O, Ricksten SE. Recombinant human atrial natriuretic peptide in ischemic acute renal failure: a randomized placebo-controlled trial. *Crit Care Med.* Jun 2004;32(6):1310–1315.
53. Arora P, Rajagopalam S, Ranjan R, et al. Preoperative use of angiotensin-converting enzyme inhibitors/angiotensin receptor blockers is associated with increased risk for acute kidney injury after cardiovascular surgery. *Clin J Am Soc Nephrol.* Sep 2008;3(5):1266–1273.
54. Benedetto U, Sciarretta S, Roscitano A, et al. Preoperative angiotensin-converting enzyme inhibitors and acute kidney injury after coronary artery bypass grafting. *Ann Thorac Surg.* Oct 2008;86(4):1160–1165.
55. Lassnigg A, Donner E, Grubhofer G, Presterl E, Druml W, Hiesmayr M. Lack of renoprotective effects of dopamine and furosemide during cardiac surgery. *J Am Soc Nephrol.* 2000;11(1):97–104.
56. Lombardi R, Ferreiro A, Servetto C. Renal function after cardiac surgery: adverse effect of furosemide. *Ren Fail.* Sep 2003;25(5):775–786.
57. Loef BG, Henning RH, Epema AH, et al. Effect of dexamethasone on perioperative renal function impairment during cardiac surgery with cardiopulmonary bypass. *Br J Anaesth.* Dec 2004;93(6):793–798.
58. Tossios P, Bloch W, Huebner A, et al. N-acetylcysteine prevents reactive oxygen species-mediated myocardial stress in patients undergoing cardiac surgery: results of a randomized, double-blind, placebo-controlled clinical trial. *J Thorac Cardiovasc Surg.* Nov 2003;126(5):1513–1520.
59. El-Hamamsy I, Stevens LM, Carrier M, et al. Effect of intravenous N-acetylcysteine on outcomes after coronary artery bypass surgery: a randomized, double-blind, placebo-controlled clinical trial. *J Thorac Cardiovasc Surg.* Jan 2007;133(1):7–12.
60. Ristikankare A, Kuitunen T, Kuitunen A, et al. Lack of renoprotective effect of i.v. N-acetylcysteine in patients with chronic renal failure undergoing cardiac surgery. *Br J Anaesth.* Nov 2006;97(5):611–616.

61. Adabag AS, Ishani A, Bloomfield HE, Ngo AK, Wilt TJ. Efficacy of N-acetylcysteine in preventing renal injury after heart surgery: a systematic review of randomized trials. *Eur Heart J.* Aug 2009;30(15):1910–1917.

62. van den Berghe G, Wouters P, Weekers F, et al. Intensive insulin therapy in the critically ill patients. *N Engl J Med.* Nov 8 2001;345(19):1359–1367.

63. Schetz M, Vanhorebeek I, Wouters PJ, Wilmer A, Van Den Berghe G. Tight blood glucose control is renoprotective in critically ill patients. *J Am Soc Nephrol.* Mar 2008;19(3):571–578.

64. Virani SS, Nambi V, Polsani VR, et al. Preoperative statin therapy decreases risk of postoperative renal insufficiency. *Cardiovasc Ther.* Apr 2010;28(2):80–86.

65. Haase M, Haase-Fielitz A, Bellomo R, et al. Sodium bicarbonate to prevent increases in serum creatinine after cardiac surgery: a pilot double-blind, randomized controlled trial. *Crit Care Med.* Jan 2009;37(1):39–47.

66. Gordon AC, Pryn S, Collin J, Gray DW, Hands L, Garrard C. Outcome in patients who require renal support after surgery for ruptured abdominal aortic aneurysm. *Br J Surg.* Jun 1994;81(6):836–838.

67. Townsend DR, Bagshaw SM, Jacka MJ, Bigam D, Cave D, Gibney RT. Intraoperative renal support during liver transplantation. *Liver Transpl.* Jan 2009;15(1):73–78.

68. Star RA. Treatment of acute renal failure. *Kidney Int.* 1998;54(6):1817–1831.

69. Chertow GM, Levy EM, Hammermeister KE, Grover F, Daley J. Independent association between acute renal failure and mortality following cardiac surgery. *Am J Med.* 1998;104(4):343–348.

70. Loef BG, Epema AH, Smilde TD, et al. Immediate postoperative renal function deterioration in cardiac surgical patients predicts in-hospital mortality and long-term survival. *J Am Soc Nephrol.* Jan 2005;16(1):195–200.

71. Thakar CV, Worley S, Arrigain S, Yared JP, Paganini EP. Improved survival in acute kidney injury after cardiac surgery. *Am J Kidney Dis.* Nov 2007;50(5):703–711.

72. Braams R, Vossen V, Lisman BA, Eikelboom BC. Outcome in patients requiring renal replacement therapy after surgery for ruptured and non-ruptured aneurysm of the abdominal aorta. *Eur J Vasc Endovasc Surg.* Oct 1999;18(4):323–327.

73. Barratt J, Parajasingam R, Sayers RD, Feehally J. Outcome of acute renal failure following surgical repair of ruptured abdominal aortic aneurysms. *Eur J Vasc Endovasc Surg.* Aug 2000;20(2):163–168.

74. Welten GMJM, Schouten O, Chonchol M, et al. Temporary worsening of renal function after aortic surgery is associated with higher long-term mortality. *Am J Kidney Dis.* 2007;50(2):219–228.

CHAPTER 35

PERIOPERATIVE PAIN

Daniel Berland and Naeem Haider

BACKGROUND

Pain is an individual experience that may be a sign of tissue damage or have no identifiable cause at all. The experience of pain is influenced by a person's cultural background, prior pain events, mood, beliefs, and current ability to cope. Anxiety, depression, pain catastrophizing, chronic pain, and previous opioid exposure are all associated with higher postoperative pain intensity and emotional response.[1] Screening for at-risk individuals, appropriate preparation, patient education, and early analgesic interventions are all essential to reduce the potential for problems with immediate postsurgical pain management as well as to minimize the potential for progression to chronic postprocedure pain or escalation of prior pain treatments.

Poorly controlled acute postoperative pain can result in harmful physiological and psychological effects as well as increase the incidence of chronic pain after surgery (see Figure 35.1). For example, acute pain may produce increases in oxygen demand or cause prolonged immobility with associated risk for a heightened incidence of venous thromboembolic phenomena. Inhibition of immune system function or increased risk for postoperative infection may also result from under treatment of postoperative pain.[2] The risk for progression to a chronic pain state is increased in patients with prior pain syndromes, intraoperative nerve injury, and psychological vulnerability.[1,3] The consequence of producing or worsening a chronic pain state may include serious and long-lasting disability and social dysfunction.[4]

The adverse effects of overtreatment of pain, particularly with opioids, are also well described. Decreased patient comfort due to nausea, vomiting, and constipation is common with opioid use. Excess sedation or respiratory depression, for example, places the patient at risk for extended hospital stay, prolonged immobilization, need for ventilator support, or pneumonia. Opioid tolerance, hyperalgesia (an exaggerated sense of pain),[5-7] relapse of addiction, or risk for opioid abstinence syndrome may be the result of excessive or extended opioid therapy.

Because both the under- or overtreatment of postoperative pain may be harmful and pain treatments require the use of pharmacological agents having a narrow

Perioperative Medicine: Medical Consultation and Co-Management, First Edition.
Edited by Amir K. Jaffer and Paul J. Grant.
© 2012 Wiley-Blackwell. Published 2012 by John Wiley & Sons, Inc.

Acute Pain

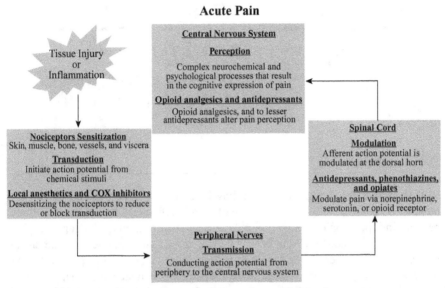

Figure 35.1. Acute pain–response mechanisms and opportunities for treatment. Mechanisms for the production by pain of physiological and psychological effects. Reproduced from Koo.[2]

therapeutic range, appropriate institutional policies and procedures should be implemented to ensure proper therapy.[8] Policies and procedures should define the training of primary service providers and nursing personnel in preoperative pain and risk assessment, perioperative analgesic techniques, opioid dosing and toxicity, monitoring of pain state, and standards for documentation of care. A role for an institutional pain service should be defined, particularly for the management of invasive pain management modalities such as epidural therapy as well as providing consultation for patients in whom over- or undertreatment is evident.[9] The use of standardized paper or computerized order sets may simplify and reduce variation in treatment, although the absence of decision support for drug selection, dosing, and monitoring can lead to continued high rates of adverse drug events when paper order entry systems are replaced with computerized systems.[10,11]

PATHOPHYSIOLOGY

Acute pain usually has a well-identified inciting event, either tissue injury or trauma. The initial transduction of this event is via peripheral nociceptors (mechanical, thermal, and polymodal) widely distributed throughout the body.[12] Damaged tissue releases prostaglandins and bradykinin that sensitizes nociceptors. This activity is tranduced through myelinated Aδ fibers and unmyelinated C fibers to the dorsal horn where synapses in laminae I–VI allow the pain signal to amplify and extend to adjacent dermatomes.[13] Following this synaptic divergence, the signal is transmitted through second-order neurons, crossing to the opposite side and ascending in the spinothalamic and spinomesencephalic tracts, targeting third-order neurons in the thalamus (pain transmission to sensory cortex) and anterior cingulate cortex (emotional aspects of pain). Descending inhibitory communication modulates the activity of the ascending Aδ and C fiber activity through chemical messengers including scrotonin, gamma aminobutyric acid, and norepinephrine.[14]

Peripheral sensitization results in the increased activity of nociceptors with a reduction in the threshold for activation and increase in both spontaneous and induced discharge. Functional alteration of response may occur with activation of other receptor subtypes (N-methyl-D-aspartate) and the maintenance of pain following resolution of the acute event, leading to a chronic pain state. The intensity of postoperative pain may also play a role in the development of such functional change. Central sensitization has been postulated to occur following surgical trauma, although functional magnetic resonance imaging (fMRI) assessment of pre- and postsurgical total knee arthroplasty patients failed to demonstrate increased pain responsiveness in a group of eight patients.[15] With the advancement of an understanding of the neuroplasticity within the nervous system, the simplistic understanding of pain conduction and perception has been replaced with a complex involvement of ascending activity, modulated at multiple synaptic locations by both descending inhibitory and excitatory signals.

PREVENTION STRATEGIES

Perioperative pain management begins with a preoperative patient evaluation that identifies physical or psychological comorbidities and controlled medication or illicit substance dependence or addiction. These elements may put an individual at risk for over- or undertreatment, with their associated complications, aberrant medication use, or evolution of chronic pain. Patient characteristics, the nature of the procedure, and anticipated postprocedure pain all require consideration prior to undertaking surgery. Occasionally, the findings from such a careful preoperative assessment will result in postponement of elective surgical procedures if there is excess risk for complications related to ongoing pain or pain management.

Many options are available for the treatment of postoperative pain, including local therapies such as regional blockade and systemic analgesics such as intravenous patient-controlled analgesia (IV-PCA). By considering the patient's preferences and making an individualized assessment of the risks and benefits of each treatment modality, the clinician can optimize the postoperative analgesic regimen for each patient. Proper assessment can lead to management strategies that minimize patient discomfort, risk for medical or psychological complications, or excessive length of stay.

Preoperative data gathering should include

- prior pain history, treatments, response, use of opioids, assessment of opioid tolerance;

- personal addiction history/risk (alcohol and substance use, arrests for driving while intoxicated, participation in substance abuse treatment programs);
- family history of addiction or chronic pain;
- uncontrolled psychiatric comorbidites that may result in the use of controlled medications for self-sedation rather than pain, for example, anxiety or depression;
- medical comorbidites.

In the past decade, the issue of pain and its relative undertreatment has received widespread attention as the "fifth vital sign." By 1999, Veteran's Administration policy required the use of a 10-point pain assessment scale, and a declaration by the Joint Commission on Accreditation of Healthcare Organizations was followed in 2001 by new standards for pain assessment and management that continue to be monitored by their surveyors. This attention has been followed by the liberalization of opioid prescribing by practitioners for many forms of chronic, nonterminal pain. With more liberal prescribing has come an increase in large dose, continuous opioid therapy, despite a lack of evidence for effectiveness of such treatment, the high risk for misuse of these medications and an increased incidence of overdose and death.[16–18] Patients currently treated with high-dose opioids require special consideration and, for elective surgical procedures, may benefit from postponement of the procedure due in part to difficult pain management or aberrant medication use that may follow the procedure. Correction of opioid prescribing based on functional measures of improvement can assist in the process of preparing the patient for postoperative rehabilitation.

High-dose opioid-treated patients may manifest substantial perioperative opioid resistance due to acquired opioid tolerance while they are simultaneously likely to suffer hyperalgesia, increased sensitivity to pain, or enhanced intensity of pain sensation.[19,20] These patients present special problems for under dosing, as their opioid requirements may be 50–300% greater than that seen in opioid naïve patients. If their chronic therapy is not able to be tapered preoperatively, these patients may be best treated with local analgesic techniques and opioid given by IV-PCA.[21,22]

Patients treated with methadone for chronic pain, opioid dependence, or addiction have ample opioid tolerance and dependence. They should generally have methadone continued to avoid opioid withdrawal state. This drug can sometimes lead to QT interval prolongation, which may put the patient at risk for *Torsades de pointes*. A QTc of greater than 500 ms is associated with a substantially increased risk.[23] A preoperative electrocardiogram must be obtained to assess the QTc and consideration made of the potential interaction between methadone and other drugs that may prolong the QT interval or slow the elimination of methadone. Because of opioid tolerance in these patients, local analgesic techniques and adequate additional opioid, often given by IV-PCA, should follow procedures expected to produce large amounts of pain.

Patients treated with buprenorphine (Suboxone®, Subutex®, Reckitt Benckiser, Berkshire, UK) also require special attention during planning for surgery.[24,25] Buprenorphine is a synthetic partial opioid agonist that acts primarily at the mu_1-opioid receptor. It is approximately 30 times as potent as morphine and has high receptor affinity, producing a long duration of activity (24–60 h) and potential receptor blockade of other opioids. Buprenorphine has proved to be a safe and effective agent in the treatment of pain, opioid dependence, and addiction. It is an effective pain treatment with a wide safety profile due to its low risk for overdose.

As a partial agonist, when high receptor occupancy has been reached, because of its very high receptor affinity, buprenorphine may block full mu_1 agonists and prove inadequate for treating acute pain. Patients treated for chronic pain or opioid dependence with smaller doses of buprenorphine ($\leq$6 mg/day) having procedures that are not expected to produce substantial pain may continue buprenorphine and be treated temporarily for additional acute pain with potent full agonists such as hydromorphone on top of the buprenorphine. Patients treated with higher doses of buprenorphine (>6 mg/day) or having procedures likely to produce substantial pain require discontinuation of buprenorphine for a minimum of 5 days with "bridging therapy" utilizing a short-acting full agonist, typically oral hydrocodone, morphine, or hydromorphone, until reinstitution of buprenorphine can take place following resolution of the acute pain state. Patients anticipated to have continuing or fluctuating pain may be better treated by conversion to methadone in divided doses with or without an additional short-acting agent. In opioid-dependent or -addicted patients, the return to buprenorphine may be more complicated.[26]

Patients with a history of excessive use of beverage alcohol, or the recent use of or addiction to prescription medications or illicit substances require careful preoperative assessment and planning as abstinence states may complicate their postoperative course.[2] When possible, these patients should be stabilized prior to surgical procedures. Consultation with an Addiction Medicine specialist may be necessary. Acute alcohol or benzodiazepine withdrawal produces a neuroexcitatory state that may be complicated by delirium or seizure. Patients at risk for alcohol withdrawal should be detoxified prior to elective surgery or prophylaxed postoperatively with benzodiazepenes to prevent withdrawal. Opioid withdrawal, though generally not life threatening, may produce severe discomfort and agitation. Benzodiazepine withdrawal may result in agitation and seizures. Opioid- and benzodiazepine-using patients require adequate replacement of these agents during the perioperative period. When a history of medication misuse is possible, patients should have urine toxicology screening using a gas chromatography–mass spectrometry test to detect prescribed agents. The use of typical enzyme-linked immunoassay urine screening test for abused drugs is inadequate to detect most prescribed controlled medications. Furthermore, there should be a check with the controlled prescription monitoring programs for prescription fills that may not have been reported by the patient. These programs are readily available online for most states and will likely become federally mandated in the future.

Patients with anxiety, depression, or another uncontrolled psychiatric illness, or those prone to catastrophizing their illness present special challenges for perioperative pain management.[1] Patients who exhibit excessive fear or anxiety require preoperative education and counseling, and need to be involved in the choice of analgesic techniques to be utilized, thereby giving them a sense of control in their treatment. This may lessen their tendency to aberrant pain medication use as a method of self-sedation. Preoperative treatment of anxiety has been shown to reduce opioid intake in the postoperative period, in addition to a reduction in the overall pain experienced.

Patients with renal dysfunction require caution in the use of medications or those with metabolites that are cleared by the kidneys. Dose or dosing interval adjustments should be made when the patient's estimated glomerular filtration rate (eGFR), most commonly estimated through the use of the modification of diet in renal disease (MDRD) equation, falls below recommended thresholds. Morphine-treated patients with an eGFR of <50 require dose reductions of 25%, while those with an eGFR of <10 require 50% dose reductions, or, may receive a more stable treatment with equianalgesic doses of hydromorphone or oxycodone.

Geriatric patients may be at risk for medication toxicity due to organ dysfunction and decreased medication clearance, or, in those with cognitive impairment, have elevated risk for postoperative delirium. For these reasons as well as communication barriers such as hearing or speech impairment, the undertreatment of geriatric patients is widespread.[8] These patients should receive care based on their size, renal function as estimated by eGFR, and comorbidites, not their age.

Pregnant or lactating women present unique issues related to medication choice. Nonsteroidal anti-inflammatory drugs (NSAIDs) increase the risk for miscarriage and should be avoided after 32 weeks' gestation. The prolonged use of opioids during pregnancy results in an increased risk of neonatal abstinence syndrome. Morphine, fentanyl, oxycodone, acetaminophen, and NSAIDs are safe in lactation.[1]

POSTOPERATIVE ASSESSMENT

The timing of postoperative pain assessment starts in the preoperative period. Allowing the patient to depart from the recovery room without an agreed upon pain treatment plan can lead to suboptimal pain care, even at institutions where an acute pain service is available on consultation.[27] At the time surgery is scheduled, consideration of postoperative pain expectations, previous pain experiences, anticipated pain, and available treatment options should be reviewed with the patient (see Table 35.1). This will allow time for the patients to make an informed choice about modalities available to them. The establishment of realistic pain management expectations can be of importance in providing the best experience possible. At no time should the absence of pain be promised. Instead, the goal is that despite pain experienced following surgery, the patient will be provided aggressive care to lower pain to a level that is tolerable. The documentation of this assessment, along with a treatment plan, will provide guidance to all medical providers in the care of the patient in the perioperative state. Research into the prediction of postoperative pain intensity to allow individualizing of pain management in select patient populations is under way utilizing validated pain assessment tools.[28–30]

Initial postoperative pain management is usually a continuum of the intraoperative pain care provided by an anesthesiology provider or by the surgeon (if no other provider is required). Pain assessment needs to involve identification of the site of pain in relationship to the surgical procedure. At times, the site of pain may

TABLE 35.1.   Pain Assessment Questions

Are you having pain now? If the answer is "Yes," then additional assessment along with immediate intervention is needed

Pain intensity—how much pain are you in now on a pain scale?

Location—where is the pain located and does it go anywhere?

Quality or pattern of pain—allow the patients to use their own words whenever possible to describe the quality of their pain

Temporal nature of pain—onset, duration, and variations

Influencing factors—alleviating and aggravating factors

Past interventions—pain management history (including past medications and their efficacy and toxicity)

Effects of pain—impact on daily life, function, sleep, appetite, emotions, concentration, and ability to perform activities

Assessment of response—clinical response to present pain management regimen in terms of efficacy and side effects

The patient's pain management goal (including pain intensity level the patient would like you to achieve and goals related to function, activities, and quality of life)

Physical assessment and observations of the pain site—direct observation of the painful site and the range of motion of the involved site will aid your final therapeutic decision. If the patient is experiencing increased back pain after a spinal procedure, and it is exacerbated by abdominal distension, then obviously you would not want to give the patient more opiates to treat the pain. Instead, you might want to try to move the patient's bowel to reduce the pressure on the spine and reduce the back pain.

Helpful questions to assess the current pain status, the patient's emotional response to pain, anticipate the patient's specific needs, and arrive at a reasonable plan of management to render the pain tolerable and maximize function. Reproduced from Koo.[2]

have no relation to the procedure performed, as in the case of headache related to caffeine withdrawal or a chronic pain state, in the case of low back pain or peripheral neuropathic pain states. A single global pain score is of little value in determining the first step in treating the postoperative acute pain patient and needs to be reviewed in conjunction with prior pain complaints as well as expected sites of pain (dressings, drains, chest tubes, etc.). Table 35.1 provides a list of questions that may be used to assess the acute pain patient, following determination that the pain is not merely an exacerbation of a chronic pain complaint.

MEDICAL MANAGEMENT

Choice of Analgesic Agent

Pain relief in the postoperative period is one of the important components in the recovery from a surgical procedure. First-line therapy for postoperative pain complaints often encompasses use of ketorolac or short- to intermediate-acting opioids by the intravenous route. Avoidance of the intramuscular route of administration is

TABLE 35.2.   Converting between Morphine and Other Opioids—Equianalgesic Dosing

Starting opioid	Target opioid	Equianalgesic ratio
Oral morphine	IV morphine	3:1
Morphine	Hydromorphone (by the same route of administration)	5:1
Oral morphine	Oxycodone (oral only)	1.5:1
Fentanyl transdermal	Oral morphine	One 25 µg/h patch: range of 50–90 mg/day morphine (use low end of range for patients on >100 µg/h fentanyl transdermal)
Methadone	Any	There are no reliable ratios for converting *from* methadone. Consider methadone-treated patients to be opioid tolerant

Reducing the target opioid dose by 25% may be appropriate, as the replacement opioid is often tolerated in a reduced dose due to the effect of cross tolerance. University of Michigan Pain Management Initiative, 2009.

recommended in order to provide rapid onset of analgesia.[31] Although fentanyl is commonly used in recovery rooms with the goal of rapid pain reduction, the inherent risk of respiratory depression with repeat loading doses makes it less than optimal following the first half to 1 h postoperatively. Though other opioids may be utilized, morphine remains the gold standard for acute postoperative pain via the intravenous route. Titrated slowly in opioid naïve patients, that is, by no more than 2–3 mg boluses every 10–15 min, it has a higher safety profile than other commonly used opioid preparations due in part to ease in dosing (low potency), high familiarity (most medical providers), and a side effect profile that is equivalent to other opioids. If another opioid is used, it is essential to understand equianalgesic potency when compared with morphine (see Table 35.2).

The first 24 h following a surgical procedure remains the highest risk period for opioid-related respiratory depressant events.[32,33] Large, frequent boluses of opioids have been reported to lead to respiratory depression at a delayed point in time and warrant use of continued respiratory monitoring either through frequent assessment, use of respiratory rate monitors, and/or the use of continuous pulse oximetry while the patient is recumbent.[34] Elderly patients (above 65 years of age); the presence of one or more comorbidities in renal, hepatic, and heart disease; sleep apnea; and use of hydromorphone were all found to incur a greater risk of respiratory depressant events in one retrospective case-control analysis.[33] Presence of comorbid medical conditions, particularly sleep apnea, should direct the choice and dose of opioid with a goal of reducing side effects from slow dose titration with a higher frequency of assessment or monitoring. Impaired renal elimination of active metabolites of morphine can result in significant respiratory depression with repeat dosing of morphine over time or in some cases with a single large bolus dose.

In patients with mild-to-moderate anticipated pain and no contraindication for its use, ketorolac may often be utilized by the intravenous route as a single agent immediately postoperatively.[35] Intravenous NSAIDs have the additional benefit of

TABLE 35.3.   Determination of Patients as Opioid Naïve or Opioid Tolerant

Morphine	≥80 mg/day
Oxycodone	≥40 mg/day
Hydromorphone	≥20 mg/day
Hydrocodone	≥80 mg/day
Codeine	≥480 mg/day
Fentanyl	≥25 µg/h
Methadone	≥15 mg/day
Buprenorphine	Surgery may require delay (see text)

Determining the patient's opioid tolerance is essential for proper dosing. Sustained treatment in the preceding 2 weeks at these doses (not necessarily equianalgesic doses due to pill sizes) determines the degree of tolerance. University of Michigan Pain Management Initiative, 2009.

rapid onset of action with side effect reduction over opioids alone.[36–38] Using morphine or another opioid in the postoperative state may have a limited effect in opioid-tolerant patients (see Table 35.3). At that point in time, rather than switching to an alternate opioid such as hydromorphone, the clinician should consider the addition of an adjuvant non-opioid analgesic such as an NSAID or acetaminophen.[39] Reduction in morphine utilization has been reported to range from 15% to 55% in one randomized, placebo-controlled trial.[40] In addition to opioid dose reduction, this study demonstrated a mild reduction in nausea and sedation attributed to opioid use, with NSAIDs offering the highest degree of analgesic benefit with an increase in risk of bleeding from 0% to 1.7% (nonselective NSAIDs).[40] The risk of bleeding in such cases needs to be weighed against the benefit of side effect reduction and improved analgesia with a multimodal approach.[41]

Due to the platelet inhibitory effect of all NSAIDs, other than cyclooxygenase-2 (COX-2) inhibitors(e.g., celecoxib), acetaminophen has been the first-choice adjuvant.[42] Reduction in morphine consumption has been reported, although a comparable reduction in morphine-related adverse effects has not been seen.[43,44] It is important to avoid the use of acetaminophen in doses above those recommended (2–3 g/day for an average adult) or in cases where liver function is impaired or expected, as in liver resection procedures or liver failure. Preemptive use of both acetaminophen and NSAIDs has been shown to reduce opioid requirements postoperatively in an attempt to minimize side effects related to opioid use, although reduction in overall pain score has not been consistently seen.[44–48] The route of administration of NSAIDs and acetaminophen may play a role in improving analgesic outcomes with the preferred method being intravenous, followed by oral and finally rectal use providing the least benefit in both adults and infants.[49–51] Planned use of multimodal analgesia in procedures with anticipated postoperative pain that is moderate to severe is recommended.[52–54]

Regional Analgesia Techniques

Despite the opioid-sparing effect of adjuvant non-opioid analgesics, the only means to eliminate opioid-related side effects perioperatively is by utilization of regional anesthetic techniques (epidural, caudal, peripheral nerve blockade, etc.) in the presence of a comprehensive non-opioid-based pain management plan. Use of regional techniques does more than simply reduce opioid-related side effects. Benefits from use of epidural analgesia in the postoperative period are wide ranging, with reduction in morbidity and mortality in high-risk patients and decreased incidence of gastrointestinal, pulmonary, and cardiac complications. Improved analgesia in conjunction with a reduction in sympathetic tone has a positive benefit on multiple organ systems. Earlier return of gastrointestional function is seen with the use of epidural local anesthetics. Effects of epidural opioid on bowel recovery after surgery are countered by the sympathetic blockade provided by local anesthetics, with the net result of improvement in return of bowel function when compared with intravenous opioid therapy (IV-PCA). Improvement in diaphramatic excursion leads to a reduction in postoperative pulmonary complications as seen in a decreased incidence of pulmonary infection rates. Reduction in hypercoagulable states, improved analgesia, and increased coronary blood flow have the net effect of decreasing myocardial infarction rates. There is evidence to support the position that aggressive perioperative analgesia using regional anesthesia can reduce the incidence of chronic pain, although the exact relationship remains unclear at this time.[14] Some well-defined neuropathic pain states (phantom limb pain) appear to manifest with a lower incidence when aggressive perioperative analgesia is utilized using regional anesthetic methods. Care must be taken to avoid a lapse in analgesia during conversion from regional analgesic modalities to oral or intravenous analgesia. Tapering of dosing regimens prior to discontinuation has been shown to improve pain management.[55] Involvement of an acute pain service can assist with the planning and preparation of patients and provides access to a team that can intervene when standardized methods of management have failed to achieve the desired response.[9]

The selection of opioid used in neuraxial analgesia can affect the side effect profile in the postoperative patient.[56] Single injection of neuraxial hydrophilic opioids (morphine, hydromorphone) can provide analgesia over the first 24 h postsurgery. Hydrophobic opioids (fentanyl) in contrast provide rapid onset of analgesia and are cleared into the systemic circulation with a resulting short duration of action that is suboptimal in the postoperative period. Patients receiving neuraxial morphine or hydromorphone are at risk for delayed respiratory depression (within the first 24 h postdose) and should be monitored with continuous pulse oximetry while recumbent as a result, along with an equivalent level of nursing care as is provided for patients on continuous epidural opioid infusions. Pruritus and urinary retention have been reported to occur at a lower incidence with use of hyromorphone and fentanyl in comparison with morphine in continuous epidural analgesia.[57] In contrast, single-dose hydromorphone offered no advantage over morphine in postcesarean section patients.[58]

Epidural analgesia via a catheter placed in concordance with the dermatomal distribution of the acute pain process, provides easy titration of dose to allow for varying degrees of response in patients. The combination of low-dose opioid (morphine 50 µg/mL or hydromorphone 10 µg/mL in adult opioid naïve patients) with low concentrations of local anesthetic (bupivicaine 0.0625%, bupivicaine 0.125%, ropivicaine 0.1%, ropivicaine 0.2%, or levobupivicaine 0.125%) provides the best depth of analgesia in rates per hour ranging from as little as 4 up to 19 total milliliters per hour as either a continuous infusion or a patient-controlled epidural analgesic (PCEA) setup, providing a bolus dose of 2–3 mL every 20 min as needed. Use of PCEA has been found to lower the total hourly rate needed by patients with no reduction in analgesia and is considered the optimal means of delivering epidural analgesia on nursing floors.[59] Patient satisfaction and quality of life are also improved when compared with IV-PCA therapy alone.[59]

Epidural catheter use may routinely be continued postoperatively until day 6, unless a fever >101.5 persists, a source of infection is identified, suspicion of deep infection is raised due to neurologic deficits, and/or signs of localized skin infection are seen at the catheter placement site.[60] Use of antibiotics during use of short-term epidural catheterization is not recommended.[61] Infectious complications are extremely rare, and the incidence for epidural catheter abscess remains low.[62–64] Repeat neurologic assessment throughout the use of an epidural catheter is recommended in order to intervene early in the development of neurologic compromise.[63,65,66]

Peripheral nerve blockade provides superior analgesia with lower incidence of side effects when compared with IV-PCA and/or epidural analgesia.[67,68] Out of all the available analgesic methods, it is regional nerve blockade that can allow for postanesthesia recovery discharge in over 98% or patients without the need for supplemental opioids. This has a significant impact in reduction in opioid-related side effects, but cannot be maintained beyond the first 24 h unless continuous catheter techniques are used.[69–71] A complication of nerve injury from regional blockade is usually transient and occurs at an incidence well below that of nerve damage from surgery itself.[72]

The use of anticoagulant therapy in the perioperative period plays a significant role in defining the timing of placement and discontinuation of regional anesthetic techniques.[73] It is important to recognize that newer agents are in development, and any guidelines in the use of anticoagulant therapy need to be constantly updated in order to maintain clinical relevance.[74] In-depth coverage of regional anesthetic-based techniques is beyond the scope of this chapter and should be discussed in the perioperative period with involvement of the patient, surgeon, anesthesia provider, and postoperative pain provider (surgeon, anesthesiologist, internist, and/or acute pain service).[75]

Role and Management of Patient-Controlled Analgesia

After the rapid establishment of adequate pain relief through repeated intermittent dosing of non-opioid and/or opioid analgesics, because of the very short half-life and duration of activity of IV push opioids, it is recommended that patients be provided with continuous access to analgesics either by scheduled oral dosing (if possible) or via utilization of IV-PCA devices. When opioids are used, several basic principles for managing opioids can produce good pain relief, minimize side effects, and maximize patient safety (see Table 35.4). Maintaining patients on one opioid at a time during dose adjustment removes guesswork for nursing staff, simplifies decision making, and permits accurate calculation of conversion between opioids or conversion from parenteral to oral routes of administration. The use of weak opioids

TABLE 35.4. Principles of Opioid Management for Acute Pain

1. Use a synergistic pain agent (NSAID or acetaminophen).
2. Use only one opioid rather than polypharmacy.
3. Morphine is the preferred agent. Hydromorphone and oxycodone are reasonable alternatives.
4. For anticipated moderate-to-severe pain, give scheduled medication rather than PRN doses.
5. The oral route is preferred over intermittent IV push dosing.
6. Dosing intervals for an oral short-acting medication should not be greater than Q4 h. For the IV route, if used, Q2 h or Q3 h is appropriate.
7. Double-range order dosing (e.g., 15–30 mg PO Q4–6 h) is ineffective and a Joint Commission violation.
8. Use PCA for severe pain not promptly controlled, especially in opioid-tolerant patients after initial achievement of analgesia with intravenous bolus doses.
9. Do not titrate long-acting medications to treat acute-on-chronic pain.
10. Conversion from parenteral to oral therapy should occur without gaps in therapy. Stop IV treatments 30 min after first oral dose is given.
11. Use agents such as senna or polyethylene glycol (MiraLax®, Merck, Memphis, TN) rather than docusate for opioid constipation prophylaxis.
12. Ondansetron is the most effective agent for nausea, vomiting, and pruritus. Prochlorperazine and promethazine are alternatives for nausea or vomiting, and nalbuphine is an alternative for pruritus. IV push diphenhydramine should not be used due to ineffectiveness and addiction risk.
13. Unless the surgery or complications dictate an extraordinary duration of pain treatment, there should be a plan to end acute treatment with short-acting medication within a week with a return to prior or no opioid treatment. Do not discharge patients with large amounts of PRN medication, particularly in patients with a known risk of substance abuse or diversion

Basic principles to follow when utilizing opioids. University of Michigan Pain Management Initiative, 2009.

(acetaminophen-containing opioid preparations) in patients where anticipated pain is moderate to high may result in inadequate analgesia and should be replaced by use of a scheduled strong opioid (morphine, oxycodone, or hydromorphone) given along with a scheduled dose of acetaminophen or NSAID with the goal of gradual titration until satisfactory analgesia is maintained. Dosing intervals for short-acting strong opioids in the acute postoperative patient may be as frequent as every 3 h, but usually no more than every 4 h. Examples of common dosing scenarios are given in Table 35.5. Failure to control pain promptly, particularly in opioid-experienced patients should prompt the use of IV-PCA.

Evidence from randomized controlled trials and meta-analyses indicate that IV-PCA therapy leads to improved pain relief, reduction in postsurgical complications and increased patient satisfaction.[76–78] The mean incidence of respiratory depression with IV-PCA therapy is reported to range from 1.2% to 11.5%.[79] Reduction in length of stay has not been observed.[76] IV PCA therapy is labor intensive and requires a standardized approach in dosing and adjustment in dosing, in order to optimize therapeutic benefit.[80,81] Understanding PCA modes of administration and the dosing variables in a structured fashion is of value in initiating and managing patients with IV-PCA therapy (see Figure 35.2).[81] Morphine is the gold standard for IV-PCA therapy.[9] If the patient's pain is not controlled after initial morphine admin-

TABLE 35.5. Typical Treatment Scenarios after General Surgical Procedures

Anticipated level of pain	Opioid-naïve patients	Opioid-tolerant patients
Mild	Acetaminophen (APAP) 650 mg PO Q4 h PRN or ibuprofen 400–600 mg Q4 h or Q6 h PRN. If NPO, ketorolac[a] 15–30 mg IV Q6 h PRN	Acetaminophen (APAP) 650 mg PO Q4 h PRN or ibuprofen 400–600 mg Q4 h or Q6 h PRN. If NPO, ketorolac[a] 15–30 mg IV Q6 h PRN
Moderate	Ketorolac[a] 30 mg IV Q6 h if NPO or APAP 325 mg/hydrocodone 10 mg or APAP 300 mg/codeine 60 mg or APAP 325 mg/oxycodone 5 mg—give one Q4 h *scheduled* while awake	Ketorolac[a] 30 mg IV Q6 h if NPO or APAP 325 mg/hydrocodone 10 mg or APAP 300 mg/codeine 60 mg or APAP 325 mg/ oxycodone 5 mg—give two Q4 h *scheduled* while awake. May combine with IV ketorolac
Severe	Ketorolac[a] 30 mg IV Q6 h *plus* morphine[b] 15 mg PO Q3 h or hydromorphone 4 mg PO Q3 h or oxycodone 10 mg PO Q3 h PRN	Ketorolac[a] 30 mg IV Q6 h *plus* morphine[b] 30 mg PO Q3 h or hydromorphone 6 mg PO Q3 h or oxycodone 20 mg PO Q3 h *scheduled*
If pain remains uncontrolled	Ketorolac[a] IV and IV-PCA morphine[c]	Ketorolac[a] IV and IV-PCA morphine[c]

Possible treatments for opioid-naïve or -tolerant patients based on anticipated pain.
[a] Ketorolac requires adjustment for weight <50 kg, age >65, Cl_{Cr} <30, and if <10 is contraindicated. Ketorolac may be contraindicated after specific orthopedic or neurosurgery procedures.
[b] Oxycodone or hydromorphone is preferred over morphine when Cl_{Cr} <30.
[c] Substitute hydromorphone if Cl_{Cr} <30.
NPO, nil per os.

istration, the morphine dose should be escalated rather than changing to an alternate opioid such as hydromorphone, unless there are side effects (nausea, emesis, pruritus) that are uncontrolled despite the use of appropriate pharmacologic intervention. Hydromorphone is an appropriate substitute, particularly in renal insufficiency patients, and is used at 20% of the morphine dose in milligrams.

Initial settings must be made with consideration for the patient's prior opioid use and should be set with a goal of gradual titration in dose with a fixed dosing interval at the lowest that the patient is expected to tolerate. Initial morphine IV-PCA dosing for adults is usually 1 mg every 6 min on demand via a bolus button with no basal rate, as this provides the best balance between optimal analgesia and minimal side effects.[81,82] This will allow access to 10 mg of morphine per hour if needed, although usual utilization should be no more than three to four button pushes per hour. If a patient is using over six button pushes on average per hour, an increase in the button bolus dose by 50% or a reduction in the time during which the patient will not receive medication despite pressing the button (lockout interval), if greater than 6 min, should be initially attempted. Bolus doses of greater than 2.5 mg of morphine in an opioid naïve patient every 6 min are usually not required and are an indication that there is minimal benefit from unimodal opioid dose increase, warranting reassessment for use of adjuvant medications or analgesic techniques

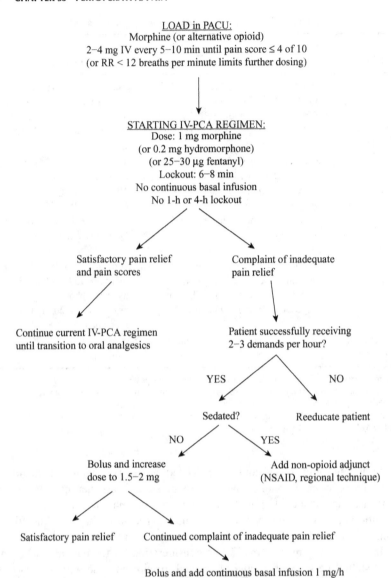

Figure 35.2. Management of intravenous patient-controlled analgesia (IV-PCA). Simplified algorithm for the management of IV-PCA in opioid-naïve patients. RR, respiratory rate; NSAID, nonsteroidal anti-inflammatory drug; PACU, postanesthesia care unit. Reproduced from Grass.[81]

(regional blockade). Lockout intervals greater than 6 min are often used with a necessary increase in the bolus dose to accommodate for the hourly dose available to the patient. In such patients, the first step in improving analgesia should be a reduction in the interval between available demand doses, that is, from 10 to 6 min, rather than an increase in the bolus dose itself. Safety from IV-PCA therapy is considered to be based in part on the inability of the patient to receive a greater than mildly sedating cumulative dose over a period of time, as long as the patient is the sole individual pushing the demand dose button (in adults only). Maintaining the lowest dose needed for maintenance of analgesia with a comparatively low lockout interval appears to provide the best means to minimize risk from respiratory depression.[82]

Opioid-tolerant patients pose a challenge in postoperative management.[83,84] Calculation of the starting dose for an IV-PCA requires knowledge of a complete history of opioid use and is best made following conversion of all currently used opioids into a single 24-h morphine equivalent dose using a conversion table.[85] It is important to recognize that the use of a conversion table is only the first step in developing an individualized treatment plan for a given patient. Equianalgesic conversion ratios for commonly prescribed opioids are provided in Table 35.2. To convert 90 mg/day oral morphine into IV morphine, use the ratio 3 mg oral morphine is equal to 1 mg IV morphine or in other words 90 mg oral morphine per day will equate to 30 mg IV morphine per day.

After obtaining the desired 24-h morphine equivalent dose following application of the principles above, the next step is to choose the opioid to be administered. In the absence of significant renal dysfunction, morphine is considered a first-choice agent due to ease of administration by any route needed (oral, intravenous, subcutaneous, epidural, intrathecal), as well as the multiple formulations available. If using PCA, provide no more than half of the calculated 24 h morphine equivalent dose in the form of a basal infusion, not to exceed 2 mg/h morphine or its equivalent or, if treatment is oral, provide as scheduled oral equivalent. The remainder of the required opioid may be provided on an as-needed basis in the form of an IV-PCA demand dose (1 mg Q6 min or 1.5 mg Q6 min) or as additional immediate-release oral morphine dosed at intervals no greater than every 4 h. Individualization of the treatment plan will need to be made for patients intolerant of morphine, in the presence of renal insufficiency, hepatic compromise, or in the presence of sleep apnea or other respiratory diseases.[84] As a matter of safety, even if opioid tolerant, rarely should a patient be started on a demand dose of greater than 2 mg of morphine (or 0.4 mg hydromorphone) every 6 min. Adjustment of the demand dose and/or addition of a small amount of continuous (morphine 0.5–2 mg/h or hydromorphone 0.1–0.4 mg/h) may follow if needed.

Novel delivery systems have been developed based on the IV-PCA model. Iontopheresis has been used to deliver fentanyl via a patient-controlled transdermal system (not to be confused with a fentanyl transdermal patch for chronic pain use).[86] Fentanyl is given via a patient-controlled transdermal delivery system that uses a needle-free device the size of a credit card containing fentanyl hydrogel acting as an anode, inert hydrogel acting as a cathode, microprocessor, battery, light-emitting diode (LED), and a drug delivery button.[87] Placement of the device on the skin of the upper arm or chest with adhesive allows the delivery of fentanyl through the epidermis to the systemic circulation via a button press that initiates an imperceptible current. The optimal dose has been found to be 40 μg of fentanyl. Lockout of the dose is limited to once every 10 min and depression of the button in that time frame does not allow additional delivery of the drug. The LED is used to calculate incremental approximations of doses delivered, and the system is deactivated within 24 h or after 80 doses have been delivered.[87] Patient satisfaction rates have been equivalent to that of conventional IV-PCA therapy, yet widespread use has not taken place due to a lack of proven safety, limited benefit over conventional IV-PCA therapy, and a risk of diversion or abuse.[88,89] So far, the use of this alternative has not become commonplace.

Conversion to oral opioids from IV-PCA follows the principles outlined above. It is preferable to ensure that the patient's pain has been optimized prior to oral conversion. Optimization of pain does not mean an absence of pain or the reduction of pain below any particular point on a visual analogue scale or verbal rating scale. Pain control is considered adequate at the point that the patient has achieved the ability to perform the rehabilitation goals needed to continue recovery or, in the case of chronic pain states, has returned to baseline or better. Understanding basic principles in opioid dosing, conversion, and management can help avoid under- as well as overdosage of opioids in most cases, providing safety in the routine management of acute pain patients.[90] Patients who reach an average of 2 mg/h total of morphine (or 0.4 mg hydromorphone) by IV-PCA or 15–30 mg Q3–4 h oral morphine (or 4–8 mg PO hydromorphone Q3–4 h) will generally do well on two tablets Q4 h of acetaminophen (APAP) 325 mg with any of hydrocodone 10 mg, codeine 60 mg, or oxycodone 10 mg.

SUMMARY

The overall goal of acute postoperative pain management is the optimization of pain relief with avoidance of side effects or escalation of any prior opioid use. Multimodal pharmacologic treatments used in conjunction with regional anesthetic techniques as part of a perioperative pain program have the highest likelihood of achieving the desired result. Opioids are commonly prescribed in high doses immediately following surgery, but are not necessarily the optimal treatment. Long-term treatment plans must include gradual dose titration downward in order to minimize risk of development of opioid-induced hyperalgesia.[91,92] Opioid dose reduction by 20% of the patients' current use can be made at intervals of 48 h, without concerns for the development of an opioid withdrawal syndrome. The use of a structured plan of care is needed for patients that continue to have pain that fails to resolve in the expected time frame. An assessment of benefit of chronic opioid therapy may be required following the acute treatment phase. Opioids should be weaned and stopped if they are not effective in achieving a functional state.[92] Various chronic pain and opioid management guidelines are available for planning that process.

REFERENCES

1. Macintyre PE, Schug SA, Scott DA, Visser EJ, Walker SM. APM:SE Working Group of the Australian and New Zealand College of Anaesthetists and Faculty of Pain Medicine, *Acute Pain Management: Scientific Evidence* (3rd edition), Melbourne: ANZCA & FPM, 2010.

2. Koo P. Acute pain management. *J Pharm Pract*. 2003;16:18.
3. Brookoff D. Chronic pain: 1. A new disease? *Hosp Pract*. 2000;35:8.
4. Williams DA, Clauw DJ. Understanding fibromyalgia: lessons from the broader pain research community. *J Pain*. 2009;10:777–791.
5. Chu L, Clark D, Angst M. Opioid tolerance and hyperalgesia in chronic pain patients after one month of oral morphine therapy: a preliminary prospective study. *J Pain*. 2006;7:6.
6. Fishbain DA, Cole B, Lewis JE, Gao J, Rosomoff RS. Do opioids induce hyperalgesia in humans? An evidence-based structured review. *Pain Med*. 2009;10:829–839.
7. Chang G, Chen L, Mao J. Opioid tolerance and hyperalgesia. *Med Clin North Am*. 2007;91:199–211.
8. Ashburn MC. Practice guidelines for acute pain management in the perioperative setting: an updated report by the American Society of Anesthesiologists Task Force on Acute Pain Management. *Anesthesiology*. 2004;100:1573–1581.
9. Momeni M, Crucitti M, De Kock M. Patient-controlled analgesia in the management of postoperative pain. *Drugs*. 2006;66:2321–2337.
10. Nebeker JR, Hoffman JM, Weir CR, Bennett CL, Hurdle JF. High rates of adverse drug events in a highly computerized hospital. *Arch Intern Med*. 2005;165:1111–1116.
11. Luchins D. The electronic medical record: optimizing human not computer capabilities. *Adm Policy Ment Health*. July 2010;37(4):375–378.
12. Basbaum AI, Bautista DM, Scherrer G, Julius D. Cellular and molecular mechanisms of pain. *Cell*. 2009;139:267–284.
13. Hodge CJ, Jr., Apkarian AV. The spinothalamic tract. *Crit Rev Neurobiol*. 1990;5:363–397.
14. Apkarian AV, Baliki MN, Geha PY. Towards a theory of chronic pain. *Prog Neurobiol*. 2009;87:81–97.
15. Kupers R, Schneider FC, Christensen R, et al. No evidence for generalized increased postoperative responsiveness to pain: a combined behavioral and serial functional magnetic resonance imaging study. *Anesth Analg*. 2009;109:600–606.
16. Trescot AM, Glaser SE, Hansen H, Benyamin R, Patel S, Manchikanti L. Effectiveness of opioids in the treatment of chronic non-cancer pain. *Pain Physician*. 2008;11:S181–S200.
17. Fields HL. Should we be reluctant to prescribe opioids for chronic non-malignant pain? *Pain*. 2007;129:233–234.
18. Ballantyne JC, LaForge KS. Opioid dependence and addiction during opioid treatment of chronic pain. *Pain*. 2007;129:235–255.
19. Berland D, Rodgers P, Green C, Harrison R, Roth R. Managing Chronic Non-Terminal Pain Including Prescribing Controlled Substances. Ann Arbor, MI: Office of Clinical Affairs, University of Michigan Health System, 2009. Available from the Agency for Healthcare Research and Quality at http://www.med.umich.edu/1info/FHP/practiceguides/pain/pain.pdf.
20. Hay JL, White JM, Bochner F, Somogyi AA, Semple TJ, Rounsefell B. Hyperalgesia in opioid-managed chronic pain and opioid-dependent patients. *J Pain*. 2009;10:316–322.
21. Rozen D, Grass GW. Perioperative and intraoperative pain and anesthetic care of the chronic pain and cancer pain patient receiving chronic opioid therapy. *Pain Pract*. 2005;5:18–32.
22. Mitra S, Sinatra RS. Perioperative management of acute pain in the opioid-dependent patient. *Anesthesiology*. 2004;101:212–227.
23. Krantz MJ, Martin J, Stimmel B, Mehta D, Haigney MC. QTc interval screening in methadone treatment. *Ann Intern Med*. 2009;150:387–395.
24. Brummett CM, Trivedi KA, Dubovoy AV, Berland DW. Dexmedetomidine as a novel therapeutic for postoperative pain in a patient treated with buprenorphine. *J Opioid Manag*. 2009;5:175–179.
25. Roberts DM, Meyer-Witting M. High-dose buprenorphine: perioperative precautions and management strategies. *Anaesth Intensive Care*. 2005;33:17–25.
26. Alford DP, Compton P, Samet JH. Acute pain management for patients receiving maintenance methadone or buprenorphine therapy. *Ann Intern Med*. 2006;144:127–134.
27. Hartog CS, Rothaug J, Goettermann A, Zimmer A, Meissner W. Room for improvement: nurses' and physicians' views of a post-operative pain management program. *Acta Anaesthesiol Scand*. Mar 2010;54(3):277–283.

28. Landau R, Kraft JC, Flint LY, et al. An experimental paradigm for the prediction of post-operative pain (PPOP). *J Vis Exp.* 2010;35.
29. Granot M. Can we predict persistent postoperative pain by testing preoperative experimental pain? *Curr Opin Anaesthesiol.* 2009;22:425–430.
30. Nielsen PR, Norgaard L, Rasmussen LS, Kehlet H. Prediction of post-operative pain by an electrical pain stimulus. *Acta Anaesthesiol Scand.* 2007;51:582–586.
31. Hutchison RW. Challenges in acute post-operative pain management. *Am J Health Syst Pharm.* 2007;64:S2–S5.
32. Taylor S, Kirton OC, Staff I, Kozol RA. Postoperative day one: a high risk period for respiratory events. *Am J Surg.* 2005;190:752–756.
33. Shapiro A, Zohar E, Zaslansky R, Hoppenstein D, Shabat S, Fredman B. The frequency and timing of respiratory depression in 1524 postoperative patients treated with systemic or neuraxial morphine. *J Clin Anesth.* 2005;17:537–542.
34. Lotsch J, Dudziak R, Freynhagen R, Marschner J, Geisslinger G. Fatal respiratory depression after multiple intravenous morphine injections. *Clin Pharmacokinet.* 2006;45:1051–1060.
35. Fiedler MA. Clinical implications of ketorolac for postoperative analgesia. *J Perianesth Nurs.* 1997;12:426–433.
36. Southworth S, Peters J, Rock A, Pavliv L. A multicenter, randomized, double-blind, placebo-controlled trial of intravenous ibuprofen 400 and 800 mg every 6 hours in the management of postoperative pain. *Clin Ther.* 2009;31:1922–1935.
37. Perttunen K, Kalso E, Heinonen J, Salo J. IV diclofenac in post-thoracotomy pain. *Br J Anaesth.* 1992;68:474–480.
38. Munro HM, Walton SR, Malviya S, et al. Low-dose ketorolac improves analgesia and reduces morphine requirements following posterior spinal fusion in adolescents. *Can J Anaesth.* 2002;49:461–466.
39. Cepeda MS, Carr DB, Miranda N, Diaz A, Silva C, Morales O. Comparison of morphine, ketorolac, and their combination for postoperative pain: results from a large, randomized, double-blind trial. *Anesthesiology.* 2005;103:1225–1232.
40. Elia N, Lysakowski C, Tramer MR. Does multimodal analgesia with acetaminophen, nonsteroidal antiinflammatory drugs, or selective cyclooxygenase-2 inhibitors and patient-controlled analgesia morphine offer advantages over morphine alone? Meta-analyses of randomized trials. *Anesthesiology.* 2005;103:1296–1304.
41. Moiniche S, Romsing J, Dahl JB, Tramer MR. Nonsteroidal antiinflammatory drugs and the risk of operative site bleeding after tonsillectomy: a quantitative systematic review. *Anesth Analg.* 2003;96:68–77, table of contents.
42. Sinatra RS, Jahr JS, Reynolds LW, Viscusi ER, Groudine SB, Payen-Champenois C. Efficacy and safety of single and repeated administration of 1 gram intravenous acetaminophen injection (paracetamol) for pain management after major orthopedic surgery. *Anesthesiology.* 2005;102:822–831.
43. Remy C, Marret E, Bonnet F. Effects of acetaminophen on morphine side-effects and consumption after major surgery: meta-analysis of randomized controlled trials. *Br J Anaesth.* 2005;94:505–513.
44. Bromley L. Pre-emptive analgesia and protective premedication. What is the difference? *Biomed Pharmacother.* 2006;60:336–340.
45. Ong CK, Lirk P, Seymour RA, Jenkins BJ. The efficacy of preemptive analgesia for acute postoperative pain management: a meta-analysis. *Anesth Analg.* 2005;100:757–773, table of contents.
46. Aubrun F, Langeron O, Heitz D, Coriat P, Riou B. Randomised, placebo-controlled study of the postoperative analgesic effects of ketoprofen after spinal fusion surgery. *Acta Anaesthesiol Scand.* 2000;44:934–939.
47. Remy C, Marret E, Bonnet F. State of the art of paracetamol in acute pain therapy. *Curr Opin Anaesthesiol.* 2006;19:562–565.
48. Montgomery JE, Sutherland CJ, Kestin IG, Sneyd JR. Morphine consumption in patients receiving rectal paracetamol and diclofenac alone and in combination. *Br J Anaesth.* 1996;77:445–447.
49. van der Marel CD, Peters JW, Bouwmeester NJ, Jacqz-Aigrain E, van den Anker JN, Tibboel D. Rectal acetaminophen does not reduce morphine consumption after major surgery in young infants. *Br J Anaesth.* 2007;98:372–379.

50. Kvalsvik O, Borchgrevink PC, Hagen L, Dale O. Randomized, double-blind, placebo-controlled study of the effect of rectal paracetamol on morphine consumption after abdominal hysterectomy. *Acta Anaesthesiol Scand.* 2003;47:451–456.
51. Beck DH, Schenk MR, Hagemann K, Doepfmer UR, Kox WJ. The pharmacokinetics and analgesic efficacy of larger dose rectal acetaminophen (40 mg/kg) in adults: a double-blinded, randomized study. *Anesth Analg.* 2000;90:431–436.
52. Kehlet H. Postoperative pain relief—what is the issue? *Br J Anaesth.* 1994;72:375–378.
53. Kehlet H. Procedure-specific postoperative pain management. *Anesthesiol Clin North Am.* 2005;23:203–210.
54. Dahl JB, Kehlet H. Treatment of postoperative pain—a status report. *Ugeskr Laeger.* 2006;168:1986–1988.
55. Brown D, O'Neill O, Beck A. Post-operative pain management: transition from epidural to oral analgesia. *Nurs Stand.* 2007;21:35–40.
56. Goodarzi M. Comparison of epidural morphine, hydromorphone and fentanyl for postoperative pain control in children undergoing orthopaedic surgery. *Paediatr Anaesth.* 1999;9:419–422.
57. Chaplan SR, Duncan SR, Brodsky JB, Brose WG. Morphine and hydromorphone epidural analgesia. A prospective, randomized comparison. *Anesthesiology.* 1992;77:1090–1094.
58. Halpern SH, Arellano R, Preston R, et al. Epidural morphine vs. hydromorphone in post-caesarean section patients. *Can J Anaesth.* 1996;43:595–598.
59. Alon E, Jaquenod M, Schaeppi B. Post-operative epidural versus intravenous patient-controlled analgesia. *Minerva Anestesiol.* 2003;69:443–446.
60. Ruppen W, Derry S, McQuay HJ, Moore RA. Infection rates associated with epidural indwelling catheters for seven days or longer: systematic review and meta-analysis. *BMC Palliat Care.* 2007;6:3.
61. Kostopanagiotou G, Kyroudi S, Panidis D, et al. Epidural catheter colonization is not associated with infection. *Surg Infect (Larchmt).* 2002;3:359–365.
62. Reynolds F. Neurological infections after neuraxial anesthesia. *Anesthesiol Clin.* 2008;26:23–52.
63. Christie IW, McCabe S. Major complications of epidural analgesia after surgery: results of a six-year survey. *Anaesthesia.* 2007;62:335–341.
64. Cameron CM, Scott DA, McDonald WM, Davies MJ. A review of neuraxial epidural morbidity: experience of more than 8000 cases at a single teaching hospital. *Anesthesiology.* 2007;106:997–1002.
65. Sendi P, Bregenzer T, Zimmerli W. Spinal epidural abscess in clinical practice. *QJM.* 2008;101:1–12.
66. Chen HC, Tzaan WC, Lui TN. Spinal epidural abscesses: a retrospective analysis of clinical manifestations, sources of infection, and outcomes. *Chang Gung Med J.* 2004;27:351–358.
67. Fowler SJ, Symons J, Sabato S, Myles PS. Epidural analgesia compared with peripheral nerve blockade after major knee surgery: a systematic review and meta-analysis of randomized trials. *Br J Anaesth.* 2008;100:154–164.
68. Singelyn FJ, Ferrant T, Malisse MF, Joris D. Effects of intravenous patient-controlled analgesia with morphine, continuous epidural analgesia, and continuous femoral nerve sheath block on rehabilitation after unilateral total-hip arthroplasty. *Reg Anesth Pain Med.* 2005;30:452–457.
69. Evans H, Steele SM, Nielsen KC, Tucker MS, Klein SM. Peripheral nerve blocks and continuous catheter techniques. *Anesthesiol Clin North America.* 2005;23:141–162.
70. Fredrickson MJ, Ball CM, Dalgleish AJ. Successful continuous interscalene analgesia for ambulatory shoulder surgery in a private practice setting. *Reg Anesth Pain Med.* 2008;33:122–128.
71. Sarnoff SJ, Sarnoff LC. Prolonged peripheral nerve block by means of indwelling plastic catheter; treatment of hiccup; note on the electrical localization of peripheral nerve. *Anesthesiology.* 1951;12:270–275.
72. Frohm RM, Raw RM, Haider N, Boezaart AP. Epidural spread after continuous cervical paravertebral block: a case report. *Reg Anesth Pain Med.* 2006;31:279–281.
73. Horlocker TT, Wedel DJ, Rowlingson JC, et al. Regional anesthesia in the patient receiving antithrombotic or thrombolytic therapy: American Society of Regional Anesthesia and Pain Medicine Evidence-Based Guidelines (Third Edition). *Reg Anesth Pain Med.* 2010;35:64–101.
74. Gogarten W. The influence of new antithrombotic drugs on regional anesthesia. *Curr Opin Anaesthesiol.* 2006;19:545–550.

75. Kehlet H. Multimodal approach to control postoperative pathophysiology and rehabilitation. *Br J Anaesth*. 1997;78:606–617.

76. Hudcova J, McNicol E, Quah C, Lau J, Carr DB. Patient controlled opioid analgesia versus conventional opioid analgesia for postoperative pain. *Cochrane Database Syst Rev*. 2006;(4):CD003348.

77. Ballantyne JC, Carr DB, Deferranti S, et al. The comparative effects of postoperative analgesic therapies on pulmonary outcome: cumulative meta-analyses of randomized, controlled trials. *Anesth Analg*. 1998;86:598–612.

78. Ballantyne JC, Carr DB, Chalmers TC, Dear KB, Angelillo IF, Mosteller F. Postoperative patient-controlled analgesia: meta-analyses of initial randomized control trials. *J Clin Anesth*. 1993;5:182–193.

79. Cashman JN, Dolin SJ. Respiratory and haemodynamic effects of acute postoperative pain management: evidence from published data. *Br J Anaesth*. 2004;93:212–223.

80. Polomano RC, Rathmell JP, Krenzischek DA, Dunwoody CJ. Emerging trends and new approaches to acute pain management. *Pain Manag Nurs*. 2008;9:S33–S41.

81. Grass JA. Patient-controlled analgesia. *Anesth Analg*. 2005;101:S44–S61.

82. Badner NH, Doyle JA, Smith MH, Herrick IA. Effect of varying intravenous patient-controlled analgesia dose and lockout interval while maintaining a constant hourly maximum dose. *J Clin Anesth*. 1996;8:382–385.

83. Patanwala AE, Duby J, Waters D, Erstad BL. Opioid conversions in acute care. *Ann Pharmacother*. 2007;41:255–266.

84. Shaheen PE, Walsh D, Lasheen W, Davis MP, Lagman RL. Opioid equianalgesic tables: are they all equally dangerous? *J Pain Symptom Manage*. 2009;38:409–417.

85. Brant JM. Opioid equianalgesic conversion: the right dose. *Clin J Oncol Nurs*. 2001;5:163–165.

86. Polomano RC, Rathmell JP, Krenzischek DA, Dunwoody CJ. Emerging trends and new approaches to acute pain management. *J Perianesth Nurs*. 2008;23:S43–S53.

87. Miaskowski C. Patient-controlled modalities for acute postoperative pain management. *J Perianesth Nurs*. 2005;20:255–267.

88. Pennington P, Caminiti S, Schein JR, Hewitt DJ, Nelson WW. Patients' assessment of the convenience of fentanyl HCl iontophoretic transdermal system (ITS) versus morphine intravenous patient-controlled analgesia (IV PCA) in the management of postoperative pain after major surgery. *Pain Manag Nurs*. 2009;10:124–133.

89. Viscusi E, Reynolds L, Chung F, Atkinson L, Khanna S. Patient-controlled transdermal fentanyl hydrochloride vs intravenous morphine pump for postoperative pain: a randomized controlled trial. *JAMA*. 2004;291(11):1333–1340.

90. Berdine HJ, Nesbit SA. Equianalgesic dosing of opioids. *J Pain Palliat Care Pharmacother*. 2006;20:79–84.

91. White JM. Pleasure into pain: the consequences of long-term opioid use. *Addict Behav*. 2004;29:1311–1324.

92. Ballantyne JC, Shin NS. Efficacy of opioids for chronic pain: a review of the evidence. *Clin J Pain*. 2008;24:469–478.

INDEX

Perioperative Medicine: Medical Consultation and Co-Management, First Edition.
Edited by Amir K. Jaffer and Paul J. Grant.
© 2012 Wiley-Blackwell. Published 2012 by John Wiley & Sons, Inc.